Metric Trends In Hominid Dental Evolution

METRIC TRENDS IN HOMINID DENTAL EVOLUTION

MILFORD H. WOLPOFF

NUMBER 2

STUDIES IN ANTHROPOLOGY
CASE WESTERN RESERVE UNIVERSITY

THE PRESS OF
CASE WESTERN RESERVE UNIVERSITY
CLEVELAND & LONDON
1971

CASE WESTERN RESERVE UNIVERSITY
STUDIES IN ANTHROPOLOGY
JAMES E. FITTING, *SERIES EDITOR*

No. 1. The Summer Island Site: A Study of Prehistoric Cultural Ecology and Social Organization in the Northern Lake Michigan Area. *By David S. Brose.* 1970.

No. 2. Metric Trends in Hominid Dental Evolution. *By Milford H. Wolpoff.* 1971.

No. 3. Life-Crisis Rituals Among the Kenuz. *By Charles Callender and Fadwa el Guindi.* Forthcoming.

Printed in the United States of America.

International Standard Book Number: 0-8295-0199-1.

Library of Congress Catalogue Card Number: 72-116388.

Preface

This work represents a very modified version of a Ph.D. thesis submitted to the University of Illinois in 1969. For this reason, the text is up to date in 1970, but the tables, and the discussions of the tables, represent the data available in 1968. Needless to say, it is gratifying to find that 2 more years of data publication necessitates no major changes.

Since the tabular information was calculated, Dr. C. L. Brace kindly made the dental dimensions which he measured on South and East African australopithecines available to me. All of the crucial calculations have been reworked using both this data and the new Lake Rudolf area australopithecine data. With australopithecine samples more than twice as large as those utilized here, the only changes discovered were in a larger number of overlapping ranges, more extensive overlap of ranges, and fewer significant differences. This, too, has been a very satisfactory discovery. While more data will be uncovered, I do not believe the major conclusions of this work will be refuted. The tendency has clearly been for additional data to fill in existing gaps and bring samples more closely together, rather than to more firmly establish differences.

A word of explanation is required with respect to the abbreviations used throughout. Most of the tables, and all of the appendix, are direct computer output. The calculations were performed on the IBM 7094 at the University of Illinois Digital Computer Laboratory. The necessary programs were written by the author. A number of abbreviations of taxonomic names were utilized in order to standardize the output. In most cases, names were restricted to either 18 or 12 character fields. While the results are obviously not taxonomically correct, the meaning is clear. I hope that the advantages of standardized output in the many rapid forms of data reduction made possible on computers outweigh the disadvantage of abbreviated designations.

I am indebted to the personnel at the Dickson Mounds Museum, the Illinois State Museum, and the Field Museum of Natural History Department of Anthropology for both the access I received to their skeletal collections and the cooperation which they kindly extended to me.

I am very grateful for the typing services extended to me by the secretarial staff of the Department of Anthropology, Case Western Reserve University.

There are a few individuals whose guidance and encouragement were indispensable to my education, and to the conception of this thesis. To these I acknowledge my sincere gratitude: Eugene Giles, Donald Lathrap, Arthur Rohn, C. Loring Brace, John T. Robinson.

I appreciate the help of J. D. Cadien, D. Brose, and J. Fitting in preparing this manuscript for publication.

My greatest debt is to my wife, Sheila. Without her love, her understanding, her cooperation, and her encouragement, this thesis would have been impossible.

The research was supported in part by U.S.P.H.S. Grant 5 Fl GM-30, 854-03.

Table of Contents

List of Tables

Metric Trends In Hominid Dental Evolution

1. Introduction

The purpose of this work is two fold. First, the presence of metric trends in hominid dental evolution will be established and the nature of the trends described. Second, a specific model of the changing hominid adaptive patterns throughout the Pleistocene, and of the mechanisms orienting the resulting changes in tooth size, will be tested against the specifics of metric dental evolution.

TRENDS

An evolutionary trend, according to Simpson (1953:245) is a "sustained, prevailing tendency in a phylogenetic progression." For a sequence of change in one predominant direction to be considered a trend, it must span at least 10^6 years (p. 259). Recognizable australopithecines are at least 2.0 to 2.5 million years old at Kanapoi (Patterson and Howells 1967) and Lothagam (Howell 1968a). Indeed, both of these may be up to 2 million years older (Maglio 1970). At Omo, the hominid bearing deposits extend to over 3.75 million years (Howell 1968b, 1969). The Kanam mandible may be as old as 4 million years (Maglio 1970). Therefore, unquestionable hominids have existed long enough for evolutionary trends to be delineated.

Trends are sought by the human paleontologist because of the fundamental insight they yield concerning the adaptive orienting factors in hominid evolution. Adaptively important and therefore taxonomically relevant characteristics are outlined and contrasted by evolutionary trends because of their sustained orientation. Establishing the presence of trends is surely not sufficient; the study of evolution goes beyond demonstrations that it has occurred. The most complete understanding of evolution comes from a detailed knowledge of the species which have evolved: their morphology, their ecology, and their behavior. Only morphology can be directly observed. Ecology and behavior must be suggested for fossil species. One source of inference stems from the functions suggested by the morphological structures. Ranges and possibilities can thus be defined. Still, the actual behavior and ecology of a species represents only a small part of the range of possible behaviors and ecologies. The determination of trends greatly limits the possibilities by establishing adaptive significance. Adaptive factors orienting evolutionary trends cannot be directly observed. However, hypotheses concerning adaptive factors can be tested against the available data. Tests of this nature become possible when the evidence of fossil material can be viewed within a framework evincing the presence of trends.

THE RELEVANCE OF TOOTH SIZE

That tooth size has an adaptive importance in extant populations is clear from a perusal of the uses to which teeth are put. In addition to mastication, teeth are utilized for grasping, holding, exerting torsion, and other manipulative functions (Dahlberg 1963a; Brace 1962a; Bailit, DeWitt, and Leigh 1968; Taylor 1963; Noble 1926; Brace and Molnar 1967; Campbell 1925; Van Reenen 1966; Brothwell 1958, 1963; Barnes

1969; Leigh 1928, 1937; Turner and Cadien 1969; Gessain 1959). Other uses observed include cutting and tearing (Keith 1915; Noble 1926; Brace 1967b), gnawing (Dahlberg 1963a), tool making (Brace 1963a, 1964a; Sollas 1924), treating leather (Waugh 1937a; Pedersen 1938), pulling (Noble 1926; Brace and Molnar 1967), prying off rusted gasoline covers (de Poncins), and the fashioning of thong, reed, and thread (Dahlberg 1963a). A variety of objects from pipes (Bailit, DeWitt, and Leigh 1968) to arrows for straightening (Sollas 1924) are commonly put in the mouth. Most of these usages affect the anterior teeth more than the posteriors (Brace 1967a; Brose and Wolpoff 1971).

Black (1895) measured a range of maximum force between the incisors from 14 kg to 80 kg in North Americans. Howell and Manly (1948) measured maximum forces ranging from 29 kg to 51 kg in only 4 individuals. A relatively great amount of force can be exerted between the incisors of extant populations (Wolpoff 1970a).

Occlusal wear, on the other hand, is best supported by the posterior teeth. Thus, factors causing occlusal wear have their greatest effect on the molars and premolars. Occlusal wear occurs from more causes than eating. Brushing with sticks, and sometimes a paste, is relatively common (Brothwell 1959; Barnes 1969; Taylor 1963). Items from betel nuts (Bailit, DeWitt, and Leigh 1968) to coca and lime-soaked tobacco are regularly chewed (Leigh 1928, 1937). Yet, mastication of food is the major function of the posterior dentition and exerts the greatest selective influence on the size of the molars and premolars. Occlusal attrition can stem from both the toughness of the food and from the presence of foreign material. It is difficult to determine which factor, if either, has the dominant effect. While it may appear that foreign particles, or grit, would exercise the greatest wear, the specialized dentition of herbivores indicates an extensive influence of tough plant fibers (Romer 1966).

Quite extensive pressures can be developed between the molars (Wolpoff 1970a). Black (1908) measured a range from 11 kg to 125 kg in a study of over 1000 North Americans. The average was 78 kg. Reports by other authors (Howell and Manly 1948; Klatsky and Fischer 1953) fall within this range. On the other hand, Waugh (1937b) measured a maximum force range from 91 kg to 158 kg in 81 Eskimo males. Twenty-eight individuals were able to exert over 136 kg. Such power is apparently developed in response to extensive dental requirements of both occlusion and manipulation. Eskimos born and raised in "White" settlements showed significantly smaller maximums (Waugh 1937a), and showed less wear (Davies and Pedersen 1938). That the relevant factor is tooth use, and not overall body size or strength, can be seen from a comparison of dental students and athletes (Brekhus, Armstrong, and Simon 1937). With identical sample sizes, and almost identical ages and heights, the weight averages were respectively 72 kg and 80 kg. The average measured biting forces were both 58 kg, in spite of weight, strength, and fitness differences. Further, Oppenheimer (1966) compared these same Minnesota athletes with 8 Middle and South American aboriginal groups. Although in all cases body size and general health is markedly inferior in the latter, the measured biting force is consistently greater, ranging from 61 kg to 84 kg.

Vegetable foods form the major bulk of the diet for most extant populations (see Lee and DeVore, eds. 1968). According to Lee (1968: 42-43): "except for the highest latitudes, where hunting contributes over half of the diet in many cases, hunted foods almost everywhere else constitute 20 to 45 percent of the diet." If we take 65% to 80% as the range of average minima of vegetable foods in the diet of extant pre-agricultural groups, and thus for pre-agricultural hominids outside of tundra or other very specialized areas, the average maxima can be determined from non-human primates. Hunting seems to account for roughly 5% of the diet for chimpanzees (van Lawick-Goodall 1967) and baboons (Dart 1963). Vegetable foods are thus delineated to constitute from 65% to 95% of the diet for various hominids.

Grit can play a significant role in occlusal wear (Greene, Ewing, and Armelagos 1967: 49-52). Grit can come from both vegetables, particularly roots (Robinson 1956), and from meat dirtied between butchering and eating (Buettner-Janusch 1966). The presence of a significant amount of grit in the diet of a number of extant groups has been established (Campbell 1925, 1939; Meggitt 1957; Tobias 1967a; Taylor 1934, 1963; Barnes 1969; Saxe 1966). Indeed, Anderson (1965) explains the obliquely worn occlusal surfaces, with multiple wear planes, observed at Tehuacan, Mexico, as the result of pulling sand-covered plant material through the teeth. Robinson has observed enamel chipping from the edge of the occlusal surface of *Homo robustus* (1954b) and relates this to chewing on particles of grit. Tobias (1967a) reports the same amount of chipping on the teeth of *H. africanus.* Turner and Cadien (1969) have observed significant amounts of pressure chipping on the teeth of Aleuts, Eskimos, and Indians, corroborating Tobias' claim that such chipping is related to grit–not necessarily to vegetables (1967a:227). Therefore, grit has been a consistent item of consumption for hominids. Other sources of grit observed in extant groups include clams (Johnston and Snow 1961), pastes made of ground bone (Leigh 1928), and grain ground on stone (Barnes 1969). Wear due to toughness of food fibers is limited to vegetable foods, while wear due to grit is not associated with any particular type of diet. It appears, to this author, almost impossible to bite down on gritty food (let alone chew it), but Australian aborigines are regularly observed doing exactly that (Campbell 1925, 1938; Begg 1954). Grit, in order to be an effective abrasive, need not be composed of large particles. Indeed, through a series of experiments, Dahlberg (1963a) discovered that fine abrasives and silts with constant stropping action wear the teeth more than rougher grit particles.

In sum, tooth size seems to be one of the major adaptive mechanisms with which hominids meet their environment. All of these dental functions are allowed by sufficient dental size, rather than groove pattern, cusp number or pattern, wrinkling, or a number of other morphological features. One would thus expect the knowledge of trends in metric variation to reflect these functions and thus be responsive to adaptive differences. Tooth size should, therefore, be a very relevant characteristic.

A number of authors have recognized this importance, and have discussed both the existence and the adaptive relevance of a general trend to the reduction of tooth size in hominid evolution (Weidenreich 1945a; Robinson 1956; Hooton 1938, 1947; Keith 1925; Arambourg 1963; Boule and Vallois 1957; Dart 1925, 1934; Gregory 1922; von Koenigswald 1958a; Le Gros Clark 1950; Piveteau 1957; Werth 1928). Dahlberg (1963a) recognizes extensive I1 and M1 reduction, but less reduction for P3. Other authors question, or even deny, the existence of any general tooth size reduction trend. Garn (1964:8) finds no true taxonomic chasm between *H. sapiens* and both *H. neanderthalensis* and *H. erectus* in tooth size. Others claim that there has been no progressive reduction of the anterior teeth relative to the posterior teeth (Garn, Lewis, and Walenga 1968d), and no systematic size reduction in modern man (Garn, Lewis, and Walenga 1969:82). Tooth size, to these authors and others (Coon 1963:351), is not morphologically significant.

Because of this disagreement, it is necessary to first demonstrate the presence of metric trends. To this end, measurements for all available fossil hominid teeth, as well as measurements for a number of extant groups (some taken from the literature and others measured directly by this author) were utilized in a comparison of hominid taxa and extant groups. In addition to dimensional comparisons of individual teeth, various summed sets of anterior and posterior teeth were utilized. Selection does not directly act on individual teeth, but rather on larger communalities (Dahlberg 1945). Individual tooth ratios, as well as tooth set ratios, were examined so that relative, as well as absolute, change could be discerned.

A SELECTION MODEL

The basis has been established for the development of a selection model of the factors acting on hominid tooth size in the Pleistocene. It is convenient to discuss the action of selection on canines, incisors, and the premolar-molar series separately.

Darwin (1859, 1874) suggested the hypothesis that canine size reduced in man when weapons replaced the defensive function of the teeth. Most authors have accepted this hypothesis in one form or another (Hooton 1947; Remane 1927; Washburn 1959, 1960, 1968a; Washburn and Avis 1958; Washburn and Howell 1960; Oppenheimer 1964, 1966, 1967; DeVore 1964; Hockett and Ascher 1964; Crook and Gartlan 1966; Brace 1962a, 1967a, 1967b). On the other hand, the hypothesis has been questioned. One of the indications used to establish the defensive nature of canines in non-human primates is the great sexual dimorphism in canine size. There is no corresponding dietary difference between male and female apes (Washburn and Avis 1958; Brace 1962a; Washburn 1968a). An alternative explanation suggested by Crook and Gartlan (1966) is that the high degree of sexual dimorphism could be due to the heightened degree of aggressive and agonistic behavioral responses within structured terrestrial primate groups. Hominids, then, would be distinguished at their origin by an intragroup behavioral shift to cooperation (Etkin 1954, 1963), leading to the reduction of sexual dimorphism and eventually of canine size (Holloway 1967:65). A number of other possibilities have been suggested as the major causes of canine size reduction. Mills (1963) would have the canines reducing from the facial shortening resulting from erect posture, a model very similar to one proposed by Weidenreich (1941) to explain the reduction of posterior teeth. According to Mills, selection for reduced canines in a short-faced primate would occur to prevent canine locking during rotary chewing. Jolly (1970), too, suggests canine reduction is the result of rotary chewing. In discussing his gelada baboon analogy of savanna-based small object feeding–presumably the initial hominid adaptation–he gives 2 possible causes for canine reduction: (1) adaptation to rotary chewing favoring crown height reductions; (2) pleiotropic effects stemming from incisor reduction resulting from hand feeding. Bailit and Friedlaender (1966:655-66) point out that in hominids, the canine roots form the piriform aperture. They thus suggest selection acts on canine size indirectly through the nose. Presumably, as man moved out of the tropics, noses became narrower and therefore canines smaller. Yet another suggestion comes from Brues (1966) who sees selection acting to reduce canines in order to allow side to side chewing as well as a sort of "balancing selection" against prognathism in erect hominids. Lastly, Prout (1964) submits that reduction in canine size could have occurred when the "biological cost" of maintaining them became too high. Many of the mechanisms suggested for canine reduction are motivated by disagreement with Darwin's initial suggestion. The reduced canines claimed for *"Ramapithecus"* (Simons 1965, 1968b, 1969) would have to mean that tool use occurred 13 million years ago, if not more. Leakey has suggested exactly that (1968c)!

However, there is some evidence indicating that *"Ramapithecus"* does not, in actuality, have particularly reduced canines. In a study of unworn pongid and hominid dentitions, Yulish (1971) relates canine area to the summed areas of the first 2 maxillary molars. This ratio is 30 for FT 1271/2. A comparable ratio, calculated from molar crown dimensions and canine socket dimensions, is identical for this African specimen and YPM 13799. The range reported for 42 *H. sapiens* specimens is 18-35 (averaging 28). Twenty-five chimpanzees range from 37 to 112 (averaging 62), and 31 gorillas range from 29 to 83 (averaging 57). If sexual dimorphism in *"Ramapithecus"* followed the gorilla model, rather than the chimpanzee model, and if defense for this fossil creature was enacted by fleeing up nearby trees (assuming a forest-edge niche), the pongid adaptive model, and the known distribution of relative canine size, would account for the *"Ramapithecus"* condition without the necessity of assuming tool use.

Indeed, the importance of primate canines in defensive action against predators seems well established (Washburn and DeVore 1961a, 1961b; DeVore 1963; DeVore and Washburn 1963; Washburn 1968a). A recent study by Bramblett (1967) indicates that canine loss and breakage in baboons is a crucial life-limiting factor. With direct evidence that defense is the most important adaptive function of canines in non-human primates, canine reduction, for whatever reason, can only occur when something else can be substituted for canines. Therefore, while many of the hypotheses discussed are not necessarily contradictory, Darwin's original hypothesis seems corroborated: the canines reduce in hominids when tools replace their defensive function. Clark (1964:155) and Livingstone (1964:150) question the effectiveness of Oldowan tools as weapons of defense. Unmodified clubs would seem much more effective in the hands of early hominids, and it is surely weapons of this type that replaced canines in the defense of early hominids (Wolpoff 1970b).

With the reduction of canines to the size and shape of incisors, it follows that further changes in canine size should be linked to changes in incisor size. However, until that point, selection acting upon the incisors and the canines should not be confused, as several authors have done (Lancaster 1968:64; Pilbeam 1967:51).

Unlike the canines, the initial reduction of incisors follows a change in feeding habits (Pilbeam and Simons 1965:242-44). While apes used their incisors in feeding (Goodall 1963; Schaller 1963) by grasping, pulling, and tearing with them, terrestrial hominoids collected food and brought it to their mouths with their hands, if they followed the pattern of terrestrial baboons (Crook and Aldrich-Blake 1968; DeVore 1963).

Jolly (1970) has identified an adaptive complex in gelada baboons which he believes is analogous to early hominids. The dental evidence he utilizes includes small incisors and incisiform canines, and expanded cheek teeth, crowded mesiodistally, with a marked molar wear gradient and extensive interstitial wear. Actually, much of the dental evidence concerned with the cheek teeth is not supported by available data (Wolpoff 1970a), although the model of hominid differentiation may be correct. The small incisors observed in gelada baboons seem to result from hand feeding of small objects. This is a reasonable model for early hominid incisor reduction. The supposed graminivorous diet of early hominids utilizing the savanna would presumably be based on the seeds of grasses and annual herbs, joined later by roots made available by using simple pointed digging tools. With the defensive adaptation resulting from club carrying (Wolpoff 1968, 1970b), early scavenging activities became possible.

From the baboon model of a graminivorous dietary adaptation, one would expect a reduction in the incisor size of early hominids. To the extent that canines approached incisors in form and function, they would also be affected by this reduction.

Another factor has had great influence on incisor size. This is the increased amount of environmental manipulation characteristic of culture bearing hominids. Until recently, the incisors, along with the incisiform canines, played a crucial role in this manipulation (Merbs 1968; Brose and Wolpoff 1971).

Brace has attempted to look at the changes in the anterior teeth as a response to selection for an efficient cutting tool (1962a). Presumably, such selection was suspended with the development of efficient cutting tools in the Upper Paleolithic (Brace and Montagu 1965), and the anterior teeth subsequently reduced in size (Brace 1963a). This interpretation is questionable for 2 reasons. First, the tooth wear on anteriors for fossil hominids is flat. Thus, as soon as the tooth begins to wear in an edge-to-edge occlusion, it can no longer cut. Second, the flakes produced in manufacturing the simplest pebble tools are effective cutting tools (Bordes 1968) and have been used quite efficiently in butchering game (Leakey 1953).

I believe that holding, grasping, and exerting torsion are the primary manipulative functions of the anterior teeth. These are functions always recognized, but only recently emphasized by Brace (1967b:812). Use of the anteriors for these purposes in extant groups has already been established. Dahlberg (1963a) presents sufficient evidence to establish these functions for the anterior teeth of fossil man. He shows extensive differential incisor wear for La Ferrassie I (the right teeth are considerably more worn) resulting in an uneven and undulating occlusal plane. Other specimens, such as Shanidar I, Ternifine 3, and Krapina J (Brace 1962a:347-48) show similar wear. Large hominid anterior teeth, particularly with great breadth, are the result of selection for gripping, holding, and exerting torsion. The reduction of these teeth did not occur until the development of large numbers of special purpose tools replacing more generalized all-purpose tools (Brose and Wolpoff 1971): it requires much more use of a vise to put a hole in a piece of wood with a knife than with a drill.

There have been only a few hypotheses suggested in explanation of the reduction in the posterior dentition. The general relationship between size and use of the posterior teeth has long been recognized (Hrdlicka 1911:7-9). Yet, only a few authors addressed themselves to the question of why reduction occurred in the course of hominid evolution. There are, in fact, only 3 major hypotheses. The first was stated in its most detailed form by Weidenreich, although both Keith (1925) and Hellman (1936) made very similar suggestions. Weidenreich saw the trend of reduction in the posterior dentition as a correlated and integral part of the general shortening of the face and mandible (1937:161-62). Weidenreich referred to this process of correlated change as "Orthogenetic" evolution (1941). There was, in his view, a compelling force contained in the enlargement of the brain due to upright posture. Facial, mandibular, and dental reduction are all part of this change. The second hypothesis is concerned with the appearance of fire. Cooking foods makes them easier to chew (Brace 1962a). In addition, this preparation will allow utilization of a wider source of foods (Dahlberg 1963b). The appearance of fire as early as the Mindel Glaciation at both Choukoutien (Oakley 1966) and Vertessollos (Kretzoi and Vertes 1965) suggests considerable antiquity for the use of fire, although not necessarily in food preparation. The third hypothesis is concerned with a dietary shift. As Weidenreich recognized (1937:161), early hominids were largely vegetarian. There was a significant dietary shift with the incorporation of large quantities of meat in the diet. This shift is, in fact, the most extensive dietary change in all known hominid evolution. While Weidenreich was emphatic in disclaiming a relationship between this dietary shift and dental reduction (p. 161-62), other authors have taken the opposite view. Chewing even uncooked meat produces much less wear than chewing vegetable foods, if for no other reason than the fact that a relatively smaller amount of meat must be ingested for equivalent food value. Therefore, the dietary shift to increased meat eating would reduce occlusal wear, and thus reduce selection for large posterior teeth (Brace 1967b:814).

Of these 3 hypotheses, the second 2 do no injustice to evolutionary thinking and are not in contradiction with each other. A combination of the dietary shift along with an increasing frequency of food preparation through cooking reduced selection for large posterior teeth.

The resulting selection model has 3 component parameters acting independently. (1) There is a reduction in canine size and sexual dimorphism, as well as a change in canine form, resulting from the substitution of defensive weapons for defensive canines. (2) The incisors, and the incisiform canines, are maintained as large (although far from pongid size), thick teeth so as to be effectively used in manipulating the environment: they grip, grasp, pull, and exert torsion as one would expect of a vise. Selection maintaining large size is reduced with the appearance of numerous special purpose tools relieving the need for extensive vise-time and power. The incisors and canines reduce in size and become narrower. (3) The shift to an omnivorous diet incorporating a significant amount of meat eating, and independently the increased frequency of cooking, reduces selection for a large posterior grinding dentition. The molars and premolars reduce in size.

THE MECHANISM OF REDUCTION

There is one common facet to the selection model proposed here: all of the parameters discussed act to reduce selection for big teeth. It has long been recognized that the reduction of selection for complex structures almost always precedes reduction of the structures themselves (Breder 1944; Emerson 1961; Huxley 1932, 1942; DeBeer 1958; Gregory 1951; Simpson 1953; Van Valen 1960; Post 1962a, 1962b, 1963, 1964, 1966a, 1966b; Hooton 1947; Garn 1964; Dahlberg 1963a). A mechanism explaining structural reduction under conditions of reduced selection has been recently proposed (Brace 1963a, 1964b) and modified (Wolpoff 1969a). The conditions necessary for reduction are met by this selection model. The mechanisms suggested by these authors derive from the necessary orientation of random changes in the genetic material. Such changes can accumulate when they are selectively neutral (Brace 1963a). In addition, they will occur when selection acting on 1 phenotype in a pleiotropic system is relaxed, and a new balance of selective forces acting on the genetic material in the system is reached. In either case, the structure for which selection was relaxed will tend to reduce in size and complexity, as well as increase in variability (Wolpoff 1969a). Reduction due to selection, from whatever sources, will not be accompanied by an increase in variability (Simpson 1953). Therefore, an analysis of variation is necessary in order to determine whether or not this mechanism explains a particular case of reduction. Such an analysis is crucial to this work, as the selective model proposed results in relaxed selection.

HOMINID PHYLOGENY AND TAXONOMY

The view of hominid phylogeny accepted by this author is essentially that proposed by Mayr (1950). The unifying concept of this framework is the "single species hypothesis" (Wolpoff 1968). Hominid evolution is viewed as unilinear, in that there is not evidence of more than 1 hominid species existing at 1 time. The rationale of this framework, and the evidence supporting it, have been discussed elsewhere (Brace 1967a; Wolpoff 1968, 1969b, 1970b; Coon 1963; Washburn 1960; Brose and Wolpoff 1971; Livingstone 1961; Buettner-Janusch 1966, 1968; Bartholomew and Birdsell 1953).

If hominid phylogeny is viewed as 1 continuous lineage, hominid taxonomy becomes simple in principle but difficult to apply. The easiest way to discuss hominid evolution is in terms of stages. Such an approach has been utilized by Arambourg (1958) and Brace (1964a, 1967a). This circumvents the problems of hominid taxonomy, but also ignores questions raised therein. It is possible to distinguish fossil taxa, and most authors have agreed on a method of delineation consistent with the new systematics (Mayr 1969; McAlester 1962; Simons 1967).

The primary criterion in the establishment of fossil species is an indication of the existence of genetic barriers (McAlester 1962). In hominid evolution there are, of course, no barriers between temporal species, and there are no synchronic species. In this instance, one must rely on other criteria which, no matter how consistent with theory, must be arbitrary in the sense that living species are non-arbitrary (Simpson 1963). For hominids, the definition of such criteria is simplified by the existence of an extant species representing the lineage. The agreed procedure is to determine the amount of variability which exists between populations in the extant species, and utilize it as a yardstick for determining the amount of variation expected in a fossil species (Mayr 1969:196-97).

Applying such a yardstick to Pleistocene hominids results in the creation of 4 or 5 temporal species, each separated by about the same amount of morphological space (Simons 1967), but each ultimately defined by a time span rather than a set of morphological characteristics. The uncertainty in species number stems from 2 sources: the number of taxa represented among the australopithecines, and the proper classification of the Neandertals.

Australopithecines have been divided into gracile and robust forms. There is widespread disagreement on both how many species each form may include, and whether or not the forms themselves are taxonomically distinct. The presence of robust teeth in the Omo deposits (Howell 1969), and the robust identification of at least 1 of the 2 Lake Rudolph crania, dated in excess of 2.6 million years (R. Leakey, personal communication), conclusively proves that robust australopithecines predate the gracile specimens at Olduvai. There is no single time sequence for the 2 groups.

I have worked all of the data treating the australopithecines as 2 separate taxa: 2 species within the genus *Homo.* The differences between the robust and gracile forms do not, in my opinion, warrant more than species distinction. Inclusion in *Homo* is justified because both groups utilize culture as their major adaptive mechanism. Thus, they occupy the same adaptive plateau as subsequent hominids.

There is some question as to whether the gracile and robust forms even represent separate species (Wolpoff 1968, 1970b; Brace 1967a; Campbell 1966; Buettner-Janusch 1968; Frisch 1965). For instance, one of the workers most familiar with the actual specimens recently stated the following with respect to the gracile and robust lines:

> The distinctness between these two lines should not be overstated: it is suggested that gene exchange between the two lines might have been possible. Such hybridizing effects might have aided the "toning down" of the extremely robust earlier *A. boisei* into the later, less robust *A. robustus;* and secondly might account for a number of *A. robustus* features in the otherwise *A. africanus* forms of Makapansgat (Tobias 1969:311-12).

Although Tobias clearly did not realize it, this description can only refer to lineages existing within 1 biological species, according to the widely accepted principles of the new systematics (Mayr 1969).

Because of these considerations, I also treated the australopithecines as 1 group for all of the calculations. By australopithecines, I refer to the group of late Pliocene and Lower Pleistocene fossils listed in Chapter 3. Later specimens are assigned to *H. erectus,* as defined by Mayr (1950) but including the recent Olduvai discoveries, ranges from about 1 million years (no definite date for Olduvai Bed II specimens is available) to the termination of the Mindel Glaciation. Subsequent hominids could be included within *H. sapiens.* Indeed, some authors have suggested the division of *Homo* into 2 species: *H. africanus* (or *H. transvaalensis* in 1 interpretation), and *H. sapiens* (Buettner-Janusch 1968; Robinson 1965b). On the other hand, authors have long recognized a "Neandertal stage" of human evolution (Hrdlicka 1927; Schwalbe 1913; Keith 1948). Morphological evidence indicates sufficient differences between the Neandertals and *H. sapiens* to maintain the former as a separate temporal species (Le Gros Clark 1964:50-87; Vlcek 1964, 1967), ancestral to anatomically modern *H. sapiens* in all geographic areas (Brace 1962b, 1964a, 1967c; Jelinek 1969; Yakimov 1969; Brose and Wolpoff 1971).

Placing all hominid species in the genus *Homo* opens up other questions. Mayr (1950) suggests that "species united in a given genus occupy an ecological situation which is different from that occupied by the species of another genus . . . a different adaptive plateau (p. 110)." A similar definition was also suggested by Simpson (1961:153). On the other hand, Simons (1967), McAlester (1962), and others view a genus in terms of morphological space, suggesting that genera are made up of groups of related species as different as such groups in extant genera (Simons 1967:313). Most human paleontologists seem to have accepted the relevance of similarity in adaptation as a uniting factor on the generic level. Such a criterion is consistent with an evolutionary framework of changes in higher categories (Rensch 1959). In the sense that Pleistocene hominids are adapted to culture as a means of survival (Bartholomew and Birdsell 1953; Bielicki 1966; Mayr 1950; Washburn 1960; Brace and Montagu 1965), they occupy a single adaptive plateau (Wolpoff 1968), and therefore are all in the genus *Homo.* They are so treated here, following Mayr (1950).

A study such as this is not designed to determine a taxonomy; indeed, taxonomic conclusions should never derive from dental evidence alone. The validity of this interpretive framework rests not upon the taxonomy suggested here, but rather upon the phylogenetic hypothesis underlying it.

2. Techniques and Methods of Collection and Analysis

DEFINITION OF THE MEASUREMENTS AND INDEXES

The mesiodistal measurement has been called a length (Hrdlicka 1952; Remane 1930; Senyurek 1939; Weidenreich 1937a; Pedersen 1949; Nelson 1938; Schuman and Brace 1954; Robinson 1956), a breadth (Martin 1928; Mijsberg 1931; de Terra 1905; Muhlreiter 1928; Selmer-Olsen 1949; Oliver 1960), a width (Seipel 1946), and a diameter (Moorrees 1957; Selmer-Olsen 1949; Tobias 1967a). By definition, the mesial surface of a tooth is that surface facing toward the central incisor, and the distal surface is that which faces away. According to Martin (1928), a length is sagittal horizontal distance. Because almost all teeth have a greater sagittal than perpendicular component to the mesiodistal measure, I feel justified in describing this measurement as a length. A breadth, then, is the perpendicular measurement.

The actual definition of mesiodistal length is of great importance. Many definitions have been used in the literature. For instance, Remane (1927, 1930) defines it in 2 ways: "mean length" is the distance between the points of contact of a tooth with its neighbors parallel to the occlusal and labial surfaces, and "greatest length" is simply the maximum mesiodistal dimension of the tooth parallel to the occlusal and labial surfaces. The latter definition is in common use and has been employed by a large number of authors (Weidenreich 1937a; Martin 1928; Pedersen 1949; Senyurek 1959; Moorrees 1957; Tobias 1967a; Korenhof 1960; Robinson 1956; Greene, Ewing, and Armelagos 1967). Additional definitions include the following: the distance between the greatest mesial and distal bulges (Hjelmman 1928; Mijsberg 1931); the maximum distance parallel to the occlusal and labial surfaces between the actual points of normal contact or the points where normal contact would occur (Selmer-Olsen 1949); the distance between points of contact measured midway on the tooth (Schuman and Brace 1954); the distance between points of contact of the tooth parallel to the labial and occlusal planes (Hrdlicka 1952; Ashton and Zuckerman 1950a; Gregory and Hellman 1926a). Breadth, on the other hand, is inevitably defined as the maximum measurement perpendicular to length and parallel to the occlusal surface. Strictly speaking, buccolingual breadth should only refer to posterior teeth, and labiolingual breadth to anteriors. I have used buccolingual throughout, as it seems a fully adequate description.

I have utilized a system of measurement essentially following that of Selmer-Olsen (1949:23-26). He defines the measuring points as *"points of contact with normal tooth position* (p. 24)." Identical or very similar definitions were utilized by Hrdlicka (1952), Ashton and Zuckerman (1950a), Gregory and Hellman (1926a), and Goose (1963). For posterior teeth, the measurement is almost at the midpoint of the tooth, and thus does not differ greatly from measurements taken by Schuman and Brace (1954) and the "Mittellange" defined by Remane

(1930). Rotation of the posterior teeth in the sockets, a not uncommon occurrence (Goose 1963:127; Selmer-Olsen 1949:23), necessitates estimation of the contact points. For posterior teeth, the measurement taken is not always the same as maximum length. In particular, measurements will differ from those taken by Korenhof (1960), Robinson (1956), and Tobias (1967a) in that maximum lengths measured along the estimated longitudinal axis of the crown will often exceed the ones I have reported.

Measurements of the anterior teeth present slightly different problems. In the maxillary incisors, the 2 contact points are often not in the same plane. The distance between them is thus misleading. I have adopted the technique of Selmer-Olsen for anterior teeth. The mesiodistal length measurement is defined as the maximum length of the tooth measured in a plane parallel to the occlusal surface (Number 4 in Figure 3 of Selmer-Olsen 1949:25). Any other definition for both incisors and canines would be difficult to reproduce. There is an extensive amount of form variation in both incisors (Taylor 1969a) and canines (Taylor 1969b). Indeed, the canines in *H. sapiens* are variable enough to include the 2 morphological forms which Robinson (1956) uses to distinguish hominid *genera* (Taylor 1969b).

Buccolingual breadth is defined in all cases as the maximum breadth perpendicular to the length. On the anterior teeth, the maximum breadth was often found at or near the base of the crown. Both length and breadth measurements were taken parallel to the occlusal plane.

These definitions were utilized for 2 reasons. First, they were easily and consistently reproducible on both human and non-human primate dentitions. Second, they seemed to best represent the average dimensions of the crown itself, regardless of its orientation in the jaw, or its irregularity in shape. Thus, the area calculated by multiplying the length by the breadth would come closest, when compared to lengths and breadths otherwise defined, to the actual cross-sectional area cut by the intersection of the crown and the occlusal plane.

All measurements were taken with Helios dial calipers. All measurements can be directly read to the nearest tenth of a millimeter, and the nearest hundredth of a millimeter can be estimated. Measurements taken by the author were recorded to the nearest hundredth of a millimeter, although such accuracy is in excess of that suggested by tests for reproducibility. The calipers were machined to points with a fine taper so that they could be inserted between teeth *in situ*.

Only 3 indexes are calculated from these dimensions. The area was found by multiplying the length by the breadth. This is the same as the robustness defined by Weidenreich (1937a), Pedersen (1949), Senyurek (1959), and others. This area measure was used because it closely approximates the actual surface area of the tooth in the occlusal plane. If the tooth was perfectly rectangular, this area measure would be an exact approximation of the actual surface area. Because of the way the measurements were defined, teeth approximating trapezoids or parallelograms will also have almost perfect area approximations. Teeth with an elliptical cross-section will yield an overestimate by a factor of 1.27 (4 divided by *pi*), or about 25%. Such an error will most consistently occur in the anterior teeth, but will affect all teeth to some extent Because the area estimates are used for comparisons, and not for the computation of actual areas as they would be if a stress analysis were attempted, it is felt that this error will not significantly influence the results.

The index of the crown, 100 times the length divided by the breadth, is a useful means for expressing the approximate shape (Goose 1963:131; Selmer-Olsen 1949:54-61; Hrdlicka 1923a, 1923b). Hrdlicka (1923a) feels that differences in this index for the first 2 molars are of taxonomic value.

The module of the crown is 1/2 the sum of the length plus the breadth. It has often been used as a convenient way of combining length and breadth measurements (Robinson 1956). It is not directly a measure of size in the sense that area is. It is rather a function of the perimeter of the crown.

Of these indexes, the index of robustness—the area—is probably of greatest use. The area, after all, is what we must mean when we refer to "size." Dental size and morphology are clearly related. Ever since Hellman's original discussion of dental patterns and their distribution (1928), patterns of morphological variation have been used as guides for phylogenetic constructions of hominid prehistory. Yet, no convincing demonstration of the direct selective value of cusp number or groove pattern has been forthcoming (Bailit, DeWitt, and Leigh 1968:285). Selection acts indirectly upon cusp number because of its relation to absolute size. Dahlberg (1961) demonstrated a significant relationship between molar mesiodistal length and cusp number. Indeed, authors for some time have been aware of the fact that populations with larger teeth tend to have more cusps (Dahlberg 1945; Jorgensen 1955; Hellman 1919; Erdbrink 1967), as well as the fact that the greatest percentage of 5 and 6 cusped lower molars appears in populations chewing "hard and tough food" (Erdbrink 1965:105; Hrdlicka 1911:7-8).

Along with the length-cusp number relationship, there has been a demonstration of a significant relationship between relative molar size and relative cusp number (Garn, Lewis, Dahlberg, and Kerewsky 1966). In addition, Davies (1968) has established a relationship between cusp number reduction in the lower first molar, and agenesis of the lower third molar. The relation of cusp number to dental size could not be clearer. In contradistinction, groove pattern, a variable independent of cusp number (Jorgensen 1955), is also independent of tooth size (Garn, Dahlberg, Lewis, and Kerewsky 1966).

GENETIC BASIS OF TOOTH SIZE

It is not my purpose to detail recent work in dental genetics, but rather I would like to indicate the relative magnitudes of genetic and environmental influences on final tooth size. In addition, the relevant parameters of a genetic model for tooth size inheritance must be delineated.

The strong genetic component of crown features and morphology has long been recognized (Hellman 1928; Korkhaus 1930), and specific genetic models for a number of features have been worked out (Dahlberg 1963c, as editor 1963; Kraus and Oka 1967; Moorrees 1962; Osborne 1967; Osborne and De George 1959; Turner 1967). The hypothesis of a strong genetic component in the development of crown size, too, has long been held (Korkhaus 1930; Dahlberg 1945, 1963a; Osborne, Horowitz, and De George 1958; Osborne and De George 1959; Garn and Shamir 1958). Dental size has long been considered relatively independent of environment (Osborne 1967:945) and a useful marker of genetic distance between populations (Garn, Lewis, and Walenga 1968b, 1968c, 1968d, 1969). A large number of twin studies (Osborne 1963) have indicated the presence of a very great genetic component, and concomitantly a very small environmental component of crown size for most teeth (Garn, Lewis, and Kerewsky 1965a; Lundstrom 1948; Osborne and De George 1959; Osborne, Horowitz, and De George 1958). The results from several family studies are corroborating (Garn, Lewis, and Kerewsky 1966d, 1967d). Using correlations to measure similarity, however, Goose (1967) has reported that the correlations in a family study are "smaller than should be expected if genetic factors were the principle factors concerned (p. 961)."

The exact proportions of the genetic and environmental components of tooth size remain unknown. The causes of variation have not been partitioned (Penrose 1954), and no estimate of heritability has been successfully attempted (Falconer 1960:165-85). There is, without doubt, at least some environmental influence upon the development of crown size (Garn, Lewis, and Walenga 1968a; Goose 1967).

One problem stems from the fact that there is no genetic model for crown size. Some attempts toward such a model have been made. Tooth size is subject, in part, to X-linked inheritance (Garn, Lewis, and Kerewsky 1965a, 1965c; Garn, Lewis, Swindler, and Kerewsky 1967; Garn and Rohmann 1962; Osborne, Horowitz, and De George 1958; Lewis and Grainger 1967). There is definite evidence for communality in the relationship of corresponding tooth size in brothers and sisters (Garn, Lewis, and Kerewsky 1967d), and for the relationship between sexual dimorphism in tooth size and body size (Garn, Lewis, and Kerewsky 1966d; Garn, Lewis, Kerewsky, and Jegart 1965). Indeed, the magnitude of sexual dimorphism in tooth size is under genetic control (Garn, Lewis, and Kerewsky 1964b, 1965a, 1966a; Garn, Lewis, Kerewsky, and Jegart 1965; Garn, Lewis, Swindler, and Kerewsky 1967). Molar size sequence is under genetic control (Garn, Lewis, and Kerewsky 1964a, 1965a).

An attempt has been made to determine whether or not there is a general size factor linking genetic control of mesiodistal and buccolingual diameters (Garn, Lewis, and Kerewsky 1968b). The correlation between the diameters was used in the determination, although one would not expect this to be a very good indicator because the area relationship between the diameters is multiplicative. Thus, the intermediate correlations are not particularly meaningful. On the other hand, correlations for the posterior teeth were significantly higher than for the anteriors. This is exactly what one would expect if selection acts on the posteriors for surface area. A difference in genetic background between anterior and posterior teeth, probably the result of the differential action of and response to selection, is indicated.

Without either models of inheritance or estimates of heritability, it will not be possible to determine the relative components of genetic and environmental influence. The complicating factor is the effect of diet and nutrition (Garn 1966). Permanent teeth could well be influenced by diet (Hunt 1960). On the other hand, type of food (oats, barley, or wheat) has a *selective* effect on mouse tooth size (Van Valen 1963). However, closely related species of *Macaca* with significant differences in tooth size have apparently identical diets (Swindler, Gavan, and Turner 1963). The results of the best controlled studies, the twin studies, probably provide the best information. These generally seem to show low nutritional and maturational but high genetic components of tooth size variation (Garn, Lewis, and Kerewsky 1965a).

TOOTH SIZE AND BODY SIZE

The possibility of a relationship between tooth size and body size must be considered. Such a relationship could complicate problems of dental comparison. A strict and direct relationship of tooth size and body size has often been assumed for fossil hominoids. Thus, *"Meganthropus"* was assumed to be a giant hominid on the basis of tooth size (Weidenreich 1945a:109-11), and *"Gigantopithecus"* was presumed even larger. Pei (1957b:836) estimated a height of 12 feet for the owner of the *"Gigantopithecus"* mandible. In a less extreme vein, the differences between the posterior dentitions of the australopithecines have often been associated with differences in body size (Robinson 1956:150, 1963b:392; Howell 1963:597; Brace 1962:345).

On the other hand, recent work questions this relationship. Garn and Lewis (1958) found no correlation between first molar size and height as well as for first incisor size and height (both jaws considered), for a sample of Ohio "Whites." Filipsson and Goldson (1963) found no relationship between incisor and canine size and stature in Swedish conscripts, as well as a very low (.2) correlation between incisor width and head width. Garn, Lewis, and Kerewsky (1968a) report low correlations between length or breadth and stature for Ohio "Whites." In this study, the correlation coefficients for all teeth ranged from r = -.24 to r = .42. Of the 56 possible correlations (both sexes were included), 17 were significant. The mean correlations for both jaws were about .12 for females and about .20 for males.

Brace and Montagu (1965) suggest a correction factor for tooth size on the basis of body size when comparing different populations (p. 300), while Bailit and Friedlaender (1966:670) cite examples indicating that no relationship exists on either the inter- or the intrapopulation basis.

The problems in both the individual level and the population level determinations are legion. Body size-tooth size comparisons between extant populations cannot be made unless all factors affecting both of these variables and the relationship between them are held constant. No study of tooth size and body size has approached this criterion. Comparisons within populations should be more fruitful. However, with the relaxation of dental selection in extant groups (Brace 1962a, 1962b; Dahlberg 1963a, 1963c), there has been an increase in dental variability due to both the accumulation of mutations (Brace 1963a, 1964b) and the differential effects of selection acting on other phenotypic expressions of those genes affecting tooth size that are pleiotropic (Wolpoff 1969a). Such an increase could be expected to be most prevalent in those populations in which selection has been reduced for the longest period of time (Post 1962a, 1962b, 1963, 1964, 1966a, 1966b). If there were a significant relationship between tooth size and body size, it would be most obscured in the very populations studied: Ohioans and Swedes.

Until populations in which selection has not been relaxed are studied in the same manner that Ohio "Whites" have been analyzed, the question of whether or not there is a relationship between tooth size and body size, and the extent of the relationship if it exists, cannot be settled.

With respect to this work, the possibility of such a relationship has an unknown effect. I am concerned with species level variation. No work has been attempted with respect to whether or not this relationship exists on the species level. In order to demonstrate a tooth size-body size relationship *on the species level,* all other variables would have to be held constant. This is probably not possible in *Homo* because there is only 1 extant species.

Indeed, if there were a relationship between tooth size and body size, it could only interfere with this study if there were a constant decrease in body size from the beginning of the Pleistocene. Otherwise, the observed trends have appeared in spite of any species level body size changes.

INTERSTITIAL WEAR

Simons (1968b:100-102) has informally advanced the suggestion that interstitial wear is a distinctively hominid characteristic. Such wear implies "a closely packed tooth row and suggests the improbability of a diastema (p. 102)." One major result is that mesiodistal shortening is a common occurrence in hominid teeth (Begg 1954). Indeed, many of the seemingly anomalous small teeth (re. SK 15 and 45, or *"Telanthropus"*) are the result of such shortening (Wolpoff 1970a).

The effect upon length can be appreciable (Robinson 1956:9; Lundstrom 1952), and a number of workers have attempted to correct for such shortening so that the true length is approximated. The difficulties in such corrections are substantial.

There have only been a few attempts to quantify the amount of loss due to interstitial wear. In an extensive study, Wolpoff (1970a) determined that the rate of wear is greater in chimpanzees than in any hominid group. A classic study was conducted by Begg (1954). Using mesiodistal length, he took measurements for a number of unworn teeth of Australian aborigines and compared them with measurements taken on the worn teeth of individuals whose third molars had not reached occlusion. The results, given in 2 tables (I and II, p. 306), indicate substantial reduction in length on both an absolute and percentage basis. The total summed average length of the tooth row (to M_2) was 62.12 mm in the unworn teeth, and 56.78 mm in the worn teeth. There was thus a total loss of 5.34 mm, or 9%. The percentage loss for individual teeth ranged from 5.2% for P_4 to 17.7% for M_1. Great contrasts appeared within both the anterior and the posterior tooth sets. For instance, the percentage loss for I_1 was 5.8%, while for I_2 it was 9.6%. It should be emphasized that these figures do not represent the total loss of tooth material throughout life, but rather represent the loss up to the approximate age of 18.

According to Begg, this loss of dental material (particularly affecting mesiodistal length) and the concomitant forward migration of teeth in the dental arch once the cusp pattern is lost through attrition, occurs constantly throughout life and results in the "normal" edge to edge occlusion of Paleolithic man (1954:298). The process begins so early that there is often interstitial loss in M_1 due to attrition against dM_2 before it is lost. The importance of interstitial wear, constant mesial migration, and prolonged vertical eruption (Taylor 1963:121-23; Begg 1954:296-98) imparts severe limitations upon mechanical attempts to simulate wear patterns and occlusions on rigid casts (Brace and Molnar 1967; Molnar 1968). Goose (1963:128) estimates that as much as 3.2 mm of the enamel may be lost from the length of the summed premolars and molars of a series of Saxons. This compares favorably with the average loss of 3.77 mm in the P_3 - M_2 series of Australian aborigines. Taylor (1963:121) observed losses up to 1 mm of enamel in individual Moriori teeth. Black (1908) notes the loss of about 1 cm from the dental arch representing about 40 years of interstitial wear.

Interstitial wear is characteristic of almost all groups of fossil men, as well as many extant groups. Using the australopithecines as an example, maxillae such as MLD 9 (a "gracile" type) and mandibulae such as SK 34 (a "robust" type) probably represent the extremes of such wear.

It is interesting to note that 1 of the few australopithecine specimens which does not exhibit interstitial wear is Olduvai Hominid (OH) 7, a specimen noted for its unusual relative narrowness in the posterior teeth. The extent of mesiodistal shortening found in most other australopithecine specimens would reduce the posterior tooth shape (L/B) indexes of this specimen to values more closely approximating the australopithecine means. Comparison of OH 7 to other australopithecine mandibles of similar chronological age is difficult. Using aging techniques developed by Mann (1968), it was found that only 5% of the available *H. africanus* specimens fall in the 10-15 year age bracket, while 20% of the *H. robustus* specimens (and 15% of all australopithecines) fall within this age range (McKinley 1971). The only published mandible of *H. africanus* which is comparable is MLD 2 (Dart 1948c) aged at 12 years (Mann 1968:145). Interstitial wear is already shown on M_1 of this specimen, on the mesial articulation with dM_2. M_2 has just erupted. Not surprisingly, the M_1 L/B ratio is about average for *H. africanus,* while the M_2 ratio is above average for *H. africanus;* in fact, it is only exceeded by the value for OH 7. OH 7, no more than a year older (McKinley 1971), shows slightly less interstitial wear on M_1. P_4 of this specimen is fully erupted, but comes far short of filling the space vacated by dM_2, and thus does not articulate mesially or distally. Comparisons with *H. robustus* are limited to SK 6 (Broom and Robinson 1952:1-3 and Plate 1) aged at 15 years (Mann 1968:139) and SK 1588 (Brain 1967:382 and Figure 3) aged at 13 years (Mann 1968:142). The former shows considerable wear between M_1 and M_2. Medial wear is not comparable because right P_4 is an anomalous misshaped tooth and left P_3 is rotated out of position (Broom and Robinson 1952:3). Mesial and distal interstitial M_1 wear of SK 1588 is considerable. Thus, the narrowness of OH 7 appears due to age.

While there is some variation among the australopithecines, all specimens show interstitial wear, and thus some degree of mesiodistal shortening. Australian aborigines only 6 years older than OH 7 already have lost almost 20% M_1 length.

There are 2 ways to look at interstitial wear. The first is to view it in terms of the error which it introduces into species descriptions. As has been indicated, this error can be considerable. Elimination of all teeth showing such attrition would exclude almost all teeth of fossil man. On the other hand, "correction" of the mesiodistal dimension can only be done 3 ways. One can simply attempt to correct for such shortening in taking the measurement (Robinson 1956; Hrdlicka 1952). One can also attempt separation of the material into age groups on the basis of wear, and then only make comparisons between corresponding age groups (Ashton and Zuckerman 1950a). Lastly, one can attempt to recompute the original dimension of the tooth. Lysell (1958) attempted such re-computation by utilizing the shape index of unworn teeth in order to estimate the original length of worn ones from their breadth. The first method is, at best, inaccurate. The second is almost impossible to apply due to difficulties in aging hominid teeth by wear (Miles 1963:207-8). The third assumes that individual shape indexes can be closely predicted from sample average indexes. The present study demonstrates that coefficients of variation for the index are regularly too high to allow such an assumption.

There is a second way to view interstitial wear which, if adopted, will circumvent the problems of correction discussed above. This view stems from the consideration of interstitial wear and mesial migration as the "normal" hominid condition (Simons 1968b) leading to "normal" occlusion in Paleolithic man (Begg 1954; Weinmann and Sicher 1955; Biggerstaff 1967). To the extent that tooth size is a factor in adaptation, its selective value is determined by the size distribution *actually present at any time,* and not by the size distribution of only unworn teeth. If size reduction is a normal facet of occlusion, and if our samples adequately represent the species from which they were drawn, these species are best compared and analyzed on the basis of both worn and unworn teeth. Tooth size phenotype is not a function of unworn size alone.

In the determination of metric trends, the measurements and indexes of all teeth can be utilized. This sample best represents the adaptive characteristics of the group from which it was drawn. Interstitial wear, then, does not introduce error in the computation of population or species level dental characteristics.

ANALYSIS OF ERROR

Physical measurements are subject to 3 types of error: (1) errors of the observer; (2) systematic errors; (3) random errors. Errors of the first type stem from mistakes and misreadings. They can occur when a caliper scale is misread, when the data is recorded, or when the data is copied. The second type of error will affect a number of measurements, if not all, in a similar manner. It stems from improper adjustment of measurement instruments, incorrect or inappropriate definition of the quantity measured, or error in an operator function or algorithm acting upon the data. The third type of error is, by definition, unpredictable. Such errors are always present to some degree in any physical data. In the gross data dealt with here, they could stem from the inability to exactly reproduce a single measurement, from differential environmental influences on tooth size and form for individuals, from errors in sampling, and from a wide variety of other sources.

Errors of the first 2 types can be reduced through careful handling of the data and checking of the analytical procedures. Such errors will, of course, never be completely eliminated. On the other hand, close and critical scrutiny of the data and procedures at all times should allow the undiscovered errors of these types to be treated as random. The random treatment of such errors is possible as long as (1) each error is only a small fraction of the observed quantity, and (2) positive and negative errors are equally likely to occur.

Random errors can be divided into errors of sampling, and "other." Errors of sampling are the result of small and/or biased samples. The following section discusses methods of determining whether or not the means of 2 samples are sufficiently different to assume their origin in 2 different parent populations. In addition, we would like a measure of the accuracy of the sample mean as an estimation of the population mean. The standard error of the mean (Parratt 1961:92-93; Margenau and Murphy 1956:510-13) is such a measure. The standard error (SE) is calculated as follows:

$$SE = \frac{SDs}{\sqrt{n}}$$

where SDs is the standard deviation of the sample, and n is the sample size. It may be pointed out that the variance of the sample is only an estimate of the population variance (Parratt 1961:88-89). The divisor for the sample variance is n minus 1. This approaches the divisor for the population variance (n) for large samples. Standard deviations used here are all *sample estimates,* as are all of the sample statistics calculated from them.

The distribution of sample means from a single parent population is normal, even if the parent population is significantly different from normal (Parratt 1961:93-94). As a result, the probability that a sample mean will differ from the mean of the parent population by "*m*" standard errors can be read from any table of values for the standard normal distribution function. For instance if $m = 1$, the probability that the sample mean differs from the parent population mean by $\pm$ 1 (m) SE is .683. Confidence limits can be constructed for the mean from the standard error. Thus, if one is willing to accept only 50% probability that the parent population falls within the range of the sample mean $\pm$ mSE, $m = .67$; for a 75% probability $m = 1.15$; for a 90% probability $m = 1.64$. Looking at it another way, $\pm$ 2 standard errors gives a confidence interval of very close to 95%; $\pm$ 2.17 standard errors gives a confidence interval of 97%; $\pm$ 2.5 standard errors falls just short of defining a 99% interval; and $\pm$ 3 standard errors gives a 99.7% interval. The great value of the standard error lies in the fact that it is distribution free; that is, these probabilities make no assumptions about the normality of the parent population.

The standard error of the mean is itself subject to error. The relative estimated probable error of the standard error is:

$$\frac{\sqrt{2}}{2n}$$

(Margenau and Murphy 1956:513; Plummer 1940:124-26). For a sample size of 2, this error is 35%. For 5, it is 14%; 7 gives an error of 10%, and 10 an error of 7%. For a sample size of 14, there is an expected relative error of 5%; a 2% error is reached for a sample size of 35; and a 1% error for 70.

The "other" category of random errors is more difficult to deal with, as the accuracy of the analysis of such error depends upon the extent to which the randomizing assumptions discussed above are met. The 2 major error sources in this dental study stem from (1) the inability to reproduce the identical measurement on different teeth, which may be estimated by a measure of the inability to reproduce the same measurements on the same tooth at different times, and (2) the more systematic errors arising from the comparison of measurements made by different authors.

The problem of comparison between authors is acute. In the hominid dental literature, one is fortunate enough to find descriptions of the measurement technique, let alone an analysis of error. There is almost no way to estimate how much of an error such comparisons introduce. Only a few purposeful comparisons have been made. Tobias (1964b:410) compared his measurements of the South African australopithecines to those of the same specimens published by Robinson (1956). He claims a mean difference of .1 mm and a maximum difference of .3 mm. However, a comparison of the measurements of the Olduvai Hominid 7 premolars between these same workers (Robinson 1965b; Tobias and von Koenigswald 1964) discloses a difference of .9 mm in the breadth of the left P_3. A comparison of Robinson's measurements to those of Leakey (1961c) shows a difference of 1.4 mm in the length. Both length and breadth measurements are on the order of magnitude of 1 cm!

Some work has been done concerning the reproducibility between and among workers on plaster casts. Richardson, Adams, and McCartney (1963) examined these differences for incisors on a set of 10 casts. The mean error between observers was calculated to be .116 ± .121 mm (Bailit, DeWitt, and Leigh 1968) for length. Hunter and Priest (1960) made similar determinations on a series of 24 casts. They report a mean difference between observers of .153 ± .026 mm. Lastly, Bailit, DeWitt, and Leigh cite an average error between observers of .05 ± .32 mm for 105 casts of Nasioi dentitions. These mean differences represent a minimum estimation because they were gathered by workers in communication attempting to use the same technique of measurement. Comparison of most measurements in the literature meet neither of these criteria The respective workers are not always attempting to utilize the same technique, and even if they are, they are almost never in a position to attempt improvement of their compatibility.

One can only hope that the errors introduced to this study as the result of using different authors' data, as well as my own, will be systematic. If so, the errors so introduced will not affect the comparisons developed. Actually, there are a number of reasons why this assumption is justified. The data for *each* of the taxa represents publications of a number of workers. The definitions of the major measurements, while not always consistent among authors, were matters of concern to most workers. Whenever possible, the data was checked against other sources. However, of probably greatest importance, the measurement techniques and definitions utilized by this author tend to neither minimize or maximize the resulting measurements. Other methods applied to the same dentitions could result in larger or smaller values. Thus, there is reason to believe that the results of divergent measurement techniques would tend to cancel each other out.

Considering the problem in another way, the failure to make an assumption of this nature renders comparative dental studies impossible.

The available studies of reproducibility seem to indicate an average error arising from comparisons of data from different observers of between .1 and .5 mm. A maximum error estimate is probably not much greater.

Lastly, then, we must consider the contribution of random errors due to measurement reproduction by 1 author. A number of authors have indicated that this error tends to be relatively low (Goose 1963; Ashton and Zuckerman 1950a). In the study by Richardson, Adams, and McCartney (1963), the mean error within observers was calculated to be .008 ± .106 mm. The Nasioi study yielded an average error among measurers of .04 ± .21 mm for 271 casts (Bailit, DeWitt, and Leigh 1968). Repeated measures attempted by Schuman and Brace (1954) produced an average error of .2 mm. Pedersen (1949) reports the same error margin, and Nelson (1938) reports an accuracy to .1 mm in repeated measurements. The maximum error reported is by Shaw (1931), claiming no accuracy better than .5 mm.

The probable error is very similar to the error of repetition for 1 author (Margenau and Murphy 1956:510-15). The probable error is defined such that 1/2 of the results of n observations are greater than it, and the other half are less. Under certain assumptions (Margenau and Murphy 1956:511), the probable error can be estimated from the standard deviation. However, this estimate is not of great value (Simpson, Roe, and Lewontin 1960:161). It is far more useful to consider the probable error equivalent to the error of reproduction for each worker, and to calculate it the same way. Reported probable errors thus range from .01 mm to .50 mm.

I followed a procedure for error estimation similar to that of other workers. Multiple measurements were taken as long as possible after the initial measurements, and in a different order. Over 500 different teeth were thus treated. By comparing the multiple measurements to each other, probable errors can be calculated for the length and breadth of each tooth. The probable error is, as a direct consequence of the definition, simply the average deviation for each set of multiple measurements. It can be calculated separately for both length and breadth and for each individual tooth.

The differences between the teeth and between the jaws did not appear to be significant. They were about the same as the differences in probable error between length and breadth measurements for all teeth.

This probable error for length was .09 ± .22 mm and for breadth .08 ± .16 mm. These are not significantly different; both length and breadth have probable errors of about .08 mm in the teeth measured by this author. This represents an average relative probable error of about 1%. While the average errors for particular teeth differed, none differed more than 25% from the mean error (1%), and no pattern was established. Thus, it seems reasonable to discuss an average probable error for all teeth, and apparently for both measurements. The maximum single error for length was 1.3 mm and for breadth 1.6 mm.

I would expect the average uncertainty introduced in this manner to be somewhat less than that resulting from the utilization of different authors' data. At least 2 other studies arrive at similar conclusions (Richardson, Adams, and McCartney 1963; Bailit, DeWitt, and Leigh 1968). Tobias' claim of a .1 mm average difference between his and Robinson's australopithecine measurements (1964b:410) would seem to indicate otherwise. Not only is the absolute error less, the relative errors for length and breadth are about 1.0% and .5% respectively. On the other hand, the performance of Leakey, Tobias, and Robinson in the measurement of 2 lower third premolars would tend to contradict a claim of consistency to 1%.

For these reasons, I believe that 1% is an underestimate of the uncertainty introduced by the utilization of data from different sources. Because 1% is close to the probable error of my own data, the probable error introduced by utilizing different sources is at least as great as that implicit in 1 source. A relative probable error of 1% is thus a minimum estimate of the uncertainty of these measurements.

The effect of the linear errors on area, L/B ratio, and module are easy to predict. If dL is the probable error in length, and dB the probable error of breadth, the probable errors in area (dA), module (dM), and L/B ratio (dR) are calculated by the following formulae (Margenau and Murphy 1956:515):

$$dA = \sqrt{(L*dB)^2 + (B*dL)^2}$$

$$dM = \tfrac{1}{2}\sqrt{(dL)^2 + (dB)^2}$$

$$dR = \frac{\sqrt{(L^2*dB^2 + B^2*dL^2)}}{B^2}$$

For the material measured by this author, the expected probable error in the area is 1.3 mm^2, or 1.9%; for the module it is .08 mm, or .9%; and for the L/B ratio it is .02, or 1.8%.

The relative uncertainty due to random errors is 1% or greater. I have calculated a range of 1% to 5% for this uncertainty. Thus, a value of 3% will be used. That is, the linear measurements will be assumed accurate to 3%. The uncertainty in area and ratio is about $\sqrt{2}$ times greater, or close to 5%. The uncertainty in module is a little less.

THE SIGNIFICANCE OF METRIC DIFFERENCES

One of the most difficult problems in human paleontology, if not in general paleontology, is concerned with the meaning of differences. In particular, this work is concerned with the taxonomic implications of metric variability, although such concern is not the primary focus. The 5 hominid taxa used as the basis of the analysis of metric trends cannot be substantiated as a result of the work, for such reasoning would be circular. On the other hand, the discussion of metric dental variability should provide a means for determining whether or not the taxa so created are reasonable–in terms of both their relation to each other and their internal consistency.

The taxonomic significance of metric differences in the dentition can be discussed in a number of ways (Simpson 1961, 1963; Sokal and Sneath 1963; Mayr 1969; Blackwelder 1967). The first level of significance is "statistical significance." One can raise the question of whether or not the nature of 2 samples allows the assumption that they come from 2 different parent populations (not *biological* populations). For single metric variables, the "*t*" test (Parratt 1961:120; Lindgren and McElrath 1959:208-9; Simpson, Roe, and Lewontin 1960:176) is sometimes applicable. However, this test assumes that the populations from which the samples stem are normal. Such an assumption is not always valid. If the sample size is sufficiently large, the assumption of normal population distributions is not necessary (Lindgren and McElrath 1959:207) as the distributions of the sample means will themselves be normal. In this case, the "*Z*" statistic may be used. However, in situations with small sample sizes when the assumption of a normal parent population is not justified, one is necessarily restricted to the use of nonparametric distribution free tests of significance which are considerably less powerful. Unfortunately, the latter case is most common when dealing with samples of fossil taxa.

If demonstrable, statistical significance is of little potential use unless differences are shown to be *non*-significant. In this event, no taxonomic distinctions are justified. On the other hand, demonstration of statistically significant differences has *no* necessary taxonomic implications. In the words of Mayr (1969:187): "To find a statistically significant difference between several populations is . . . only of minor interest to the taxonomist; he takes it for granted." Populations, samples of populations, or just samples of species are bound to be different. Mayr (1969:190) will allow 90% *non*-overlap between subspecies of the same species. Species is not a concept of morphology, but of breeding behavior.

The existence of taxonomic significance in differences cannot be inferred from statistical significance. Taxonomically significant differences at the species level must be determined in other ways. For fossil groups, this determination is ultimately untestable (Wolpoff 1968:477). Mayr (1969:193-97) discusses various types of evidence which are used in deciding whether 2 taxonomically distinct groups are subspecies or allopatric species if they are allochronic, or whether they are subspecies or species on the same lineage if they are not allochronic. This determination is of particular relevance here, as the author believes that the hominid taxa discussed are on the same lineage, and in fact are members of the same genus (*Homo*). When direct proof of breeding behavior is unavailable, several sorts of evidence can be used to help infer the taxonomic status of samples (Mayr 1969:197). The most valid criteria which are applicable stem from 2 considerations: (1) the degree of difference between related sympatric species, and (2) the degree of difference between intergrading subspecies within related widespread species. With respect to the latter, Mayr (1969:197) states: "The amount of morphological difference between the most divergent subspecies of species in the same genus indicates how much morphological difference may evolve without aquisition of reproductive isolation." When dealing with fossil hominids, the first criterion is of limited use. There are no sympatric species within *Homo* to form the basis for such a comparison. The 2 species of *Pan* could, perhaps, be used. However, (1) it is not clear that they are sympatric, and (2) because they are in another genus the comparison is of limited value. On the other hand, the second criterion can be applied to any hominid species by comparison to any other hominid species, extinct or extant. In addition, the most extreme difference between extant hominid groups should give an indication of how much morphological divergence can exist within a hominid species without implying reproductive isolation.

Thus, at the species level, the question of how much difference between the groups represented by samples is necessary to infer reproductive isolation can be partially answered by comparison with corresponding differences between extant groups within *H. sapiens.* Even after making such a comparison, Mayr (1969:197) reminds us: "It is preferable for several reasons to treat allopatric populations of doubtful rank as subspecies," rather than as species.

In this work, a number of different comparisons between the hominid species are attempted. Statistical significance to the differences in means for various measurements is calculated. When the sample size is sufficient, the "*Z*" statistic was used. When the frequency distribution of the samples appears normal and sample size is small, a "*t*" test was attempted. In *non*-normal small samples, limited information was gathered by use of the "Sign Test" and the "Median Test" (Lindgren and McElrath 1959:210-14).

Linear differences of less than 3%, and area or module differences of less than 5% are not significant as they fall within the range of uncertainty represented by the probable error. This range is probably minimum. In addition, the difference between the means is considered as a function of the standard error of the mean of each sample (Parratt 1961:92-93; Margenau and Murphy 1956:510-13). In these ways, the question of whether or not the observed differences between samples could have arisen through either random error or sampling error can be considered. The lack of significant difference allows the treatment of the parent populations as identical. The confidence interval thus established cannot exceed 97% for linear measurements, and 95% for areas. This much uncertainty is already established in the probable error. Thus, a range of ± 2.15 standard errors for linear measurements, and ± 2.50 standard errors for area measurements, defines the minimum acceptable width of appropriate confidence intervals.

The question of taxonomic significance on the species level is approached by several methods. For each measurement, differences between taxa are compared to differences between extant group means. Whereas living groups represent a greater geographical spread, in compensation the time span is far less. Not only taxonomic differences, but also the significance of general trends occurring through time can be approached in this manner. This is probably the best measure of significance available. Finally, the amount of overlap between specimens, as well as the expected overlap of the groups from which the specimens were sampled, is examined.

METRIC TRENDS

Metric trends, then, can be discussed on a variety of levels. There will always be differences between the hominid taxa considered here. If these differences all fall within the actual range of variation of extant groups, there has clearly been no trend. That is, trends are only apparent when significant change can be discerned. Because hominid evolution is viewed as species changes on the same lineage, and within 1 genus, the significance necessary to establish trends must be taxonomic significance on the species level.

The problem is somewhat more difficult when the actual values for hominid taxa fall outside the extant group range of variation. In this case, the problem of taxonomic significance to trends can be approached by comparing degree of change due to the proposed trend to the maximum amount of variation which exists among extant groups. Evolutionary change exceeding the maximum difference among extant groups clearly represents a taxonomically significant trend, although the converse is not necessarily true.

Trends can also be established by the demonstration of non-overlap between ranges of variation.

In sum, the procedure for identifying trends is purposefully conservative in that some possible trends may be missed, although no spurious ones will be identified.

3. The Material Studied

ORIGIN OF THE INDIVIDUAL MEASUREMENTS

This study is based on the measurements of some 47,650 individual teeth. Of these, 5,315, or about 11%, were measured directly by the author. Data for the remainder in the form of either individual measurements or group statistics were taken from the literature.

The Appendix lists every individual measurement used, arranged by jaw, tooth, and hominid species. Eight columns of information are given. From left to right, the first column gives the popular name, museum number, or other designation by which the individual represented by the particular tooth is known. This corresponds to the N_1 level of the naming set suggested by Simpson (1963:1-3) and has no taxonomic status. It is simply a designation of the specimen. The second column gives, when possible, the side of the jaw from which the tooth comes. The third column, labeled N, gives a number which I have assigned to each designated specimen. As such, it is partially redundant with the information in the first column. It represents, however, an unequivocable way of referring to specimens not otherwise designated in Column 1, and provides a means of unambiguous and shorthand reference. When used in the text, these numbers will be written as "#2", "#1401", etc. The fourth column, labeled L(M-D), gives the mesiodistal length in millimeters, and the fifth, labeled B(B-L) gives the buccolingual, or labiolingual, breadth. The sixth through eighth columns are calculated from the fourth and fifth. The sixth column gives the area, which is the length multiplied by the breadth (L*B). The seventh column gives the dental index, which is the length divided by the breadth and multiplied by 100 (L/B). The eighth column gives the module, half the sum of the length plus the breadth (L+B)/2.

There are 2 groups of hominoids which were not considered hominids in this study, although in both cases the classification is ambiguous–some authors feel that each of these represents a truly hominid genus. The first group is represented by the "*Gigantopithecus*" material from Asia. A number of teeth of this megadont form were discovered in Chinese drugstores (von Koenigswald 1952, 1957c; Walter 1954; Weidenreich 1945a; Weinert 1950). Many additional teeth and 3 mandibles were found *in situ* in Pleistocene deposits (Pei 1957a, 1957b; Pei and Li 1958; Pei and Woo 1956; Woo 1962, 1963). The original teeth were interpreted both as pongid (von Koenigswald 1952, 1957c; Remane 1952b) and as hominid (Weidenreich 1945a; Weinert 1950). The later discovery of the mandibles did not seem to clarify the situation.

In spite of the simian shelf, diastema, large canines, and marked wear on the posterior side of the canine (Pei and Li 1958), some authors still view the specimens as megadont prehominids (Dart 1960a; von Koenigswald 1968b, 1963; Woo 1962, 1963). On the other hand, numerous authors judge the mandibles and teeth as anthropoid (Pei and Woo 1956; Pei 1957c; Remane 1960). In their preliminary revision of the Dryopithecinae, Simons and Pilbeam (1965) regard "*Gigantopithecus*" as one of the 3 valid dryopithecine genera. With the discovery of a fourth mandible

(Simons 1970) of Pliocene age, the lineage leading to "*Gigantopithecus blacki*" is better understood. Pilbeam (1970) derives the lineage from *Dryopithecus indicus,* a late Miocene form. The trends evinced by the lineage include size increase, tooth crowding and interstitial wear, molarization of the premolars, and smaller incisors (p. 517). Many of these features suggested hominid ancestry, or at least close relation, to some workers. Simons (1970) and Pilbeam (1970) explain the trends as the result of effective savanna adaptation to a graminivorous diet, thus paralleling the early hominids (Jolly 1970). However, many of the dental features upon which this interpretation rests come closer to duplication in chimpanzees than they do in australopithecines (Wolpoff 1970a). If the suggested adaptation actually occurred, better evidence must be found. I believe the available evidence does not support the hominid interpretation for both morphological reasons and because a hominid line is already known for part of the period of its existence.

The case of "*Ramapithecus*" is somewhat more ambiguous. A number of recent summaries concerned with the long history of taxonomic confusion associated with this genus (Simons and Pilbeam 1965) have been published (Pilbeam 1966; Pilbeam and Simons 1965; Simons 1963, 1964a, 1965, 1967, 1968a, 1968b, 1968c) and thus need not be repeated here. The major specimens include both maxillary (Simons 1961, 1965) and mandibular (Simons 1964b) fragments from India, as well as maxillary (Leakey 1961a, 1967) and mandibular (Leakey 1968a, 1968b) pieces from East Africa. Other specimens from both Europe and Asia have been included in this genus (Simons 1967, 1968b). Leakey has given a separate generic name (1961a) to all the East African material, and divided it into 2 temporally distinct species (1967, 1968a). He further suggests that the later taxon, "*Kenyapithecus wickeri,*" may have used tools (1968c). However, Simons asserts that there are insufficient grounds for either specific or generic separation of the late Miocene/early Pliocene African and Indian specimens (1963, 1964a, 1967), and Pilbeam has attacked the validity of the early Miocene African species (1968).

There is thus evidence for a small Miocene and Pliocene ape taxon. Unfortunately for taxonomic clarity, many of the "hominid" features of this taxon, such as the facial foreshortening and tooth crowding, are the result of its small size (Giles 1956; Washburn 1968b). The most important dental features, small conical canines projecting only slightly above the tooth row, appear quite regularly in the Hamann *Pan gorilla* collection at Case Western Reserve University. They are thus of dubious phyletic valence (Robinson 1967). All of these features may be the result of adaptation to a savanna-based graminivorous diet, as Jolly (1970) suggests. Still, the primate is not necessarily at the base of the hominid lineage.

The taxonomic difficulties stem from the fact that if there were a small (between chimpanzee and gibbon size) primate in a forest-edge niche at this time, it would have been replaced by true hominids whether or not it was ancestral to them. The available taxonomic evidence is equivocal because the distinctive early hominid dental features appear in the anterior dentition. Of these, incisor reduction seems closely tied to diet. However, canine reduction comes as the result of the primary hominid locomotive adaptation (Washburn 1963; Dart 1925, 1957; Brace 1962a, 1967a; Wolpoff 1968). For "*Ramapithecus,*" there is absolutely no indication of the type of locomotion in the available material. Thus the question of whether the morphological similarities of this taxon to the early hominids represents the hominid adaptation of a taxon within the lineage leading to Pleistocene hominids, or whether these similarities rather exist irrespective of possible hominid ancestry as in the case with *Oreopithecus* (Straus 1963), is still completely open.

That an effective means of defense is necessary in a savanna adaptation for early hominid-sized primates is illustrated by the fact that the giant Villafranchian baboon males found at Olduvai, many larger than gorillas (Leakey 1964, 1965), have large canines. Yet, as has been indicated, the canines of both YPM 13799 and FT 1271/2 are not particularly larger, in relative size, than those of female gorillas.

The distribution of incisor size, too, indicates overlap of "*Ramapithecus*" and modern pongids. Simons (1969:450) very clearly indicates that incisor reduction in FT 1271/2 is measured by the incisor height. A recent study relating the height of unworn incisors in chimpanzees, gorillas, modern men, and FT 1271/2 to the summed length of the first 2 maxillary molars (Yulish 1971) gives a ratio of 47 for the "*Ramapithecus*" specimen. While this overlaps with *H. sapiens* (range 44-61), it also overlaps with gorillas (range 42-58). In fact, the gorilla range can be included in the *H. sapiens* range. One wonders whether there is evidence for *any* incisor height reduction in hominid evolution, let alone whether FT 1271/2 is a reduced incisor form.

Given the paucity of actual "*Ramapithecus*" specimens, there is still some basis for taxonomic judgment. This stems from the hypothesis that attaining erect posture and efficient bipedal locomotion was fairly rapid (Washburn 1960, 1963, 1968a, 1968b). If so, there are 2 lines of evidence which suggest that our ancestors became erect, diverging from the pongid line, within the last 5 to 6 million years. The first is purely biochemical (Sarich 1968; Sarich and Wilson 1967a, 1967b; King and Jukes 1969). The second derives from the fact that while the early hominids are not completely erect (Robinson 1969; Le Gros Clark 1967; Tobias 1967a), there is an evolutionary tendency toward the attainment of progressively more erect and more efficient bipedal locomotion among them (Zuckerman 1966) culminating in the *H. erectus* condition (Brace 1967a; Brace and Montagu 1965). If bipedal locomotion developed rapidly, and if the australopithecines represent the final stages of this development, then the beginning of the development surely did not predate them by 12 million years (Washburn 1963, 1968b.) Thus, even if "*Ramapithecus*" is ancestral to hominids, it cannot itself be considered a hominid should these considerations be correct. Contrary to Pilbeam (1968), the denial of hominid status to "*Ramapithecus*" does not at all mean "none of the *Dryopithecus* species can be ancestral to any living pongids (p. 1338)."

For these reasons, the dentitions of the "*Ramapithecus*" specimens cannot, without further evidence, be taken to represent the ancestral hominid condition.

The specimens numbered from 1 to 399 are australopithecines. A large number of these specimens, particularly those from the South African sites, have been measured by Robinson (1956). For consistency, his measurements will be used unless another worker has taken more measurements at a specific site. Sources for almost all of the African fossil hominid specimens are given in a recent catalog edited by Oakley and Campbell (1967).

A large number of teeth, as well as some mandibles and crania, have been reported from East Africa, both east and north of Lake Rudolf, since this manuscript was originally prepared. Howell (1969) has given a detailed report of his discoveries, and 1 of the several mandibles recovered by the French expedition has been published (Arambourg and Coppens 1967, 1968; Arambourg, Chavaillon, and Coppens 1967). An expedition directed by Richard Leakey has recovered several mandibles and 2 crania from areas east of Lake Rudolf (personal communication). Patterson discovered a mandibular fragment at Lothagam (Simons 1968e) with a deciduous second molar, and the roots of M_1 - M_2. Finally, recent dating may place the Kanam mandible in the basal Pleistocene, as old as 4 million years (Maglio 1970). All of these discoveries were published after the statistics were computed and the original manuscript prepared. They could not be included in the final version.

The child from Taung (#2) has been the subject of a large number of works concerned with the origin of the human dentition (Dart 1925, 1934; Broom 1925, 1929; Abel 1930; Adloff 1931a, 1939; Bronowski and Long 1951, 1952, 1953; Ergartner 1949; Keith 1931; Remane 1927; Weidenreich 1937a). The dentition of the specimen was completely described in the monograph by Abel (1930) and again by Dart (1934). In addition, Broom (1929) described a few of the unerupted permanent teeth. I have used the measurements given by Robinson (1956). These are almost identical to Dart's (1934).

The Makapansgat australopithecines, ascribed to *H. africanus* (Robinson 1954a, 1954b, 1954c), have been discussed in a large number of papers (Broom 1950; Ergartner 1950; Heberer 1956, 1966; Krug 1952; Remane 1952a). The best dental measurements come from a series of publications by Dart and Bone. Because this is the most recent and consistent set, they are incorporated in this work.

Almost all of the specimens were recovered from the dumps outside of the main site (Brain 1958). Most of the material comes from the grey (lower phase I) breccia, also yielding the "Osteodontokeratic" cultural remains (Dart

1957). Two specimens come from overlying breccia horizons. A calvarium, MLD 37/38 comes from the pink breccia (upper phase I) immediately overlying the grey which also yielded the remains of a "pebble culture" (Dart 1962a). A maxilla (#3) MLC 1 (Dart 1955b) comes from the brown breccia (lower phase II) which overlies the pink. The remaining specimens come from the grey breccia. These include (#4) MLD 2 (Dart 1948c), (#5) MLD 5 (1949a), (#6) MLD 6 (1949a), (#7) MLD 9 (1949b), (#8) MLD 11/23 (Robinson 1956; Tobias 1967a), (#9) MLD 18 (Dart 1954, 1962b), (#10) MLD 19 (Bone 1955, 1957), and (#11 - #13) MLD 22, 24, and 40 (Dart 1962b).

Robinson (1962) published 3 of the permanent teeth from the Sterkfontein Extention site: Se 255 (#14), Se 1508 (#15), Se 1937 (#16). This site is stratigraphically the same as the middle breccia at the main site (Robinson 1962, Brain 1958; Mason 1962).

Most of the material reportedly from the lower breccia at Sterkfontein was published by Robinson (1952, 1956). This includes the earlier material with TM museum numbers (#17 - #29) and the later material with STS numbers (#30 - #59).

A number of the earlier specimens were described by Broom (1939a, 1939b; Broom and Schepers 1946; Broom, Robinson, and Schepers 1950), providing the basis for much of the early discussion on the dentition of *H. africanus* (Adloff 1939; Ergartner 1950; Gregory and Hellman 1939; Heberer 1956; von Koenigswald 1942, 1957a; Le Gros Clark 1947, 1949, 1950, 1951a, 1951b; Montandon 1939; Remane 1952b, 1954b, 1957; Senyurek 1941; Weidenreich 1937a; Weinert 1944, 1950, 1951c). Thus, there are descriptions of (what Broom referred to as) Skulls 1 (#17, TM 1511), 2 (#18, TM 1512), 3 (#19, TM 1514), and 4 (#20, TM 1515) by Broom and Schepers (1946), as well as Skulls 5 (#34, STS 5 and STS 6), 6 (#39, STS 17), 7 (STS 71), and 8 (STS 19 and STS 58) by Broom, Robinson, and Schepers. Where measurements are not given by Robinson (1956) but are given in 1 of Broom's publications, the latter are incorporated. Robinson (1956) gives measurements for all additional material, labeled with "STS" museum numbers, presumably from the lower breccia.

In a report concerned with recent excavations at Sterkfontein, and the re-evaluation of proveniences reported earlier, Tobias and Hughes (1969) positively identified the site of discovery of STS 5–in the *middle breccia.* Therefore, it is clearly associated with the lithic industry. The question of whether any specimens actually came from the lower breccia has now been raised, but is far from solution. There are some indications that the lower breccia is simply a filled crack.

The remaining specimens assigned to *H. africanus* are from East Africa. A number of these, originally placed in "*H. habilis*" (Leakey, Tobias, and Napier 1964) come from Bed I, Olduvai Gorge (Robinson 1965a, 1965b, 1965c, 1966b, 1967; Bielicki 1966; Heberer 1965; Le Gros Clark 1967; Pilbeam and Simons 1965; Simons 1967, 1968a, 1968b; Wolpoff 1968). Olduvai Hominid 4 (OH 4) from MK I (#303) was described by Leakey, Tobias, and Napier (1964). OH 6 (#304) from FLK I, the "*Zinjanthropus*" yielding site, has been provisionally included in *H. africanus* as a paratype of "*H. habilis*" (Leakey, Tobias, and Napier 1964). The measurements can be inferred from data given by Tobias (Tobias and von Koenigswald 1964; Tobias 1966a). OH 7a (#306) is possibly the same individual as OH 6. The measurements of this specimen were given by Tobias (1966a). OH 7 (#305) was first described by Leakey (1960b, 1961c). The measurements of the post canine dentition were published by Tobias (Tobias and von Koenigswald 1964), replacing earlier measurements by Leakey (1961c). Both Leakey (1966) and Robinson (1965b, 1966b, 1967) took exception to the measurements of PM_3 made by Tobias. Indeed, the measurements were different enough to place the hominid in 2 different *genera,* as defined by the above authors (Leakey, Tobias, and Napier 1964). For consistency with the rest of the dentition, I have used the measurements published by Tobias. Measurements for the canines and incisors have not as yet been published for this specimen. I have used measurements taken from a number of the published scaled photographs (Leakey 1961b; Leakey and Leakey 1964; Tobias 1965c).

The final *H. africanus* specimen (#1) is a maxillary fragment from Garusi near Lake Eyassi (Kohl-Larsen 1943; Hennig 1948). The specimen was once suggested to be the maxilla corresponding to "*Meganthropus*" mandibles in Java

(Weinert 1950, 1951b, 1952), and was correspondingly named *"Meganthropus africanus."* Robinson (1953c, 1955) convincingly demonstrated its close affinites to *H. africanus.* Although later contested by Remane (1951, 1952a, 1954a), Robinson's placement of the specimen with *H. africanus* is in line with the available evidence (especially in the light of *H. africanus* specimens discovered at a later time in East Africa), and is accepted here. His measurements (1953c) are incorporated.

The dentition of *H. robustus* has been the subject of a large number of publications, most of which involved a comparison with *H. africanus* (Adloff 1949; Broom 1939b; Broom and Robinson 1952; Broom and Schepers 1946; Ergartner 1950; Ferembach 1964; Kustaloglu 1961; Montandon 1939; Robinson 1952, 1954b, 1956, 1960b, 1968; Senyurek 1941; Tobias 1967a; Weinert 1952).

Two of the *H. robustus* specimens come from East Africa. The mandible (#108) from Lake Natron (Leakey and Leakey 1964; Isaac 1965, 1967) was measured by Tobias (1964). Olduvai Hominid 5 (#109) from FLK I, preliminarily described and measured by Leakey (1959), was the subject of an extensive monograph by Tobias (1967a). While some criticisms have been raised of these analyses (Robinson 1960b, 1968), the measurements published by Tobias remain unchallenged and are subsequently used here.

There are a number of specimens attributed to *H. robustus* outside of Africa. The most important of these are the 3 Javanese mandibles from Djetis faunal beds attributed first to the genus *"Meganthropus"* (von Koenigswald 1954a, 1956, 1957b, 1962a, 1962b, 1963, 1965a; Remane 1951, 1954a; Weidenreich 1945a), and later to the advanced stages of *"H. habilis"* (Tobias and von Koenigswald 1964; Tobias 1967b). Le Gros Clark does not believe that *"Meganthropus"* can be specifically separated from *H. erectus* in the Djetis fauna of Java (1964; see also Piveteau 1957). On the other hand, Robinson has persuasively argued that the 3 *"Meganthropus"* specimens are robust australopithecines (1953c, 1954a, 1954c, 1955, 1961b, 1961c).

The first *"Meganthropus"* (#105) specimen is the mandible found in 1941 (von Koenigswald 1954a, 1956, 1957b, 1962a). This mandible was subsequently described by Weidenreich (1945a). The dental measurements used here were published by Tobias and von Koenigswald (1964). The measurements given by Weidenreich were taken on a cast. The second specimen (#106) was discovered in 1939 (von Koenigswald 1950) but was not described until recently (Tobias and von Koenigswald 1964).

The third specimen (#107) was discovered in 1952 (Marks 1953). It consists of the greater part of a shattered mandible. There are a number of secondary sources reporting the association of this mandible with Trinil fauna (Robinson 1961b:127). However, Marks, in the single primary description, clearly states that it was discovered by a native, most likely in a river deposit, associated with Djetis faunal elements (1953:26). The mandible is thus either of Djetis age or was washed out of a deposit of even earlier age. The dental measurements were reported by Marks.

A number of hominid teeth from China were originally placed in the genus *"Hemianthropus"* (subsequently changed to *"Hemanthropus"*) by von Koenigswald (1957c). The australopithecine identity of these teeth is clear (Tobias 1967a; Le Gros Clark 1964; Simons 1968d:57). Following the original comparison made by von Koenigswald (1957c), I have included them in *H. robustus* (#308 - #315).

The remaining specimens of *H. robustus* come from Kromdraai and Swartkrans in South Africa. The dentition of the best preserved specimen from Kromdraai (#101, TM 1517) was described in a number of papers (Broom and Schepers 1946; Gregory and Hellman 1939; Robinson 1956). Robinson's measurements are used when possible. TM 1536 (#102), a mandible, was also described by Broom and Schepers (1946). Robinson's measurements are used (1956). Measurements for TM 1600 (#203) were given by Tobias (1966a, 1967a).

Two mandibles (SK 15, SK 45) and a maxilla (SK 80) at Swartkrans were originally described as representing a more advanced hominid contemporary with *H. robustus* (Robinson 1953a, 1953b; Broom and Robinson 1950, 1952). However, a number of authors immediately denied the taxonomic distinction of this *"Telanthropus"* material (Le Gros Clark 1949, 1964, 1967; Straus 1950; Dart 1955a). The inclusion of these specimens in *H. robustus* is reasonably indicated (Wolpoff 1968, 1970b). The measurements for

SK 15 (#301) were given by Robinson (Broom and Robinson 1952) as were the measurements for SK 45 (#302), the smaller of the 2 mandibles (Robinson 1953b).

The other skeletal remains from Swartkrans were described in a monograph by Broom and Robinson (1952). The dental measurements for SK 1 through SK 846 (#110 - #204) are Robinson's (1956), and those of SK 1587 and SK 1588 (#205 - #206) were taken from Brain (1967).

Tobias (1966a, 1967a) gives or uses dental measurements from maxillae he measured at Sterkfontein, Makapansgat, and Swartkrans. When measurements were taken or derived from Tobias' works which were not presented by Robinson, the former were incorporated. In addition, some supplementary measurements of otherwise unpublished teeth were taken from the scaled photographs in the Transvaal Museum Memoirs, and in Mann's thesis (1968).

The *H. erectus* materials from Java include 4 mandibles, 1 maxilla, and a small number of isolated specimens. The first mandible (#401), "Pithecanthropus A" or "Kedung Brubus," was measured by Tobias (1966e). Weidenreich (1945a) measured the second mandible (#407) "Pithecanthropus B" (Dubois 1924; von Koenigswald 1937, 1962b). The measurements given by Tobias and von Koenigswald (1964) are used here. "Pithecanthropus C" (#408) was described by both Saronto (1961) and Jacob (1967a). Measurements given by the former are used here. The fourth mandible (#411), the Sangiran mandible of 1939 (see Coon 1963), was described and measured by Weidenreich (1945a). There was also an isolated lower canine (#410) from Sangiran (von Koenigswald and Weidenreich 1939). All of this mandibular material, with the exception of mandible A, come from the underlying Djetis beds.

The maxilla of "Pithecanthropus IV" (#407) from the Djetis beds (von Koenigswald and Wiedenreich 1939; von Koenigswald 1958a, 1962b; Weidenreich 1945a) was most recently measured by Tobias (Tobias and von Koenigswald 1964). The measurements are used, along with those of several incisors attributed to the maxilla (von Koenigswald and Weidenreich 1939; von Koenigswald 1958a).

There are a number of studies which compare the dentition of these Javanese *H. erectus* specimens with that of the australopithecines (Dart 1960b; von Koenigswald 1953a, 1953b, 1954a, 1954b). Lastly, several other teeth found in Java were once attributed to *H. erectus* (Dubois 1924; Weinert 1928). These teeth are most likely those of extant *H. sapiens* mixed within the fossil teeth (von Koenigswald 1956, 1962a; Le Gros Clark 1964).

A number of East African *H. erectus* specimens were found in Olduvai Bed II (Tobias 1965a, 1965b, 1967b). OH 13 (#406 from MNK II), although once referred to the species "*H. habilis*" as a Bed II representative (Leakey, Tobias, and Napier 1964; Leakey 1966), is considered to be *H. erectus* by most authors (Robinson 1965b; Howell 1965a; Howells 1966; Tobias 1966a). Tobias and von Koenigswald (1964) published measurements for the posterior dentition. I have taken the measurements of the anterior dentition from a number of published, scaled photographs (Leakey and Leakey 1964; Tobias and von Koenigswald 1964; Tobias 1965c).

OH 16 (#307) from FLK II (Leakey and Leakey 1964) was initially described as an australopithecine (Tobias and von Koenigswald 1964; Tobias 1965b, 1966c). Leakey (1966) recently recognized the specimen as a "Protopithecanthropine", and Howell has long denied its initial australopithecine designation (1965). The dentition was measured from the photographs published in the original description (Leakey and Leakey 1964).

OH 3 from BK II is represented by a deciduous canine and a molarized tooth (Leakey 1958). Whether the molarized tooth represents a deciduous second mandibular molar (Leakey 1958, 1960a) or a permanent maxillary molar (Dahlberg 1960a; Robinson 1960a; von Koenigswald 1960, 1963, 1967) has been the subject of some debate. Difficulties in the interpretation of both the morphology and stratigraphic position (Leakey 1964, 1965; M. Leakey 1967; Tobias 1965a, 1965b) make it impossible to classify the specimen.

There are 3 sources of North African *H. erectus* dental specimens. The first is the Rabat cranium (#409) from Morocco (Marcais 1934). Neither the dating nor the morphology of the badly shattered specimen can unequivocably place it in either *H. erectus* or *H. neanderthalensis.* Thus a number of authors describe the specimen as Neandertal (Vallois 1945, 1959; Briggs 1948, 1955; Vallois and Roche 1958) and date it within Wurm (Briggs 1968); others feel that both the date and the morphology indicate inclusion within *H. erectus* (Howell 1960, 1961; Arambourg 1957, 1963). The dental measurements were taken from Day (1965) and Arambourg (1963).

The Casablanca mandible (#413) from Sidi Abderrahman (Arambourg 1957; Arambourg and Biberson 1956) has been dated in the period just after the end of the Mindel/Riss Interglacial (Biberson 1963; Briggs 1968). The measurements used here were given by Arambourg (1963).

The Ternifine site in Algeria has yielded a number of *H. erectus* specimens. Among these are 3 mandibles: (#470) Ternifine I (Arambourg 1954, 1955a), (#471) Ternifine II (Arambourg 1955b, 1955c), and (#472) Ternifine III (Arambourg 1956, 1957). These mandibles and 7 isolated teeth (#459 - #461 and #473 - #476) were described in detail by Arambourg (1963). Measurements from this monograph were used here.

The Ubeidiya fragments from Israel (#463, #464) were treated as *H. erectus* on the basis of morphology (Tobias 1966b) and dating (Molleson and Oakley 1966; Hooijer 1962).

In Europe there are only a few specimens of *H. erectus* teeth. The remains from Vertessollos (Thoma 1966) include only deciduous teeth (Thoma 1967).

The Mauer mandible (#404) was first described by Schoetensack (1908). The dentition of this specimen was measured in the monograph (the measurements appear to be maximum). A variety of other dental measurements for the mandible have appeared over the years (Gorjanovic-Kramberger 1910; Hrdlicka 1923b, 1924; Klaatsch 1909a; Howell 1960; Wust 1950). Klaatsch's data is used here.

Within *H. erectus,* the teeth from Pekin represent the largest and best studied sample (Adloff 1938; Montandon 1938; Weidenreich 1936, 1937a, 1937b, 1943). Dental measurements for the pre-1941 specimens (#414 - #416, #419 - #450) were taken from Weidenreich's publications (1936, 1937a, 1943). Several other measurements for mandible G1 (#433) and maxilla O1, or Skull 13, (#447) were taken from available casts. A number of additional specimens attributed to "*Sinanthropus pekinensis*" were discovered after the Second World War (Chang 1962; Kurth 1965; Pei 1954). These include an almost complete mandible (#417), AN 16 (Woo and Chao 1959; Woo 1964a), and 6 additional teeth belonging to 3 individuals (#418, #451, and #452) published by Woo (1954; Woo and Chia 1954). In addition, a mandible (#402) and cranial fragments of an older hominid, "*Sinanthropus lantianensis,*" attributed to *H. erectus* have also been reported (Tang 1964; Woo 1964a, 1964b, 1965, 1966).

Lastly, there are some isolated teeth taken from drugstores (#456 - #458), "*Sinanthropus officinalis,*" (Walter 1954; von Koenigswald 1952; Tobias 1967a) attributed to *H. erectus.* Measurements given by von Koenigswald are employed here.

Only a few publications have been concerned with the general characteristics of the Neandertal dentition (Bay 1958; Hrdlicka 1930; Boule and Vallois 1957; Patte 1959, 1960a, 1961; Brace 1962, 1964a, 1967b, 1967c; Coon 1963). Of these, the works of Patte include some individual measurements for the better-known Wurm European specimens. These are incorporated in this study.

The Krapina Neandertals have been the subject of a large number of works, most of which are placed in historical context by Ozegovic (1958). Measurements for the Maxillae A through F (#501 - #506), and the mandibles A through I (#507 - #515) were given by Garjanovic-Kramberger (1901, 1902, 1904, 1905, 1906). These measurements were checked against those made by other authors (Hrdlicka 1923a, 1923b, 1924, 1930; Kallay 1955; De Terra 1903). Gorjanovic-Kramberger gave a number of different averages for sets of isolated teeth in the publications cited above. The individual dental measurements used here (#516 - #663), clearly not representing all of the available material, were taken from these publications as well as additional ones by Gorjanovic-Kramberger (1907, 1908, 1910) and others (Adloff 1907, 1908, 1909; Kallay 1949; De Terra 1903).

Of the early European Neandertal specimens, the earliest (Steinheim) could probably as well be included within *H. erectus* (Brace 1964a). The cranium was briefly described by Berckhemer (1933, 1937), and in more detail by Weinert (1936) and Howell (1960). The dental measurements were given by Weinert (1936) and checked on the available cast. The Montmaurin mandible (Baylac *et al.* 1950) was described by Vallois (1955, 1956, 1957). Howell's measurements (1960) are used here (#579).

There is some dental material representing the pre-Wurm Neandertals. A right lower canine and left upper incisor were found in an evolved Acheulean deposit of the Lazaret Cave, dating from the period between Riss II and Riss III (Piveteau 1967). Descriptions of these teeth have not been published. Eemian Interglacial specimens come from both southern and eastern Europe. Excellent descriptions and measurements of the dentitions of both (#767) Saccopastore I (Sergi 1944) and (#768) Saccopastore II (Sergi 1948) are available. From Germany, measurements are available for both the child (#722) and the adult (#723) Ehringsdorf mandibles (Schwalbe 1914; Legoux 1966; H. Virchow 1914, 1916, 1920; McCurdy 1924). There are 2 Chinese specimens from this interglacial not included in this study. These are the finds from Ting-Ts'un (Movius 1956; Chang 1962) and Changyang (Chia 1957; Chang 1962).

Of the Neandertals from within the last 120,000 years, the measurements of only a few published specimens were not included. A single molar from Bombarral, Portugal, was excluded because its exact identity was not established (Ferembach 1965b). The single tooth from the Florisbad specimen (Dreyer 1935) was not included because of the extreme ambiguity of its dating (Coon 1963; Tobias 1962; Cooke 1963). Lastly, the dentitions of the excellent Neandertal cranium from the Chalcidique Peninsula in Greece (Kokkoros and Kamellis 1960; Bostanci 1964), of the Kulna maxilla (Jelinek 1966, 1969), of La Ferrassie II (Heim 1968), and of La Quina H4 and H17 (Henri-Martin 1923) remain undescribed.

The African specimens range from North to South Africa. The Haua Fteah mandibles from Libya were described most recently by McBurney (1967). Measurements for the first mandible (#727) were taken from Wells (in McBurney, Trevor, and Wells 1953). The 1967 publication shows a different set of measurements for the first, as well as the measurements for the single third molar of the second. The information was received too late for inclusion in this work. There are 2 crania from Jebel Irhound in Morocco. The second (Ennouchi 1968; Jullien 1965) is a calvarium. On the other hand, the first (#728) is an almost complete cranium containing some teeth (Arambourg 1965; Ennouchi 1962, 1963). An additional Moroccan find, the Tangier specimens from Mugharet el-Aliya (#805 and #806) has been described (Senyurek 1940; Briggs (1948). An Ethopian mandible, Diredawa (#721) was published by Vallois (1951; Coon 1963). East Africa is represented by the Lake Eyasi finds (#701 - #705) once attributed to "*Africanthropus njarasensis*" (see Tobias 1962; Wells 1957). Dental measurements are available for a number of these specimens (Weinert 1939; Remane 1954a). Lastly, from Southern Africa come the Rhodesian specimens. There is a complete cranium (#765) with most of the dentition (Carter 1928; Clark *et al.* 1947), and (#766) a portion of a smaller maxilla (Wells 1947). A mandible from Makapansgat (#749) was associated with the final hand axe industry (Dart 1948a; Tobias 1966d).

A large number of Neandertal specimens have been found in the Near East. There is a single tooth (#724) from El Wad (McCown and Keith 1939). A maxilla (#730) comes from level 15 (Emiran) at Ksar' Akil (Ewing 1963). A single tooth (#763) from Ras-el-Kelb was described by Vallois (1962). There are 2 teeth (#775) from the Shukbah Cave (Keith 1931; Patte 1960a). The Kafzeh (Boule and Vallois 1957) lower third premolars for skeletons 5, 6, and 7 (#908 - #910) have been published (Vallois 1962). The specimens from the Shanidar Cave include (#771) a juvenile (Senyurek 1957a, 1957b, 1959), and the adults (#772) Shanidar I (Solecki 1960; Stewart 1958a, 1958b), (#773) Shanidar II (Solecki 1960; Stewart 1961a, 1961b), and (#774) Shanidar IV (Stewart 1963). Lastly, from the Mt. Carmel Cave of Et Tabun there is a cranium with a mandible (#783), an additional mandible (#784), and a large number of isolated teeth (#785 - #804). The dental measurements for this material were published by McCown and Keith (1939). For #783 and #784 I have supplemented these measurements with additional ones taken from the excellent published photographs and drawings as well as from the available casts.

The remaining Neandertal material comes from Europe and European Russia. From Arcy-Sur-Cure (Leroi-Gourhan 1958) come the remains of 2 mandibles (#706 and #707), a maxilla (#708), and a number of additional teeth (#709

#715). All of the material comes from level 20, an "Old" Mousterian layer except for #714, a molar from the "Evolved" Mousterian from level 15. Measurements are available for the Italian specimens (#717) Circeo 2 (Sergi 1954), (#718) Circeo 3 (Sergi and Ascenzi 1955), and (#719) Circeo 4 (Blanc 1954; Sergi 1958). There are dental measurements available for a larger number of Neandertal children. These include (#716) Chateauneuf-Sur (Patte 1957), (#720) Combe Grenal (Piveteau 1957; Legoux 1966), the Gibraltar child (Buxton 1928; Hrdlicka 1930; Keith 1931) from Devil's Tower (#725), (#731) Salento (Blanc 1958a, 1960), (#733) La Chaise (David and Bordes 1950; David 1960; Legoux 1966; Patte 1961; Piveteau 1957), (#741) the child from La Quina (Henri-Martin 1926; Legoux 1966; Hrdlicka 1930), (#751 - #753) Meridonale A, B, and C (Palma di Cesnola and Messeri 1967), (#761) Pech de l'Aze (Patte 1957), (#770) Salemas (Ferembach 1965a), (#779) Staroselje (Roginskii 1954; Ulrich 1956a; Vleck 1956c), (#781) Subaluk child (Thoma 1964), (#808) the second Taubach tooth (Nehring 1895; H. Virchow 1917), and (#809) the juvenile from Teshik Tash (Okladnikov, *et al.* 1949; Ulrich 1956b). The adult Neandertals include (#726) Gibraltar (Keith 1915, 1925), (#729) Jersey (Keith 1912, 1913), (#732) L'Hortus (Piveteau, de Lumley, and Mme. de Lumley 1963), (#734) La Chapelle (Boule 1913; Ewing 1963), (#735 - #739) the 6 teeth from La Croze del Dua (Genet-Varcin 1962, 1966), (#740) La Ferrassie I (Boule 1913; Piveteau 1957; Werth 1928), (#742 and #743) La Quina adults H5 (Henri-Martin 1923; Hrdlicka 1930; Werth 1928) and H9 (Henri-Martin 1923; Piveteau 1964), (#744) La Verrerie (Piveteau 1951), (#745) La Vienne (Patte 1960b), (#747) Le Placard (Genet-Varcin 1962), (#750) Malta (Keith 1924), (#754) Meridonale D (Palma di Cesnola and Messeri 1967), (#755 - #758) Monsempron B, C, D, and H (Vallois 1952), (#760) Ochoz (Jelinek 1962), (#762) Petit-Puymoyen (Siffre 1908; Piveteau 1964), (#764) Regourdou (Piveteau 1963, 1964, 1966), (#769) the St. Brais incisor (Koby 1956; Bay 1958) from La Grotte d'Isturitz (R. de Saint-Perrier 1950), (#776) Spika (R. Virchow 1882), (#777 and #778) Spy I and II (Fraipont and Lohest 1887; Hrdlicka 1923a, 1923b, 1924, 1930; Werth 1928), (#782) Subalyuk adult (Jelinek 1962), (#807) the Taubach molar (Nehring 1895; H. Virchow 1917), and (#810 - #813) the teeth from Vergisson (Piveteau 1957; Genet-Varcin 1962).

The specimen from Le Moustier (#746) is of particular interest. This is the only reasonably complete adult Neandertal find associated with the Mousterian of Acheulean tradition (Bordes 1958; Oakley 1966). There is a large literature concerned with the discovery (Klaatsch and Hauser 1909a) and anatomy (Klaatsch 1909a, 1909b; Weinert 1925; Werth 1928) of the specimen. A number of works discuss and measure the dentition (Dieck 1923, 1925; Klaatsch and Huaser 1909a; Weinert 1925). The measurements used here are those given by Klaatsch (quoted in Patte 1959, 1960a, 1961).

The 10 hominids from the es Skhul Cave (#901 - #907) have a more recent date than any of the Neandertals already discussed (Higgs 1961a, 1961b; Solecki 1963; Oakley 1966). These specimens form a transition between the Neandertals and *H. sapiens* in morphology as well as date (Brace 1962b, 1964a, 1967a, 1967c; Howell 1965b; Howells 1967). The dental measurements used here were taken from the original monograph (McCown and Keith 1939). Because in some cases only 1 side of the jaw is given, the published measurements are, when possible, supplemented by additional ones taken from photographs and the available casts of Skhul 5.

H. sapiens was divided into a number of different types of groups, and was also considered as a whole. The first group consists of skeletal material from Europe and European Russia, the Near East, and North Africa dating from the upper Paleolithic to the present. This entire sample is referred to as "Caucasoid."

The Upper Paleolithic series begins with material (#1000 - #1006) from the Chattelperonian layers C-8 to C-10 at Arcy-Sur-Cure (Leroi-Gourhan 1958), and (#1017) the possibly Chattelperonian (Brace 1964a; Narr 1962) skeleton from Combe Capelle (Klaatsch and Hauser 1909b). Material from Aurignacian deposits include (#1056) Salemas (Ferembach 1965a), (#1106) Abri Blachard (Ferembach 1958), (#1120 - #1122) Isturitz (Ferembach 1957), (#1021 - #1023) La Rochette A, B, and C (Elsner 1913), (#1024 and #1025) Le Rois mandibles A and B as well as (#1026 - #1055) a number of individual teeth (Vallois 1958a,

1958b), and the Szeletian find at Klaty Kun (Vleck 1956a). There is also some Aurignacian-associated skeletal material (Oakley 1966) from Lautsch (Szombathy 1902) and Barma Grande (Verneau 1899). The Dolni Vestonice skeletons (Maly 1939; Jelinek 1964) are associated with Pavlovian, an Eastern Gravettian (Oakley 1966). Measurements of the complete maxillary and mandibular dentition of Dolni Vestonice III (#1057) were published by Jelinek (1953). The Predmost material was associated with an Eastern Gravettian (Oakley 1966). I was able to find published dental measurements (#1007 - #1016, #1058 - #1061) for 14 of the 46 available specimens (Matiegka 1938; Hrdlicka 1924; Jelinek 1953; Kriz 1903; Maska 1886; Schlaginhaufen 1925). There is a skeleton from Pavlov (Vleck 1961) also associated with the Eastern Gravettian. A "Proto-Magdalenian" skeleton associated with a Venus comes from Abri Pataud (Movius and Vallois 1959). The Magdalenian specimens include (#1104 and #1105) the Saint-Vincent material at Arlay (Ferembach 1954), (#1110) Cap Blanc (von Bonin 1935), (#1111) Chancelade (Vallois 1941), (#1114 and #1115) Farincourt 2 and 3 (Sauter 1957), (#1128) Lafaye (Genet-Varcin and Miquel 1967), and Obercassel I (Verworn, Bonnet, and Steinmann 1919; Werth 1928). There is additional material from Obercassel, as well as a skeleton from Bichon (Sauter 1956). Other less well associated Upper Paleolithic dental remains include (#1019) the Grimaldi "Negroid" adolescent (Verneau 1906; Gregory 1922), along with a large number of other remains from the Grimaldi Caves (Verneau 1906; Werth 1928; Boule and Vallois 1957), (#1018) Brno 3 (Matiegka 1929), Biscordine (Montandon 1936), (#1125 - #1127) 3 mandibles from Lachaud (Ferembach 1957), (#1143) Silicka Brezova (Vleck 1956b), (#1129) Les Vachons (Ferembach 1954), and (#1145 and #1146) Terrasson A and B (Ferembach 1954). It should be pointed out that these constitute almost all of the well-dated or associated early Upper Paleolithic dental specimens known. The only additional ones are from China: (#2203) Changyang (Chia 1957; Chang 1962), and (#2206) Ting Ts'un (Movius 1956; Chang 1962; Woo 1956).

The more recent specimens from Europe include (#1101) the A Culoz cranium and mandible (Genet-Varcin and Vilain 1963), (#1102 and #1103) Alamann 5 and 1288 (Schwertz 1917), (#1108 and #1109) Buggisen 1 and 2 (Schwertz 1914), (#1112) Egolzwil (Schlaginhaufen 1925), (#1116) Galley Hill (Klaatsch 1903), (#1117) Gardar 7 (Broste *et al.* 1944), (#1118 and #1119) Hohlerfels A and C (Elsner 1917), (#1124) Koerhuisbeek (Vallois 1943), (#1134 - #1137) Pas Estret 3, 4, 9, and 8 (Ampoulange 1959); (#1138 - #1141) Pritzerber 3 - 6 (Reche 1928), (#1142) Rhunda (Jacobshagen 1957), (#1144) Svaerdborg (Berlin 1956), (#1149) a Frenchman (Gregory 1922), (#1150 and #1151) Europeans 344c and AJ 2 (Elsner 1917), and (#1152 - #1176) a series of "Whites" from the American Museum collection measured and photographed by Gregory and Hellman (1926a). There are dental descriptions for other European archaeological materials at Matelles (Brabrant, Sahly, and Bouyssou 1961), Prussa (Perret 1943), Rouffignac (Sahly, Brabrant, and Bouyssou 1962), Coxyde (Twiesselmann and Brabrant 1960), and Jebel Shaqadud (Zuhrt 1967).

The recent specimens from the Near East and North Africa are represented by the following: (#1183 - #1187) Alaca Hoyuk 2, 3, 8, 15, and 17 (Senyurek 1950, 1952), a Bedouin specimen (#1188) from the American Museum (Gregory and Hellman 1926a), (#1189) parts of an individual from the Belt Cave in Iran (Coon 1957), (#1113) a tooth from the Elementeita finds (Leakey 1935), Goungou A and C (#1975 and #1976) collected in Mauritania by Patrick Munson (University of Illinois, Urbana) and measured by the author, (#1193 - #1195) Jarmo (Dahlberg 1960b), (#1147 and #1148) 2 specimens marked "Kaffir" at the American Museum (Gregory and Hellman 1926a), (#1130) Masat 3 (Senyurek 1946), (#1131) Mechta (Ennouchi 1953), (#1133) Okuzini (Senyurek 1958), (#1190 - #1192) Sialk (Dahlberg 1962), and (#1196 - #1214) Wadi Halfa (Greene, Ewing, and Armelagos 1967).

The Australoid group includes material from both Australia and Tasmania, as well as the fossil Wadjak crania (#1701 and #1702) from Java (Dubois 1922 for measurements and scaled photographs). The fossil, or semi-fossil, material from Australia includes (#1704) Talgai (Smith 1918; Brothwell 1959), (#1703) Keilor (Wunderly, Adam, and Mahony 1943; W. Adam 1943; Weidenreich 1945c), and (#1705) Cohuna

(Keith 1931; T. Campbell 1941). The single possibly fossil specimen from Tasmania (#1753) was found by the Jones expedition (Macintosh and Barker 1965). The modern specimens from Australia used here comprise the following: (#1706 and #1707) 2 specimens from the Leipzig collection (Klaatsch 1909a), (#1708) a "Scottish" specimen (Turner 1908), (#1709 - #1721, #1730 - #1732) a series from the American Museum (Gregory and Hellman 1926a), (#1722 - #1724) 3 specimens measured by Elsner (1917), (#1725) a specimen from the Field Museum measured by the author, (#1732) measured by Burkitt (1928), (#1726 and #1727) measured from the description by Boule and Vallois (1957), and (#1728 and #1729) measured from the description by Werth (1928).

The Tasmanian specimens are much more limited (Macintosh and Barker 1965). Nicholls (1914) published the measurements for the only large series, but unfortunately these were not available. Published measurements used here come from the following sources: #1751 by Klaatsch (1903), #1752 by Turner (1909), #1754 by Basedow (1910), #1755 by Macintosh and Barker (1965), and #1756 to #1760 by Wood-Jones and Campbell (1924). Number 1761 to #1763 are specimens from the Field Museum measured by the author.

The group from Sub-Saharan Africa includes some fossil and sub-fossil material such as (#1903) Asselar (Boule and Vallois 1932), (#1902) Boskop (Galloway 1937), (#1904) Cape Flats (Drennan 1929b), (#1901) Florisbad (Dreyer 1935), (#1972) Fish Hoek (Coon 1963), and (#1123) Kabua 1 (Whitworth 1966). Measurements for "Negro" dentitions in the literature include (#1905 and #1906) 2 by Boule and Vallois (1957), (#1914) 1 by Galloway (1937), (#1915 and #1916) 2 by Keene (1967), and (#1907 - #1913) by Gregory and Hellman (1926a). Abel (1933) published measurements for "Negroes" (#1917 - #1925), a Bushman (#1973), a Hottentot (#1974), and a number of "mixed" specimens (#1943 - #1949). Two Bushmen (#1967 and #1968), and 3 Hottentots (#1969 - #1971) from the American Museum collections were published by Gregory and Hellman (1926a). Galloway (1937) described the dentitions of the skeletal remains from Mapungubwe (#1951 - #1956) and (1959) from Bambandyanlo (#1957 - #1965).

The specimens from Dickson Mound (#1502 - #1634) near Havana, Illinois, on the Illinois River, were measured by the author. The Dicksons began excavation of this site in 1927 (Cole and Deuel 1937:120), leaving the skeletons in an *in situ* exhibit (Throop 1928:47-55). A very preliminary description of the skeletal material was published by Neumann (1937:250-5). Recent excavations have resulted in the recovery of over 800 burials (Hall 1967a:268, 1968:537). Description of this material, although attempted (Hall 1967b), has never been published. The cultural provenience of these burials is the Middle Spoon River phase of the late Middle Mississippian (Wray 1952:157), although there seems to be a Woodland component at the site (Hall 1966). Food production on a considerable scale is indicated (Caldwell 1959:33). The material measured was sampled from the 565 burials not on exhibition. This represents the extent of the excavations as of June, 1968.

Another group of Illinois Indians (#1426 - #1437), mostly from Pike County, was measured by the author. The remaining sample (#1401 - #1425) of American aboriginal remains is mixed. The Eskimos include (#1402) a specimen from the Hunterian collection (Klaatsch 1903), and 3 individuals (#1403 - #1405) from East Greenland (Pedersen 1949). Two of the earlier remains include (#1419) the Minnesota specimen (Jenks 1936), and (#1420) the Punin cranium from Equador (Sullivan and Hellman 1925). There is a Delaware Indian (#1401) measured by Hrdlicka (1916), and (#1406) a Haida measured by the author. A number of specimens from the American Museum of Natural History (#1407 - #1418), 4 of which were from New Mexico (#1421 - #1425), were described by Gregory and Hellman (1926a).

The "Malay" sample consists of 2 groups. The first (#2001 - #2021) comes from Gol ba It (Snell 1948b) and the second (#2022 - #2151) from Melolo (Snell 1948a).

There is a series (#1801 - #1865) consisting only of molar measurements from the Harappa excavations in India (Gupta, Dutta, and Basu 1962).

A sample of New Britain islanders (#1301 - #1346) was measured by the author at the Field Museum of Natural History in Chicago.

Finally, there are a few miscellaneous remains.

There is (#2208) a "Hindu" measured by the author from the collection at the University of Illinois, and (#2201 - #2202) 2 others from the American Museum (Gregory and Hellman 1926a). From Paleolithic China come the specimens from Ting Ts'un (#2206) described by Chang (1962; Movius 1956) and (#2203) Changyang (Chia 1957). There are 2 (#2204 - #2205) specimens from St. Cruz (Speiser), and lastly the possibly Wurm (Harrisson 1959) specimen from the great Niah Cave (#2207) in Borneo (Brothwell 1959; Howells 1967).

ORIGIN OF THE COMPILED GROUP MEASUREMENTS

The group statistics for many of the samples of extant groups were taken from the extensive literature concerned with the metrics of dental variation. The literature considered here gives information about the group means, sample size, variability, and range for at least some of the teeth in the human dentition. Dahlberg (1960b) published data for a sample of Chicago "Whites." Indeed, a large number of other American "White" samples have been described (Black 1902; Moorrees and Chadha 1962; Moorrees, Thomsen, Jensen, and Yen 1957; Sicher 1952; Sillman 1964). Data for Ohio "Whites" (Garn, Lewis, and Kerewsky 1964b, 1966a; Garn, Lewis, Swindler, and Kerewsky 1967), as well as for American "Whites" (Moorrees 1959; Moss, Chase, and Howes 1967) are incorporated in this work. There is a large amount of material available for European or European-derived groups. A number of studies of European "Whites" have been published (Brabrant 1965; Miyabara 1916; Seipel 1946; DeTerra 1905). Great Britain is represented by British (Dolamore 1908, Lavelle 1968), and Irish (Dockrell 1956) material. There are reports of dental metric variation for Swedish nationals (Seipel 1946; Lysell 1957), Lapps (Kajava 1912), Finns (Hjelmann 1928), Germans (Kantorowicz 1931; Mühlreiter and de Jonge-Cohen 1928), French (Choquet 1908; Marseillier 1945), French and Belgians (Brabrant 1963a), Swiss Alamannen (Schwertz 1917), Rumanians (Boboc 1965), and Hungarians (Hillebrand 1909). I have used data for the Swedish (Moorrees 1957), Lapps (Selmer-Olsen 1949), English (Goose 1963), and English-derived inhabitants of Tristan da Cunha (Thomsen 1955)–an island off the west coast of South Africa. Appropriate data is available for both Chinese (Hosaka 1936) and Japanese (Gonda 1959; Ono 1960; Yamada 1932). I have used Miyabara's Japanese data (1916).

Of the American aborigines, I have used dental statistics for Aleuts (Moorrees 1957), East Greenland Eskimos (Pedersen 1949), and Indians of the Pecos Pueblo (Nelson 1938). Some data for Canadian Eskimos is also available (Ritchie 1923). Goaz and Miller (1966) published data for Peruvian Indians.

Much relevant work has been published for both Tasmanians (Nicholls 1914; Macintosh and Barker 1965) and Australian aborigines (Begg 1954; Janzer 1927; Nicholls 1914). The Australian aborigine sample used here incorporates data taken from several sources (Campbell 1925; Gabriel 1955; Barrett, Brown, and Macdonald 1963).

There is a great amount of published material available for African and African-derived groups. "Negroes" in general (Galloway 1937; DeTerra 1905), and specifically Bantu (Shaw 1931; Abel 1933) are well represented. Particular groups include the Hutu of Rwanda (Brabrant 1963b), the Teso of Uganda (Barnes 1969), and the ancient inhabitants of Bambandyanalo (Galloway 1959), and Mapungubwe (Galloway 1937). In addition, there are reports for central African Pygmies (Brabrant 1965), Bushmen (Galloway 1937), and Bushmen, Hottentots, and mixed South African aborigines (Abel 1933). I have used data for American Negroes of Liberian descent (Moss, Chase, and Howes 1967), and for Bushmen (Drennan 1929a). I have used data for 5 groups from the Near East and North Africa. These include Jews from Yemen and Cochin (Rosenzweig and Zilberman 1967), a Mesolithic population from Wadi Halfa (Greene, Ewing, and Armelagos 1967) in the Sudan, and ancient Natufians, and the inhabitants of Jarmo (Dahlberg 1960b).

In Southeast Asia and the regions southward, a number of populations have been sampled. Janzer (1927) published material for New Pomerania and for natives of the Gazelle Peninsula in New Guinea. The teeth of the Nasioi, again from New Guinea, have been described (Bailit, DeWitt, and Leigh 1968). The molar teeth of the New Britain islanders have received some attention (Stein and Epstein 1934), and some of the material from Buggisen in the Celebes is available (Schwertz 1914).

There is data for St. Cruz in the Philippines (Speiser 1923). I have incorporated the statistics for Javanese (Mijsberg 1931) and for a group from Gilimanuk, Bali, Indonesia (Jacob 1967b).

ORIGIN OF THE NON-HUMAN PRIMATE GROUP DENTAL MATERIAL

There have been a reasonable number of general studies of the primate dentition yielding metric data (Adloff 1908, 1927; Hrdlicka 1923b, 1924; James 1960; Remane 1961). Some studies of fossil primates are particularly complete for both *Cercopithecus* (Freedman 1957, 1960, 1961) and *Dryopithecus* (Gregory 1966a; Hrdlicka 1924), although the sample sizes for both taxa are too small to be of use in this work.

Data for a number of species are used as comparative material. The sources of this material are as follows: *Pan gorilla* (Ashton and Zuckerman 1950a; Gregory and Hellman 1926a; Hrdlicka 1923b; James 1960; Remane 1961); *Pan troglodytes* (Ashton and Zuckerman 1950a; Gregory 1922; Gregory and Hellman 1926a; Hrdlicka 1923b; James 1960; Remane 1961; Schuman and Brace 1954); *Hylobates* (Frisch 1963, 1965); *Cercopithecus aethiops* (Swindler, Gavan, and Turner; Ashton and Zuckerman 1950b); *Macaca mulatta* and *Macaca speciosa* (Biggerstaff 1966); *Cercopithecus nictitans buttikoferi, Cercopithecus mona cambelli,* and *Cercopithecus diana* (Lampel 1963); *Cercopithecus ascanius* and *Cercocebus albigena* (Swindler, Gavan, and Turner 1963); *Alouatta caraya* (Zingeser 1967). A recent publication by Vogel (1966) provided the basis for additional morphological comparisons.

4. Individual Teeth

LOWER CENTRAL INCISOR

Figures for the length of the first lower incisor are given in Table I. The greatest average length for a hominid taxon is reached by *H. erectus* (6.13 mm). While the Krapina Neandertals have an even greater average length of 6.21 mm, this is surpassed by the Australoid average of 6.40 mm. In addition, the average for Neandertals as a taxon (5.70 mm) is virtually identical to that of *H. sapiens* (5.68 mm). There is thus an apparent length maximization in the pre-Wurm Mid-Pleistocene hominids. These data, however, show no significant trend. Not only does the range for *H. sapiens* include all known fossil hominid teeth, but the range of the averages for the *H. sapiens* groups includes the averages of the 4 fossil hominid taxa. Indeed, the values for *H. robustus* and all but 7% of *H. erectus* can be included in the range of variation for *H. africanus* (Table III). The ranges of all 3 of these taxa are included within the *H. neanderthalensis* range, and the ranges of all taxa fit within *H. sapiens.* Thus, trends of lower central incisor length change are not significant.

The coefficients of variation for the 5 hominid taxa range between 18.2 for *H. africanus* and 2.4 for *H. robustus.* The very high value for *H. africanus* is more a function of small sample size than of unusual range. Indeed, the actual range of *H. africanus* is less than that of both the Neandertals and modern man. This relationship can be seen in Table III. The very low value for *H. robustus* presents more of an anomaly. Yet, the coefficients of variation for the *H. sapiens* groups range almost as greatly, from 14.5 to 4.4, and these groups represent a considerably smaller time span. When the australopithecines are treated together as a single group, the coefficient of variation of this group is 11.5–identical to the value for *H. sapiens* and in line with the values for the other hominid taxa. The frequency distribution of length for the australopithecines treated as a single group (Table III) is unimodal, and its range is compatible with the other taxa.

The length coefficient of variation for the Liberian chimpanzee (Table LXXXI) is 6.5, and the value for 50 Howler monkeys was calculated from Zingeser's data (1967:976) as 7.6. With the exception of *H. robustus,* all the taxa of *Homo,* as well as the australopithecines taken as a single taxon, are more variable than these non-human primates.

While the average length for *H. africanus* is slightly larger than that of *H. robustus,* the difference is small compared to differences between groups within *H. sapiens.* The difference between the *H. africanus* and the *H. robustus* means is less than 1/2 of 1 standard error of the *H. africanus* mean. Therefore, the probability that this difference is the result of small sample size is greater than 70% based on the available data.

Unlike length, the maximum breadth of the first lower incisor is reached in *H. neanderthalensis* (7.40 mm), and of the groups within this taxon the Krapina Neandertals attain the maximum group average for *Homo* of 8.17 mm. In *H. sapiens* the average value for breadth is 5.89 mm, and the group averages range from 6.67 to 5.20 mm. The Mt. Carmel Neandertals

TABLE I. Lower First Incisor Length and Breadth: Mean, Standard Error of the Mean (SE(M)), Range, Sample Size (N), and Coefficient of Variation (CV).

LOWER I1	LENGTH(M-D)					BREADTH(B-L)				
	MEAN	SE(M)	RANGE	N	CV	MEAN	SE(M)	RANGE	N	CV
H. AFRICANUS	5.73	.47	4.00 - 6.70	6	18.2	6.75	.56	6.00 - 8.10	4	14.3
H. ROBUSTUS	5.50	.05	5.20 - 5.60	9	2.4	6.30	.16	5.50 - 6.90	9	7.1
H. ERECTUS	6.13	.18	5.00 - 7.15	13	10.1	6.57	.15	5.80 - 7.10	10	6.8
H. NEANDERTAL	5.70	.14	4.50 - 7.50	31	13.9	7.40	.11	6.40 - 8.20	22	6.8
H. SAPIENS	5.68	.04	3.80 - 7.80	245	11.5	5.89	.05	3.70 - 7.85	226	11.9
AUSTRALOPITHECINES	5.59	.17	4.00 - 6.70	15	11.5	6.44	.19	5.50 - 8.10	13	10.0
KRAPINA	6.21	.31	5.30 - 7.50	8	13.3	8.17	.04	8.10 - 8.20	3	.7
NEANDERTAL	5.68	.16	4.50 - 6.90	17	11.6	7.39	.09	7.00 - 8.00	15	4.4
MT CARMEL	5.10	.34	4.50 - 6.50	6	14.7	6.90	.34	6.40 - 7.70	4	8.6
AUSTRALOID	6.40	.12	6.00 - 6.90	7	4.4	6.67	.31	6.00 - 7.20	4	8.1
AUSTR. ABORIGINE	6.00	.00	5.00 - 7.00	43	.0	6.30	.00	5.50 - 7.50	77	.0
SUB SAHARAN	5.88	.13	4.50 - 7.40	28	11.5	6.40	.16	4.20 - 7.50	24	11.7
WADI HALFA MESOL.	5.70	.00	5.40 - 6.00	4	.0	6.30	.00	6.10 - 6.50	4	.0
NEW BRITAIN	5.67	.09	4.60 - 6.90	30	8.8	6.15	.08	5.50 - 7.10	29	6.7
GILIMANUK (INDON.)	5.60	.00	4.60 - 6.90	28	.0	6.10	.00	5.00 - 7.80	42	.0
DICKSON MOUND	5.59	.05	4.50 - 7.20	103	8.2	5.75	.05	3.75 - 6.80	95	8.5
MALAY	5.53	.43	5.00 - 6.20	3	11.0	5.80	.23	5.50 - 6.60	5	7.9
TRISTANITES	5.52	.03		286	9.2					
PECOS PUEBLO	5.52	.03	4.87 - 6.33	84	4.9	5.87	.04	4.99 - 6.93	84	6.0
JAVANESE	5.48	.04		165	8.8	5.81	.04		167	8.6
SWEDES	5.47	.01		998	5.9					
INDIAN	5.47	.15	4.50 - 6.10	11	8.7	6.06	.18	5.20 - 6.80	10	8.9
NATUFIANS	5.37	.13		10	7.1	6.21	.17		10	8.2
OHIO WHITES	5.34	.02		462	7.3					
AMERICAN WHITES(1)	5.33	.03	4.30 - 6.10	172	6.4					
JAPANESE	5.30	.02		173	4.9					
JARMO	5.30	.00		3	.0	5.80	.00		3	.0
LAPPS	5.27	.02	4.40 - 6.20	246	5.7	5.74	.02	4.70 - 6.80	358	7.0
COCHINI JEWS	5.23	.04		58	5.7					
YEMEN JEWS	5.20	.05		60	7.1					
ALEUTS	5.17	.03	3.70 - 6.40	171	7.2					
CAUCASOID	5.16	.12	3.80 - 6.50	37	14.5	6.32	.12	5.10 - 7.85	33	10.6
BUSHMEN	5.00	.00	4.30 - 6.00	22	.0	5.20	.00	5.00 - 6.00	22	.0

TABLE II. Lower First Incisor Area (L*B), Index (100L/B), and Module ((L+B)/2): Mean, Range, and Coefficient of Variation (CV).

LOWER I1	L*B			100L/B			(L+B)/2		
	MEAN	RANGE	CV	MEAN	RANGE	CV	MEAN	RANGE	CV
H. AFRICANUS	35.9	27.2 - 47.8	25.8	79.6	58.8 - 103.3	23.5	6.0	5.4 - 7.0	12.3
H. ROBUSTUS	34.6	29.7 - 38.6	7.3	87.7	77.6 - 98.2	7.8	5.9	5.4 - 6.2	3.9
H. ERECTUS	40.2	35.5 - 44.2	6.6	94.2	70.4 - 115.5	14.7	6.3	6.0 - 6.6	3.0
H. NEANDERTAL	42.6	31.2 - 61.5	19.6	77.4	56.2 - 92.0	12.9	6.6	5.6 - 7.8	9.0
H. SAPIENS	33.2	16.9 - 51.8	16.9	97.3	61.3 - 173.0	18.0	5.8	4.1 - 7.2	8.3
AUSTRALOPITHECINES	35.0	27.2 - 47.8	14.6	85.2	58.8 - 103.3	13.6	5.9	5.4 - 7.0	7.1
KRAPINA	57.5	50.2 - 61.5	10.9	86.1	76.5 - 91.5	9.6	7.6	7.1 - 7.8	5.1
NEANDERTAL	41.4	36.0 - 51.7	10.9	76.3	56.2 - 92.0	13.5	6.5	6.2 - 7.2	4.6
MT CARMEL	36.2	31.2 - 50.0	25.6	75.2	64.3 - 84.4	11.2	6.0	5.6 - 7.1	11.6
AUSTRALOID	41.7	36.0 - 44.6	9.5	94.0	86.1 - 100.0	7.5	6.5	6.0 - 6.7	5.0
SUB SAHARAN	38.2	18.9 - 51.8	20.1	92.9	76.0 - 107.1	9.4	6.2	4.3 - 7.2	10.6
NEW BRITAIN	34.7	26.2 - 44.8	11.9	92.3	69.0 - 119.0	10.4	5.9	5.1 - 6.7	5.9
MALAY	33.4	28.5 - 40.9	19.8	92.1	87.7 - 94.7	4.2	5.8	5.3 - 6.4	9.7
INDIAN	33.2	29.6 - 37.8	8.2	91.7	67.2 - 115.1	16.0	5.8	5.4 - 6.1	3.8
CAUCASOID	32.8	20.8 - 50.0	22.9	81.5	61.3 - 100.0	12.1	5.7	4.6 - 7.1	11.2
DICKSON MOUND	31.8	16.9 - 41.6	12.1	96.6	74.6 - 120.0	9.6	5.6	4.1 - 6.4	6.2

TABLE III. Lower First Incisor Length: Frequency Distribution in Percentiles.

FREQUENCY DISTRIBUTICN OF LOWER I1 L(M-D)

	3.7	4.0	4.3	4.6	4.9	5.2	5.5	5.8	6.1	6.4	6.7	7.0	7.3	7.6	7.9
H.AFRICAN.		16			16			16	16	16	16				
H.ROBUSTUS						22	77								
H.ERECTUS					7		23	15	23		23	7			
H.NEANDER.			9	3	16	12	12	19	6	9	3		6		
H.SAPIENS	1	1	2	4	9	19	19	19	9	8	3	2	1	1	
AUSTRALOP.		6			6	13	46	6	6	6	6				
KRAPINA						25		37	12				25		
NEANDERTAL			13	4	21	8	17	13	4	13	4				
MT CARMEL			33	16	16	16				16					
CAUCASOID	5	8	8	10	21	8	13	16	2	5					
INDIAN			9	9		18	36	18	9						
AUSTRALOID								14	28	42	14				
NEW BRITAI				3	9	16	29	19	9	6	3				
DICKSON MD			1	3	7	31	21	24	4	3		1			
MALAY					33	33			33						
SUB SAHARA			3		10	14	17	10	10	21	7		3		

TABLE IV. Lower First Incisor Breadth: Frequency Distribution in Percentiles.

FREQUENCY DISTRIBUTICN OF LOWER I1 B(B-L)

	3.6	4.0	4.4	4.8	5.2	5.6	6.0	6.4	6.8	7.2	7.6	8.0	8.4	8.8	9.2
H.AFRICAN.							50		25			25			
H.ROBUSTUS					11	11	33	33	11						
H.ERECTUS						9	19	29	39						
H.NEANDER.								9	18	40	9	22			
H.SAPIENS	1	2	2	7	16	24	22	14	7	1	1				
AUSTRALOP.					7	7	38	23	15			7			
KRAPINA												99			
NEANDERTAL								10	21	47	10	10			
MT CARMEL								50	25		25				
CAUCASOID				3	3	15	45	9	12	6	6				
INDIAN					19	19	19	29	9						
AUSTRALOID							25	25	25	25					
NEW BRITAI					6	27	34	24	6						
DICKSON MD	1			8	24	36	18	8	2						
MALAY					39	39		19							
SUB SAHARA		4			12	4	8	37	29	4					

TABLE V. Lower First Incisor Area (L*B): Frequency Distribution in Percentiles.

FREQUENCY DISTRIBUTION OF LOWER I1 L*B

	16	20	24	28	32	36	40	44	48	52	56	60	64	68	72
H.AFRICAN.			25	25		25		25							
H.ROBUSTUS				11	66	22									
H.ERECTUS					9	39	39	9							
H.NEANDER.				13		40	9	13	13			9			
H.SAPIENS	1	2	9	32	29	12	7	3	1						
AUSTRALOP.			7	15	46	23		7							
KRAPINA									33			66			
NEANDERTAL						59	13	19	6						
MT CARMEL				75					25						
CAUCASOID		15	6	30	21	9	9	3	6						
INDIAN				39	39	19									
AUSTRALOID						25	25	50							
NEW BRITAI			3	28	25	35	3	3							
DICKSON MD	1		12	38	37	6	3								
SUB SAHARA	4		4	12	16	12	29	16	4						
MALAY				99											
HARAPPA															

show their affinities with an average breadth of 6.9 mm. Although the ranges of variation within all taxa overlap one another, the range within *H. sapiens* does *not* include all fossil teeth. In contrast to their near identity in length, the difference in breadth between *H. neanderthalensis* and *H. sapiens* is marked and significant. Indeed, while the differences between the values for *H. africanus, H. robustus,* and *H. erectus* are small enough to be accounted for by small sample size, all 3 taxa are significantly smaller than the Neandertals.

The frequency distributions for breadth (Table IV) show that while the ranges for *H. robustus* and *H. erectus* overlap almost completely, those of *H. africanus* and *H. neanderthalensis* (while being almost identical to each other) extend to greater values. Thus about 1/4 of the australopithecines do not overlap, and only about 30% of the *H. erectus* values overlap into the range for *H. neanderthalensis.* Indeed, 22% of the latter fall outside the range for *H. sapiens.*

The breadth difference between *H. robustus* and *H. erectus* is less than that between the Dickson Mound Indians and Pike County Illinois Indians, and the difference between *H. robustus* and *H. africanus* far less than that between Lapps and Caucasoids. The difference between *H. africanus* and *H. robustus* is less than 1 standard error of the *H. africanus* mean. On the other hand, the difference between *H. sapiens* and *H. neanderthalensis* is greater than that among any extant groups.

The coefficients of variation for the fossil taxa range from 14.3 for *H. africanus* to 6.8 for *H. erectus* and *H. neanderthalensis.* A similar range is encountered within *H. sapiens.* The incisor breadth coefficient of variation for 50 Howler monkeys is 8.1 (Zingeser 1967:976). Both *H. sapiens* and *H. africanus* are more variable than these non-human primates, to the extent that this coefficient can be taken as a comparative index of variation.

The area of the lower central incisor (Table II) increases from the australopithecines through *H. erectus,* culminating in a maximum value for

H. neanderthalensis. The value for *H. sapiens* is smaller than the value for any other taxa, although not significantly smaller than the australopithecine values. The size difference between *H. neanderthalensis* and *H. sapiens* is on the order of the maximum size difference between 2 extant groups. The Neandertal value is barely greater than the maximum size in an extant group. Thus, while there is a great size difference between *H. neanderthalensis* and *H. erectus,* the essential continuity between these taxa is preserved in the variation of extant group averages right up to the average for *H. neanderthalensis.* On the other hand, the 2 australopithecine taxa lie closer together than do the 2 groups of Illinois Indians. In terms of area, then, the size of the lower central incisor has undergone steady increase through the Middle Paleolithic, and has significantly decreased in the Upper Paleolithic. These changes are more a function of changes in breadth than in length which has not varied significantly throughout the Pleistocene.

From Table V one can see that unlike the mean value, the modal area reached its peak with *H. erectus,* and has subsequently decreased. Both *H. robustus* and *H. erectus* lie within the range of variation for *H. africanus,* and only 11% of the *H. robustus* specimens lie outside the range for *H. erectus.* The continuity and overlap of the taxa ranges indicate the absence of really significant change between any of the taxa. There is, however, a total tendency for reduction in area.

The L/B index (Table II) shows no consistent pattern of change. Its variation among the taxa is approximately the same as its variation among extant groups in both range and absolute values. The module varies almost exactly as does the area.

UPPER CENTRAL INCISOR

The length of the first upper incisor (Table VI) undergoes a steady increase, reaching its maximum value for a taxon with *H. erectus* (10.06 mm). The Krapina Neandertals have the maximum group average of 10.19 mm. However, from *H. erectus* to *H. sapiens* there is a consistent decrease in average length. The *H. sapiens* group value most closely approaching that of *H. neanderthalensis,* differing by only .05 mm, belongs to the Mesolithic remains from Wadi Halfa. However, the sample size is only 5. Australian aborigines, with a sample size of 56, have the next highest mean (9.37 mm), differing from the *H. neanderthalensis* value (9.85 mm) by .48 mm. The aborigine value is also surpassed by the value for the transitional Mt. Carmel Neandertals of 9.42 mm.

The averages for the australopithecine taxa are different, the value for H. robustus is .36 mm greater (2-1/2 times the standard error of the mean) than that of *H. africanus.* The latter is represented, however, by only 2 teeth from 1 individual (STS 52). In any event, this difference lies within the range of differences in extant groups. There is only slightly less difference between the 2 groups of Illinois Indians. The difference between *H. robustus* and *H. erectus* is similar.

Even without including the Wadi Halfa value, variation among *H. sapiens* groups is as great as that among the species of *Homo.* On the other hand, averages for *H. erectus* and *H. neanderthalensis* are greater than the averages for any *H. sapiens* group, and some individual teeth in these fossil taxa extend outside of the extant species range of variation.

There is, therefore, a significant trend to the increase in upper central incisor length which culminates in a maximum value for the Krapina Neandertals. Other Neandertals show decreasing length. This trend continues through such transitional forms as the Mt. Carmel population, and results in a decrease of over 20% for the taxon *H. sapiens.*

The length distributions are unimodal for almost all taxa and for the australopithecines taken as a single taxon (Table VIII). The distribution for *H. neanderthalensis* is bimodal. The ranges of all the taxa overlap greatly.

While the coefficient of variation is not the same for the 5 hominid species, there is no consistent trend in its variation. Compared to the 5.7 value for the Liberian chimpanzee (Table LXXXI), and that of 5.3 for the Howler monkeys (Zingeser 1967:976), all of the hominid species with reasonable sample sizes are more variable, and only 7 out of 19 extant hominid groups have lower coefficients of variation.

The breadth of the upper central incisor undergoes no consistent pattern of change.

TABLE VI. Upper First Incisor Length and Breadth: Mean, Standard Error of the Mean (SE(M)) Range, Sample Size (N), and Coefficient of Variation (CV).

UPPER 11	LENGTH(M-D)					BREADTH(B-L)				
	MEAN	SE(M)	RANGE	N	CV	MEAN	SE(M)	RANGE	N	CV
H. AFRICANUS	9.40	.14	9.30 - 9.50	2	1.5	8.25	.07	8.20 - 8.30	2	.9
H. ROBUSTUS	9.76	.17	8.30 - 10.90	9	5.3	7.70	.09	7.30 - 8.10	8	3.2
H. ERECTUS	10.06	.48	7.20 - 11.80	9	11.7	7.78	.13	7.50 - 8.20	7	3.7
H. NEANDERTAL	9.85	.15	8.00 - 12.00	41	9.8	8.59	.12	7.50 - 10.60	34	8.2
H. SAPIENS	8.92	.05	6.00 - 11.00	254	8.6	7.44	.05	5.50 - 10.60	244	9.6
AUSTRALOPITHECINES	9.69	.19	8.30 - 10.90	11	6.4	7.81	.32	7.30 - 8.30	10	12.1
KRAPINA	10.19	.13	9.40 - 11.00	15	4.8	8.87	.17	8.00 - 9.50	13	6.5
NEANDERTAL	9.73	.27	8.00 - 12.00	20	12.0	8.54	.20	8.00 - 10.60	16	8.9
MT CARMEL	9.42	.42	8.40 - 10.90	6	10.0	8.02	.26	7.50 - 8.70	5	6.4
WADI HALFA MESOL.	9.80		7.20 - 10.30	5		7.30		5.50 - 8.10	5	
AUSTR. ABORIGINE	9.37		8.50 - 10.60	56		7.90		7.00 - 9.00	93	
AUSTRALOID	9.31	.44	7.50 - 11.00	9	13.3	8.34	.53	6.20 - 10.60	9	17.9
SUB SAHARAN	9.30	.19	7.50 - 10.60	21	9.3	7.91	.20	6.00 - 9.50	20	11.3
NEW BRITAIN	9.00	.08	7.80 - 10.00	28	4.9	7.58	.08	6.70 - 8.80	30	5.9
DICKSON MOUND INDIAN	8.92	.05	7.85 - 9.95	116	5.4	7.33	.05	6.10 - 8.75	108	7.0
NATUFIANS	8.92	.19		9	6.1	7.26	.15		8	5.5
MALAY	8.84	.28	8.20 - 9.50	5	6.4	7.64	.28	6.90 - 8.20	5	7.3
JARMO	8.80			2		6.60			2	
SWEDES	8.73	.02		973	7.1					
TRISTANITES	8.70	.03		283	5.7					
GILIMANUK (INDON.)	8.70		8.00 - 10.00	32		7.40		5.90 - 8.20	36	
PECOS PUEBLO	8.67	.04	7.56 - 9.84	105	4.1	7.30	.03	6.22 - 8.53	105	4.8
OHIO WHITES	8.62	.03		472	6.6					
AMERICAN WHITES (1)	8.59	.04	7.10 - 10.00	174	5.8					
INDIAN	8.58	.11	8.00 - 9.10	11	4.0	7.47	.08	7.10 - 8.05	11	3.4
JAVANESE	8.51	.05		164	8.1	7.29	.04		166	7.5
CAUCASOID	8.44	.19	6.00 - 10.50	38	13.9	7.57	.11	6.40 - 9.10	35	8.3
JAPANESE	8.40	.03		117	3.8					
LAPPS	8.31	.03	7.40 - 9.50	229	5.7	6.88	.03	5.60 - 8.30	316	7.0
BUSHMEN	8.30		8.00 - 9.50	25		6.50		6.00 - 7.50	27	
ALEUTS	8.30	.04	7.10 - 9.50	162	5.4					
YEMEN JEWS	8.24	.08		60	7.5					
COCHINI JEWS	8.24	.07		60	6.8					

TABLE VII. Upper First Incisor Area (L*B), Index (100L/B), and Module ((L+B)/2): Mean, Range, and Coefficient of Variation (CV).

UPPER 11	L*B			100L/B			(L+B)/2		
	MEAN	RANGE	CV	MEAN	RANGE	CV	MEAN	RANGE	CV
H. AFRICANUS	77.5	77.2 - 77.9	.6	114.0	112.0 - 115.9	2.4	8.8	8.8 - 8.9	.5
H. ROBUSTUS	75.4	64.7 - 82.9	7.4	127.6	106.4 - 143.4	5.9	8.8	8.1 - 9.3	4.0
H. ERECTUS	75.8	54.0 - 86.7	13.9	126.4	96.0 - 144.0	12.8	8.8	7.4 - 9.4	7.6
H. NEANDERTAL	84.8	63.0 - 117.7	15.6	115.0	94.1 - 150.0	9.7	9.2	7.9 - 10.8	7.8
H. SAPIENS	66.7	42.0 - 98.8	15.3	120.6	83.8 - 157.1	10.0	8.2	6.5 - 9.9	7.6
AUSTRALOPITHECINES	75.8	64.7 - 82.9	10.2	123.4	106.4 - 143.4	7.8	8.8	8.1 - 9.3	5.1
KRAPINA	90.5	76.1 - 104.5	10.5	115.1	106.4 - 123.7	5.3	9.5	8.7 - 10.2	5.1
NEANDERTAL	83.1	68.0 - 117.7	17.3	114.2	94.1 - 150.0	13.3	9.1	8.2 - 10.8	8.4
MT CARMEL	75.8	63.0 - 94.8	17.6	117.0	112.0 - 125.3	5.3	8.7	7.9 - 9.8	9.0
AUSTRALOID	78.1	51.2 - 95.4	23.9	114.0	84.9 - 138.7	17.6	8.8	7.2 - 9.8	12.6
SUB SAHARAN	74.5	48.0 - 98.8	17.5	119.2	106.5 - 143.5	9.7	8.6	7.0 - 9.9	8.9
NEW BRITAIN	68.9	54.6 - 83.6	8.1	118.1	107.5 - 131.6	6.6	8.3	7.4 - 9.1	4.0
MALAY	67.8	57.3 - 77.9	13.4	115.8	113.7 - 120.3	2.3	8.2	7.6 - 8.8	6.8
DICKSON MOUND INDIAN	65.3	49.4 - 82.2	10.9	121.8	105.3 - 142.1	6.1	8.1	7.1 - 9.1	5.4
CAUCASOID	64.1	42.0 - 84.0	18.3	111.8	83.8 - 142.9	14.1	8.0	6.5 - 9.2	9.5
INDIAN	64.0	58.7 - 68.2	5.0	115.0	105.0 - 125.4	5.5	8.0	7.7 - 8.3	2.5

TABLE VIII. Upper First Incisor Length: Frequency Distribution in Percentiles.

FREQUENCY CISTRIBUTICN OF UPPER I1 L(M-D)

	5.8	6.3	6.8	7.3	7.8	8.3	8.8	9.3	9.8	10.3	10.8	11.3	11.8	12.3	12.8
H.AFRICAN.								99							
H.ROBUSTUS						11	11	55	11		11				
H.ERECTUS			12						37	25	12	12			
H.NEANDER.					7	4	17	14	21	9	19	2	2		
H.SAPIENS	1	1	1	1	9	22	32	19	6	3	1				
AUSTRALOP.						9	9	63	9		9				
KRAPINA								13	46	19	19				
NEANDERTAL					11	7	26	15	7	3	19	3	3		
MT CARMEL						33	16	16	16		16				
CAUCASOID	5	7	7	5	7	23	18	13	5	5					
INDIAN					18	45	36								
AUSTRALOID				11	11	11	22		22		22				
NEW BRITAI					3	21	46	25	3						
DICKSON MD					10	25	38	22	2						
MALAY					19	19	39	19							
SUB SAHARA				4	9	9	14	28	23	9					

TABLE IX. Upper First Incisor Breadth: Frequency Distribution in Percentiles.

FREQUENCY CISTRIBUTICN OF UPPER I1 B(B-L)

	5.3	5.7	6.1	6.5	6.9	7.3	7.7	8.1	8.5	8.9	9.3	9.7	10.1	10.5	10.9
H.AFRICAN.								99							
H.ROBUSTUS						50	37							12	
H.ERECTUS						50	16	33							
H.NEANDER.						5	14	29	20	8	14		2	2	
H.SAPIENS	1	2	4	8	25	25	19	7	3	1	1		1	1	
AUSTRALOP.						39	29	19						9	
KRAPINA							7	23	7	23	38				
NEANDERTAL						9	19	33	28				4	4	
MT CARMEL						39		39	19						
CAUCASOID			2	8	28	17	25	8	5	2					
INDIAN					27	63	9								
AUSTRALOID			22			11	11		22	11			11	11	
NEW BRITAI				3	19	29	39	3	3						
DICKSON MD			5	13	27	28	15	7	1						
MALAY					39		39	19							
SUB SAHARA		4		4	14	9	14	29	9		9				

TABLE X. Upper First Incisor Area (L*B): Frequency Distribution in Percentiles.

FREQUENCY DISTRIBUTION OF UPPER I1 L*B

	41	47	53	59	65	71	77	83	89	95	101	107	113	119	125
H.AFRICAN.							99								
H.ROBUSTUS				14	28	14	28				14				
H.ERECTUS			16			16	33	33							
H.NEANDER.				5	5	29	17	2	20	2	8	2	2		
H.SAPIENS	3	5	11	22	25	16	7	4	1	1					
AUSTRALOP.				11	22	11	44				11				
KRAPINA						7	30		38		23				
NEANDERTAL					12	50	6	6	6	6		6	6		
MT CARMEL				39		19	19		19						
CAUCASOID	11	11	8	11	31	14	2	8							
INDIAN			9	54	35										
AUSTRALOID		11	22					33	22	11					
NEW BRITAI			3	15	57	15	3	3							
DICKSON MD		3	14	32	25	19	3								
SUB SAHARA		9	4	9	4	14	29	14	4	4					
MALAY			19	19		39	19								
HARAPPA															

Indeed, even the greatest differences among hominid taxa are exceeded by a number of differences among extant groups. Thus, the difference between *H. neanderthalensis* and *H. sapiens,* the maximum between hominid taxa, is surpassed by that between Bushmen and a sample of all Sub-Saharan Africans. Of the taxa, *H. africanus* and *H. neanderthalensis* have large mean breadths, with that of the latter being maximum. *H. robustus* and *H. erectus* have smaller, almost identical, values, and the mean for *H. sapiens* is miminum. Of the hominid groups, the Krapina Neandertals have the maximum value.

The breadth coefficient of variation increases consistently from *H. africanus* and *H. robustus* to *H. sapiens.*

The combination of length and breadth in the area (or module) of the tooth (Table VII) shows a specific pattern. The earlier 3 taxa have almost identical means; the *H. neanderthalensis* value is larger and that for *H. sapiens* is minimum. The difference between the last 2 taxa is significant, exceeding the maximum difference between extant groups.

The Krapina Neandertals have the largest upper central incisor of all groups. Still, reduction of this tooth to the condition which appears in *H. sapiens* seems to begin in the Wurm Neandertals. The tooth is larger in the Mt. Carmel Neandertals than it is in any extant group except the Australoids, and it may be pointed out that the value for the Australoids exceeds that of all hominid taxa.

The distribution of area (Table X) is bimodal for *H. robustus* and *H. neanderthalensis.* There is no bimodality in any of the extant groups. The distributions for *H. robustus* and *H. erectus* are almost identical. *H. africanus,* represented by the 2 teeth of STS 52, falls within this range. In turn, almost all the specimens of these 3 taxa fall within the range of *H. neanderthalensis.* Upper central incisor size clearly reaches a maximum with the latter, and subsequently shows significant decrease to the *H. sapiens* range and mean value.

The coefficient of variation for area and

module follows a consistent pattern of increase from the australopithecines to *H. sapiens.* In comparison, the breadth coefficient for 47 Howler monkeys is 7.0 (Zingeser 1967:976). This value is surpassed by the values for *H. erectus, H. neanderthalensis,* and *H. sapiens,* as well as by 7 out of 11 extant groups within the taxon *H. sapiens.*

There is a moderate amount of variation in the L/B ratio among the hominid taxa. The teeth in *H. robustus* and *H. erectus* are longest with respect to breadth: the upper central incisor L/B ratio for these species is greater than in any other hominid taxon or extant group. Ratios in other taxa are matched by ratios in extant groups. Indeed, the difference between Indians from Dickson Mound and Pike County Illinois is greater than that between *H. sapiens* and *H. neanderthalensis.*

LOWER LATERAL INCISOR

Compared to the distribution in modern human groups, there has been very little change in lower lateral incisor length from *H. africanus* to *H. sapiens* (Table XI). The maximum difference between human groups is 1.33 mm, while between species it is only .61 mm. The maximum average for a modern group comes within .01 mm of the maximum for a hominid species. On the other hand, longer teeth appear in the fossil record than any reported for *H. sapiens* (Table XIII).

The difference between the 2 australopithecine groups is exceeded by that between Illinois Indians and Indians of the Pecos Pueblo. Indeed, Table XIII shows that the distribution for *H. robustus* fits neatly within the distribution for *H. africanus.*

Generally the length distribution of this tooth is the same as that of its medial counterpart, although the differences in the former are not as great. Trends in the fossil record are visible, but do not clearly represent *significant* changes in view of their magnitude. This conclusion is similarly justified by the distribution of the modal (Table XIII), as well as the mean, incisor length value.

The coefficient of variation for the Liberian chimpanzee is 5.1 (Table LXXXI) and for the Howler monkeys 6.0 (Zingeser 1967:976). Of the 5 hominid taxa, 4 show greater variation, and the variability of the 5th (*H. robustus*) is comparable to that of the non-human primates. Two-thirds of the extant groups are more variable than the non-human primates.

The lower lateral incisor is more variable than the lower central incisor in 3 out of 5 hominid species, and in 5 out of 18 living groups. It has greater variability in the Liberian chimpanzee. Thus, in hominids, central incisor length is more variable in about 70% of the sample. On the other hand, the lateral incisor is inevitably the larger of the 2 teeth. Lower central incisor breadth is more variable than lower lateral incisor breadth in about the same percentage, although not necessarily with the same species and groups. In terms of area, the lower central incisor is the more variable of the 2, in 2 out of 5 species and in 5 out of 6 extant groups (Table XII).

As in the case of the lower central incisor, breadth shows a much greater variation than does length (Table XI). A maximum value is reached in *H. neanderthalensis,* and within that species the sample from Krapina has the largest average, as well as maximum, breadth. The increase from the australopithecines through *H. erectus* and *H. neanderthalensis* is steady. The average breadth in *H. sapiens* is, however, the smallest among the hominid species although individual teeth of this species are as broad as almost any in the fossil record.

The breadth coefficient of variation for 50 Howler monkeys, calculated from Zingeser's data (1967:976), is 6.7. Thus all but 1 hominid taxon (*H. robustus* with a coefficient of variation of 5.7), and all but 1 of 11 extant groups, are more variable in lower lateral incisor breadth than this non-human primate.

When compared with the distribution and variation of lower lateral incisor breadth in *H. sapiens,* significant changes become apparent between the fossil species. The difference between mean values for *H. africanus* and *H. erectus* is not as great as the difference between the mean values of some diverse modern groups, and is only 68% of the largest such difference. On the other hand, 3 out of 4 values for *H. africanus* fall outside of the *H. robustus* range of variation (Table XIV). Four out of 6 values for *H. robustus* fall within the range of variation for *H. africanus.*

The increase in breadth from *H. erectus* to *H. neanderthalensis* is greater. It is exceeded by only

TABLE XI. Lower Second Incisor Length and Breadth: Mean, Standard Error of the Mean (SE(M)), Range, Sample Size (N), and Coefficient of Variation (CV).

LOWER I2	LENGTH(M-D)					BREADTH(B-L)				
	MEAN	SE(M)	RANGE	N	CV	MEAN	SE(M)	RANGE	N	CV
H. AFRICANUS	6.73	.49	5.20 - 7.80	6	16.3	7.67	.34	6.80 - 8.10	4	7.8
H. ROBUSTUS	6.33	.14	5.90 - 6.70	6	5.0	6.77	.17	6.40 - 7.50	6	5.7
H. ERECTUS	6.94	.23	5.60 - 8.80	15	12.4	7.03	.15	5.60 - 7.80	14	7.9
H. NEANDERTAL	6.73	.10	5.50 - 8.60	42	9.4	8.11	.12	7.00 - 10.00	30	8.2
H. SAPIENS	6.45	.04	4.30 - 7.85	259	9.0	6.36	.04	4.30 - 9.80	249	11.0
AUSTRALOPITHECINES	6.53	.24	5.20 - 7.80	12	12.2	7.13	.22	6.40 - 8.10	10	9.1
KRAPINA	7.05	.24	6.10 - 8.60	11	10.6	8.62	.44	7.10 - 10.00	6	11.5
NEANDERTAL	6.66	.11	5.50 - 7.80	26	8.6	8.07	.10	7.50 - 9.00	21	5.7
MT CARMEL	6.44	.25	6.00 - 7.20	5	7.7	7.37	.39	7.00 - 8.00	3	7.5
AUSTRALOID	6.93	.11	6.70 - 7.40	6	3.6	6.90	.32	6.30 - 7.60	4	7.9
AUSTR. ABORIGINE	6.70	.00	6.00 - 7.80	51	.0	6.60	.00	6.00 - 7.50	92	.0
INDIAN	6.56	.07	6.15 - 7.00	11	3.6	6.36	.12	5.80 - 7.05	11	5.9
DICKSON MOUND	6.53	.04	5.60 - 7.70	101	5.8	6.30	.04	5.20 - 7.15	99	6.8
SUB SAHARAN	6.46	.09	5.20 - 7.50	32	7.9	6.73	.21	4.30 - 9.80	26	15.4
NEW BRITAIN	6.33	.09	5.50 - 7.60	34	7.7	6.48	.09	5.30 - 7.80	35	8.0
WADI HALFA MESOL.	6.20	.00	6.10 - 6.40	3	.0	6.60	.00	6.50 - 6.70	3	.0
JAVANESE	6.18	.04		172	8.6	6.35	.04		172	7.7
PECOS PUEBLO	6.14	.03	5.50 - 6.78	74	4.6	6.06	.04	5.22 - 6.68	74	5.2
GILIMANUK (INDON.)	6.10	.00	5.20 - 7.20	31	.0	6.30	.00	5.20 - 7.70	45	.0
TRISTANITES	6.08	.03		287	8.4					
SWEDES	6.04	.00		0	.0					
ALEUTS	6.01	.03	4.70 - 6.70	172	5.8					
JARMO	6.00	.00		3	.0	6.10	.00		3	.0
CAUCASOID	5.99	.12	4.30 - 7.85	46	13.8	6.73	.10	5.60 - 8.50	43	9.9
MALAY	5.97	.33	5.60 - 6.50	3	7.9	6.22	.28	5.90 - 7.20	5	8.9
NATUFIANS	5.95	.17		13	9.7	6.61	.12		13	6.5
OHIO WHITES	5.93	.02		474	6.9					
JAPANESE	5.90	.02		187	4.6					
LAPPS	5.87	.02	5.00 - 7.40	348	6.6	6.11	.02	5.00 - 7.10	407	6.2
AMERICAN WHITES(1)	5.86	.03	4.70 - 6.90	172	6.5					
COCHINI JEWS	5.74	.05		58	6.8					
YEMEN JEWS	5.61	.06		60	8.0					
BUSHMEN	5.60	.00	5.00 - 7.00	24	.0	5.60	.00	5.00 - 6.50	23	.0

TABLE XII. Lower Second Incisor Area (L*B), Index (100L/B), and Module ((L+B)/2): Mean, Range, and Coefficient of Variation (CV).

LOWER I2	L*B			100L/B			(L+B)/2		
	MEAN	RANGE	CV	MEAN	RANGE	CV	MEAN	RANGE	CV
H. AFRICANUS	47.9	40.6 - 57.5	15.4	82.6	66.7 - 107.4	23.0	7.0	6.5 - 7.6	6.7
H. ROBUSTUS	42.9	37.8 - 48.7	9.0	93.7	86.7 - 100.0	5.5	6.5	6.1 - 7.0	4.6
H. ERECTUS	46.8	31.4 - 52.5	12.3	95.4	76.9 - 101.5	8.0	6.8	5.6 - 7.2	6.6
H. NEANDERTAL	54.8	42.6 - 86.0	17.2	83.3	67.1 - 97.3	9.8	7.4	6.5 - 9.3	8.1
H. SAPIENS	41.0	22.4 - 67.6	14.8	102.6	61.4 - 148.1	14.8	6.4	4.7 - 8.3	7.2
AUSTRALOPITHECINES	44.9	37.8 - 57.5	12.9	89.3	66.7 - 107.4	14.5	6.7	6.1 - 7.6	6.2
KRAPINA	64.5	46.9 - 86.0	20.4	86.6	76.9 - 93.0	6.6	8.0	6.8 - 9.3	10.2
NEANDERTAL	52.8	45.1 - 64.8	11.1	81.4	67.1 - 97.3	10.8	7.3	6.8 - 8.1	5.2
MT CARMEL	48.3	42.6 - 57.6	16.8	88.6	84.5 - 91.4	4.1	6.9	6.5 - 7.6	8.2
AUSTRALOID	47.4	43.5 - 51.7	7.1	100.2	89.5 - 109.5	8.7	6.9	6.6 - 7.2	3.6
SUB SAHARAN	43.8	22.4 - 67.6	21.5	97.2	70.4 - 120.9	10.6	6.6	4.7 - 8.3	11.1
INDIAN	41.5	35.7 - 46.9	7.9	102.7	94.3 - 111.7	5.7	6.4	6.0 - 6.8	3.9
DICKSON MOUND	41.1	30.9 - 50.8	9.5	104.1	86.2 - 128.8	8.5	6.4	5.6 - 7.1	4.7
NEW BRITAIN	41.0	32.4 - 57.0	11.4	98.2	74.4 - 134.0	11.7	6.4	5.7 - 7.5	5.6
CAUCASOID	40.3	28.0 - 64.4	21.7	89.3	61.4 - 108.6	10.9	6.3	5.3 - 8.0	10.4
MALAY	38.6	33.6 - 46.8	18.5	92.9	90.3 - 95.1	2.6	6.2	5.8 - 6.8	9.2

TABLE XIII. Lower Second Incisor Length: Frequency Distribution in Percentiles.

FREQUENCY DISTRIBUTION OF LOWER I2 L(M-D)

	4.2	4.6	5.0	5.4	5.8	6.2	6.6	7.0	7.4	7.8	8.2	8.6	9.0	9.4	9.8
H.AFRICAN.			16	16				33	16	16					
H.ROBUSTUS					33	33	33								
H.ERECTUS				6	6	19	13	39				13			
H.NEANDER.				2	21	14	26	21	7	4		2			
H.SAPIENS	1	1	4	7	13	28	27	11	4	1					
AUSTRALOP.			8	8	16	16	16	16	8	8					
KRAPINA					9	18	18	18	18	9		9			
NEANDERTAL				3	25	12	29	22	3	3					
MT CARMEL					39	19	19	19							
CAUCASOID	2	2	21	17	19	10	4	17	2	2					
INDIAN					9	27	54	9							
AUSTRALOID							66	16	16						
NEW BRITAI				11	26	29	23	5	2						
DICKSON MD				2	11	41	31	9	1						
MALAY				33	33	33									
SUB SAHARA			3	9	12	31	34	3	6						

TABLE XIV. Lower Second Incisor Breadth: Frequency Distribution in Percentiles.

FREQUENCY DISTRIBUTION OF LOWER I2 B(B-L)

	4.2	4.6	5.0	5.4	5.8	6.2	6.6	7.0	7.4	7.8	8.2	8.6	9.0	9.4	9.8
H.AFRICAN.							25			75					
H.ROBUSTUS						33	50		16						
H.ERECTUS				7		7	14	50	14	7					
H.NEANDER.								9	16	29	23		16	3	
H.SAPIENS	1	1	7	6	21	29	16	12	3	1	1			1	
AUSTRALOP						19	39		9	29					
KRAPINA								16			33		33	16	
NEANDERTAL								8	20	37	20		12		
MT CARMEL								66		33					
CAUCASOID				2	18	23	20	16	9	4	4				
INDIAN					36	27	27	9							
AUSTRALOID						25	25	25	25						
NEW BRITAI			2		22	37	22	5	5	2					
DICKSON MD			2	9	23	41	15	9							
MALAY					79			19							
SUB SAHARA	3		3	7	7	15	15	30	7	3				3	

TABLE XV. Lower Second Incisor Area (L*B): Frequency Distribution in Percentiles.

FREQUENCY DISTRIBUTION OF LOWER I2 L*B

	21	26	31	36	41	46	51	56	61	66	71	76	81	86	91
H.AFRICAN.				25	25	25		25							
H.ROBUSTUS				33	50	16									
H.ERECTUS			7	7	15	38	30								
H.NEANDER.					10	32	21	7	21		3		3		
H.SAPIENS	1	3	14	35	28	13	2	2	1	1					
AUSTRALOP.				29	39	19		9							
KRAPINA						16		16	33		16		16		
NEANDERTAL					5	42	31		21						
MT CARMEL					66			33							
CAUCASOID		14	19	33	9	9	4	7	2						
INDIAN			9	29	50	9									
AUSTRALOID					25	50	25								
NEW BRITAI			12	40	37	6		3							
DICKSON MD		1	7	40	37	14									
SUB SAHARA	3	3	15	11	26	23	7	3		3					
MALAY															
HARAPPA															

the maximum difference between average values in extant groups. The decrease in breadth between *H. neanderthalensis* and *H. sapiens* exceeds the maximum difference within *H. sapiens.* This decrease surely represents a drastic and significant reversal of the breadth increase in the Middle and Lower Pleistocene hominid species.

Within *H. neanderthalensis,* the population represented by the Krapina material has the largest mean and maximum breadth of all hominid groups. Breadth in subsequent early-Wurm Neandertals decreases, and this decrease continues through the slightly later Neandertals at Mt. Carmel. The mean value for the Mt. Carmel specimens still, however, greatly exceeds the maximum average value for an extant group.

There are trends in the evolutionary changes of length and breadth common to the upper central incisor and the lower central and lateral incisors. In some instances, the changes are of great enough magnitude for the trends to be significant. In these 3 teeth *H. erectus* has the greatest average length. The average decreases in the subsequent hominid species. Average breadth, on the other hand, increases to a maximum in *H. neanderthalensis,* and reduces to a minimum in *H. sapiens.*

The maximum area for the lower lateral incisor is reached in *H. neanderthalensis* (Table XII). The minimum area is found in *H. sapiens.* The difference between these 2 species is about 1 1/2 times as great as the maximum difference between living groups, and thus is clearly of significance. Among the Neandertals, the Krapina specimens have the largest teeth of any hominid group. The teeth in other Neandertal groups decrease as a function of time, although in the most recent group, the Mt. Carmel specimens, the average is still slightly greater than in the living group with the largest average area.

Differences in area between the 2 australopithecine groups, or between either of these and *H. erectus,* are less than the greatest difference among living groups. Both *H. africanus* and *H. erectus,* however, have average areas greater than that of any extant group.

There is a general pattern of increase in the L/B index with the exception of *H neanderthalensis.* The lower Neandertal value serves to underline the great absolute as well as relative breadth of these teeth. The distribution of the module follows that of area.

UPPER LATERAL INCISOR

With respect to the 5 hominid taxa, both length and breadth of the upper lateral incisor follow the same pattern of change (Table XVI). The means are minimum for all taxa in *H. africanus.* They increase steadily through *H. erectus,* and then decrease steadily to *H. sapiens.* Within the extant human groups, however, groups with the greater mean lengths do not necessarily have greater mean breadths, and vice versa.

The incisor length variation is not clearly significant. The greatest difference between taxa averages is somewhat less than the greatest difference between averages in living groups. The difference between the australopithecine means, for instance, is only slightly greater than the difference between means for Indians from Pecos Pueblo and from Dickson Mound. Again, the mean value for a sample from Sub-Saharan Africa differs from the mean of a Bushman sample by more than twice the difference which exists between the australopithecines. Indeed, the average for the Sub-Saharan group approaches that of *H. erectus,* the maximum for hominid taxa.

Variation in incisor breadth, on the other hand, exhibits significant directions of change. Both *H. erectus* and *H. neanderthalensis* have mean values far outside the range of variation in extant groups. There is more variation among the hominid taxa than there is among the extant groups. The largest difference between temporally adjacent taxa occurs for *H. neanderthalensis* and *H. sapiens,* and the maximum difference among taxa is yet greater.

As with the other anterior teeth, the greatest mean length and breadth for a subspecific group is found in the Krapina Neandertals.

The coefficient of variation for upper lateral incisor length is 6.2 in the Liberian chimpanzee (Table LXXXI), and 5.8 in a sample of 50 Howler monkeys (Zingeser 1967:976). These values are exceeded by the values for all but 1 of 17 extant groups. The breadth coefficient of variation for the Howler monkeys is 5.1. This is exceeded by the value for all 10 extant groups with appropriate data.

The continuity between the hominid taxa is illustrated by the fact that no taxon lies completely outside the range of variation of any other taxon for both length and breadth (Tables XVIII and XIX).

Area of the upper lateral incisor varies as does both length and breadth (Table XVII). With the exception of *H. erectus* and *H. neanderthalensis,* the difference in mean area between temporally adjacent taxa exceeds the maximum difference between living groups—thus underlining the significance of the change. The pattern for the upper lateral incisor is different from that of the other 3 incisors in that the maximum area value for a taxon in the former is found in *H. erectus,* while in the latter it is found in *H. neanderthalensis.* This is also true for average incisor breadth. In that the breadth and area variation of the anterior teeth seems to be more significant than the length variation, the former represents a clear and consistent pattern of evolutionary change. While maximization in the upper lateral incisor may appear to be a minor exception, the difference between *H. erectus* and *H. neanderthalensis* is not significant. This is quite apparent in the frequency distribution for area (Table XX).

LOWER CANINE

Length and breadth variation in the lower canine are shown in Table XXI. *H. africanus* has the largest canines in any hominid taxon, although there is size overlap with every hominid taxon. Not all the early hominids do have canines as large. *H. robustus* canines are smaller than those of *H. erectus* and *H. neanderthalensis* in average length and breadth, as well as area (Table XXII). The canines of all the australopithecines taken together as a single taxon are longer than, although not quite as broad as, those of *H. erectus.* The average area for this taxon also exceeds that for *H. erectus.* In terms of the coefficient of variation, variability of this taxon exceeds that of all other hominid taxa, while coefficients of *H. africanus* and *H. robustus* taken separately are exceeded by all other hominid taxa.

The difference between the mean length for *H. africanus* and *H. robustus* is 1.39 mm,

TABLE XVI. Upper Second Incisor Length and Breadth: Mean, Standard Error of the Mean (SE(M)), Range, Sample Size (N), and Coefficient of Variation (CV).

UPPER 12	LENGTH(M-D)					BREADTH(B-L)				
	MEAN	SE(M)	RANGE	N	CV	MEAN	SE(M)	RANGE	N	CV
H. AFRICANUS	6.72	.38	5.80 - 7.30	4	9.7	6.42	.40	5.60 - 7.00	4	10.8
H. ROBUSTUS	7.31	.28	5.90 - 9.20	9	11.4	7.09	.16	6.30 - 7.60	9	6.8
H. ERECTUS	8.18	.39	6.80 - 10.00	6	11.6	8.64	.50	8.00 - 10.40	5	11.6
H. NEANDERTAL	7.86	.15	6.00 - 9.00	36	11.1	8.42	.19	6.00 - 11.20	31	12.6
H. SAPIENS	7.47	.05	4.90 - 10.30	237	10.7	6.69	.05	4.40 - 9.40	235	11.6
AUSTRALOPITHECINES	7.14	.26	5.80 - 9.20	13	13.5	6.88	.32	5.60 - 7.60	13	16.0
KRAPINA	8.44	.07	8.20 - 9.00	12	2.9	8.90	.39	6.00 - 11.20	11	14.0
NEANDERTAL	7.72	.21	6.00 - 9.00	19	11.4	8.47	.19	7.50 - 9.95	15	8.3
MT CARMEL	7.04	.52	6.20 - 8.80	5	14.7	7.26	.34	6.20 - 8.00	5	9.4
SUB SAHARAN	8.04	.21	6.70 - 10.30	20	11.6	7.26	.20	6.00 - 9.40	20	11.9
AUSTR. ABORIGINE	7.65		6.50 - 9.60	78		6.91		6.00 - 8.50	126	
WADI HALFA MESOL.	7.60		6.90 - 8.10	5		6.80		6.50 - 7.40	5	
DICKSON MOUND INDIAN	7.52	.05	6.00 - 9.00	108	7.1	6.69	.05	5.60 - 7.92	107	7.0
INDIAN	7.46	.32	4.90 - 8.40	10	12.8	6.50	.25	4.40 - 7.20	11	11.9
NEW BRITAIN	7.31	.09	6.10 - 8.20	34	7.3	6.76	.07	5.90 - 7.50	33	5.5
AUSTRALOID	7.29	.46	6.00 - 8.90	9	17.8	7.47	.34	6.00 - 8.80	10	13.7
ALEUTS	7.20	.04	6.10 - 8.10	147	7.4					
PECOS PUEBLO	7.06	.04	6.17 - 8.00	84	5.5	6.46	.04	5.58 - 7.69	84	5.9
JAPANESE	7.00			167						
JAVANESE	6.93	.05		169	9.7	6.61	.04		169	7.6
GILIMANUK (INDON.)	6.80		5.00 - 8.10	31		6.80		5.40 - 7.60	39	
LAPPS	6.73	.03	5.30 - 8.30	271	8.0	6.13	.02	5.00 - 7.40	332	5.9
SWEDES	6.72	.02		945	9.1					
TRISTANITES	6.71	.04		277	10.0					
BUSHMEN	6.70		6.00 - 8.50	24		6.00		5.30 - 6.80	26	
JARMO	6.70			4		6.00			4	
NATUFIANS	6.67	.16		8	6.3	6.82	.18		8	7.0
CAUCASOID	6.66	.18	5.00 - 8.85	30	14.8	7.01	.16	6.00 - 8.70	28	12.1
OHIO WHITES	6.58	.03		451	9.6					
AMERICAN WHITES (1)	6.55	.05	4.50 - 8.50	170	9.6					
COCHINI JEWS	6.47	.06		60	7.1					
YEMEN JEWS	6.29	.09		56	10.3					
MODERN ENGLISH	6.28			14		6.29			13	

TABLE XVII. Upper Second Incisor Area (L*B), Index (100L/B), and Module ((L+B)/2): Mean Range, and Coefficient of Variation (CV).

UPPER 12	L*B			100L/B			(L+B)/2		
	MEAN	RANGE	CV	MEAN	RANGE	CV	MEAN	RANGE	CV
H. AFRICANUS	43.5	32.5 - 51.1	19.4	104.8	100.0 - 111.5	4.6	6.6	5.7 - 7.1	10.0
H. ROBUSTUS	53.2	38.4 - 69.9	15.5	101.5	90.8 - 121.1	11.7	7.3	6.2 - 8.4	7.7
H. ERECTUS	72.2	54.4 - 104.0	23.2	93.5	85.0 - 101.2	8.4	8.5	7.4 - 10.2	11.0
H. NEANDERTAL	66.8	44.6 - 100.8	20.5	94.5	77.8 - 141.9	14.1	8.1	6.7 - 10.1	10.2
H. SAPIENS	50.1	21.6 - 85.5	17.8	113.1	73.2 - 188.9	15.3	7.1	4.6 - 9.2	8.8
AUSTRALOPITHECINES	50.2	32.5 - 69.9	21.2	102.5	87.4 - 123.3	10.0	7.1	5.7 - 8.4	11.3
KRAPINA	75.0	49.2 - 100.8	15.9	96.4	80.4 - 136.7	15.5	8.6	7.1 - 10.1	8.1
NEANDERTAL	66.2	51.0 - 89.5	18.4	91.7	77.8 - 100.0	5.8	8.1	7.2 - 9.5	9.0
MT CARMEL	50.7	44.6 - 54.6	8.1	98.7	83.1 - 141.9	25.1	7.1	6.7 - 7.5	4.5
SUB SAHARAN	58.9	40.2 - 85.5	20.9	111.3	96.8 - 149.3	10.0	7.6	6.3 - 9.2	10.6
AUSTRALOID	55.0	36.0 - 71.3	28.7	98.3	85.2 - 117.1	11.7	7.4	6.0 - 8.4	14.9
DICKSON MOUND INDIAN	50.4	34.5 - 63.8	12.1	112.6	98.6 - 137.8	7.0	7.1	5.9 - 8.0	6.1
NEW BRITAIN	49.5	40.9 - 56.9	9.5	108.6	89.7 - 124.2	9.2	7.0	6.4 - 7.5	4.8
INDIAN	49.2	21.6 - 56.5	21.0	114.6	107.0 - 126.3	6.1	7.0	4.6 - 7.5	12.3
CAUCASOID	47.4	30.0 - 77.0	25.6	95.5	73.2 - 119.1	11.4	6.8	5.5 - 8.8	12.4

TABLE XVIII. Upper Second Incisor Length: Frequency Distribution in Percentiles.

FREQUENCY CISTRIBUTICN OF UPPER I2 L(M-D)

	4.8	5.2	5.6	6.C	6.4	6.8	7.2	7.6	8.0	8.4	8.8	9.2	9.6	10.0	10.4
H.AFRICAN.			25			50	25								
H.ROBUSTUS			9		27	27		9	9		18				
H.ERECTUS				19					59					19	
H.NEANDER.				8	2	13	13		25	22	13				
H.SAPIENS	1	1		6	5	16	22	19	17	4	2	1	1	1	
AUSTRALOP			13		19	33	6	6	6		13				
KRAPINA									50	41	8				
NEANDERTAL				12	4	20	20		12	12	16				
MT CARMEL				19	19	39					19				
CAUCASOID	3	13		29	9	13	13	6	3	3	3				
INDIAN	9						29	39	9	9					
AUSTRALOID				44			11	11		11	22				
NEW BRITAI				5	2	32	29	14	14						
DICKSON MD				1	8	14	28	26	15	2	1				

TABLE XIX. Upper Second Incisor Breadth: Frequency Distribution in Percentiles.

FREQUENCY CISTRIBUTICN OF UPPER I2 B(B-L)

	4.3	4.8	5.3	5.8	6.3	6.8	7.3	7.8	8.3	8.8	9.3	9.8	10.3	10.8	11.3
H.AFRICAN.			25	25		50									
H.ROBUSTUS					33	22	33						11		
H.ERECTUS								59	19				19		
H.NEANDER.				6		6	9	25	3	35	6	3		3	
H.SAPIENS	1	3	2	17	29	28	7	6	1	1	1				
AUSTRALOP			7	7	23	30	23						7		
KRAPINA				9				9	9	45	18			9	
NEANDERTAL				4		9	14	34		29		4			
MT CARMEL				19		39	19	19							
CAUCASOID				25	25	21	3	17	7						
INDIAN	9			9	36	45									
AUSTRALOID				19	9	9	9	29		19					
NEW BRITAI				9	42	39	9								
DICKSON MD			1	19	35	32	9	1							

TABLE XX. Upper Second Incisor Area (L*B): Frequency Distribution in Percentiles.

FREQUENCY DISTRIBUTION OF UPPER I2 L*B

	21	27	33	39	45	51	57	63	69	75	81	87	93	99	105
H.AFRICAN.		25		25	25	25									
H.ROBUSTUS			11	33		22	11	11				11			
H.ERECTUS					19			59						19	
H.NEANDER.				3	9	22	9	3	19	22	3	3		3	
H.SAPIENS	1	1	5	20	28	28	6	5	2	1	1				
AUSTRALOP.		7	7	30	7	23	7	7				7			
KRAPINA					9			9	36	36				9	
NEANDERTAL						33	19		13	19	6	6			
MT CARMEL				19	39	39									
CAUCASOID		10	14	28	14	14	3	7	3	3					
INDIAN	9				39	50									
AUSTRALOID			22	22				33	22						
NEW BRITAI				15	43	40									
DICKSON MD			2	14	36	32	9	3							
SUB SAHARA				14	9	19	14	19	9	4	4				
MALAY															
HARAPPA															

exceeding by .08 mm or 5.8% the maximum difference between extant groups. Given the probable time span represented by the australopithecines, the difference between the 2 taxa is surely comparable to that within *H. sapiens.* The difference between the mean value for *H. africanus* and *H. erectus* is .88 mm while for *H. robustus* and *H. erectus* this value is .51 mm. Additional data deprives these differences of statistical significance (Wolpoff 1970b).

While there is an evident trend for canine reduction from the australopithecines to *H. sapiens,* the actual pattern of change reflects changes in selective pressures acting upon the canines which were not always consistent with the general trend. The same pattern of variation exists in the other 2 lower anterior teeth (Tables I, II, XI, XII), although the relative differences are minimal compared with those among average canine sizes (Table XXI and XXII).

Unlike the lower incisors, lower canine length in *H. robustus* is greater than in *H. sapiens.* Breadth for all the lower anterior teeth is greater in *H. robustus* than it is in *H. sapiens.* Area variation follows the latter pattern.

Relative difference between average breadths (Table XXI) and areas (Table XXII) for the hominid taxa is not as great. Yet, changes in breadth and area are generally more significant for the other anterior teeth. Thus, the maximum difference in average breadth among extant groups exceeds the difference between the australopithecine taxa. In breadth, the mean value for *H. erectus* lies closer to that for *H. africanus* than *H. robustus.*

Next to *H. africanus, H. erectus* has the largest lower canines. The values for *H. neanderthalensis* are only slightly smaller than *H. erectus.* The latter difference is less than that between *H. neanderthalensis* and *H. sapiens.* The size difference between *H. erectus* and *H. sapiens* exceeds that between *H. erectus* and either of the australopithecine taxa.

In terms of length (Table XXIII), breadth (Table XXIV), and area (Table XXV) the ranges of variation for both *H. africanus* and *H.*

TABLE XXI. Lower Canine Length and Breadth: Mean, Standard Error of the Mean (SE(M)), Range, Sample Size (N), and Coefficient of Variation (CV).

LOWER C	LENGTH(M-D)					BREADTH(B-L)				
	MEAN	SE(M)	RANGE	N	CV	MEAN	SE(M)	RANGE	N	CV
H. AFRICANUS	9.07	.17	8.30 - 10.50	12	6.4	10.05	.29	9.00 - 12.10	12	9.5
H. ROBUSTUS	7.68	.16	6.90 - 8.50	11	6.5	8.04	.19	7.20 - 9.20	11	7.6
H. ERECTUS	8.19	.18	7.00 - 10.00	18	9.2	9.24	.20	7.80 - 11.00	21	9.7
H. NEANDERTAL	7.83	.10	5.00 - 9.10	50	8.5	8.99	.12	7.00 - 10.50	46	9.0
H. SAPIENS	7.39	.04	5.00 - 10.00	311	8.8	7.85	.05	5.00 - 10.00	318	10.9
AUSTRALOPITHECINES	8.41	.19	6.90 - 10.50	23	10.5	9.09	.28	7.20 - 12.10	23	14.3
KRAPINA	8.11	.07	7.60 - 8.50	13	3.0	9.04	.24	7.90 - 10.30	13	9.1
NEANDERTAL	7.75	.13	5.00 - 8.60	30	9.2	9.14	.15	7.50 - 10.50	27	8.2
MT CARMEL	7.70	.37	6.40 - 9.10	7	11.8	8.25	.32	7.00 - 9.00	6	8.8
AUSTRALOID	7.77	.25	6.80 - 8.40	6	7.1	9.12	.34	8.00 - 9.90	6	8.3
AUSTR. ABORIGINE	7.60	.00	7.00 - 9.00	88	.0	8.30	.00	7.00 - 10.00	120	.0
WADI HALFA MESOL.	7.40	.00	6.90 - 8.50	4	.0	8.10	.00	7.70 - 8.30	4	.0
SUB SAHARAN	7.39	.10	6.45 - 8.50	35	8.3	7.95	.15	6.00 - 9.00	34	10.6
DICKSON MOUND	7.38	.04	6.15 - 8.50	123	6.1	7.93	.05	6.60 - 9.55	124	7.7
INDIAN	7.34	.12	6.30 - 8.30	18	6.5	8.09	.24	6.75 - 10.00	17	11.8
NEW BRITAIN	7.32	.05	6.40 - 8.10	44	4.9	8.06	.10	7.20 - 9.60	47	8.4
PECOS PUEBLO	7.27	.05	6.30 - 8.30	94	6.1	7.71	.05	6.72 - 8.94	94	6.6
GILIMANUK (INDON.)	7.20	.00	6.10 - 8.40	39	.0	7.40	.00	6.20 - 8.90	43	.0
E.GREENLAND ESKIMO	7.13	.00	6.90 - 7.40	7	.0	7.70	.11	7.00 - 8.40	14	5.3
MALAY	7.12	.12	6.50 - 7.80	12	5.7	7.42	.17	6.50 - 9.20	16	8.8
JAVANESE	7.11	.04		181	7.3	7.74	.04		181	6.3
JARMO	7.10	.00		4	.0	7.70	.00		4	.0
SWEDES	7.06	.01		996	4.5					
NATUFIANS	7.03	.12		13	5.7	7.91	.12		13	5.4
TRISTANITES	7.02	.03		256	6.8	8.74	.07		97	7.9
ALEUTS	6.98	.03	5.90 - 8.30	165	6.0	7.78	.05	6.60 - 9.60	131	7.1
JAPANESE	6.90	.02		194	4.1	7.60	.03		194	5.5
CAUCASOID	6.87	.12	5.00 - 8.50	42	11.3	8.12	.10	7.00 - 9.90	43	8.3
BUSHMEN	6.80	.00	6.00 - 8.30	29	.0	7.00	.00	6.00 - 8.00	28	.0
OHIO WHITES	6.74	.02		461	6.1					
AMERICAN WHITES(1)	6.71	.03	5.80 - 8.10	171	5.1					
LAPPS	6.65	.02	5.00 - 8.00	499	6.3	7.23	.02	5.90 - 8.60	488	7.6
COCHINI JEWS	6.58	.06		59	6.8					
YEMEN JEWS	6.46	.05		54	5.1					

TABLE XXII. Lower Canine Area (L*B), Index (100L/B), and Module ((L+B)/2): Mean, Range, and Coefficient of Variation (CV).

LOWER C	L*B			100L/B			(L+B)/2		
	MEAN	RANGE	CV	MEAN	RANGE	CV	MEAN	RANGE	CV
H. AFRICANUS	92.6	75.6 - 127.0	15.8	89.9	83.6 - 101.1	5.6	9.6	8.7 - 11.3	7.8
H. ROBUSTUS	61.9	49.7 - 75.6	12.6	95.8	84.8 - 103.7	6.0	7.9	7.0 - 8.7	6.4
H. ERECTUS	76.5	59.7 - 110.0	17.6	88.5	70.0 - 98.8	10.4	8.7	7.7 - 10.5	8.6
H. NEANDERTAL	70.7	37.5 - 87.7	13.2	87.9	66.7 - 130.0	11.8	8.4	6.2 - 9.4	6.9
H. SAPIENS	57.9	36.5 - 80.5	14.5	95.6	68.5 - 160.0	15.5	7.6	6.1 - 9.0	7.2
AUSTRALOPITHECINES	77.2	49.7 - 127.0	25.2	92.9	83.6 - 103.7	6.5	8.7	7.0 - 11.3	12.5
KRAPINA	73.4	63.1 - 87.5	10.9	90.3	80.0 - 103.8	8.3	8.6	7.9 - 9.4	5.6
NEANDERTAL	71.2	37.5 - 87.7	13.4	85.4	66.7 - 100.0	10.3	8.4	6.2 - 9.4	7.1
MT CARMEL	63.1	52.5 - 73.9	13.4	93.9	78.0 - 130.0	19.8	8.0	7.3 - 8.6	6.5
AUSTRALOID	70.7	64.0 - 79.8	8.2	86.0	69.4 - 100.0	13.2	8.4	8.0 - 8.9	4.0
INDIAN	59.7	42.5 - 80.5	16.5	91.7	70.0 - 107.1	9.5	7.7	6.5 - 9.0	8.3
SUB SAHARAN	59.0	40.8 - 76.5	16.9	93.4	77.8 - 113.3	8.5	7.7	6.4 - 8.7	8.6
NEW BRITAIN	59.0	50.3 - 73.5	10.3	91.5	69.8 - 108.0	9.0	7.7	7.1 - 8.6	5.2
DICKSON MOUND	58.6	42.4 - 79.9	12.4	93.5	76.4 - 106.0	6.0	7.6	6.5 - 8.9	6.3
CAUCASOID	55.6	36.5 - 77.2	16.8	85.2	68.5 - 102.4	10.0	7.5	6.1 - 8.8	8.3
MALAY	52.0	44.2 - 71.8	14.0	98.3	84.8 - 105.7	6.7	7.2	6.6 - 8.5	6.8

TABLE XXIII. Lower Canine Length: Frequency Distribution in Percentiles.

FREQUENCY DISTRIBUTION OF LOWER C L(M-D)

	4.8	5.2	5.6	6.0	6.4	6.8	7.2	7.6	8.0	8.4	8.8	9.2	9.6	10.0	10.4
H.AFRICAN.									8	16	41	25		8	
H.ROBUSTUS						18	27	27	18	9					
H.ERECTUS						11	5	16	22	22	16			5	
H.NEANDER.	1				1	11	11	9	45	13	1				
H.SAPIENS	1	1	1	3	8	21	33	15	11	3	1	1	1	1	
AUSTRALOP.						8	13	13	13	13	21	13		4	
KRAPINA								15	69	15					
NEANDERTAL	2				2	16	16	8	37	13	2				
MT CARMEL					14	14	14	14	28		14				
CAUCASOID	4	2	2	14	14	30	14	4	9	2					
INDIAN				5		22	38	22	11						
AUSTRALOID						16	16	16	33	16					
NEW BRITAI					4	27	45	18	4						
DICKSON MD				2	6	16	46	19	7	1					
MALAY					16	41	25	16							
SUB SAHARA					14	28	19	11	17	8					

TABLE XXIV. Lower Canine Breadth: Frequency Distribution in Percentiles.

FREQUENCY DISTRIBUTION OF LOWER C B(B-L)

	4.8	5.3	5.8	6.3	6.8	7.3	7.8	8.3	8.8	9.3	9.8	10.3	10.8	11.3	11.8
H.AFRICAN.									33	8	16	25	8	8	
H.ROBUSTUS					9	18	45	9	18						
H.ERECTUS							19	9	23	19	9	4	9		
H.NEANDER.					2	2	15	19	19	17	19	4			
H.SAPIENS	1	1	3	4	11	26	19	19	8	3	1				
AUSTRALOP					4	8	21	4	26	4	8	13	4	4	
KRAPINA							15	38		15	23	7			
NEANDERTAL					3	3	15	12	27	18	18	3			
MT CARMEL					16		33	16	33						
CAUCASOID					11	18	27	25	11	2	2				
INDIAN				5	17	29		23	5	11	5				
AUSTRALOID							16	16	16	16	33				
NEW BRITAI					4	34	27	17	6	10					
DICKSON MD				1	13	29	22	24	6	2					
MALAY				12	25	43	12		6						
SUB SAHARA			2	8	8	20	14	20	23						

TABLE XXV. Lower Canine Area (L*B): Frequency Distribution in Percentiles.

FREQUENCY DISTRIBUTION OF LOWER C L*B

	35	42	49	56	63	70	77	84	91	98	105	112	119	126	133
H.AFRICAN.						9	27	9	27	18				9	
H.ROBUSTUS			18	36	27	18									
H.ERECTUS				6	37	18	12	12	6		6				
H.NEANDER.	2		2	10	26	36	17	4							
H.SAPIENS	1	13	27	27	21	6	1								
AUSTRALOP.			9	18	13	13	13	4	13	9				4	
KRAPINA					53	7	30	7							
NEANDERTAL	3			11	14	51	14	3							
MT CARMEL			16	33	16	33									
CAUCASOID	7	17	24	24	19	4	2								
INDIAN		11	29	29	11	5	11								
AUSTRALOID					50	33	16								
NEW BRITAI			41	37	13	6									
DICKSON MD		12	23	33	24	4	1								
SUB SAHARA	2	14	20	17	29	14									
MALAY		50	50												
HARAPPA															

robustus can be almost completely included within the range of *H. erectus.*.

The L/B ratio has not changed consistently or significantly for the hominid taxa (Table XXII). There is more variation between extant groups.

Variation in the dimensions of the lower canine is of some interest. It is not possible to sex fossil hominids with any degree of certainty. For this reason, all of the samples considered in this study are of pooled sex. Yet, some light may be shed upon the evolution of sexual dimorphism in canine size.

Sexual dimorphism in the canines of the Great apes is well established. A decrease in sexual dimorphism should lead to a decrease in both the range and the variability of the canine dimensions, and a progressive clouding of the pongid bimodal distribution.

Calculated from the data given by Lampel (1963:23), the length coefficients of variation for *Cercopithecus nictitans buttikoferi, C. mona cambelli,* and *C. diana* are respectively 8.4, 4.9, and 5.8. The value for *Alouatta caraya* is 7.4 (Zingeser 1967:976), and also 7.4 for the Liberian chimpanzee (Table LXXXI). The values for the non-human primates considered here thus range between 4.9 and 8.4.

Of the fossil hominid species, the coefficients of variation for the australopithecines taken as separate taxa fall within the range for non-human primates. The value for the australopithecines taken as a single taxon, as well as those for the other fossil and extant hominid taxa exceeds this range. On the other hand, the values for only 3 of 19 extant groups fall outside of the non-human primate range and of these, only 1 exceeds the range. Clearly, then, canine length in hominid species is more variable than in non-human primate species. This is particularly interesting in light of the greater sexual dimorphism for canine length in the non-human primates.

The frequency distribution for lower canine length (Table XXIII) is unimodal for the australopithecines taken as separate taxa, as it is for them lumped as a single taxon. The distribution for *H. erectus* is slightly bimodal. If the smaller size mode is taken to represent females, only 3 of 22 *H. erectus* specimens are female (Maur, Ternifine 2, and Casablanca), an unlikely eventuality. The distribution for *H. neanderthalensis* is also bimodal, with 18 of 50 possible specimens in the smaller size mode. On this basis alone, the bimodality of the distribution is much more likely to be an indication of sexual dimorphism in canine length than it is in any other hominid species. The distribution for *H. sapiens* is unimodal. Within 7 extant groups, all of the distributions are unimodal.

The breadth coefficient of variation for the Liberian chimpanzee is 9.9 (Table LXXXI), and 5.9 for the Howler (*Alouatta caraya*), calculated from data given by Zingeser (1967:976). In comparison, only *H. sapiens* and the australopithecines taken as a single taxon exceed this range of variation. Five of the 15 extant groups fall outside of the range of variation for the non-human primates, although only 2 of these exceed this range. Variation in canine breadth is, therefore, more comparable between the human and non-human primate species.

The frequency distributions for canine breadth are only bimodal in the earlier hominid species. The distributions for *H. africanus* and *H. robustus* are both bimodal (Table XXIV), while that for the australopithecines taken as a single taxon is *tri*modal! The distribution for *H. erectus* is *also* trimodal, although not strongly so, as the mode for greatest breadth can probably be ignored. The mode for smallest breadth is made up of 4 out of 21 possible specimens and has absolutely no overlap with those specimens in the small mode for canine length.

The frequency distributions for lower canine area (Table XXV) are only bimodal for *H. africanus* (and for the australopithecines taken together as a single taxon). With respect to the establishment of sexual dimorphism, the area distributions show the greatest internal consistency, the greatest consistency with the length and breadth distributions, and follow most closely our other conceptions of the evolution of sexual dimorphism. In the distribution for *H. africanus,* the modes are of approximately equal size. Individuals in the small area mode are almost entirely the same as those in the small length and breadth modes. Using area as the most important distinguishing attribute, the only hominid species with pronounced sexual dimorphism in the form of a bimodal distribution is the earliest species—*H. africanus.* This species is not significantly more or less variable than any other hominid species with respect to lower canine area. Indeed, variability of this characteristic is about the same in all hominid species (Table XXII).

UPPER CANINE

The distributions for length and breadth of the maxillary canine (Table XXVI) are somewhat different. In length, *H. africanus* has the maximum value for a hominid taxon, whereas in breadth *H. erectus* is maximum. For length, the *H. robustus* value is less than both *H. africanus* and *H. erectus* (the second largest). The decrease after *H. erectus* continues through the subsequent 2 taxa. The pattern therefore is one of decrease, increase, and final decrease. None of the changes are as great as the differences which can be found among extant groups. For breadth, on the other hand, the changes are more consistent, although if anything less significant. Here, there is a breadth increase from the australopithecines (with almost identical values) to *H. erectus,* and then a decrease to *H. sapiens.* Again, the differences are well surpassed by differences among living groups, and indeed, Australian aborigines have broader canines than any fossil taxon except *H. erectus.* The value for the latter is great enough to exceed the Krapina average.

The area of the tooth (Table XXVII) follows the distribution of length in terms of changes, but of breadth in terms of magnitude. Thus the pattern is to decrease, increase, and decrease, while the maximum value is found in *H. erectus.* Module follows the same pattern. The magnitude of these changes is within the range of variation of the magnitude of changes among extant groups. Thus the only discernable pattern which borders on significance is the final reduction of canine size in *H. sapiens.*

There is no significant pattern of change for the L/B ratio among the taxa (Table XXVII).

While variability in maxillary canine length and area does not differ significantly, the variability in breadth shows a steady increase through time.

For reasons discussed with respect to the mandibular canine, a decrease in sexual

TABLE XXVI. Upper Canine Length and Breadth: Mean, Standard Error of the Mean (SE(M)), Range, Sample Size (N), and Coefficient of Variation (CV).

UPPER C	LENGTH(M-D)					BREADTH(B-L)				
	MEAN	SE(M)	RANGE	N	CV	MEAN	SE(M)	RANGE	N	CV
H. AFRICANUS	9.59	.17	8.80 - 10.20	8	4.7	9.52	.20	8.70 - 9.90	6	4.7
H. ROBLSTUS	8.66	.15	8.10 - 10.60	17	7.0	9.57	.19	8.40 - 11.10	17	8.0
H. ERECTUS	9.38	.16	8.50 - 10.50	11	5.6	10.31	.27	8.90 - 11.90	11	8.4
H. NEANDERTAL	8.43	.14	6.50 - 10.50	42	10.3	9.71	.14	8.00 - 11.30	39	8.6
H. SAPIENS	8.38	.04	6.00 - 11.00	283	8.1	8.57	.05	6.10 - 11.50	285	10.7
AUSTRALOPITHECINES	8.96	.14	8.10 - 10.60	25	7.9	9.56	.15	8.40 - 11.10	23	7.2
KRAPINA	9.12	.21	8.00 - 10.50	11	7.2	10.15	.22	9.30 - 11.30	10	6.4
NEANCERTAL	8.11	.17	6.50 - 10.00	25	10.4	9.67	.18	8.00 - 11.20	23	8.7
MT CARMEL	8.50	.28	7.50 - 9.20	6	7.4	9.10	.33	8.00 - 10.00	6	8.2
AUSTRALOID	8.95	.23	7.80 - 10.40	16	9.8	10.07	.34	7.40 - 11.50	15	12.5
AUSTR. ABORIGINE	8.43	.00	6.50 - 9.60	116	.0	9.00	.00	7.50 - 11.00	159	.0
NEW BRITAIN	8.39	.07	7.40 - 9.20	43	5.6	8.67	.11	7.60 - 10.50	44	8.0
DICKSCN MOUND	8.37	.04	7.10 - 9.40	113	5.6	8.57	.05	7.45 - 10.15	113	6.7
INCIAN	8.36	.09	7.80 - 9.00	18	4.4	8.70	.16	7.80 - 9.85	19	8.0
JARMC	8.30	.00		5	.0	8.40	.00		5	.0
SUB SAHARAN	8.28	.20	6.00 - 9.30	18	10.2	8.96	.20	6.80 - 9.80	18	9.3
MALAY	8.13	.47	7.70 - 8.90	3	8.2	8.73	.53	8.30 - 9.60	3	8.6
PECOS PUEBLO	8.05	.05	7.00 - 9.17	86	5.7	8.36	.06	7.09 - 9.68	86	6.3
JAVANESE	7.93	.04		178	6.9	8.33	.04		179	6.7
SWECES	7.92	.01		936	3.9					
GILIMANUK (INDON.)	7.90	.00	6.20 - 9.40	38	.0	8.00	.00	6.10 - 9.20	42	.0
ALEUTS	7.88	.04	6.80 - 9.00	138	5.6	8.34	.05	7.10 - 9.90	109	5.6
E.GREENLAND ESKIMO	7.87	.04	7.00 - 8.40	16	2.0	8.38	.04	7.50 - 9.10	21	2.1
CAUCASOID	7.86	.10	6.90 - 9.35	42	8.5	8.64	.11	7.40 - 10.50	43	8.5
TRISTANITES	7.84	.03		244	6.0	9.19	.06		129	7.4
NATUFIANS	7.72	.14		10	5.3	8.61	.18		9	5.9
JAPANESE	7.70	.02		194	3.6	8.20	.03		194	5.1
OHIO WHITES	7.70	.02		422	5.7					
MODERN ENGLISH	7.61	.08		25	5.4	8.32	.10		24	6.0
WADI HALFA MESOL.	7.60	.00	7.20 - 8.00	4	.0	8.50	.00	7.90 - 8.90	4	.0
LAPPS	7.59	.02	6.50 - 9.20	448	5.5	7.92	.03	6.50 - 9.80	440	7.2
BUSHMEN	7.50	.00	7.00 - 7.30	26	.0	7.80	.00	7.00 - 8.80	26	.0
COCHINI JEWS	7.45	.05		59	4.7					
YEMEN JEWS	7.39	.10		40	8.4					
AMERICAN WHITES(1)	6.85	.03	6.60 - 9.00	172	5.8					

TABLE XXVII. Upper Canine Area (L*B), Index (100L/B), and Module ((L+B)/2): Mean, Range, and Coefficient of Variation (CV).

UPPER C	L*B			100L/B			(L+B)/2		
	MEAN	RANGE	CV	MEAN	RANGE	CV	MEAN	RANGE	CV
H. AFRICANLS	90.5	81.8 - 98.0	8.2	99.9	93.6 - 108.0	4.9	9.5	9.0 - 9.9	4.1
H. ROBUSTLS	83.2	68.0 - 110.2	14.1	90.8	83.0 - 101.9	5.7	9.1	8.2 - 10.5	7.0
H. ERECTLS	96.8	83.3 - 113.0	11.3	91.5	79.8 - 105.6	8.4	9.8	9.1 - 10.7	5.8
H. NEANCERTAL	82.9	56.0 - 118.6	15.2	88.1	60.7 - 108.7	10.2	9.1	7.5 - 10.9	7.5
H. SAPIENS	71.9	40.8 - 119.6	14.8	98.8	73.4 - 156.2	13.7	8.5	6.4 - 10.9	7.2
AUSTRALOPITHECINES	85.1	68.0 - 110.2	13.0	93.1	83.0 - 108.0	7.0	9.2	8.2 - 10.5	6.5
KRAPINA	93.9	78.1 - 118.6	11.6	91.0	84.8 - 100.0	5.3	9.7	8.8 - 10.9	5.7
NEANDERTAL	79.5	56.0 - 110.0	14.5	85.3	60.7 - 100.0	10.7	8.9	7.5 - 10.5	7.2
MT CARMEL	77.4	67.5 - 92.0	11.6	94.0	83.3 - 108.7	11.4	8.8	8.2 - 9.6	5.7
AUSTRALOIC	90.1	57.7 - 119.6	19.8	89.0	73.4 - 106.7	10.4	9.5	7.6 - 10.9	10.2
SUB SAHARAN	74.7	40.8 - 90.2	17.5	92.5	78.9 - 102.4	6.2	8.6	6.4 - 9.5	9.3
NEW BRITAIN	73.0	59.3 - 92.0	11.4	97.1	77.5 - 109.6	7.3	8.5	7.7 - 9.6	5.7
INCIAN	72.5	61.6 - 88.2	11.1	97.0	88.3 - 108.1	6.5	8.5	7.8 - 9.4	5.5
CICKSON MOUND	71.9	52.9 - 93.2	10.7	97.9	80.6 - 115.7	6.0	8.5	7.3 - 9.7	5.4
MALAY	71.4	63.9 - 85.4	17.1	93.2	92.7 - 94.0	.8	8.4	8.0 - 9.2	8.4
CAUCASOIC	68.5	52.5 - 97.7	15.5	90.9	77.8 - 112.3	7.2	8.3	7.2 - 9.9	7.6

TABLE XXVIII. Upper Canine Length: Frequency Distribution in Percentiles.

FREQUENCY DISTRIBUTION OF UPPER C L(M-D)

	5.8	6.2	6.6	7.0	7.4	7.8	8.2	8.6	9.0	9.4	9.8	10.2	10.6	11.0	11.4
H.AFRICAN.								12	12	25	37	12			
H.ROBUSTUS						11	41	29	11				5		
H.ERECTUS							9	9	18	54		9			
H.NEANDER.		2	2	4	14	16	9	11	30		4	2			
H.SAPIENS	1		1	5	9	21	25	18	13	2	2	1		1	
AUSTRALOP						7	27	23	11	7	11	3	3		
KRAPINA						9	9	9	54		9	9			
NEANDERTAL		3	3	6	19	19	9	12	22		3				
MT CARMEL					16	16		50	16						
CAUCASOID			2	26	9	33	9	11	7						
INDIAN						33	33	27	5						
AUSTRALOID						31	12		25	12	6	12			
NEW BRITAI					11	16	37	18	16						
DICKSON MD				1	9	22	31	26	7	1					
MALAY					33	33		33							
SUB SAHARA	5				22	11	27		33						

TABLE XXIX. Upper Canine Breadth: Frequency Distribution in Percentiles.

FREQUENCY DISTRIBUTION OF UPPER C B(B-L)

	5.9	6.4	6.9	7.4	7.9	8.4	8.9	9.4	9.9	10.4	10.9	11.4	11.9	12.4	12.9
H.AFRICAN.						16		50	33						
H.ROBUSTUS						29	11	11	35	5	5				
H.ERECTUS							9	18	27	27		9	9		
H.NEANDER.					5	10	20	10	30	12	10				
H.SAPIENS	1	2	4	8	27	21	18	10	1	3	1	1			
AUSTRALOP						26	8	21	34	4	4				
KRAPINA							19	9	19	39	9				
NEANDERTAL					6	13	20	10	34	3	10				
MT CARMEL					16	16	16	33	16						
CAUCASOID				9	27	23	27	4		6					
INDIAN				5	36	15	15	26							
AUSTRALOID				13			13		13	26	19	13			
NEW BRITAI				6	31	31	13	9	2	4					
DICKSON MD				9	31	24	25	7	1						
MALAY					66			33							
SUB SAHARA		5		5	11	22	5	50							

TABLE XXX. Upper Canine Area (L*B): Frequency Distribution in Percentiles.

FREQUENCY DISTRIBUTION OF UPPER C L*B

	39	45	51	57	63	69	75	81	87	93	99	105	111	117	123
H.AFRICAN								33	16	50					
H.ROBUSTUS					5	23	11	23	23		5	5			
H.ERECTUS								27	18	9	18	9	18		
H.NEANDER			2		10	15	15	20	20	7	2	2		2	
H.SAPIENS	1		3	15	23	22	17	9	4	2	1		1	1	
AUSTRALOP					4	17	8	26	21	13	4	4			
KRAPINA							9	19	19	29	9			9	
NEANDERTAL			4		13	21	13	21	21			4			
MT CARMEL					16	16	33	16	16						
CAUCASOID			14	16	23	23	7	7	2	4					
INDIAN				5	38	16	16	16	5						
AUSTRALOID				13		13		6	13	33	6		6	6	
NEW BRITAI				11	27	23	13	13	4						
DICKSON MD			1	12	23	25	26	7	1	1					
SUB SAHARA	5			11	11	27	11	11	22						
MALAY					66			33							
HARAPPA															

dimorphism in hominid evolution should lead to a decrease in size variability as well as to a clouding of the non-human primate bimodal distribution. As a basis for comparison, the following length and breadth coefficients of variation are shown by other primates: Liberian chimpanzee (Table LXXXI), 7.1 and 11.9; Howler monkey (Zingeser 1967:976), 6.70 and 7.47. Length coefficients of variation exist for 3 species of *Cercopithecus* (Lampel 1963:23): *C. nictitans* with 9.26; *C. mona* with 5.39; and *C. diana* with 6.49. Of the hominid taxa only *H. africanus* is less variable than the non-human primates in length and breadth. The australopithecines, taken as a single taxon, are more variable than are the non-human primates considered here. For length, only 5 of 21 relevant extant groups are less variable than the least variable non-human primate, and only 2 are more variable than the most variable primate species. For breadth, only 1 out of 16 extant groups exceeds the maximum non-human primate species in variability, while a much larger number (10) are smaller than the minimum. Thus there is great overlap in ranges of variabilities.

With respect to the frequency distributions, length (Table XXVIII) is only bimodal for *H. neanderthalensis*. The modes are of about equal size. A number of extant groups are also bimodal: Caucasoids, Australoids, and Sub-Saharan Africans.

It may be pointed out that the range of variation in this tooth for *H. africanus* can be completely encompassed within the range of variation for *H. robustus* in terms of length, breadth, and area (Tables XXVIII - XXX).

LOWER THIRD PREMOLAR

The trend of change for this tooth is one of almost complete reduction in length and breadth (Table XXXI). For length, the australopithecine values are almost identical. In breadth, the *H. robustus* average value is only .46 mm greater than that of *H. africanus* (the maximum difference between extant groups is 1.8 mm). In both length and breadth, the averages for the subsequent taxa decrease to *H. sapiens* in about equal steps. Indeed, the length differences between hominid taxa is rivaled by that between the 2 groups of American "Whites."

The Krapina Neandertals have the highest average length of any recent group. For breadth, however, the maximum for a recent or extant group belongs to the Mt. Carmel group, clearly demonstrating their Neandertal affinites.

The coefficients of variation show a slight increase in variability for breadth, but the opposite for length, in the 5 taxa. Although the teeth are not strictly comparable, length and breadth coefficients of variation for *Alouatta caraya* (mixed sex) calculated from Zingeser (1967:976) are 4.3 and 5.6. The corresponding values are 4.8 and 9.8 for *Cercopithecus nictitans,* 7.7 and 6.2 for *Cercopithecus mona,* and 5.6 and 6.9 for *Cercopithecus diana* (Lampel 1963:27). These values exceed all hominid taxa and all but a few extant groups of *H. sapiens.*

The tooth shows almost no tendency toward sexual dimorphism. The frequency distribution for length (Table XXXIII) is bimodal for *H. africanus* and *H. erectus,* but the breadth distribution (Table XXXIV) is bimodal for *H. africanus* only. The australopithecine ranges for length are identical. However for breadth (Table XXXIV), 1/4 of the *H. africanus* specimens fall outside the *H. robustus* range of variation.

The statistics for area and module (Table XXXII) show almost no difference between the australopithecines, but a big drop between these hominids and *H. erectus,* and again between *H. neanderthalensis* and *H. sapiens.* The drop between *H. erectus* and *H. neanderthalensis* is more gradual, the difference falling within the range of variation of difference among extant groups. *H. neanderthalensis* clearly has a larger mandibular third premolar than does *H. sapiens.*

The frequency distribution for area (Table XXXV) shows identical ranges for the 2 australopithecine taxa. About 40% of the *H. erectus* specimens are below the australopithecine range of variation, but all of the former are included within the *H. neanderthalensis* range.

The data for the L/B ratio is of some interest. The group averages show no significant change until *H. sapiens* (where the ratio increases). The variation of this ratio in hominid evolution only slightly exceeds that among extant groups. Thus the claim of an early (Mid-Pleistocene) trend increasing the L/B ratio as a significant factor in hominid evolution, raised by certain authors in the definition of a new taxon (Leakey, Tobias, and Napier 1964; Leakey 1966; Tobias 1966a, 1966c, 1967b), is not supported by the evidence.

UPPER THIRD PREMOLAR

In both length and breadth (Table XXXVI), dimensions for the upper third premolar are maximum for *H. robustus.* The average value for *H. africanus* is less, followed by *H. erectus, H. neanderthalensis,* and finally *H. sapiens.* This pattern of size variation among the hominid taxa is consistent for all remaining posterior teeth with respect to length, breadth, area, and module (Tables XXXVI - LXXX).

The maximum length difference among extant groups is 1.45 mm. No difference between 2 temporally adjacent taxa is this great. The largest difference—between *H. robustus* and *H. erectus*—is 1.34 mm. However, the greatest extreme among hominid taxa is 2.28 mm. Thus, while the variation of this tooth between species is not taxonomically significant, the total reduction in length between the australopithecines and *H. sapiens* is. While the Krapina Neandertals have the greatest length for a recent group, both Australian aborigines and Sub-Saharan Africans exceed the other Neandertal groups.

The breadth variation follows the same pattern, but the differences are greater. Thus, the differençe between *H. africanus* and *H. robustus* is almost identical to the maximum difference among extant groups (1.86 mm), and the difference between *H. robustus* and *H. erectus* (2.38 mm) exceeds this. Other differences between hominid taxa are significantly less. Both the Mt. Carmel and the Krapina Neandertals exceed the maximum value for extant groups. Therefore, reduction of the breadth of this tooth from the australopithecines to *H. erectus,* and subsequently to *H. sapiens* is significant.

The breadth difference between the australopithecines borders on significance. The frequency distribution for breadth (Table

TABLE XXXI. Lower Third Premolar Length and Breadth: Mean, Standard Error of the Mean (SE(M)), Range, Sample Size (N), and Coefficient of Variation (CV).

LOWER P3	LENGTH(M-D)					BREADTH(B-L)				
	MEAN	SE(M)	RANGE	N	CV	MEAN	SE(M)	RANGE	N	CV
H. AFRICANUS	9.70	.22	8.50 - 11.50	12	7.7	11.47	.41	9.30 - 14.00	12	11.9
H. ROBUSTUS	9.80	.13	8.60 - 11.30	22	6.1	11.93	.22	10.30 - 13.50	20	7.9
H. ERECTUS	8.58	.17	5.00 - 10.00	30	10.4	9.88	.14	8.40 - 11.20	28	7.3
H. NEANDERTAL	7.83	.11	5.00 - 10.00	55	10.5	9.04	.11	7.00 - 11.30	54	8.9
H. SAPIENS	7.38	.04	5.80 - 10.00	390	9.9	8.04	.04	5.60 - 10.20	390	9.9
AUSTRALOPITHECINES	9.77	.11	8.50 - 11.50	34	6.6	11.76	.20	9.30 - 14.00	32	9.6
KRAPINA	8.22	.20	7.00 - 9.20	13	8.6	8.97	.18	8.10 - 10.00	12	6.7
NEANDERTAL	7.75	.14	5.00 - 10.00	34	10.5	9.02	.15	7.00 - 11.30	34	9.4
MT CARMEL	7.52	.35	5.80 - 8.90	8	12.2	9.20	.37	7.70 - 10.50	8	10.6
JARMO	8.00	.00		3	.0	7.40	.00		3	.0
AMERICAN NEGROS	7.80	.22	6.80 - 8.40	9	7.9	8.50	.25	6.90 - 9.30	9	8.2
MALAY	7.75	.14	7.10 - 8.30	8	4.7	8.44	.15	8.00 - 9.30	10	5.2
SUB SAHARAN	7.64	.11	6.00 - 9.60	53	10.5	8.53	.12	6.00 - 10.20	52	10.2
WADI HALFA MESOL.	7.60	.00	7.30 - 7.90	5	.0	8.90	.00	8.30 - 9.50	5	.0
AUSTR. ABORIGINE	7.60	.00	7.00 - 9.00	93	.0	8.80	.00	7.00 - 10.00	120	.0
GILIMANUK (INDON.)	7.50	.00	6.30 - 8.40	49	.0	8.10	.00	7.00 - 9.00	48	.0
AMERICAN WHITES(2)	7.40	.10	6.70 - 8.20	18	5.5	8.10	.08	7.60 - 8.70	18	4.3
AUSTRALOID	7.37	.11	6.50 - 8.50	21	6.7	8.57	.11	7.80 - 9.30	22	5.9
NEW BRITAIN	7.31	.07	6.40 - 8.30	42	6.6	8.55	.10	7.10 - 9.60	44	7.7
DIXON MOUND INDIAN	7.28	.04	5.92 - 8.70	126	6.7	8.01	.04	6.70 - 8.95	126	6.2
JAVANESE	7.25	.04		175	6.9	8.08	.04		174	7.2
SWEDES	7.22	.02		306	4.8					
INDIAN	7.21	.12	6.00 - 8.45	30	9.3	7.84	.14	6.40 - 9.10	26	9.1
PECOS PUEBLO	7.15	.04	5.79 - 8.33	105	5.7	7.91	.05	6.93 - 9.04	105	6.6
OHIO WHITES	7.11	.02		454	6.0					
E.GREENLAND ESKIMO	7.10	.00	6.80 - 7.30	12	.0	7.68	.16	6.90 - 8.70	15	7.6
JAPANESE	7.10	.02		192	3.9	7.90	.02		192	3.5
TRISTANITES	7.09	.03		255	6.8	8.75	.05		125	6.4
NATUFIANS	7.06	.13		16	7.4	7.82	.11		16	5.6
CAUCASOID	7.00	.07	5.80 - 9.00	75	8.9	7.91	.07	6.50 - 9.00	75	7.4
AMERICAN WHITES(1)	6.97	.03	5.90 - 8.10	172	5.3					
ALEUTS	6.95	.03	5.90 - 8.30	158	5.9	7.73	.05	6.30 - 9.30	135	7.1
BUSHMEN	6.90	.00	6.30 - 7.50	27	.0	7.60	.00	6.30 - 9.00	26	.0
COCHINI JEWS	6.76	.07		58	8.0	7.24	.08		58	8.0
YEMEN JEWS	6.65	.08		55	8.4	7.11	.07		55	7.5
LAPPS	6.65	.02	5.60 - 8.00	511	6.5	7.25	.02	5.60 - 8.90	504	7.2

TABLE XXXII. Lower Third Premolar Area (L*B), Index (100L/B), and Module ((L+B)/2): Mean, Range, and Coefficient of Variation (CV).

LOWER P3	L*B			100L/B			(L+B)/2		
	MEAN	RANGE	CV	MEAN	RANGE	CV	MEAN	RANGE	CV
H. AFRICANUS	111.6	86.0 - 149.5	16.8	85.4	70.8 - 99.5	11.6	10.6	9.3 - 12.2	8.4
H. ROBUSTUS	116.0	88.6 - 141.0	10.6	81.8	68.1 - 92.8	7.8	10.8	9.4 - 11.9	5.5
H. ERECTUS	85.3	42.0 - 106.0	14.5	87.3	59.5 - 97.8	9.9	9.2	6.7 - 10.3	7.5
H. NEANDERTAL	71.0	35.0 - 113.0	16.7	86.9	70.0 - 113.6	10.3	8.4	6.0 - 10.6	8.3
H. SAPIENS	59.4	36.0 - 96.0	14.7	92.8	66.7 - 163.3	15.5	7.7	6.0 - 9.8	7.3
AUSTRALOPITHECINES	114.4	86.0 - 149.5	13.0	83.1	68.1 - 99.5	9.6	10.7	9.3 - 12.2	6.7
KRAPINA	74.0	64.4 - 92.0	12.8	92.0	76.1 - 113.6	10.0	8.6	8.1 - 9.6	6.2
NEANDERTAL	70.3	35.0 - 113.0	17.8	86.2	71.4 - 100.0	9.4	8.4	6.0 - 10.6	8.8
MT CARMEL	69.6	44.7 - 81.9	18.4	82.1	70.0 - 96.7	11.7	8.4	6.7 - 9.0	9.7
MALAY	65.9	56.8 - 74.4	9.7	91.4	86.0 - 97.5	4.0	8.1	7.5 - 8.6	4.9
SUB SAHARAN	65.8	36.0 - 96.0	19.3	89.8	77.8 - 107.1	7.2	8.1	6.0 - 9.8	9.8
AUSTRALOID	63.1	52.0 - 76.5	11.1	86.2	77.8 - 95.5	6.0	8.0	7.2 - 8.7	5.5
NEW BRITAIN	62.9	46.9 - 76.4	10.8	85.4	68.7 - 103.9	9.0	7.9	6.8 - 8.7	5.4
DICKSON MOUND	58.4	41.2 - 70.3	10.9	91.1	79.3 - 115.9	6.6	7.6	6.4 - 8.4	5.6
INDIAN	56.8	38.7 - 75.6	16.0	92.4	76.9 - 113.6	10.0	7.5	6.2 - 8.7	8.1
CAUCASOID	55.4	42.0 - 72.0	12.3	88.9	66.7 - 138.5	11.1	7.4	6.5 - 8.5	6.2

TABLE XXXIII. Lower Third Premolar Length: Frequency Distribution in Percentiles.

FREQUENCY DISTRIBUTION OF LOWER P3 L(M-D)

	4.8	5.3	5.8	6.3	6.8	7.3	7.8	8.3	8.8	9.3	9.8	10.3	10.8	11.3	11.8
H.AFRICAN.								8	25	16	41			8	
H.ROBUSTUS								4	13	27	36	13		4	
H.ERECTUS	3					3	26	16	36	6	6				
H.NEANDER.	1		1	1	14	23	29	16	9		1				
H.SAPIENS			4	13	28	27	15	4	2	2	1				
AUSTRALOP.								5	17	23	38	8		5	
KRAPINA					7	15	30	23	23						
NEANDERTAL	2		2	2	16	26	28	14	4		2				
MT CARMEL			12		25	25	25		12						
CAUCASOID			10	27	25	26	7		1						
INDIAN			9	19	9	43	9	6							
AUSTRALOID				4	47	23	19	4							
NEW BRITAI				9	45	21	21	2							
DICKSON MD			1	11	36	34	12	2							
MALAY					12	25	50	12							
SUB SAHARA			3	5	24	26	20	9	3	5					

TABLE XXXIV. Lower Third Premolar Breadth: Frequency Distribution in Percentiles.

FREQUENCY DISTRIBUTION OF LOWER P3 B(B-L)

	5.4	6.0	6.6	7.2	7.8	8.4	9.0	9.6	10.2	10.8	11.4	12.0	12.6	13.2	13.8
H.AFRICAN							8	16	8	8	25	8	16	8	
H.ROBUSTUS									9	19	19	25	9	14	
H.ERECTUS						10	25	25	28	10					
H.NEANDER.			1	1	11	25	37	16	1	3					
H.SAPIENS	1	3	7	20	32	21	11	1	1						
AUSTRALOP.							3	6	9	15	21	18	12	12	
KRAPINA					8	41	33	16							
NEANDERTAL			2	2	11	21	38	16	2	4					
MT CARMEL				12	12		37	25	12						
CAUCASOID		1	9	29	34	18	6								
INDIAN		3	11	30	34	11	7								
AUSTRALOID					31	27	40								
NEW BRITAI			2	13	27	22	27	6							
DICKSON MD			4	28	37	29									
MALAY					59	29	9								
SUB SAHARA		3	1	11	23	23	28	5	1						

TABLE XXXV. Lower Third Premolar Area (L*B): Frequency Distribution in Percentiles.

FREQUENCY DISTRIBUTION OF LOWER P3 L*B

	34	42	50	58	66	74	82	90	98	106	114	122	130	138	146
H.AFRICAN.							8	8	33	16	8	8		16	
H.ROBUSTUS							4	4	4	29	25	19	4	4	
H.ERECTUS	3				7	28	25	21	14						
H.NEANDER.	1	1	3	25	31	25	1	3	1	1					
H.SAPIENS	1	12	30	36	14	3	1	1							
AUSTRALOP.							6	6	15	25	18	15	3	9	
KRAPINA				33	16	33		16							
NEANDERTAL	2		2	29	38	17	2		2	2					
MT CARMEL		12	12		25	50									
CAUCASOID		22	41	30	5										
INDIAN	3	23	19	42	7	3									
AUSTRALOID			23	38	33	4									
NEW BRITAI		2	23	47	19	7									
DICKSON MD	1	8	34	42	12										
SUB SAHARA	3	3	23	17	28	13	3	5							
MALAY					99										
HARAPPA															

XXXIX), however, shows a 67% overlap between *H. africanus* and *H. robustus.* The overlap for length (Table XXXVIII) is 100%. The distributions for both length and breadth are unimodal for all hominid taxa and all extant groups.

On the other hand, the frequency distribution for area (Table XL) shows an overlap of *H. africanus* within the range of *H. robustus* of 87%. Similarly, all but 16% of *H. erectus* specimens fall within the range of *H. neanderthalensis.* The distributions are bimodal for both of the australopithecine taxa.

The variability for both length and breadth (Table XXXVI) increases from the australopithecines to *H. sapiens.* The coefficients of variability for length and breadth in *Alouatta caraya* (Zingeser 1967:976) are 7.7 and 4.7. As calculated from data given by Lampel (1963:27), the corresponding values are 5.7 and 5.9 for *Cercopithecus nictitans,* 4.7 and 6.0 for *Cercopithecus mona,* and 4.8 and 4.9 for *Cercopithecus diana.* These values are exceeded by the coefficients of variation for *H. sapiens.* However, the values for only a few of the extant groups are less than or greater than the ranges for non-human primates.

Both area and module (Table XXXVII) show the common pattern of posterior dental variation. The difference between the australopithecines exceeds the maximum difference among extant groups, as does the difference between *H. erectus* and *H. neanderthalensis.* The Mt. Carmel Neandertals fall within the range of extant groups.

The L/B ratio remains constant for all hominid taxa except *H. sapiens,* for which it is 13% higher.

LOWER FOURTH PREMOLAR

Length and breadth variation among the hominid taxa in the lower fourth premolar follows the common posterior pattern with the exception of length variation between the last 2

TABLE XXXVI. Upper Third Premolar Length and Breadth: Mean, Standard Error of the Mean (SE(M)), Range, Sample Size (N), and Coefficient of Variation (CV).

UPPER P3	LENGTH(M-D)					BREADTH(B-L)				
	MEAN	SE(M)	RANGE	N	CV	MEAN	SE(M)	RANGE	N	CV
H. AFRICANUS	8.88	.08	8.50 - 9.40	15	3.5	12.47	.22	10.70 - 13.90	15	6.5
H. ROBUSTUS	9.88	.15	8.30 - 10.90	23	7.1	14.35	.24	13.10 - 17.00	22	7.8
H. ERECTUS	8.54	.18	7.40 - 9.80	12	6.9	11.97	.21	10.50 - 13.20	13	6.2
H. NEANDERTAL	7.64	.12	6.20 - 9.00	35	9.3	10.49	.11	9.00 - 12.00	35	6.3
H. SAPIENS	7.60	.06	4.50 - 12.00	315	12.9	9.61	.06	5.30 - 12.30	315	11.8
AUSTRALOPITHECINES	9.48	.12	8.30 - 10.90	38	8.0	13.59	.23	10.70 - 17.00	37	10.0
KRAPINA	8.18	.09	8.00 - 8.50	6	2.4	10.92	.35	10.10 - 12.00	6	7.2
NEANDERTAL	7.49	.14	6.30 - 9.00	24	9.1	10.37	.13	9.00 - 12.00	24	6.2
MT CARMEL	7.74	.49	6.20 - 8.70	5	12.6	10.56	.23	10.00 - 11.20	5	4.4
AUSTRALOID	7.95	.20	6.00 - 9.60	21	11.2	10.40	.24	8.00 - 12.30	22	10.5
AUSTR. ABORIGINE	7.81	.00	7.00 - 9.00	124	.0	10.30	.00	8.50 - 12.00	163	.0
SUB SAHARAN	7.74	.18	6.20 - 9.00	23	11.0	9.98	.26	6.80 - 11.70	22	11.7
WADI HALFA MESOL.	7.60	.00	7.40 - 8.30	9	.0	9.70	.00	8.10 - 10.90	9	.0
AMERICAN NEGROS	7.60	.09	7.20 - 8.20	15	4.6	10.10	.14	8.90 - 10.90	15	5.3
GILIMANUK (INDON.)	7.60	.00	6.70 - 8.40	40	.0	8.70	.00	8.60 - 10.90	43	.0
NEW BRITAIN	7.56	.07	6.30 - 9.00	55	6.9	10.19	.07	9.10 - 11.20	56	4.9
MALAY	7.55	.15	6.50 - 8.10	11	6.1	9.85	.23	8.20 - 10.70	11	7.4
E.GREENLAND ESKIMO	7.52	.07	6.60 - 8.60	15	3.6	9.19	.14	6.80 - 10.50	20	6.9
JARMO	7.50	.00		2	.0	9.50	.00		2	.0
DIXON MOUND INDIAN	7.45	.05	5.90 - 8.60	103	6.7	9.80	.05	8.70 - 11.50	102	5.5
JAVANESE	7.45	.04		172	7.0	9.71	.05		171	6.2
PECOS PUEBLO	7.43	.04	6.54 - 8.42	82	5.4	9.89	.06	8.78 - 11.00	82	5.6
INDIAN	7.42	.15	6.35 - 9.30	21	9.3	9.70	.18	8.60 - 11.50	21	8.3
AMERICAN WHITES(2)	7.40	.13	6.00 - 9.70	30	9.3	9.40	.15	6.20 - 10.50	30	8.5
JAPANESE	7.30	.02		186	3.7	9.50	.03		186	4.3
SWEDES	7.11	.02		259	4.5					
ALEUTS	7.08	.05	5.80 - 8.00	114	6.9	9.28	.04	8.00 - 10.50	110	5.0
NATUFIANS	7.01	.08		13	4.1	9.44	.14		13	5.3
OHIO WHITES	7.00	.02		451	6.1					
TRISTANITES	6.99	.04		244	8.9	9.74	.06		124	6.9
AMERICAN WHITES(1)	6.93	.03	5.80 - 8.20	171	5.8					
COCHINI JEWS	6.84	.06		59	6.1	8.78	.06		59	4.8
YEMEN JEWS	6.83	.07		57	7.2	8.54	.09		57	7.6
BUSHMEN	6.80	.00	6.00 - 7.80	27	.0	8.60	.00	7.80 - 9.50	25	.0
CAUCASOID	6.77	.12	4.50 - 8.50	46	12.3	9.37	.12	8.00 - 11.00	46	8.3
LAPPS	6.65	.02	5.30 - 8.00	502	6.8	8.63	.02	6.80 - 10.40	464	5.0
MODERN ENGLISH	6.50	.05		54	5.7	8.77	.09		52	7.0

TABLE XXXVII. Upper Third Premolar Area (L*B), Index (100L/B), and Module ((L+B)/2): Mean, Range, and Coefficient of Variation (CV).

UPPER P3	L*B			100L/B			(L+B)/2		
	MEAN	RANGE	CV	MEAN	RANGE	CV	MEAN	RANGE	CV
H. AFRICANUS	110.8	93.1 - 126.9	8.5	71.5	65.4 - 81.3	6.3	10.7	9.7 - 11.5	4.6
H. ROBUSTUS	142.1	109.6 - 185.3	14.0	68.9	61.2 - 74.5	5.9	12.1	10.7 - 13.9	6.9
H. ERECTUS	103.2	77.7 - 129.4	12.4	70.9	66.1 - 75.7	3.8	10.3	8.9 - 11.5	6.1
H. NEANDERTAL	81.1	56.7 - 102.0	13.5	72.9	60.2 - 82.9	7.0	9.1	7.6 - 10.2	6.6
H. SAPIENS	73.0	36.4 - 108.0	17.5	80.6	55.6 - 169.4	22.4	8.6	6.3 - 10.5	8.7
AUSTRALOPITHECINES	129.4	93.1 - 185.3	17.4	69.9	61.2 - 81.3	6.3	11.5	9.7 - 13.9	8.8
KRAPINA	89.4	80.8 - 102.0	9.0	75.2	70.2 - 79.4	5.9	9.5	9.0 - 10.2	4.8
NEANDERTAL	78.7	56.7 - 99.6	13.4	72.2	63.6 - 81.8	6.3	9.0	7.6 - 10.1	6.5
MT CARMEL	81.9	63.9 - 91.8	15.2	73.2	60.2 - 82.9	11.2	9.1	8.2 - 9.7	7.0
AUSTRALOID	83.5	55.2 - 108.0	19.3	76.7	57.1 - 95.7	10.5	9.2	7.4 - 10.5	9.7
SUB SAHARAN	78.5	42.2 - 104.4	21.4	78.1	71.4 - 91.2	5.7	8.9	6.5 - 10.3	11.0
NEW BRITAIN	77.2	59.2 - 94.5	10.6	74.3	66.7 - 85.7	5.4	8.9	7.8 - 9.7	5.2
MALAY	74.7	53.3 - 86.7	12.8	76.8	74.3 - 81.1	2.6	8.7	7.3 - 9.4	6.8
DICKSON MOUND	73.3	51.9 - 92.6	10.9	76.2	67.0 - 85.5	5.2	8.6	7.3 - 9.8	5.4
INDIAN	72.4	57.1 - 106.0	17.1	76.7	68.6 - 85.4	6.2	8.6	7.7 - 10.3	8.2
CAUCASOID	63.9	36.4 - 89.2	19.2	72.3	55.6 - 86.0	9.3	8.1	6.3 - 9.5	9.2

TABLE XXXVIII. Upper Third Premolar Length: Frequency Distribution in Percentiles.

FREQUENCY DISTRIBUTION OF UPPER P3 L(M-D)

	4.4	5.0	5.6	6.2	6.8	7.4	8.0	8.6	9.2	9.8	10.4	11.0	11.6	12.2	12.8
H.AFRICAN.							13	66	19						
H.ROBUSTUS							8	4	30	30	26				
H.ERECTUS						8	50	25	8	8					
H.NEANDER.				14	14	25	39	5							
H.SAPIENS	1	1	4	9	30	26	19	3	1		2	1	1		
AUSTRALOP.							10	28	26	18	15				
KRAPINA							99								
NEANDERTAL				17	17	31	27	6							
MT CARMEL				19		19	39	19							
CAUCASOID	2	2	23	23	23	13	10								
INDIAN				14	42	28	9		4						
AUSTRALOID			4		23	19	28	19	4						
NEW BRITAI				3	32	41	19	1							
DICKSON MD			1	6	39	33	17	1							
MALAY				9	18	63	9								
SUB SAHARA				8	34	4	30	21							

TABLE XXXIX. Upper Third Premolar Breadth: Frequency Distribution in Percentiles.

FREQUENCY DISTRIBUTION OF UPPER P3 B(B-L)

	5.1	5.9	6.7	7.5	8.3	9.1	9.9	10.7	11.5	12.3	13.1	13.9	14.7	15.5	16.3
H.AFRICAN.								6	33	39	13	6			
H.ROBUSTUS											36	31	22	9	
H.ERECTUS							7	15	38	30	7				
H.NEANDER.					2	8	57	25	5						
H.SAPIENS	1	2	1	4	11	33	33	9	1	1					
AUSTRALOP.								2	13	16	27	21	13	5	
KRAPINA							50	33	16						
NEANDERTAL					3	10	58	24	3						
MT CARMEL							59	39							
CAUCASOID				13	23	34	21	6							
INDIAN					33	19	38	4	4						
AUSTRALOID				4	9	18	22	31	9	4					
NEW BRITAI						26	58	14							
DICKSON MD					4	53	35	4	1						
MALAY				9		36	45	9							
SUB SAHARA			4		18	22	18	27	9						

TABLE XL. Upper Third Premolar Area (L*B): Frequency Distribution in Percentiles.

FREQUENCY DISTRIBUTION OF UPPER P3 L*B

	35	46	57	68	79	90	101	112	123	134	145	156	167	178	189
H.AFRICAN.						13	53	13	19						
H.ROBUSTUS							4	4	31	13	22	13		9	
H.ERECTUS				8		25	50	8	8						
H.NEANDER.		2	8	32	32	20	2								
H.SAPIENS	1	8	26	31	23	6	2								
AUSTRALOP.						5	24	8	27	8	13	8		5	
KRAPINA					50	33	16								
NEANDERTAL		4	8	43	30	13									
MT CARMEL			19	19	19	39									
CAUCASOID	2	30	36	15	15										
INDIAN			42	38	9	4	4								
AUSTRALOID		4	14	23	19	19	19								
NEW BRITAI			14	41	38	5									
DICKSON MD		1	29	43	24	1									
SUB SAHARA	4		36	9	18	22	9								
MALAY		9	9	36	45										
HARARPA															

taxa (Table XLI). *H. neanderthalensis* has a slightly smaller length than does *H. sapiens* (this is also true of the maxillary tooth). The difference is .06 mm, or a little over 1 standard error of the *H. sapiens* mean. The difference is thus not significant. In both length and breadth, variation between the australopithecines is less than the maximum difference among extant groups. On the other hand, variation between *H. robustus* and *H. erectus* exceeds this value.

The Krapina Neandertals have maximum size for a recent group. In length, the Mt. Carmel Neandertals fall within the range of variation of extant group average values. In breadth, however, the value for the Mt. Carmel group exceeds the extant group maximum.

The frequency distribution for length (Table XLII) places the differences among the hominid taxa in a slightly different light. All of the values for *H. africanus* lie within the *H. robustus* range of variation. Similarly, all of the values for *H. erectus* fall within the range of variation of *H. neanderthalensis.* All of the distributions are unimodal.

In terms of breadth (Table XLIII), the frequency distributions overlap almost as completely. Here, too, the distributions have only a single mode.

The coefficients of variation for length and breadth (Table XLI) show a significant trend for increased variability beginning with the australopithecines and reaching a maximum with *H. sapiens.* In comparison, the length and breadth coefficients for the Liberian chimpanzee (Table LXXXI) are 6.6 and 6.9. These are less than the coefficients for any hominid taxa. Coefficients for other cercopithecoid species (Lampel 1963:31), similarly of small dimensions, are as follows: *Cercopithecus nictitans,* 4.9 and 7.0; *Cercopithecus mona,* 4.1 and 4.9; *Cercopithecus diana,* 5.3 and 5.8. About 1/2 of the extant groups exceed the primate species in length and about 1/3 in breadth.

Area and module (Table XLII) follow the common posterior dental pattern in variation between the taxa. With the exception of the

TABLE XLI. Lower Fourth Premolar Length and Breadth: Mean, Standard Error of the Mean (SE(M)), Range, Sample Size (N), and Coefficient of Variation (CV).

LOWER P4	LENGTH(M-D) MEAN	SE(M)	RANGE	N	CV	BREADTH(B-L) MEAN	SE(M)	RANGE	N	CV
H. AFRICANUS	10.09	.24	9.00 - 11.30	11	7.4	11.87	.36	10.70 - 14.00	9	8.5
H. ROBUSTUS	11.10	.23	8.50 - 14.50	24	10.1	13.08	.21	11.40 - 15.20	22	7.4
H. ERECTUS	8.79	.15	7.20 - 9.90	23	8.0	10.07	.21	8.00 - 12.00	24	9.9
H. NEANDERTAL	7.58	.13	5.50 - 10.50	56	12.8	9.10	.13	6.50 - 11.40	56	10.3
H. SAPIENS	7.64	.04	6.00 - 11.30	409	11.6	8.48	.04	5.60 - 11.90	410	10.1
AUSTRALOPITHECINES	10.78	.19	8.50 - 14.50	35	10.3	12.73	.20	10.70 - 15.20	31	8.7
KRAPINA	8.08	.19	7.00 - 9.20	14	8.3	9.50	.17	8.40 - 11.00	14	6.6
NEANDERTAL	7.35	.17	5.50 - 10.50	37	13.9	9.01	.17	6.50 - 11.40	37	11.5
MT CARMEL	7.59	.16	7.20 - 7.85	4	3.7	8.75	.21	8.30 - 9.10	4	4.2
JARMO	8.30	.00		3	.0	8.60	.00		3	.0
NEW BRITAIN	7.88	.15	6.30 - 11.30	52	13.2	9.04	.10	7.80 - 11.20	52	7.9
AUSTRALOID	7.80	.12	7.00 - 9.30	25	7.5	8.97	.13	7.50 - 10.10	25	6.9
SUB SAHARAN	7.73	.11	6.10 - 10.50	51	10.5	8.80	.13	6.50 - 11.90	50	10.3
MALAY	7.72	.16	7.00 - 8.90	12	7.0	8.58	.15	7.30 - 9.50	14	6.4
WADI HALFA MESOL	7.70	.00	6.70 - 8.10	5	.0	9.20	.00	8.00 - 10.20	5	.0
AMERICAN NEGROS	7.70	.27	6.80 - 8.70	8	9.2	8.90	.20	8.00 - 9.60	8	6.0
AUSTR. ABORIGINE	7.70	.00	6.50 - 9.00	79	.0	8.90	.00	7.00 - 10.00	109	.0
DICKSON MOUND	7.59	.05	6.40 - 10.75	120	7.7	8.50	.05	7.00 - 10.30	120	6.8
AMERICAN WHITES(2)	7.50	.19	6.80 - 8.40	10	7.6	8.50	.19	7.80 - 9.50	10	6.8
PECOS PUEBLO	7.42	.05	6.26 - 8.27	91	6.2	8.42	.05	7.16 - 9.74	91	6.0
SWEDES	7.30	.03		220	6.0					
GILIMANUK (INDON.)	7.30	.00	6.30 - 8.50	50	.0	8.50	.00	6.90 - 9.70	51	.0
JAVANESE	7.25	.04		173	7.9	8.43	.04		173	6.5
NATUFIANS	7.18	.09		14	4.7	8.24	.42		14	18.2
TRISTANITES	7.17	.03		228	6.3	9.19	.08		1	.5
AMERICAN WHITES(1)	7.15	.04	6.20 - 9.60	165	6.4					
INDIAN	7.15	.12	6.00 - 8.80	34	9.3	8.38	.10	7.50 - 9.45	34	6.8
CAUCASOID	7.14	.09	6.00 - 10.50	79	11.5	8.44	.07	7.00 - 10.10	79	7.1
OHIO WHITES	7.13	.02		414	6.0					
ALEUTS	7.11	.04	5.90 - 8.40	137	6.3	8.31	.06	6.50 - 9.90	121	7.5
JAPANESE	7.10	.02		185	3.8	8.30	.03		185	4.9
E.GREENLAND ESKIMO	7.08	.09	6.50 - 7.80	19	5.5	8.21	.10	6.90 - 9.00	24	6.0
BUSHMEN	7.00	.00	6.30 - 8.00	30	.0	7.80	.00	7.00 - 9.00	30	.0
YEMEN JEWS	6.97	.09		42	8.5	7.91	.08		42	6.6
COCHINI JEWS	6.90	.06		57	6.5	7.70	.06		57	6.0
LAPPS	6.66	.02	5.60 - 8.30	508	6.2	7.61	.02	5.90 - 9.20	503	6.4

TABLE XLII. Lower Fourth Premolar Area (L*B), Index (100L/B), and Module ((L+B)/2): Mean, Range, and Coefficient of Variation (CV).

LOWER P4	L*B MEAN	RANGE	CV	100L/B MEAN	RANGE	CV	(L+B)/2 MEAN	RANGE	CV
H. AFRICANUS	120.5	108.9 - 140.0	8.8	86.4	71.4 - 103.7	12.8	11.0	10.5 - 12.0	4.5
H. ROBUSTUS	147.8	116.6 - 220.4	15.9	86.0	74.5 - 95.6	5.8	12.2	10.8 - 14.8	7.6
H. ERECTUS	89.3	69.0 - 107.9	12.5	87.4	74.0 - 123.7	12.9	9.5	8.3 - 10.4	6.3
H. NEANDERTAL	69.5	35.7 - 118.6	20.4	83.6	65.5 - 112.2	11.8	8.3	6.0 - 10.9	10.1
H. SAPIENS	64.9	39.6 - 126.6	17.0	91.0	66.7 - 157.8	16.5	8.1	6.3 - 11.2	8.2
AUSTRALOPITHECINES	139.9	108.9 - 220.4	17.1	86.1	71.4 - 103.7	8.2	11.8	10.5 - 14.8	8.2
KRAPINA	77.0	65.1 - 96.8	13.9	85.1	75.3 - 92.9	6.3	8.8	8.1 - 9.9	6.8
NEANDERTAL	66.8	35.7 - 118.6	22.9	81.9	65.5 - 112.2	12.7	8.2	6.0 - 10.9	11.1
MT CARMEL	66.4	61.9 - 70.6	6.9	86.8	83.7 - 91.6	4.1	8.2	7.9 - 8.4	3.4
NEW BRITAIN	71.6	52.3 - 126.6	19.4	87.2	75.9 - 119.8	11.0	8.5	7.3 - 11.2	9.1
AUSTRALOID	70.0	53.9 - 86.2	11.8	87.2	75.8 - 106.7	8.7	8.4	7.3 - 9.3	5.8
SUB SAHARAN	68.4	39.6 - 107.1	18.9	88.0	75.6 - 108.7	8.5	8.3	6.3 - 10.4	9.4
MALAY	66.4	54.0 - 77.4	11.5	90.1	78.7 - 102.3	7.9	8.1	7.3 - 8.8	5.8
DICKSON MOUND	64.7	45.8 - 99.4	13.1	89.5	76.7 - 116.2	6.2	8.0	6.8 - 10.0	6.5
CAUCASOID	60.4	45.5 - 99.7	15.9	84.5	66.7 - 117.6	10.7	7.8	6.7 - 10.0	7.6
INDIAN	60.2	46.2 - 83.2	15.0	85.3	75.3 - 96.1	6.4	7.8	6.8 - 9.1	7.3

TABLE XLIII. Lower Fourth Premolar Length: Frequency Distribution in Percentiles.

FREQUENCY DISTRIBUTICN OF LOWER P4 L(M-D)

	5.3	6.0	6.7	7.4	8.1	8.8	9.5	10.2	10.9	11.6	12.3	13.0	13.7	14.4	15.1
H.AFRICAN.						18	36	27	18						
H.ROBUSTUS					4		4	37	33	8	8			4	
H.ERECTUS			4	8	26	43	17								
H.NEANDER.	7	8	21	33	17	8		1							
H.SAPIENS		8	32	35	13	3	3	1	1						
AUSTRALOP.					2	5	14	34	28	5	5			2	
KRAPINA			14	28	35	21									
NEANDERTAL	9	11	23	35	11	4		2							
MT CARMEL			25	75											
CAUCASOID		25	48	18	3		2	1							
INDIAN		23	44	20	3	2									
AUSTRALOID			23	51	15	7									
NEW BRITAI		1	30	42	13	3		1	5						
DICKSON MD		2	33	44	19			1							
MALAY			16	66	8	8									
SUB SAHARA		3	27	45	13	5	1	1							

TABLE XLIV. Lower Fourth Premolar Breadth: Frequency Distribution in Percentiles.

FREQUENCY DISTRIBUTION OF LOWER P4 B(B-L)

	5.4	6.1	6.8	7.5	8.2	8.9	9.6	10.3	11.0	11.7	12.4	13.1	13.8	14.5	15.2
H.AFRICAN.								22	22	33	11		11		
H.ROBUSTUS									4	13	36	27	4	13	
H.ERECTUS.				4	8	8	41	20	8	8					
H.NEANDER.		1		16	16	33	25	1	5						
H.SAPIENS	1	3	5	20	38	23	6	1	1	1					
AUSTRALOP.								6	9	19	29	19	6	9	
KRAPINA					7	42	42.		7						
NEANDERTAL		2		21	19	30	19	2	4						
MT CARMEL					50	50									
CAUCASOID			6	25	44	21	2								
INDIAN				41	38	20									
AUSTRALOID				7	23	55	11								
NEW BRITAI				9	32	32	19	3	1						
DICKSON MD			3	26	48	17	3	1							
MALAY			7	14	50	28									
SUB SAHARA		1	3	11	33	27	17			1					

TABLE XLV. Lower Fourth Premolar Area (L*B): Frequency Distribution in Percentiles.

FREQUENCY DISTRIBUTION OF LOWER P4 L*B

	34	47	60	73	86	99	112	125	138	151	164	177	190	203	216
H.AFRICAN.						22	55	11	11						
H.ROBUSTUS							13	22	36	9	9	4		4	
H.ERECTUS			8	30	34	26									
H.NEANDER.	3	14	46	25	8		1								
H.SAPIENS	1	32	47	14	1	1		1							
AUSTRALOP.						6	25	19	29	6	6	3		3	
KRAPINA			42	35	21										
NEANDERTAL	5	21	43	21	5		2								
MT CARMEL			99												
CAUCASOID	2	52	38	3	1	1									
INDIAN	5	50	35	8											
AUSTRALOID		11	51	31	3										
NEW BRITAI		11	53	26	1	3		1							
DICKSON MD	1	32	53	11	1	1									
SUB SAHARA	3	15	51	21	1	3									
MALAY				99											
HARAPPA															

difference between *H. sapiens* and *H. neanderthalensis* in area (4.6 mm^2), the differences among the other hominid taxa exceed the maximum difference among extant groups (11.4 mm^2). The indicated changes in tooth size are thus significant.

The frequency distribution for area (Table XLV) shows a relatively great amount of overlap for the australopithecines; all but 22% of the *H. africanus* specimens fit within the range of variation for *H. robustus.* On the other hand, there is no overlap at all between *H. robustus* and *H. erectus.* The latter falls within the range of variation of both *H. neanderthalensis* and *H. sapiens.* None of the distributions are bimodal.

Variation of the L/B index shows only a very slight tendency toward increase (relative elongation). The differences among taxa are only slightly greater than the differences among extant groups.

UPPER FOURTH PREMOLAR

Length and breadth of the upper fourth premolar (Table XLVI) follow the same posterior dental pattern of variation among taxa as does the mandibular tooth, with the same exception! Length is .1 mm greater in *H. sapiens* than it is in *H. neanderthalensis.* This difference is only slightly greater than 1 standard error of the *H. sapiens* mean, and thus could well be the result of sampling error.

On the other hand, the length difference between the australopithecines is much more extensive. It is greater than the maximum difference in length found among extant groups (1.41 mm). About 35% of the *H. robustus* specimens lie outside of the *H. africanus* range of variation (Table XLVIII). The frequency distribution is bimodal for *H. africanus, H. erectus,* and the extant groups for Sub-Saharan Africans.

The Krapina Neandertals have the longest average length of a recent group, and the Mt. Carmel Neandertals fall well within the range of variation for extant groups.

Breadth variation is similar to that of length. The only exception is that the value for

TABLE XLVI. Upper Fourth Premolar Length and Breadth: Mean, Standard Error of the Mean (SE(M)), Range, Sample Size (N), and Coefficient of Variation (CV).

UPPER P4	LENGTH(M-D)					BREADTH(B-L)				
	MEAN	SE(M)	RANGE	N	CV	MEAN	SE(M)	RANGE	N	CV
H. AFRICANUS	8.67	.29	6.00 - 10.50	16	12.7	12.89	.13	12.20 - 13.90	15	3.9
H. RCBLSTUS	10.77	.18	9.20 - 12.20	23	7.7	15.64	.22	13.70 - 18.00	23	6.5
H. ERECTUS	7.94	.15	7.00 - 8.85	17	7.7	11.58	.20	10.30 - 13.80	17	7.0
H. NEANCERTAL	7.23	.14	6.00 - 9.00	36	11.3	10.41	.13	8.40 - 11.70	35	7.5
H. SAPIENS	7.32	.06	4.60 - 12.00	319	13.6	9.50	.07	5.10 - 11.70	318	12.6
AUSTRALOPITHECINES	9.91	.23	6.00 - 12.20	39	14.2	14.55	.26	12.20 - 18.00	38	11.0
KRAPINA	8.13	.12	7.60 - 8.60	7	3.7	10.90	.22	10.20 - 11.60	7	4.9
NEANCERTAL	6.97	.16	6.00 - 9.00	25	11.4	10.29	.15	9.00 - 11.70	24	7.1
MT CARMEL	7.27	.18	7.00 - 7.60	4	4.4	10.24	.71	8.40 - 11.00	4	12.0
AMERICAN NEGROS	7.80	.17	6.80 - 8.70	10	6.5	9.80	.21	8.80 - 10.80	9	6.1
JARMC	7.80	.00		3	.0	9.80	.00		2	.0
AUSTRALOID	7.68	.10	7.00 - 8.60	21	5.8	10.54	.19	8.95 - 11.50	20	8.0
SUB SAHARAN	7.50	.20	6.20 - 9.30	22	12.4	9.86	.24	7.00 - 11.50	22	11.0
WADI HALFA MESOL.	7.40	.00	6.50 - 8.00	8	.0	10.00	.00	9.00 - 10.90	8	.0
NEW BRITAIN	7.23	.07	6.20 - 9.30	59	7.9	10.12	.07	9.20 - 11.30	58	5.5
AUSTR. ABORIGINE	7.23	.00	6.50 - 8.30	89	.0	10.14	.00	8.50 - 12.00	168	.0
DIXON MOUND INDIAN	7.11	.05	5.50 - 8.11	108	7.6	9.58	.06	7.98 - 11.35	109	7.0
GILIMANUK (INDON.)	7.10	.00	6.20 - 8.20	41	.0	9.50	.00	8.50 - 10.60	42	.0
MALAY	7.09	.08	6.80 - 7.50	11	3.8	9.32	.16	8.30 - 10.20	12	5.8
INCIAN	7.09	.23	6.00 - 9.85	20	14.3	9.63	.20	8.30 - 11.60	20	9.0
PECOS PUEBLO	7.01	.05	6.32 - 7.96	88	6.8	9.18	.05	8.12 - 9.95	88	4.8
JAVANESE	6.98	.04		169	7.4	9.58	.05		169	6.4
SWECES	6.91	.03		240	6.7					
AMERICAN WHITES(2)	6.90	.10	6.30 - 7.30	11	4.6	9.20	.26	7.70 - 10.80	12	9.2
NATUFIANS	6.85	.09		15	5.1	9.53	.13		15	5.2
E.GREENLAND ESKIMO	6.80	.08	5.60 - 7.40	17	4.9	9.21	.11	7.70 - 10.00	21	5.4
JAPANESE	6.80	.03		186	6.0	9.30	.03		186	4.4
AMERICAN WHITES(1)	6.72	.03	5.20 - 7.80	167	6.0					
CAUCASOID	6.72	.14	4.60 - 9.85	45	14.3	9.59	.14	7.00 - 11.70	44	9.8
OHIO WHITES	6.71	.02		427	6.4					
ALEUTS	6.63	.05	5.10 - 8.10	99	7.5	9.10	.06	7.40 - 10.90	99	7.0
TRISTANITES	6.62	.02		230	4.5	9.91	.06		106	6.3
YEMEN JEWS	6.55	.09		49	9.0	8.74	.10		49	8.1
COCHINI JEWS	6.52	.05		58	6.1	8.56	.08		58	7.5
BUSHMEN	6.50	.00	5.80 - 7.30	28	.0	8.50	.00	7.30 - 9.30	26	.0
MODERN ENGLISH	6.44	.05		58	5.9	9.17	.08		56	6.2
LAPPS	6.39	.02	5.30 - 7.70	515	6.7	8.60	.03	6.10 - 10.10	468	7.1

TABLE XLVII. Upper Fourth Premolar Area (L*B), Index (100L/B), and Module ((L+B)/2): Mean, Range, and Coefficient of Variation (CV).

UPPER P4	L*B			100L/B			(L+B)/2		
	MEAN	RANGE	CV	MEAN	RANGE	CV	MEAN	RANGE	CV
H. AFRICANUS	112.3	78.0 - 145.9	13.8	67.7	46.2 - 78.6	13.4	10.8	9.5 - 12.2	5.7
H. ROBUSTUS	169.0	127.4 - 212.4	13.3	68.9	63.0 - 75.8	5.0	13.2	11.5 - 14.9	6.6
H. ERECTUS	92.3	74.2 - 122.1	13.6	68.7	63.2 - 75.7	5.8	9.8	8.7 - 11.3	6.7
H. NEANDERTAL	75.9	57.0 - 99.8	16.2	69.9	57.9 - 89.3	9.9	8.8	7.7 - 10.1	7.8
H. SAPIENS	69.5	38.5 - 109.8	18.4	78.9	48.4 - 165.6	24.2	8.4	6.2 - 10.5	9.2
AUSTRALOPITHECINES	146.6	78.0 - 212.4	23.4	68.4	46.2 - 78.6	9.1	12.2	9.5 - 14.9	11.6
KRAPINA	88.7	82.6 - 99.8	7.2	74.7	67.9 - 79.4	5.0	9.5	9.1 - 10.1	3.7
NEANDERTAL	72.5	57.0 - 99.0	16.4	68.2	57.9 - 81.8	9.0	8.6	7.7 - 10.0	7.9
MT CARMEL	74.3	63.0 - 81.7	10.8	72.1	63.6 - 89.3	16.4	8.8	7.9 - 9.2	6.3
AUSTRALOID	81.3	65.2 - 98.0	13.0	73.2	67.0 - 81.6	5.7	9.1	8.1 - 10.0	6.7
SUB SAHARAN	74.7	43.4 - 104.2	21.7	76.3	66.7 - 90.6	8.5	8.7	6.6 - 10.2	10.9
NEW BRITAIN	72.9	57.0 - 89.9	11.5	71.1	63.4 - 82.0	5.1	8.6	7.7 - 9.6	5.7
INDIAN	68.9	49.8 - 109.6	22.7	73.6	64.0 - 93.4	9.4	8.4	7.1 - 10.5	10.5
DICKSON MOUND	68.4	47.1 - 90.1	13.3	74.3	62.5 - 85.7	6.0	8.3	6.9 - 9.6	6.7
MALAY	66.1	58.1 - 75.7	8.7	76.3	71.6 - 84.3	5.3	8.2	7.6 - 8.8	4.5
CAUCASOID	65.2	38.5 - 109.8	22.1	70.9	48.4 - 88.3	10.9	8.2	6.2 - 10.5	10.4

TABLE XLVIII. Upper Fourth Premolar Length: Frequency Distribution in Percentiles.

FREQUENCY DISTRIBUTION OF UPPER P4 L(M-D)

	4.5	5.1	5.7	6.3	6.9	7.5	8.1	8.7	9.3	9.9	10.5	11.1	11.7	12.3	12.9
H.AFRICAN.			6		6	18	12	18	25	6	6				
H.ROBUSTUS								4	8	13	39	17	17		
H.ERECTUS					35	17	29	17							
H.NEANDER			13	22	22	25	13	2							
H.SAPIENS	1	1	6	22	32	22	5	1	1	1	2		1		
AUSTRALOP			2		2	7	5	10	15	10	25	10	10		
KRAPINA						28	71								
NEANDERTAL			17	27	27	24		3							
MT CARMEL					50	50									
CAUCASOID	4	6	17	28	19	17	2		2						
INDIAN			19	29	29	9			9						
AUSTRALOID					33	42	23								
NEW BRITAI			1	30	35	25	5		1						
DICKSON MD		1	5	25	39	27	1								
MALAY				27	54	18									
SUB SAHARA			9	18	27	9	22	9	4						

TABLE XLIX. Upper Fourth Premolar Breadth: Frequency Distribution in Percentiles.

FREQUENCY DISTRIBUTION OF UPPER P4 B(B-L)

	4.9	5.8	6.7	7.6	8.5	9.4	10.3	11.2	12.1	13.0	13.9	14.8	15.7	16.6	17.5
H.AFRICAN.									53	39	6				
H.ROBUSTUS										4	17	34	30	13	
H.ERECTUS							29	41	23	5					
H.NEANDER.				2	8	19	54	14							
H.SAPIENS	1	3	2	3	29	36	16	5							
AUSTRALOP.									21	18	13	21	18	7	
KRAPINA						14	42	42							
NEANDERTAL				3	10	21	57	7							
MT CARMEL				25			75								
CAUCASOID			4		40	31	20	2							
INDIAN				9	34	25	25	4							
AUSTRALOID					9	25	34	29							
NEW BRITAI					6	56	29	6							
DICKSON MD				3	42	43	8	2							
MALAY				8	50	41									
SUB SAHARA			4		31	27	18	18							

TABLE L. Upper Fourth Premolar Area (L*B): Frequency Distribution in Percentiles.

FREQUENCY DISTRIBUTION OF UPPER P4 L*B

	37	49	61	73	85	97	109	121	133	145	157	169	181	193	205
H.AFRICAN.				6	6	19	46	13		6					
H.ROBUSTUS								4	8	17	17	17	21	13	
H.ERECTUS				35	23	35		5							
H.NEANDER.		14	28	31	19	5									
H.SAPIENS	5	16	38	27	7	1	1								
AUSTRALOP.				2	2	7	18	7	5	13	10	10	13	7	
KRAPINA				28	57	14									
NEANDERTAL		20	37	25	12	4									
MT CARMEL			25	75											
CAUCASOID	6	37	27	20	2	2	2								
INDIAN		34	34	19		4	4								
AUSTRALOID			34	19	39	4									
NEW BRITAI		3	48	41	6										
DICKSON MD	3	16	46	28	4										
SUB SAHARA	4	18	27	22	22	4									
MALAY		27	54	18											
HARAPPA															

H. neanderthalensis is greater than the value for *H. sapiens*–similar to the case of the lower fourth premolar. The differences between *H. africanus* and *H. robustus,* and between *H. robustus* and *H. erectus* exceed the maximum difference among extant groups (2.04 mm). The change between *H. neanderthalensis* and *H. sapiens,* on the other hand, is only about 1/2 as great. Thus a full 50% of the *H. africanus* specimens lie outside the range of variation (Table XLIX) of *H. robustus.* Of the *H. erectus* specimens, 70% lie outside the range of variation of *H. africanus,* and 83% outside the range of variation of *H. robustus.* Specimens of *H. neanderthalensis,* however, lie completely within the range of *H. sapiens.* Unlike length, no distributions of breadth are bimodal.

The broadest tooth average of a recent group belongs to the Krapina Neandertals. The Neandertals from Mt. Carmel, on the other hand, have an average breadth which fits within the extant group range of variation.

Variability in breadth clearly increases from *H. africanus* to *H. sapiens* (Table XLVI). However, this is not true for length. The values of the coefficient of variation for length are almost the same for these 2 species. The other hominid taxa have lower values. Coefficients of variation for area (Table XLVII) show an increase from the australopithecines to *H. sapiens.* The length and breadth coefficients of variation for the Liberian chimpanzee (Table LXXXI) are 7.9 and 5.6. For 3 cercopithecoid species (Lampel 1963: 30) they are 4.7 and 5.5 (*Cercopithecus nictitans*), 4.2 and 4.7 (*Cercopithecus mona*), and 4.9 and 3.9 (*Cercopithecus diana*). *H. sapiens* is more variable than any of the non-human primates in length and breadth.

In terms of area and module (Table XLVII), the maximum difference among extant groups is less than the differences between all temporally adjacent hominid taxa except *H. neanderthalensis* and *H. sapiens.* Indeed, only 4% of the *H. robustus* specimens overlap with *H. africanus.* These same 4% also overlap uniquely with *H. erectus.* On the other hand, all but 5%

of the *H. erectus* specimens overlap with *H. neanderthalensis,* and the latter is completely included within *H. sapiens* (Table L).

The area frequency distribution for *H. erectus* is slightly bimodal. Those of the other taxa and extant groups are unimodal.

The L/B index is relatively unchanged for most of the hominid taxa, but increases by over 10% for *H. sapiens* (Table L).

LOWER FIRST MOLAR

The pattern of variation for the lower first molar (Table LI) follows the common posterior relationship. The difference in length between *H. robustus* and *H. africanus,* however, is less than that between the 2 groups of American "Whites." The length differences between *H. neanderthalensis* and either *H. sapiens* or *H. erectus* are about the same, and are a little greater than the difference between the 2 samples mentioned above. Yet even the differences between these 2 taxa fall well within the range of variation of differences among extant groups. Even the most extreme difference between temporally adjacent taxa—that between *H. robustus* and *H. erectus*—is about the same as the maximum difference among extant groups. However, the maximum difference among any hominid taxa exceeds the maximum among extant groups. Thus, while the changes in length between taxa are relatively small (less than the expected variation within the taxa), the total reduction of length for this tooth in hominid evolution is significant. As one would expect, the average tooth length for both Neandertal groups and for the taxon as a whole falls within the range of variation of extant groups.

The same relations both within and among taxa hold for breadth of the lower first molar. Thus the difference between the australopithecines lies far within the range of variation for extant group differences. Even the most extreme difference between temporally adjacent taxa (*H. robustus* and *H. erectus*) falls within this range. Only the maximum difference between any 2 taxa falls outside of it. Thus as with length, the changes among taxa are not great compared with the ranges of variation within the taxa, although the total reduction of the tooth is quite significant. Neandertal groups and the taxon, again, fall within the range of variation of extant groups.

There do not seem to be any significant trends in the variability of either length or breadth. The coefficients of length and breadth variation for the Liberian chimpanzee are 4.4 and 5.0 (Table LXXXII) and are thus somewhat smaller than are those of the hominid taxa as well as most of the extant groups. On the other hand, the coefficients for species of *Macacca, Cercopithecus,* and *Cercocebus* (Table LXXXII) range from 4.5 to 12.6 for length and from 5.9 to 13.1 for breadth. They thus encompass the upper part of the range for hominids. In comparison to *Pan,* the hominid taxa show consistently greater variability.

The frequency distribution for first lower molar length (Table LIII) is bimodal for *H. africanus, H. robustus,* and *H. neanderthalensis.* Both *H. africanus* and *H. neanderthalensis* are split into about equal-sized groups. These groups are surprisingly consistent with those which could be constructed from lower canine length. In *H. neanderthalensis,* only 1 of the specimens clearly assigned to a mode for canine length was not clearly assigned to the same mode on the basis of lower first molar length.

The frequency distribution for breadth (Table LIV) is bimodal for *H. africanus, H. robustus,* and *H. erectus.* Of these, only the distribution for *H. erectus* is about evenly split. The agreement of *H. erectus* molar breadth modes with those of the lower canine, however, is not very good.

Both area and module (Table LII) vary with the common posterior pattern. The difference between the australopithecines is about 1/2 the maximum difference among extant groups, and thus is not of great significance. The only difference between temporally adjacent taxa which exceeds the maximum difference among extant groups is between *H. erectus* and *H. robustus.* The maximum difference among hominid taxa also exceeds that among extant groups. Thus, while the size reduction of the lower first molar was relatively gradual, the total reduction from the australopithecines to *H. sapiens* is quite significant.

The frequency distribution for area (Table LV) is bimodal for both *H. africanus* and *H. erectus.* There is about 75% agreement between the relatively clear assignments to modes for lower canine area and lower first molar area for *H. erectus.*

TABLE LI. Lower First Molar Length and Breadth: Mean, Standard Error of the Mean (SE(M)), Range, Sample Size (N), and Coefficient of Variation (CV).

LOWER M1	LENGTH(M-D) MEAN	SE(M)	RANGE	N	CV	BREADTH(B-L) MEAN	SE(M)	RANGE	N	CV
H. AFRICANUS	13.87	.32	11.60 - 16.50	16	9.0	13.04	.25	11.30 - 15.00	15	7.1
H. ROBUSTUS	14.57	.20	11.80 - 16.40	32	7.6	13.77	.17	11.50 - 15.50	32	6.9
H. ERECTUS	12.74	.18	9.90 - 14.70	30	7.7	12.02	.16	10.10 - 13.70	29	7.2
H. NEANDERTAL	11.69	.13	8.00 - 14.00	75	9.3	11.13	.08	9.00 - 12.70	74	6.5
H. SAPIENS	11.55	.04	9.00 - 14.10	558	7.5	10.99	.03	8.30 - 13.00	558	7.2
AUSTRALOPITHECINES	14.34	.17	11.60 - 16.50	48	8.3	13.53	.15	11.30 - 15.50	47	7.4
KRAPINA	12.30	.20	11.00 - 13.80	23	7.5	11.44	.15	10.20 - 12.60	23	6.2
NEANDERTAL	11.41	.16	8.00 - 14.00	46	9.5	10.97	.11	9.00 - 12.70	46	6.5
MT CARMEL	11.56	.36	10.50 - 13.00	6	7.0	11.18	.20	10.50 - 11.50	5	3.7
AUSTR. ABORIGINE	12.30	.00	11.00 - 14.00	139	.0	11.90	.00	10.00 - 13.50	186	.0
WADI HALFA MESOL.	12.10	.00	10.90 - 13.20	9	.0	11.50	.00	10.10 - 12.70	9	.0
PECOS PUEBLO	11.96	.07	10.78 - 13.01	67	4.6	10.74	.06	9.46 - 11.92	67	4.4
AMERICAN WHITES(2)	11.90	.35	10.10 - 13.20	10	8.9	10.60	.21	9.60 - 11.40	10	5.8
AMERICAN NEGROS	11.90	.17	10.60 - 13.40	19	6.1	10.80	.13	9.80 - 11.90	19	5.2
AUSTRALOID	11.87	.19	10.00 - 13.70	31	8.6	11.76	.11	10.70 - 13.00	31	5.3
E.GREENLAND ESKIMO	11.81	.10	10.60 - 12.60	29	4.6	11.32	.10	10.10 - 12.50	33	5.0
SUB SAHARAN	11.77	.13	9.50 - 14.10	63	8.4	11.16	.11	8.80 - 13.00	62	7.5
NEW BRITAIN	11.75	.08	10.00 - 13.60	77	6.0	11.36	.07	10.10 - 12.60	76	5.4
MALAY	11.71	.13	10.70 - 12.50	14	4.0	10.68	.10	10.10 - 11.60	18	3.7
INDIAN	11.68	.12	10.00 - 13.30	39	6.6	11.28	.12	10.00 - 12.45	38	6.4
DIXON MOUND INDIAN	11.65	.06	9.90 - 13.10	134	5.7	11.17	.05	9.80 - 12.85	134	5.1
GILIMANUK (INDON.)	11.60	.00	10.00 - 13.40	49	.0	11.00	.00	9.60 - 12.20	47	.0
NATUFIANS	11.52	.12		16	4.2	10.76	.07		16	2.6
ALEUTS	11.45	.07	10.10 - 12.80	67	5.2	10.50	.04	9.20 - 11.30	65	3.4
JAVANESE	11.43	.05		150	5.4	10.93	.05		152	5.8
JARMO	11.40	.00		6	.0	10.50	.00		6	.0
CAUCASOID	11.21	.08	9.80 - 13.00	115	7.4	10.74	.06	9.20 - 12.70	115	6.1
SWEDES	11.12	.04		268	5.8					
TRISTANITES	11.12	.04		255	5.8	11.15	.05		210	6.5
JAPANESE	11.10	.03		189	3.7	10.80	.03		189	3.8
OHIO WHITES	11.01	.03		361	5.8					
AMERICAN WHITES(1)	10.95	.04	9.40 - 12.70	160	4.7					
BUSHMEN	10.90	.00	10.00 - 12.00	33	.0	10.20	.00	9.00 - 11.30	33	.0
COCHINI JEWS	10.89	.08		58	5.3	10.11	.07		58	5.5
LAPPS	10.80	.03	9.20 - 12.80	576	5.6	10.22	.02	8.30 - 12.20	602	5.3
YEMEN JEWS	10.79	.08		60	5.5	10.16	.05		60	3.8
HARAPPA, INDIA	10.57	.09	9.00 - 12.50	49	5.7	10.33	.11	8.50 - 12.00	48	7.5

TABLE LII. Lower First Molar Area (L*B), Index (100L/B), and Module ((L+B)/2): Mean, Range, and Coefficient of Variation (CV).

LOWER M1	L*B MEAN	RANGE	CV	100L/B MEAN	RANGE	CV	(L+B)/2 MEAN	RANGE	CV
H. AFRICANUS	182.0	150.3 - 247.5	15.1	106.7	89.2 - 117.7	7.5	13.5	12.3 - 15.7	7.4
H. ROBUSTUS	201.5	135.7 - 250.9	13.7	105.8	100.0 - 114.8	3.5	14.2	11.6 - 15.8	7.1
H. ERECTUS	153.6	100.0 - 182.0	13.1	106.0	93.4 - 118.2	4.8	12.4	10.0 - 13.5	6.7
H. NEANDERTAL	130.8	85.5 - 176.4	14.1	105.3	74.1 - 119.0	7.6	11.4	9.2 - 13.3	7.1
H. SAPIENS	127.3	83.6 - 179.2	12.6	105.3	78.3 - 147.0	7.8	11.3	9.1 - 13.4	6.3
AUSTRALOPITHECINES	195.2	135.7 - 250.9	14.8	106.1	89.2 - 117.7	5.1	13.9	11.6 - 15.8	7.5
KRAPINA	141.3	112.2 - 171.4	13.3	107.5	100.9 - 114.8	3.6	11.9	10.6 - 13.1	6.7
NEANDERTAL	125.4	85.5 - 176.4	13.6	104.2	74.1 - 119.0	9.0	11.2	9.2 - 13.3	6.9
MT CARMEL	131.6	121.8 - 145.6	6.6	105.4	98.3 - 116.1	7.2	11.5	11.0 - 12.1	3.3
AUSTRALOID	140.0	112.3 - 174.1	12.8	100.9	87.0 - 115.4	6.8	11.8	10.6 - 13.2	6.4
NEW BRITAIN	134.0	103.0 - 170.1	10.1	103.6	92.6 - 117.0	5.3	11.6	10.1 - 13.0	5.1
INDIAN	132.2	108.0 - 162.3	12.0	103.8	86.6 - 118.7	5.3	11.5	10.4 - 12.7	6.0
SUB SAHARAN	131.6	83.6 - 179.2	14.5	105.3	90.8 - 118.9	5.6	11.4	9.1 - 13.4	7.3
DICKSON MOUND	130.4	99.0 - 165.8	9.7	104.4	94.0 - 124.6	4.9	11.4	9.9 - 12.9	4.8
MALAY	126.1	112.3 - 145.0	6.9	108.9	101.9 - 113.2	3.3	11.2	10.6 - 12.0	3.5
CAUCASOID	120.8	90.2 - 158.7	12.0	104.5	85.5 - 120.0	6.4	11.0	9.5 - 12.6	6.0
HARAPPA, INDIA	109.2	90.0 - 143.7	9.5	102.9	78.3 - 129.4	9.7	10.4	9.5 - 12.0	4.6

TABLE LIII. Lower First Molar Length: Frequency Distribution in Percentiles.

FREQUENCY DISTRIBUTION OF LOWER M1 L(M-D)

	7.8	8.4	9.0	9.6	10.2	10.8	11.4	12.0	12.6	13.2	13.8	14.4	15.0	15.6	16.2
H.AFRICAN.							6	6	18	12	25	12	12	6	
H.ROBUSTUS							6		3	6	15	37	12	18	
H.ERECTUS				3		6	9	16	33	16	9	3			
H.NEANDER.	1	1	1	2	3	29	15	27	7	5	2				
H.SAPIENS			1	6	11	24	24	22	8	2	1				
AUSTRALOP.							6	2	8	8	18	29	12	14	
KRAPINA						26	8	26	17	17	4				
NEANDERTAL	1	1	1	3	5	30	19	28	3		1				
MT CARMEL					16	16	50		16						
CAUCASOID				10	21	26	15	21	4						
INDIAN				2	7	25	25	25	10	2					
AUSTRALOID				3	9	16	25	22	9	12					
NEW BRITAI				1	2	32	25	20	14	2					
DICKSON MD				1	6	24	32	26	7						
MALAY					7	14	42	35							
SUB SAHARA			1	4	9	15	23	26	9	4	3				
HARAPPA			2	32	26	28	8	2							

TABLE LIV. Lower First Molar Breadth: Frequency Distribution in Percentiles.

FREQUENCY DISTRIBUTION OF LOWER M1 B(B-L)

	8.1	8.6	9.1	9.6	10.1	10.6	11.1	11.6	12.1	12.6	13.1	13.6	14.1	14.6	15.1
H.AFRICAN.							6		26	26	13	19		6	
H.ROBUSTUS							6	3		9	15	31	12	21	
H.ERECTUS					3	10	13	27	6	34		3			
H.NEANDER.		1		5	17	29	20	14	6	4					
H.SAPIENS	1	1	3	8	15	26	22	15	6	1					
AUSTRALOP.							6	2	8	14	14	27	8	17	
KRAPINA					13	26	13	21	21	4					
NEANDERTAL		1		7	19	31	23	11		3					
MT CARMEL					19		79								
CAUCASOID			5	11	23	37	11	9	1	1					
INDIAN				5	13	23	15	23	18						
AUSTRALOID						19	25	29	12	12					
NEW BRITAI					13	19	28	22	14	1					
DICKSON MD				4	8	26	37	16	5	1					
MALAY					33	50	11	5							
SUB SAHARA		3	3	3	9	20	30	20	4	3					
HARAPPA	2	8	6	31	22	18	6	4							

TABLE LV. Lower First Molar Area (L*B): Frequency Distribution in Percentiles.

FREQUENCY DISTRIBUTION OF LOWER M1 L*B

	81	93	105	117	129	141	153	165	177	189	201	213	225	237	249
H.AFRICAN.						19	13	13	6	19	19			6	
H.ROBUSTUS					3	6		3	12	21	21	15	6	9	
H.ERECTUS		3		3	14	32	14	21	10						
H.NEANDER.	4	1	14	28	24	17	2	6							
H.SAPIENS	1	6	21	24	27	12	4	1	1						
AUSTRALOP.					2	10	4	6	10	21	21	10	4	8	
KRAPINA			8	30	8	26	8	17							
NEANDERTAL	6	2	19	26	30	13		2							
MT CARMEL				39	39	19									
CAUCASOID	1	12	33	23	19	8	1								
INDIAN			23	18	28	18	10								
AUSTRALOID			6	22	29	19	9	12							
NEW BRITAI		1	6	26	38	14	9	2							
DICKSON MD		1	12	30	37	13	3	1							
SUB SAHARA	4	1	14	22	25	19	6	3	1						
MALAY					99										
HARAPPA	4	25	58	8	2	2									

The average lower first molar area for *H. neanderthalensis* falls within the range of variation for extant groups of *H. sapiens.* Of the Neandertal groups, Mt. Carmel falls within the extant group range, while Krapina exceeds it slightly.

The L/B ratio (Table LII) undergoes no change whatsoever either between the hominid taxa or within the extant groups of *H. sapiens.*

UPPER FIRST MOLAR

Both length and breadth of the upper first molar (Table LVI) follow the common posterior dental pattern of variation between taxa. Paralleling the first lower molar, the difference between the australopithecines in both length and breadth is much less than the maximum difference among extant groups. The difference between the molar length for *H. robustus* and *H. erectus* (2.00 mm) slightly exceeds the maximum difference among extant groups (1.71 mm), while the molar breadth difference between these 2 taxa (1.95 mm) is less than the maximum breadth difference among extant groups (2.26 mm). Thus relative variation among the taxa is even less than is the case for its lower counterpart. For both length and breadth, on the other hand, the maximum difference among taxa exceeds that among extant groups. The eventual reduction of this tooth from the australopithecines to *H. sapiens* can be regarded as significant.

The Krapina Neandertals fall outside of the extant group range of variation for length, although not for breadth. Both average values for the Mt. Carmel Neandertals fall within the extant group.

The frequency distributions for length (Table LVIII) are all unimodal. The close size relationships among the taxa are shown by the fact that all but 4% of the australopithecines fall within the *H. sapiens* range of variation. The breadth distributions (Table LIX) are not as consistent; *H. erectus* is bimodal. About 30% of the australopithecine sample, both *H. robustus* and *H. africanus* specimens, falls outside of the *H. sapiens*

TABLE LVI. Upper First Molar Length and Breadth: Mean, Standard Error of the Mean (SE(M)), Range, Sample Size (N), and Coefficient of Variation (CV).

UPPER M1	LENGTH(M-D) MEAN	SE(M)	RANGE	N	CV	BREADTH(B-L) MEAN	SE(M)	RANGE	N	CV
H. AFRICANUS	12.40	.16	10.90 - 14.00	22	5.8	13.66	.13	12.60 - 15.10	22	4.3
H. ROBUSTUS	13.68	.19	11.80 - 15.20	22	6.2	14.89	.27	12.70 - 17.70	22	8.2
H. ERECTUS	11.68	.26	10.00 - 13.50	17	8.9	12.94	.25	11.70 - 14.70	16	7.4
H. NEANDERTAL	11.33	.15	7.20 - 14.00	66	10.7	12.08	.10	9.30 - 15.00	66	6.8
H. SAPIENS	10.82	.05	6.00 - 14.75	488	9.9	11.64	.05	7.00 - 14.50	492	9.6
AUSTRALOPITHECINES	13.11	.15	10.90 - 15.20	42	7.4	14.32	.18	12.60 - 17.70	42	7.9
KRAPINA	11.98	.27	10.00 - 13.40	14	8.2	12.44	.28	10.70 - 15.00	14	8.2
NEANDERTAL	11.14	.20	7.20 - 14.00	43	11.7	11.97	.12	9.30 - 13.70	43	6.5
MT CARMEL	11.24	.26	9.90 - 12.40	9	6.5	12.07	.19	11.20 - 12.50	9	4.4
AUSTRALOID	11.61	.15	10.45 - 12.70	22	5.9	12.86	.16	10.80 - 14.50	25	6.3
AUSTR. ABORIGINE	11.43	.00	10.00 - 13.00	198	.0	12.84	.00	11.50 - 14.75	255	.0
NEW BRITAIN	11.35	.08	9.70 - 13.00	79	6.2	12.17	.07	11.10 - 13.80	79	5.2
WADI HALFA MESOL.	11.30	.00	10.10 - 12.10	8	.0	12.30	.00	11.30 - 13.00	8	.0
SUB SAHARAN	11.06	.21	9.00 - 13.10	26	9.4	11.88	.19	10.00 - 13.00	24	7.6
INDIAN	10.94	.13	9.90 - 12.30	24	5.6	12.08	.15	10.50 - 13.50	24	5.9
NATUFIANS	10.87	.19		14	6.2	12.30	.09		14	2.8
GILIMANUK (INDON.)	10.80	.00	9.50 - 12.60	40	.0	11.50	.00	10.00 - 13.10	40	.0
DIXON MOUND INDIAN	10.75	.06	9.20 - 13.00	140	6.8	11.92	.06	10.00 - 13.83	140	5.5
PECOS PUEBLO	10.74	.06	9.60 - 11.90	67	4.5	11.54	.05	10.27 - 12.63	68	3.6
JAVANESE	10.73	.05		170	6.0	11.66	.04		171	5.0
E.GREENLAND ESKIMO	10.68	.07	9.60 - 11.90	57	5.0	11.62	.07	10.00 - 12.50	60	4.6
AMERICAN WHITES(1)	10.66	.04	9.40 - 12.40	168	5.1					
AMERICAN WHITES(2)	10.60	.20	9.30 - 12.50	16	7.2	11.50	.12	10.50 - 12.40	16	3.9
SWEDES	10.59	.03		299	4.9					
TRISTANITES	10.58	.03		267	4.6	11.99	.05		174	5.5
AMERICAN NEGROS	10.50	.45	7.50 - 12.30	9	12.2	12.10	.36	10.90 - 14.30	9	8.4
MODERN ENGLISH	10.40	.06		96	5.4	11.31	.06		97	5.0
CAUCASOID	10.39	.13	7.70 - 13.00	53	9.1	11.76	.12	9.80 - 13.30	54	7.6
MALAY	10.33	.19	8.80 - 11.70	19	7.9	11.33	.15	10.20 - 12.40	22	6.2
COCHINI JEWS	10.32	.07		58	5.0	10.72	.07		58	4.7
YEMEN JEWS	10.28	.08		60	5.9	10.90	.09		60	6.5
ALEUTS	10.24	.07	9.00 - 12.00	89	6.2	11.30	.07	10.10 - 12.80	65	4.7
JAPANESE	10.20	.03		211	4.3	11.30	.03		211	3.9
LAPPS	10.09	.02	8.00 - 11.90	633	5.7	10.97	.02	9.20 - 12.80	580	5.5
HARAPPA, INDIA	10.00	.12	6.00 - 11.50	90	11.4	10.83	.13	7.00 - 12.50	89	11.6
OHIO WHITES	9.97	.03		469	5.5					
BUSHMEN	9.90	.00	8.50 - 11.30	33	.0	10.60	.00	9.50 - 11.30	33	.0

TABLE LVII. Upper First Molar Area (L*B), Index (100L/B), and Module ((L+B)/2): Mean, Range, and Coefficient of Variation (CV).

UPPER M1	L*B MEAN	RANGE	CV	100L/B MEAN	RANGE	CV	(L+B)/2 MEAN	RANGE	CV
H. AFRICANUS	169.5	148.7 - 203.0	8.5	90.8	79.6 - 100.0	5.8	13.0	12.2 - 14.2	4.1
H. ROBUSTUS	204.7	166.4 - 269.0	12.9	93.1	77.6 - 106.1	6.8	14.3	12.9 - 16.4	6.3
H. ERECTUS	150.7	117.0 - 198.4	15.0	89.6	81.0 - 100.0	6.3	12.3	10.8 - 14.1	7.4
H. NEANDERTAL	137.1	86.4 - 189.0	14.2	94.1	60.0 - 140.9	11.9	11.7	9.6 - 13.8	6.9
H. SAPIENS	126.3	42.0 - 184.1	15.4	93.8	59.7 - 164.0	12.5	11.2	6.5 - 13.6	8.0
AUSTRALOPITHECINES	188.3	148.7 - 269.0	14.4	92.2	77.6 - 106.1	6.1	13.7	12.2 - 16.4	7.0
KRAPINA	149.4	116.0 - 189.0	14.1	96.7	84.0 - 115.0	8.9	12.2	10.8 - 13.8	7.0
NEANDERTAL	133.4	86.4 - 189.0	14.2	93.5	60.0 - 140.9	13.4	11.5	9.6 - 13.7	6.9
MT CARMEL	135.6	115.8 - 150.0	8.0	93.3	84.6 - 109.7	7.8	11.6	10.8 - 12.2	4.0
AUSTRALOID	149.5	122.0 - 184.1	10.6	91.0	80.8 - 106.9	7.4	12.2	11.0 - 13.6	5.3
NEW BRITAIN	138.3	111.9 - 179.4	10.0	93.3	82.2 - 106.6	5.6	11.8	10.6 - 13.4	4.9
SUB SAHARAN	132.4	94.5 - 162.4	14.1	93.8	80.0 - 111.4	9.3	11.5	9.7 - 12.7	7.2
INDIAN	132.2	116.4 - 151.2	8.3	90.9	80.6 - 109.5	8.3	11.5	10.8 - 12.3	4.2
DICKSON MOUND	128.5	92.0 - 170.3	11.3	90.2	78.5 - 101.3	5.1	11.3	9.6 - 13.1	5.6
CAUCASOID	122.6	90.0 - 169.0	14.4	88.5	59.7 - 101.5	8.7	11.1	9.5 - 13.0	7.0
MALAY	116.2	94.9 - 145.1	11.4	92.2	72.1 - 100.0	8.2	10.8	9.7 - 12.0	5.7
HARAPPA, INDIA	109.3	42.0 - 137.5	19.3	92.7	78.3 - 121.1	8.3	10.4	6.5 - 11.7	10.9

TABLE LVIII. Upper First Molar Length: Frequency Distribution in Percentiles.

FREQUENCY DISTRIBUTION OF UPPER M1 L(M-D)

	5.8	6.5	7.2	7.9	8.6	9.3	10.0	10.7	11.4	12.1	12.8	13.5	14.2	14.9	15.6
H.AFRICAN.								9	22	40	22	4			
H.ROBUSTUS									9		36	27	18	9	
H.ERECTUS							23	17	17	23	11	5			
H.NEANDER.			1	1		7	15	24	22	18	7	1			
H.SAPIENS	1	1	1		3	9	29	28	16	7	3		1		
AUSTRALOP.								2	14	21	30	16	9	4	
KRAPINA							7	21	21	28	21				
NEANDERTAL			1	1		9	17	25	23	15	3	1			
MT CARMEL						11		55	22	11					
CAUCASOID			1		7	15	45	13	11	3	1				
INDIAN						4	37	33	16	8					
AUSTRALOID							9	27	40	22					
NEW BRITAI						3	10	39	30	13	2				
DICKSON MD					2	15	26	34	17	3	1				
MALAY					10	21	31	26	10						
SUB SAHARA					3	7	30	19	19	15	3				
HARAPPA	1	6			6	7	50	24	3						

TABLE LIX. Upper First Molar Breadth: Frequency Distribution in Percentiles.

FREQUENCY DISTRIBUTION OF UPPER M1 B(B-L)

	6.8	7.6	8.4	9.2	10.0	10.8	11.6	12.4	13.2	14.0	14.8	15.6	16.4	17.2	18.0
H.AFRICAN.								22	36	36	4				
H.ROBUSTUS								4	9	31	36	4	4	9	
H.ERECTUS							37	18	31	12					
H.NEANDER.				1	1	24	36	28	6		1				
H.SAPIENS	1	1	1	2	8	28	31	20	3	1					
AUSTRALOP.								11	21	35	21	2	2	4	
KRAPINA					7	7	35	28	14		7				
NEANDERTAL				1		28	36	28	3						
MT CARMEL						22	33	44							
CAUCASOID				1	12	35	18	27	3						
INDIAN					4	25	33	33	4						
AUSTRALOID						7	15	43	23	7					
NEW BRITAI						15	48	29	7						
DICKSON MD					2	25	47	21	2						
MALAY					22	40	27	9							
SUB SAHARA					16	16	25	41							
HARAPPA	4	3	5		15	51	16	2							

TABLE LX. Upper First Molar Area (L*B): Frequency Distribution in Percentiles.

FREQUENCY DISTRIBUTION OF UPPER M1 L*B

	41	57	73	89	105	121	137	153	169	185	201	217	233	249	265
H.AFRICAN.							13	31	45	4	4				
H.ROBUSTUS								4	19	33	23	4	4	9	
H.ERECTUS					6	31	12	31	12	6					
H.NEANDER			1	3	16	25	40	4	4	3					
H.SAPIENS	1		1	7	29	33	21	5	1						
AUSTRALOP							4	17	34	19	14	2	2	4	
KRAPINA					7	21	42		21	7					
NEANDERTAL			2	4	18	32	32	6		2					
MT CARMEL					22		77								
CAUCASOID				9	47	20	16	3	1						
INDIAN					20	41	37								
AUSTRALOID						23	38	28	9						
NEW BRITAI					11	40	34	12	1						
DICKSON MD				3	27	39	25	2	1						
SUB SAHARA				12	3	33	33	12							
MALAY				21	47	26	5								
HARAPPA	7		1	17	43	26	2								

range of variation, as well as the range of variation for *H. erectus.*

There do not seem to be great differences in variability for either length or breadth (Table LVI). The slight tendency for increasing length variability just borders on significance. Compared to the coefficients of variation for the Liberian chimpanzee (Table LXXXII) of 5.0 and 4.1, the values for all hominid taxa are high. Indeed, only 4 of 24 available extant groups have a lower coefficient for length, and 4 of 21 for breadth (Table LVI). Other non-hominoid primate species range from 3.5 to 10.4 in coefficient of length variability, and from 4.7 to 10.2 in coefficient of breadth variability (Table LXXXII).

Both area and module (Table LVII) follow the common posterior pattern of variation, as could be expected. The difference between *H. africanus* and *H. robustus* is less than the maximum difference among extant groups. The only difference between temporally adjacent taxa which exceeds the australopithecine difference is between *H. robustus* and *H. erectus.* The frequency distribution for area (Table LX) shows that only about 13% of the 2 australopithecine taxa do not overlap with each other. A greater percentage, 40%, of the *H. robustus* specimens do not overlap with *H. erectus.* Thus, it seems clear that most differences among taxa border on significance while the total pattern of reduction is quite significant.

The L/B index does not undergo any significant change among the hominid taxa. There is more variation among extant groups (Table LVII).

LOWER SECOND MOLAR

Length and breadth variation (Table LXI), as well as area and module (Table LXII) follows the common posterior pattern. The length and breadth differences between temporally adjacent hominid taxa are, even at maximum, within the range of variation for extant groups. Indeed, the difference in length between the australopithecines is less than that between 1 group of American "Whites" and Ohio "Whites." On the other hand, the maximum difference

TABLE LXI. Lower Second Molar Length and Breadth: Mean, Standard Error of the Mean (SE(M)), Range, Sample Size (N), and Coefficient of Variation (CV).

LOWER M2	LENGTH(M-D)					BREADTH(B-L)				
	MEAN	SE(M)	RANGE	N	CV	MEAN	SE(M)	RANGE	N	CV
H. AFRICANUS	15.34	.23	14.30 - 16.80	14	5.5	14.29	.19	13.20 - 15.30	15	5.0
H. ROBUSTUS	15.78	.27	13.30 - 17.40	23	8.1	14.67	.24	12.30 - 16.20	23	7.8
H. ERECTUS	12.89	.14	11.30 - 14.20	27	5.6	12.46	.17	11.10 - 14.30	26	6.7
H. NEANDERTAL	11.78	.11	9.50 - 13.70	65	7.7	11.18	.08	9.90 - 12.60	67	5.6
H. SAPIENS	11.22	.05	8.70 - 15.40	531	9.3	10.63	.04	7.00 - 13.20	529	8.7
AUSTRALOPITHECINES	15.61	.19	13.30 - 17.40	37	7.3	14.52	.17	12.30 - 16.20	38	6.9
KRAPINA	11.97	.24	10.30 - 13.60	16	7.7	11.24	.16	9.90 - 12.50	16	5.6
NEANDERTAL	11.83	.13	10.10 - 13.70	43	6.9	11.21	.09	10.00 - 12.60	45	5.6
MT CARMEL	10.92	.51	9.50 - 12.60	6	10.4	10.87	.27	10.00 - 11.65	6	5.6
AUSTR. ABORIGINE	12.50	.00	10.00 - 14.25	152	.0	11.70	.00	10.00 - 13.50	184	.0
AMERICAN NEGROS	12.00	.22	10.30 - 13.60	17	7.4	10.90	.22	9.60 - 12.20	17	8.2
WADI HALFA MESOL.	11.80	.00	9.90 - 13.40	8	.0	11.50	.00	9.50 - 13.20	8	.0
AUSTRALOID	11.78	.15	10.00 - 14.00	37	7.9	11.34	.10	10.40 - 12.60	37	5.3
SUB SAHARAN	11.64	.15	9.50 - 15.40	60	10.0	10.97	.11	9.00 - 13.20	61	8.0
DICKSON MOUND	11.51	.07	9.60 - 13.50	118	6.9	10.83	.06	9.65 - 12.60	117	5.9
E.GREENLAND ESKIMO	11.44	.10	10.30 - 12.80	34	5.1	10.85	.11	8.50 - 12.00	35	6.0
PECOS PUEBLO	11.41	.06	10.27 - 12.85	62	4.0	10.47	.06	9.49 - 11.71	62	4.5
NEW BRITAIN	11.27	.10	9.20 - 13.10	67	7.2	10.96	.08	9.50 - 12.50	65	5.9
ALEUTS	11.17	.10	9.50 - 12.80	79	7.6	10.45	.07	8.70 - 11.60	82	6.2
MALAY	11.16	.16	9.50 - 12.20	17	5.6	10.33	.12	9.60 - 11.60	19	4.9
INDIAN	11.10	.15	9.00 - 12.70	31	7.4	10.87	.12	9.50 - 12.30	32	6.3
GILIMANUK (INDON.)	11.10	.00	9.50 - 12.60	50	.0	10.70	.00	9.20 - 11.90	50	.0
NATUFIANS	11.05	.11		16	4.0	10.62	.08		16	3.0
JARMO	11.00	.00		6	.0	10.10	.00		6	.0
SWEDES	10.91	.03		516	6.2					
JAPANESE	10.90	.03		186	3.8	10.40	.03		186	3.9
AMERICAN WHITES(2)	10.90	.10	10.40 - 11.40	13	3.2	10.10	.13	9.50 - 11.20	13	4.5
CAUCASOID	10.87	.09	8.70 - 13.30	109	8.5	10.59	.07	8.70 - 12.50	108	7.2
JAVANESE	10.79	.06		170	6.7	10.43	.05		171	6.3
TRISTANITES	10.65	.05		200	6.7	11.05	.06		152	6.7
BUSHMEN	10.60	.00	9.30 - 11.50	32	.0	10.10	.00	8.50 - 11.30	32	.0
AMERICAN WHITES(1)	10.55	.07	9.20 - 12.50	106	6.4					
OHIO WHITES	10.38	.04		294	5.9					
LAPPS	10.31	.03	8.60 - 12.50	558	6.7	9.83	.03	8.00 - 11.60	576	6.1
HARAPPA, INDIA	9.92	.10	9.00 - 11.50	53	7.2	9.59	.17	7.00 - 12.00	51	12.5
YEMEN JEWS	9.90	.10		41	6.6	9.61	.08		41	5.5
COCHINI JEWS	9.67	.09		46	6.0	9.45	.07		46	4.8

TABLE LXII. Lower Second Molar Area (L*B), Index (100L/B), and Module ((L+B)/2): Mean, Range, and Coefficient of Variation (CV).

LOWER M2	L*B			100L/B			(L+B)/2		
	MEAN	RANGE	CV	MEAN	RANGE	CV	MEAN	RANGE	CV
H. AFRICANUS	218.9	188.8 - 257.0	9.9	107.7	98.0 - 115.6	3.9	14.8	13.7 - 16.0	4.9
H. ROBUSTUS	232.8	163.6 - 281.9	15.2	107.6	101.4 - 117.2	3.9	15.2	12.8 - 16.8	7.7
H. ERECTUS	160.9	129.9 - 201.6	10.7	103.8	96.0 - 125.0	6.8	12.7	11.4 - 14.2	5.3
H. NEANDERTAL	132.1	99.7 - 169.9	11.9	105.4	90.5 - 119.4	6.3	11.5	10.0 - 13.0	6.0
H. SAPIENS	119.9	67.5 - 203.3	15.7	106.0	79.2 - 153.5	9.3	10.9	8.2 - 14.3	7.9
AUSTRALOPITHECINES	227.5	163.6 - 281.9	13.8	107.7	98.0 - 117.2	3.8	15.1	12.8 - 16.8	6.9
KRAPINA	134.9	102.0 - 160.8	11.9	106.6	94.4 - 119.3	5.4	11.6	10.1 - 12.7	6.1
NEANDERTAL	132.9	102.0 - 169.9	11.1	105.7	95.2 - 119.4	6.1	11.5	10.1 - 13.0	5.6
MT CARMEL	119.0	99.7 - 146.8	14.5	100.4	90.5 - 113.0	9.1	10.9	10.0 - 12.1	7.1
AUSTRALOID	134.0	106.0 - 175.0	11.8	103.9	84.9 - 117.9	6.2	11.6	10.3 - 13.2	6.0
SUB SAHARAN	128.7	90.0 - 203.3	17.6	105.9	95.7 - 116.7	5.1	11.3	9.5 - 14.3	8.7
DICKSON MOUND	125.1	95.1 - 170.1	11.9	106.3	91.7 - 123.8	5.0	11.2	9.7 - 13.0	6.0
NEW BRITAIN	123.8	91.2 - 163.7	12.1	102.8	89.0 - 115.9	5.1	11.1	9.5 - 12.8	6.1
INDIAN	121.0	94.0 - 153.7	12.9	102.3	86.1 - 113.6	5.4	11.0	9.7 - 12.4	6.5
CAUCASOID	115.7	75.7 - 158.7	14.1	103.0	79.2 - 123.1	6.9	10.7	8.7 - 12.6	7.1
MALAY	115.4	96.9 - 129.8	8.7	108.2	93.1 - 119.6	6.2	10.7	9.8 - 11.4	4.4
HARAPPA, INDIA	95.5	67.5 - 132.0	17.1	104.8	81.8 - 142.9	12.3	9.7	8.2 - 11.5	8.3

TABLE LXIII. Lower Second Molar Length: Frequency Distribution in Percentiles.

FREQUENCY DISTRIBUTION OF LOWER M2 L(M-D)

	8.5	9.1	9.7	10.3	10.9	11.5	12.1	12.7	13.3	13.9	14.5	15.1	15.7	16.3	16.9
H.AFRICAN.										21	21	35		21	
H.ROBUSTUS									13	4	13	13	13	43	
H.ERECTUS					3	7	33	29	11	14					
H.NEANDER.		1	3	10	18	30	21	7	6						
H.SAPIENS	3	3	10	16	24	22	11	4	2	1		1			
AUSTRALOP.									8	10	16	21	8	35	
KRAPINA				12	18	18	31	6	12						
NEANDERTAL		2	4	10	18	34	18	8	4						
MT CARMEL		16	16	16	16	16	16								
CAUCASOID	1	7	17	20	27	15	7	2	1						
INDIAN	3	3	9	22	19	38		3							
AUSTRALOID			2	16	16	35	13	10	2	2					
NEW BRITAI		4	2	20	29	22	16	2							
DICKSON MD		1	6	11	26	28	20	4	1						
MALAY		5		11	47	29	5								
SUB SAHARA		1	4	21	21	19	16	3	4	3		1			
HARAPPA	26	7	39	9	15	1									

TABLE LXIV. Lower Second Molar Breadth: Frequency Distribution in Percentiles.

FREQUENCY DISTRIBUTION OF LOWER M2 B(B-L)

	6.8	7.5	8.2	8.9	9.6	10.3	11.0	11.7	12.4	13.1	13.8	14.5	15.2	15.9	16.6
H.AFRICAN.										26	26	39	6		
H.ROBUSTUS								4	4	8	21	30	4	26	
H.ERECTUS							23	19	38	15	3				
H.NEANDER.					11	11	56	14	4						
H.SAPIENS	1	1	2	8	19	29	27	10	1	1					
AUSTRALOP.								2	2	15	23	34	5	15	
KRAPINA					12	6	68	6	6						
NEANDERTAL					11	13	52	17	3						
MT CARMEL					16	33	50								
CAUCASOID			2	3	30	24	30	6	1						
INDIAN				3	15	37	28	15							
AUSTRALOID						18	48	27	5						
NEW BRITAI				3	9	33	38	13	1						
DICKSON MD					19	40	29	10	1						
MALAY					47	42	10								
SUB SAHARA				3	21	22	31	14	4	1					
HARAPPA	1	11	3	39	9	19	7	5							

TABLE LXV. Lower Second Molar Area (L*B): Frequency Distribution in Percentiles.

FREQUENCY DISTRIBUTION OF LOWER M2 L*B

	66	81	96	111	126	141	156	171	186	201	216	231	246	261	276
H.AFRICAN.									21	42	7	7	21		
H.ROBUSTUS							4	8	8	4	26	8	13	26	
H.ERECTUS					7	26	46	11	3	3					
H.NEANDER.			9	30	29	24	6								
H.SAPIENS	1	8	21	32	22	9	2	1		1					
AUSTRALOP.							2	5	13	18	18	8	16	16	
KRAPINA			12	18	31	31	6								
NEANDERTAL			4	34	30	23	6								
MT CARMEL			33	33	16	16									
CAUCASOID	1	10	32	30	17	7	1								
INDIAN		6	22	32	25	12									
AUSTRALOID			8	27	29	27	5	2							
NEW BRITAI		3	15	43	24	10	3								
DICKSON MD		1	17	39	27	12	2								
SUB SAHARA		3	15	26	31	8	6	4		1					
MALAY				99											
HARAPPA	15	47	19	9	7										

between any 2 taxa far exceeds the extant maximum. Thus, for both length and breadth the differences among taxa are not taxonomically significant, while the general reduction trend is.

For both these diameters, *H. neanderthalensis* falls within the range of variation of extant groups, as do the Krapina Neandertals.

With respect to area (Table LXII), the difference between the australopithecines falls within the extant group range of variation. However, the difference between *H. robustus* and *H. erectus* is almost double this range. Thus, these 2 taxa show a significant difference. *H. neanderthalensis* falls within the extant group range of variation, and the Krapina Neandertals exceed this range by only .9 mm^2. The reduction trend in area is quite significant. Module varies in a similar manner. On the other hand, there is almost no variation of the L/B index either among taxa or extant groups.

For both length and breadth (Tables LXIII and LXIV), the frequency distributions of *H. robustus* are bimodal. In both cases, *H. africanus* falls completely within the range of variation for *H. robustus* *H. erectus* falls further outside this range: only 17% overlap in length, although there is a 75% overlap in breadth. *H. africanus* is also bimodal for breadth.

The distribution for area (Table LXV) is bimodal for *H. africanus* and *H. robustus.* The agreement of specimen placement with lower canine area (Table XXV) and first lower molar length (Table LV) is quite good. There is an 83% overlap between the area distributions of the 2 australopithecine taxa. Although the average areas of *H. robustus* and *H. erectus* are significantly different, 56% of the *H. robustus* specimens fall within the *H. erectus* range of variation. *H. erectus,* in turn, falls completely within the range of variation for *H. neanderthalensis.*

Variability for both length and breadth (Table LXI) shows a slight tendency for increase. The length and breadth coefficients of variation for the Liberian chimpanzee are 5.3 and 4.2 (Table LXXXIII). With the exception of length in *H. africanus,* the values for every other hominid taxon exceed these. The hominids are thus significantly more variable than this chimpanzee sample. Coefficients for other non-human primate samples vary from 3.5 to 10.4 in length, and 4.8 to 9.8 in breadth. This range exceeds that of the hominid taxa, as well as that of almost all of the extant groups.

UPPER SECOND MOLAR

The common posterior dental pattern is followed by length and breadth (Table LXVI) as well as area and module (Table LXVII) for the second upper molar. For length and breadth, the differences between the australopithecines fall well within the range of variation for extant groups. However, the differences between *H. robustus* and *H. erectus* is mean value exceed this range, although in breadth this excess is very slight.

The values for *H. neanderthalensis* fall within the extant group range of variation, as do the values for the 3 groups within this taxon. The total reduction of both length and breadth in this tooth is quite significant.

These patterns are reflected in the frequency distributions. The distribution for length (Table LVIII) shows *H. africanus* overlapping *H. robustus* by 80%, while the overlap of *H. erectus* with the latter is only 9%. The breadth overlaps are more extensive (Table LXIX). *H. africanus* falls completely within the *H. robustus* range, although 66% of the *H. erectus* sample falls outside of the australopithecine range. Breadth for *H. africanus, H. robustus,* and *H. erectus* is slightly bimodal. On the other hand, the sizes of the modes are by no means equal within each taxon.

For area and module (Table LXVII), the difference between the australopithecines is significantly less than the greatest difference among extant groups. However, the latter is exceeded by the difference between *either* australopithecine group and *H. erectus. H. neanderthalensis,* and the sample groups which individually comprise it, falls within the range of variation for extant groups. The area frequency distribution (Table LXX) shows the complete inclusion of *H. africanus* within the range of variation of *H. robustus. H. erectus,* on the other hand, has a 20% overlap with the latter. The other 80% overlaps with the range of *H. neanderthalensis.* Of these distributions, *H. erectus* shows a slight bimodality.

The L/B index (Table LXVII) does not vary greatly within the hominid taxa. There is greater variation of this index within extant groups.

Changes in variability for both length and breadth (Table LXVI) are not consistent. Compared with the non-human primates, however, the hominid taxa are generally more variable (Table LXXXIII). The coefficients of variation for the Liberian chimpanzee length and breadth are 5.8 and 5.1. These exceed the values for all hominid taxa, except length for *H. africanus* (5.2). Most extant groups are also exceeded by these values. The ranges of the coefficient for other primates represented are 3.5 to 10.4 in length, and 4.7 to 10.2 in breadth. Consequently, almost all of the extant group values fall within these ranges.

LOWER THIRD MOLAR

Length, breadth, area, and module (Tables LXXI and LXXII) follow the common posterior pattern of variation. The differences between taxa are greatest for length. The difference between the australopithecine taxa is less than the maximum among extant groups (2.31 mm). However, the difference between either australopithecine taxon and *H. erectus* exceeds the maximum extant group difference. The frequency distribution for length (Table LXXIII) shows that all but 9% of the *H. africanus* specimens fall within the *H. robustus* range of variation. However, only 26% of the *H. erectus* specimens fall within this range, and only 33% fall within the range for *H. africanus. H. neanderthalensis,* and all of the groups within this taxon, falls inside of the extant group range of variation for length as well as breadth.

The breadth differences among taxa are slightly less, although they follow the same pattern. Thus, the frequency distribution for breadth (Table LXXIV) shows a complete overlap between the australopithecines. Over 45% of the *H. erectus* specimens fall within the range of variation for *H. robustus.*

Area and module (Table LXXII) vary greatly among taxa. The difference between the australopithecines is less than the maximum between either australopithecine taxon and *H. erectus,* and exceeds the modern maximum difference. The frequency distribution for area (Table LXXV)

TABLE LXVI. Upper Second Molar Length and Breadth: Mean, Standard Error of the Mean (SE(M)), Range, Sample Size (N), and Coefficient of Variation (CV).

UPPER M2	LENGTH(M-D) MEAN	SE(M)	RANGE	N	CV	BREADTH(B-L) MEAN	SE(M)	RANGE	N	CV
H. AFRICANUS	13.71	.17	12.70 - 15.10	19	5.2	15.36	.23	13.80 - 17.10	19	6.2
H. ROBUSTUS	14.86	.21	13.60 - 17.20	22	6.5	16.31	.38	14.20 - 21.00	22	10.8
H. ERECTUS	11.33	.34	10.00 - 13.60	15	11.1	13.45	.37	11.90 - 16.30	15	10.3
H. NEANDERTAL	10.61	.14	8.35 - 13.00	51	9.6	12.49	.14	10.00 - 14.50	50	7.7
H. SAPIENS	10.25	.05	7.00 - 16.00	450	10.5	11.51	.06	7.00 - 14.75	456	11.7
AUSTRALOPITHECINES	14.33	.16	12.70 - 17.20	41	7.2	15.87	.24	13.80 - 21.00	41	9.5
KRAPINA	10.66	.34	8.35 - 12.00	11	10.1	12.46	.33	10.60 - 14.00	11	8.4
NEANDERTAL	10.72	.17	9.00 - 13.00	32	8.7	12.65	.18	10.00 - 14.50	31	7.8
MT CARMEL	10.09	.47	8.60 - 12.20	8	12.3	11.87	.16	11.10 - 12.30	8	3.5
WADI HALFA MESOL.	11.10	.00	9.70 - 11.70	9	.0	12.30	.00	11.20 - 13.20	9	.0
AMERICAN NEGROS	11.00	.22	9.70 - 13.20	19	8.5	12.20	.16	10.60 - 13.30	19	5.5
SUB SAHARAN	10.99	.26	9.50 - 14.10	25	11.6	12.20	.23	10.00 - 14.30	26	9.3
AUSTR. ABORIGINE	10.93	.00	10.00 - 12.50	168	.0	13.10	.00	11.00 - 16.00	241	.0
AUSTRALOID	10.92	.14	9.60 - 12.10	24	6.2	13.03	.24	10.30 - 14.50	28	9.6
NATUFIANS	10.52	.17		11	5.0	12.14	.13		11	3.3
AMERICAN WHITES(2)	10.40	.22	9.70 - 12.00	9	6.1	11.20	.39	8.60 - 12.30	9	9.7
NEW BRITAIN	10.36	.08	8.40 - 11.80	70	6.7	12.18	.10	10.75 - 14.00	70	6.9
SWEDES	10.24	.03		327	5.3					
JARMO	10.20	.00		5	.0	11.40	.00		5	.0
DICKSON MOUND	10.20	.07	7.90 - 12.00	119	7.5	11.88	.08	10.00 - 14.75	119	7.0
E.GREENLAND ESKIMO	10.18	.07	8.70 - 11.50	55	5.1	11.54	.09	10.00 - 12.50	53	5.7
AMERICAN WHITES(1)	10.12	.05	8.30 - 11.80	115	5.7					
INDIAN	10.11	.16	8.80 - 11.80	24	7.8	11.93	.17	10.75 - 13.40	24	6.9
GILIMANUK (INDON.)	10.00	.00	8.10 - 12.20	46	.0	11.40	.00	9.50 - 12.60	45	.0
PECOS PUEBLO	9.94	.05	8.88 - 10.83	79	4.8	11.24	.07	9.88 - 12.60	79	5.6
ALEUTS	9.93	.07	8.00 - 11.50	92	6.3	11.33	.09	9.90 - 13.20	69	6.5
TRISTANITES	9.91	.06		205	8.7	12.20	.07		131	6.6
JAVANESE	9.90	.05		164	7.0	11.51	.06		164	6.2
OHIO WHITES	9.81	.03		351	6.1					
MALAY	9.81	.19	8.30 - 11.10	17	7.6	11.43	.15	10.20 - 12.40	18	5.3
CAUCASOID	9.76	.16	7.00 - 11.50	44	10.6	11.52	.16	9.00 - 13.30	44	9.0
BUSHMEN	9.70	.00	8.80 - 10.80	30	.0	10.60	.00	9.80 - 12.00	30	.0
JAPANESE	9.70	.03		198	4.3	11.40	.03		198	3.7
HARAPPA, INDIA	9.62	.09	7.00 - 11.50	92	8.9	10.52	.12	7.00 - 12.50	92	11.1
COCHINI JEWS	9.50	.08		47	6.0	10.39	.09		47	6.0
YEMEN JEWS	9.46	.14		31	7.9	10.42	.15		31	7.8
MODERN ENGLISH	9.42	.06		83	5.7	11.32	.08		85	6.8
LAPPS	9.13	.03	7.10 - 11.00	585	6.9	10.64	.03	8.60 - 12.70	548	7.0

TABLE LXVII. Upper Second Molar Area (L*B), Index (100L/B), and Module ((L+B)/2): Mean, Range, and Coefficient of Variation (CV).

UPPER M2	L*B MEAN	RANGE	CV	100L/B MEAN	RANGE	CV	(L+B)/2 MEAN	RANGE	CV
H. AFRICANUS	210.9	180.8 - 258.2	10.5	89.4	83.1 - 95.4	4.8	14.5	13.4 - 16.1	5.2
H. ROBUSTUS	243.8	194.5 - 361.2	17.5	91.6	81.9 - 103.5	6.2	15.6	13.9 - 19.1	8.4
H. ERECTUS	153.5	119.0 - 214.1	20.3	84.4	71.9 - 100.0	8.5	12.4	10.9 - 14.7	9.8
H. NEANDERTAL	132.5	94.4 - 182.0	14.4	85.0	70.6 - 113.0	9.9	11.5	9.8 - 13.5	7.1
H. SAPIENS	118.1	56.0 - 195.9	17.6	90.3	65.6 - 171.4	16.5	10.9	7.5 - 14.0	8.8
AUSTRALOPITHECINES	228.6	180.8 - 361.2	16.7	90.6	81.9 - 103.5	5.7	15.1	13.4 - 19.1	7.9
KRAPINA	133.5	94.4 - 168.0	16.3	85.7	73.9 - 97.2	8.8	11.6	9.8 - 13.0	8.1
NEANDERTAL	135.4	100.8 - 182.0	13.3	84.8	70.6 - 113.0	10.0	11.7	10.1 - 13.5	6.6
MT CARMEL	119.8	103.2 - 146.4	13.1	85.0	71.7 - 101.7	12.3	11.0	10.2 - 12.1	6.1
AUSTRALOID	142.2	105.6 - 174.2	14.2	84.8	74.6 - 107.5	10.5	11.9	10.3 - 13.2	7.4
SUB SAHARAN	135.0	95.0 - 195.9	20.3	90.3	79.2 - 102.9	6.8	11.6	9.7 - 14.0	9.9
NEW BRITAIN	126.5	102.3 - 165.2	11.8	85.1	65.6 - 96.6	6.9	11.3	10.1 - 12.9	5.9
DICKSON MOUND	121.7	88.0 - 177.0	13.6	86.0	70.5 - 102.5	5.5	11.0	9.4 - 13.4	6.8
INDIAN	120.8	94.6 - 149.9	11.6	85.0	73.6 - 106.3	9.0	11.0	9.8 - 12.2	5.8
CAUCASOID	113.2	63.0 - 149.0	17.3	84.9	67.2 - 107.4	8.3	10.6	8.0 - 12.2	8.9
MALAY	112.3	88.7 - 129.9	10.8	85.9	74.1 - 96.4	7.4	10.6	9.4 - 11.4	5.4
HARAPPA, INDIA	101.5	56.0 - 132.0	16.2	92.2	68.2 - 122.2	12.0	10.1	7.5 - 11.5	8.4

TABLE LXVIII. Upper Second Molar Length: Frequency Distribution in Percentiles.

FREQUENCY DISTRIBUTION OF UPPER M2 L(M-D)

	6.8	7.5	8.2	8.9	9.6	10.3	11.0	11.7	12.4	13.1	13.8	14.5	15.2	15.9	16.6
H.AFRICAN.									21	31	31	15			
H.ROBUSTUS										9	22	40	18	9	
H.ERECTUS					26	19	19	6	13	13					
H.NEANDER.			3	13	19	21	25	13	1						
H.SAPIENS	1	1	4	17	28	24	14	4	1	1	1			1	
AUSTRALOP.									9	19	26	29	9	4	
KRAPINA			9		27	18	27	18							
NEANDERTAL			2	17	17	22	25	12	2						
MT CARMEL			12	25	25	12	12	12							
CAUCASOID	2	4	11	11	36	22	11								
INDIAN			4	20	45	12	8	8							
AUSTRALOID					20	20	50	8							
NEW BRITAI			1	11	32	28	24	1							
DICKSON MD		1	2	17	26	40	8	3							
MALAY			17	11	47	17	5								
SUB SAHARA				3	27	23	19	7	7	3	3				
HARAPPA	1	4	7	39	27	9	10								

TABLE LXIX. Upper Second Molar Breadth: Frequency Distribution in Percentiles.

FREQUENCY DISTRIBUTION OF UPPER M2 B(B-L)

	6.8	7.8	8.8	9.8	10.8	11.8	12.8	13.8	14.8	15.8	16.8	17.8	18.8	19.8	20.8
H.AFRICAN								26	47	10	15				
H.ROBUSTUS								22	4	50	13			9	
H.ERECTUS						33	33	13	6	13					
H.NEANDER				3	19	33	31	9							
H.SAPIENS	1	3	3	14	32	28	12	3							
AUSTRALOP								24	24	31	14			4	
KRAPINA				9	18	18	45	9							
NEANDERTAL				2	20	38	28	10							
MT CARMEL					37	62									
CAUCASOID			6	13	29	38	11								
INDIAN				4	41	37	16								
AUSTRALOID				10	7	7	50	25							
NEW BRITAI				1	32	41	17	7							
DICKSON MD				8	39	39	10	1							
MALAY				16	55	27									
SUB SAHARA				15	15	34	30	3							
HARAPPA	2	7	5	35	38	10									

TABLE LXX. Upper Second Molar Area (L*B): Frequency Distribution in Percentiles.

FREQUENCY DISTRIBUTION OF UPPER M2 L*B

	54	75	96	117	138	159	180	201	222	243	264	285	306	327	348
H.AFRICAN.							42	31	15	10					
H.ROBUSTUS							9	22	22	31	4			9	
H.ERECTUS				33	39	6		19							
H.NEANDER.		1	21	35	29	7	1								
H.SAPIENS	1	11	33	38	11	2	1								
AUSTRALOP.							24	26	19	21	2			4	
KRAPINA		9	18	27	36	9									
NEANDERTAL			16	38	32	9	3								
MT CARMEL			50	37	12										
CAUCASOID	4	15	27	45	6										
INDIAN		4	33	50	12										
AUSTRALOID			12	25	41	20									
NEW BRITAI			27	50	10	2									
DICKSON MD		5	33	45	14	1									
SUB SAHARA		3	23	35	19	7	7								
MALAY		11	47	41											
HARAPPA	6	28	46	18											

shows a complete overlap between the australopithecine taxa. There is a 25% overlap of *H. erectus* with the australopithecines.

There is a clear reductive difference among the australopithecines and for the subsequent taxa. The overall trend for reduction is significant. Indeed, of all the mandibular teeth, the lower third molar shows the greatest reduction in length, breadth, and area.

The L/B index is almost identical for all the hominid taxa and extant groups, with the exception of *H. robustus*. In the latter, the index is significantly higher, indicating a relatively longer tooth. It might be pointed out that *H. robustus* is the only taxon for which the average for the third mandibular molar exceeds that for the second in all dimensions.

The distributions are bimodal for *H. robustus* in length, breadth, and area (Tables LXXIII LXXV). Indeed, the area distribution is actually *tri*modal. There is a slight bimodality for length in *H. erectus*.

With respect to the coefficient of variation, there is no consistent pattern of variability increase in length (Table LXXI). Both *H. erectus* and *H. sapiens* are more variable than the other taxa. Breadth, on the other hand, shows a smoother, although less significant, increase in variability. In comparison, the coefficients for other primates are less variable (Table LXXXIV). For the Liberian chimpanzee, the length and breadth values are 6.0 and 5.3. Every hominid taxon is more variable, as is almost every extant group in both dimensions.

UPPER THIRD MOLAR

Length and breadth (Table LXXVI), as well as area and module (Table LXXVII) of the upper third molar follow the common posterior pattern. For both length and breadth, the difference between the australopithecines is less than the maximum among extant groups. The difference between *H. robustus* and *H. erectus*, however, greatly exceeds this maximum extant

TABLE LXXI. Lower Third Molar Length and Breadth: Mean, Standard Error of the Mean (SE(M)), Range, Sample Size (N), and Coefficient of Variation (CV).

LOWER M3	LENGTH(M-D)					BREADTH(B-L)				
	MEAN	SE(M)	RANGE	N	CV	MEAN	SE(M)	RANGE	N	CV
H. AFRICANUS	15.17	.28	13.50 - 17.10	15	6.9	13.89	.22	12.70 - 15.70	15	6.0
H. ROBUSTUS	16.64	.33	13.90 - 18.80	20	8.6	14.42	.31	12.30 - 16.50	20	9.2
H. ERECTUS	12.56	.30	10.00 - 15.20	25	11.6	11.76	.21	10.00 - 14.60	25	8.6
H. NEANDERTAL	11.56	.14	8.30 - 13.60	55	8.7	10.87	.14	8.00 - 13.00	54	9.3
H. SAPIENS	11.11	.05	7.50 - 14.60	450	10.4	10.43	.05	6.50 - 13.50	448	10.5
AUSTRALOPITHECINES	16.01	.25	13.50 - 18.80	35	9.2	14.20	.20	12.30 - 16.50	35	8.2
KRAPINA	11.99	.19	11.10 - 13.60	15	6.1	10.88	.15	9.90 - 12.00	14	4.9
NEANDERTAL	11.47	.19	8.30 - 13.00	35	9.5	10.95	.20	8.00 - 13.00	35	10.8
MT CARMEL	10.94	.29	10.30 - 11.70	5	5.4	10.31	.21	9.90 - 10.95	5	4.1
AMERICAN NEGROS	12.00	.20	10.40 - 13.40	17	6.7	10.80	.16	9.30 - 12.00	17	6.0
AUSTR. ABORIGINE	11.90	.00	9.00 - 14.00	136	.0	11.10	.00	8.00 - 13.00	152	.0
WADI HALFA MESOL.	11.80	.00	10.90 - 13.50	6	.0	11.50	.00	10.70 - 12.40	6	.0
AUSTRALOID	11.62	.16	10.00 - 13.00	33	7.7	11.30	.16	9.80 - 13.30	33	7.9
NEW BRITAIN	11.52	.11	9.30 - 14.00	63	7.7	10.93	.08	9.60 - 12.50	60	6.0
E.GREENLAND ESKIMO	11.36	.13	10.10 - 12.80	27	6.0	10.81	.13	9.60 - 12.40	27	6.3
INDIAN	11.32	.17	9.30 - 13.50	32	8.6	10.88	.13	9.35 - 12.30	32	6.6
DICKSON MOUND	11.32	.10	8.65 - 13.90	101	9.1	10.58	.08	8.10 - 12.90	101	7.6
AMERICAN WHITES(2)	11.30	.20	9.20 - 12.60	22	8.1	10.10	.19	8.30 - 12.00	22	8.7
ALEUTS	11.22	.15	9.20 - 12.80	35	7.7	10.30	.11	9.00 - 11.60	30	5.6
SUB SAHARAN	11.15	.17	8.50 - 14.60	54	11.3	10.67	.15	8.00 - 12.90	52	9.7
SWEDES	11.14	.10		63	7.1					
PECOS PUEBLO	11.13	.08	9.97 - 12.24	62	5.9	10.10	.07	9.07 - 11.28	62	5.3
JARMO	11.10	.00		2	.0	10.80	.00		2	.0
NATUFIANS	10.90	.12		14	4.1	10.40	.16		13	5.2
GILIMANUK (INDON.)	10.90	.00	8.10 - 13.20	38	.0	10.40	.00	6.90 - 12.20	40	.0
JAVANESE	10.86	.07		126	6.7	10.35	.06		128	6.7
CAUCASOID	10.78	.11	7.70 - 13.00	80	9.4	10.35	.11	7.80 - 13.50	80	9.2
TRISTANITES	10.60	.09		88	7.9	11.30	.12		27	5.5
MALAY	10.30	.36	9.60 - 12.20	7	8.5	10.32	.14	9.70 - 11.20	11	4.3
JAPANESE	10.00	.06		114	6.4	10.00	.04		114	4.3
BUSHMEN	9.90	.00	8.00 - 11.00	33	.0	9.60	.00	8.00 - 10.50	33	.0
LAPPS	9.74	.04	6.50 - 12.20	356	8.3	9.36	.04	6.80 - 11.00	353	7.6
HARAPPA, INDIA	9.69	.13	7.50 - 12.00	45	9.0	9.26	.16	7.00 - 11.50	44	11.3

TABLE LXXII. Lower Third Molar Area (L*B), Index (100L/B), and Module ((L+B)/2): Mean, Range, and Coefficient of Variation (CV).

LOWER M3	L*B			100L/B			(L+B)/2		
	MEAN	RANGE	CV	MEAN	RANGE	CV	MEAN	RANGE	CV
H. AFRICANUS	211.3	174.0 - 268.5	11.9	109.2	97.2 - 116.2	5.2	14.5	13.2 - 16.4	5.9
H. ROBUSTUS	241.6	171.0 - 306.4	17.1	115.5	106.6 - 124.0	4.6	15.5	13.1 - 17.5	8.6
H. ERECTUS	148.6	100.0 - 214.6	17.9	106.9	91.6 - 138.2	9.8	12.2	10.0 - 14.6	9.0
H. NEANDERTAL	126.0	70.5 - 160.0	15.6	106.3	88.5 - 121.5	6.8	11.2	8.4 - 12.6	8.1
H. SAPIENS	116.4	59.5 - 188.3	17.9	107.2	77.8 - 187.7	11.7	10.8	7.7 - 13.7	9.0
AUSTRALOPITHECINES	228.6	171.0 - 306.4	16.6	112.8	97.2 - 124.0	5.5	15.1	13.1 - 17.5	8.3
KRAPINA	129.4	109.9 - 156.0	9.2	109.3	101.8 - 115.5	3.8	11.4	10.5 - 12.5	4.6
NEANDERTAL	126.5	70.5 - 160.0	17.8	105.1	88.5 - 121.5	8.0	11.2	8.4 - 12.6	9.3
MT CARMEL	113.0	104.0 - 128.1	9.3	106.1	102.0 - 108.6	2.3	10.6	10.2 - 11.3	4.6
AUSTRALOID	131.7	98.0 - 169.0	13.7	103.1	88.8 - 118.2	6.7	11.5	9.9 - 13.0	6.9
NEW BRITAIN	126.2	95.0 - 168.0	11.3	105.7	82.3 - 135.4	7.8	11.2	9.7 - 13.0	5.6
INDIAN	123.7	90.2 - 162.0	13.8	104.1	89.4 - 116.8	6.3	11.1	9.5 - 12.7	6.9
DICKSON MOUND	120.2	73.1 - 168.2	14.7	107.2	84.5 - 137.6	8.0	10.9	8.5 - 13.0	7.4
SUB SAHARAN	119.2	76.0 - 188.3	20.0	104.1	86.5 - 125.0	7.2	10.9	8.7 - 13.7	9.9
CAUCASOID	112.1	60.1 - 151.0	16.3	104.5	77.8 - 135.5	8.1	10.6	7.7 - 12.3	8.3
MALAY	104.4	94.1 - 130.5	11.8	101.7	95.0 - 114.0	5.9	10.2	9.7 - 11.4	5.8
HARAPPA, INDIA	90.2	59.5 - 126.0	17.2	105.5	81.8 - 129.4	10.7	9.5	7.7 - 11.2	8.6

TABLE LXXIII. Lower Third Molar Length: Frequency Distribution in Percentiles.

FREQUENCY DISTRIBUTION OF LOWER M3 L(M-D)

	7.3	8.1	8.9	9.7	10.5	11.3	12.1	12.9	13.7	14.5	15.3	16.1	16.9	17.7	18.5
H.AFRICAN.								6	19	26	33	6	6		
H.ROBUSTUS									9		29	14	14	29	
H.ERECTUS				7	11	11	31	7	11	15					
H.NEANDER.		1	1	9	25	34	14	12							
H.SAPIENS	1	1	8	18	25	26	12	4	1	1					
AUSTRALOP.								2	14	11	31	11	11	17	
KRAPINA					19	39	26	13							
NEANDERTAL		2	2	12	27	32	9	12							
MT CARMEL				19	39	39									
CAUCASOID	1		8	27	36	16	8	1							
INDIAN			6	9	31	34	12	6							
AUSTRALOID				9	30	30	15	15							
NEW BRITAI			1	9	17	52	11	6	1						
DICKSON MD		1	2	17	26	27	16	3	2						
MALAY			14	71			14								
SUB SAHARA		1	11	18	29	16	16	1		3					
HARAPPA	4	8	35	28	17	4									

TABLE LXXIV. Lower Third Molar Breadth: Frequency Distribution in Percentiles.

FREQUENCY DISTRIBUTION OF LOWER M3 B(B-L)

	6.3	7.0	7.7	8.4	9.1	9.8	10.5	11.2	11.9	12.6	13.3	14.0	14.7	15.4	16.1
H.AFRICAN.										26	26	26	13	6	
H.ROBUSTUS									9	14	14	9	19	29	
H.ERECTUS						7	19	23	35	7		3			
H.NEANDER.			1	3	5	12	44	14	9	7					
H.SAPIENS	1	1	2	7	10	23	33	12	5	1	1				
AUSTRALOP.									5	19	19	17	17	19	
KRAPINA						14	64	14	7						
NEANDERTAL			2	4	7	12	37	14	9	9					
MT CARMEL						59	39								
CAUCASOID			1	1	23	32	28	7	3		1				
INDIAN					6	18	43	21	9						
AUSTRALOID						15	39	21	12	9	3				
NEW BRITAI					1	19	39	28	9						
DICKSON MD			1	2	6	33	37	10	4	1					
MALAY					9	54	27	9							
SUB SAHARA			5		11	15	40	15	7	3					
HARAPPA		9	2	45	15	9	15	2							

TABLE LXXV. Lower Third Molar Area (L*B): Frequency Distribution in Percentiles.

FREQUENCY DISTRIBUTION OF LOWER M3 L*B

	58	75	92	109	126	143	160	177	194	211	228	245	262	279	296
H.AFRICAN.							13		46	19	6	6	6		
H.ROBUSTUS							4	4	19	9	14	9	9	25	
H.ERECTUS			7	7	27	27	11	11		3					
H.NEANDER.	1	3	14	24	33	20	1								
H.SAPIENS	1	9	24	30	24	7	1	1							
AUSTRALOP.							8	2	31	14	11	8	8	14	
KRAPINA				28	64	7									
NEANDERTAL	2	5	14	22	22	28	2								
MT CARMEL			59	19	19										
CAUCASOID	1	11	31	31	13	6									
INDIAN		3	12	40	31	9	3								
AUSTRALOID			12	27	30	24	6								
NEW BRITAI			9	39	39	8	1								
DICKSON MD	1	1	24	34	29	5	1								
SUB SAHARA		11	21	32	19	11		3							
MALAY															
HARAPPA	11	45	29	11	2										

difference. In length, the difference between *H. africanus* and *H. erectus* also exceeds the extant maximum difference, while in breadth the difference between these taxa is within the modern extant range. Variation of the third maxillary molar among taxa is the greatest of all the maxillary molars, and its subsequent size reduction is consequently greatest. Although *H. neanderthalensis* falls within the range of variation of *H. sapiens* groups, the Krapina Neandertals fall outside this range for both length and breadth.

The frequency distribution of length (Table LXXVIII) shows 27% of the *H. africanus* specimens outside the range of *H. robustus* variation, and all specimens of *H. erectus* fall outside this range. *H. erectus,* however, falls completely within the *H. neanderthalensis* range of variation. None of the length distributions are bimodal. The breadth distribution (Table LXXIX) shows only 9% of the *H. erectus* specimens falling outside this range, but within the range of *H. neanderthalensis.* No breadth distributions are bimodal.

Area and module (Table LXXVII) variation between the australopithecines, and between either australopithecine taxon and *H. erectus,* greatly exceeds the maximum among extant groups (34.4 mm^2). The significance of the reduction in upper third molar size is most visible using area as a measure. The frequency distribution for area (Table LXXX) shows 20% of the *H. robustus* specimens outside the range of *H. africanus* variation, while 81% of the *H. erectus* specimens fall outside this range, but within the range for *H. neanderthalensis.* There is absolutely no overlap between *H. robustus* and *H. erectus.* None of the area distributions are significantly bimodal.

The L/B index (Table LXXVII) does not vary significantly among the hominid taxa or among the extant groups.

The variability for length clearly increases to the maximum value in *H. sapiens.* With respect to breadth, the trend of increasing variability is also present. However, coefficients of variation for both *H. erectus* and *H. sapiens* are maximum.

TABLE LXXVI. Upper Third Molar Length and Breadth: Mean, Standard Error of the Mean (SE(M)), Range, Sample Size (N), and Coefficient of Variation (CV).

UPPER M3	LENGTH(M-D)					BREADTH(B-L)				
	MEAN	SE(M)	RANGE	N	CV	MEAN	SE(M)	RANGE	N	CV
H. AFRICANUS	13.14	.33	11.60 - 15.20	11	7.8	15.14	.41	12.75 - 17.90	11	8.6
H. ROBUSTUS	15.23	.21	12.80 - 17.00	24	6.7	17.10	.30	15.10 - 21.40	24	8.3
H. ERECTUS	10.22	.23	8.70 - 12.00	18	9.1	12.59	.44	10.40 - 16.90	18	14.5
H. NEANDERTAL	9.90	.18	8.30 - 13.00	39	11.3	11.72	.17	9.00 - 14.00	40	8.8
H. SAPIENS	9.49	.07	7.00 - 15.00	331	13.5	10.84	.08	5.00 - 14.40	336	14.1
AUSTRALOPITHECINES	14.54	.24	11.60 - 17.00	36	9.6	16.49	.28	12.75 - 21.40	35	10.0
KRAPINA	10.52	.47	10.00 - 12.20	5	9.0	12.40	.11	12.00 - 12.50	5	1.8
NEANDERTAL	9.80	.22	8.30 - 13.00	28	11.4	11.61	.22	9.00 - 14.00	29	9.9
MT CARMEL	9.87	.58	8.60 - 11.90	6	13.1	11.70	.29	11.00 - 12.50	6	5.5
JARMO	10.40	.00		1	.0	10.70	.00		1	.0
SUB SAHARAN	10.05	.37	8.00 - 13.30	20	15.9	11.43	.36	8.00 - 13.10	17	12.6
AUSTR. ABORIGINE	10.03	.00	8.00 - 13.00	142	.0	12.33	.00	10.00 - 15.00	193	.0
AUSTRALOID	9.99	.24	8.00 - 11.40	22	11.0	12.33	.29	9.40 - 14.40	24	11.2
AMERICAN NEGROS	9.80	.30	7.60 - 13.40	18	12.6	11.50	.30	9.70 - 14.10	18	10.8
E.GREENLAND ESKIMO	9.60	.15	8.00 - 11.10	35	9.3	11.13	.13	8.30 - 13.00	35	6.9
AMERICAN WHITES(2)	9.60	.24	7.70 - 11.90	23	11.7	10.90	.27	8.10 - 13.20	23	11.7
INDIAN	9.44	.27	7.40 - 10.70	14	10.1	11.03	.27	9.30 - 12.60	14	9.0
NEW BRITAIN	9.43	.11	7.80 - 12.00	52	8.3	11.65	.12	10.00 - 13.60	55	7.5
WADI HALFA MESOL.	9.40	.00	8.30 - 10.70	10	.0	11.80	.00	10.60 - 13.40	10	.0
GILIMANUK (INDON.)	9.40	.00	7.00 - 11.30	33	.0	11.30	.00	9.30 - 12.60	33	.0
MALAY	9.36	.39	8.50 - 10.20	5	8.4	11.13	.25	10.40 - 12.00	7	5.5
PECOS PUEBLO	9.36	.07	7.89 - 10.70	84	6.4	10.57	.06	9.24 - 12.49	84	5.4
NATUFIANS	9.34	.28		8	7.9	11.30	.26		8	6.0
SWEDES	9.28	.14		40	9.6					
JAVANESE	9.18	.08		127	10.1	11.08	.09		127	8.8
DICKSON MOUND	9.17	.10	7.20 - 11.80	88	9.8	11.07	.10	8.90 - 13.80	89	8.1
ALEUTS	9.10	.12	7.10 - 11.20	42	8.2	10.75	.17	7.30 - 12.50	31	8.5
CAUCASOID	8.93	.18	7.30 - 11.50	38	12.1	11.14	.20	9.00 - 14.00	38	10.8
HARAPPA, INDIA	8.93	.11	7.00 - 11.00	61	9.8	9.97	.17	6.50 - 12.50	61	12.8
TRISTANITES	8.88	.07		119	8.6	11.96	.14		52	8.4
MODERN ENGLISH	8.71	.11		49	8.6	10.99	.12		34	6.5
JAPANESE	8.70	.06		102	7.0	10.60	.06		102	5.8
BUSHMEN	8.20	.00	7.00 - 9.80	26	.0	10.30	.00	9.30 - 12.00	26	.0
LAPPS	7.95	.04	5.00 - 10.40	366	9.7	9.69	.05	5.30 - 11.90	355	9.9

TABLE LXXVII. Upper Third Molar Area (L*B), Index (100L/B), and Module ((L+B)/2): Mean, Range, and Coefficient of Variation (CV).

UPPER M3	L*B			100L/B			(L+B)/2		
	MEAN	RANGE	CV	MEAN	RANGE	CV	MEAN	RANGE	CV
H. AFRICANUS	199.7	171.7 - 272.1	15.5	87.0	78.4 - 105.9	8.0	14.1	13.1 - 16.5	7.4
H. ROBUSTUS	260.9	224.2 - 336.0	12.1	89.5	70.3 - 107.3	8.8	16.2	15.0 - 18.5	6.0
H. ERECTUS	130.0	90.5 - 194.3	23.2	81.8	68.0 - 91.6	7.2	11.4	9.5 - 14.2	11.7
H. NEANDERTAL	115.6	81.6 - 146.4	14.5	85.5	70.5 - 144.4	14.9	10.8	9.0 - 12.1	7.3
H. SAPIENS	102.6	45.5 - 172.9	20.1	89.8	62.9 - 224.5	24.8	10.1	6.7 - 13.1	10.0
AUSTRALOPITHECINES	241.7	171.7 - 336.0	17.5	88.7	70.3 - 107.3	8.6	15.5	13.1 - 18.5	8.8
KRAPINA	130.3	125.0 - 146.4	7.0	85.0	80.0 - 101.7	11.0	11.5	11.2 - 12.1	3.1
NEANDERTAL	113.0	81.6 - 139.1	14.5	85.8	70.5 - 144.4	16.3	10.7	9.0 - 11.8	7.4
MT CARMEL	115.8	94.6 - 140.4	16.3	84.3	74.4 - 100.8	11.4	10.8	9.8 - 11.8	7.9
AUSTRALOID	123.9	88.0 - 164.2	19.4	81.8	63.1 - 110.7	14.3	11.2	9.5 - 12.9	9.9
SUB SAHARAN	113.4	72.0 - 172.9	25.5	86.4	69.2 - 120.0	13.7	10.6	8.5 - 13.1	12.6
NEW BRITAIN	110.3	87.4 - 150.0	13.2	81.0	66.9 - 96.6	8.4	10.5	9.4 - 12.2	6.4
INDIAN	104.6	68.8 - 127.3	16.0	85.8	73.0 - 100.5	9.5	10.2	8.3 - 11.3	8.3
MALAY	102.3	94.6 - 109.0	5.5	85.9	70.8 - 98.1	12.9	10.2	9.8 - 10.4	2.6
DICKSON MOUND	102.2	64.1 - 162.8	16.8	82.8	67.8 - 101.3	6.9	10.1	8.0 - 12.8	8.2
CAUCASOID	100.2	67.5 - 133.9	19.7	80.6	62.9 - 105.6	11.7	10.0	8.2 - 11.6	9.8
HARAPPA, INDIA	89.5	45.5 - 132.0	18.7	90.7	68.0 - 114.3	12.9	9.4	6.7 - 11.5	9.6

TABLE LXXVIII. Upper Third Molar Length: Frequency Distribution in Percentiles.

FREQUENCY DISTRIBUTION OF UPPER M3 L(M-D)

	6.8	7.5	8.2	8.9	9.6	10.3	11.0	11.7	12.4	13.1	13.8	14.5	15.2	15.9	16.6
H.AFRICAN.							9	18	27	27	9		9		
H.ROBUSTUS									4		25	12	33	25	
H.ERECTUS			5	16	33	22	11	11							
H.NEANDER.			17	28	25	10	7	7	2						
H.SAPIENS	1	11	18	29	19	7	6	2	1	1	1	1			
AUSTRALOP.							2	5	11	11	19	8	25	16	
KRAPINA					79			19							
NEANDERTAL			20	32	17	11	8	5	2						
MT CARMEL			16	50			16	16							
CAUCASOID	2	26	21	23	7	15	2								
INDIAN	7	7	7	21	35	21									
AUSTRALOID		9	9	9	22	22	27								
NEW BRITAI		1	21	36	30	3	3	1							
DICKSON MD	2	12	21	38	17	2	3	2							
MALAY			39	19	39										
SUB SAHARA		4	19	14	25	9	4	4	9	4					
HARAPPA	3	18	22	36	14	3	1								

TABLE LXXIX. Upper Third Molar Breadth: Frequency Distribution in Percentiles.

FREQUENCY DISTRIBUTION OF UPPER M3 B(B-L)

	4.8	6.0	7.2	8.4	9.6	10.8	12.0	13.2	14.4	15.6	16.8	18.0	19.2	20.4	21.6
H.AFRICAN.							9		72	9	9				
H.ROBUSTUS									4	41	37	8		8	
H.ERECTUS					11	27	38	5	5	5	5				
H.NEANDER.				2	9	34	44	7							
H.SAPIENS	1	2	4	9	24	38	16	3	1						
AUSTRALOP.							2		25	31	28	5		5	
KRAPINA							99								
NEANDERTAL				2	11	39	37	8							
MT CARMEL						66	33								
CAUCASOID				13	21	39	23	2							
INDIAN				14	14	64	7								
AUSTRALOID				4	8	20	41	20	4						
NEW BRITAI					14	52	25	7							
DICKSON MD				2	33	51	10	2							
MALAY					28	57	14								
SUB SAHARA			5	5	11	35	41								
HARAPPA		3	6	24	39	18	8								

TABLE LXXX. Upper Third Molar Area (L*B): Frequency Distribution in Percentiles.

FREQUENCY DISTRIBUTION OF UPPER M3 L*B

	44	64	84	104	124	144	164	184	204	224	244	264	284	304	324
H. AFRICAN.							45	18	18	9		9			
H. ROBUSTUS										37	29	12	12	8	
H. ERECTUS			16	38	16	11	5	11							
H. NEANDER.		2	25	33	35	2									
H. SAPIENS	2	14	40	28	11	1	1								
AUSTRALOP.							14	5	5	28	19	11	8	5	
KRAPINA					79	19									
NEANDERTAL		3	28	39	28										
MT CARMEL			33	33	33										
CAUCASOID		21	42	15	21										
INDIAN		14	28	50	7										
AUSTRALOID			23	26	28	14	4								
NEW BRITAI			44	36	17	1									
DICKSON MD		12	46	32	6	1									
SUB SAHARA		17	29	17	23		11								
MALAY			59	39											
HARAPPA	6	27	47	16	1										

Comparison with the non-human primates (Table LXXXIV) shows the coefficients of variation for the Liberian chimpanzee to be significantly less than those of any hominid taxa, and less than those of almost all extant groups. The other primates, although more varied, are still generally less variable than most of the hominids.

METRIC TRENDS IN INDIVIDUAL TEETH

It is convenient to summarize trends for the individual teeth by morphological group. A distinction will be maintained between the lack of statistically significant difference and the lack of morphologically significant difference.

a) Incisors

There is very little statistically significant difference between the mean values calculated for the incisor dimensions. Considering, for instance, the lower incisors, the only significant difference between the australopithecine taxa is in breadth of the lateral incisor. While the breadth for *H. robustus* is significantly smaller, only 33% of the specimens fall outside of the *H. africanus* range of variation (Table XIV). Taxonomic relevance is thus not indicated. Comparison of these taxa individually with *H. erectus*, or together as 1 taxon, indicates that the larger size of the incisors of *H. erectus* is barely, if at all, significant. Morphologically, incisor size does not distinguish these taxa. The differences in size between *H. erectus* and *H. neanderthalensis*, again; border on statistical significance and are not morphologically significant; the same is true for the length differences between *H. neanderthalensis* and *H. sapiens*. There is a significant decrease in mandibular incisor breadth and area between the last 2 taxa. Yet even here there is extensive overlap in the ranges of variation, with about 10% of the *H. neanderthalensis* exceeding the *H. sapiens* maximum. On the other hand, the breadth difference between these 2 taxa exceeds the maximum difference among extant groups. Generally, one may conclude the following: (1) There are no significant trends for mandibular incisor length or area; (2) there is a gradual, although not statistically significant, trend for breadth increase culminating in the *H. neanderthalensis* maximum and then showing a significant decrease to the *H. sapiens* value.

The maxillary incisors vary in much the same manner. Between the australopithecines the only difference of statistical significance is the slightly narrower central incisor of *H. robustus.* Indeed, "statistical significance" is misleading here, as *H. africanus* is represented by 2 incisors from 1 individual. When the australopithecines are compared with *H. erectus,* the lateral incisors are significantly larger in *H. erectus.* In turn, when *H. erectus* is compared with *H. neanderthalensis* the latter has significantly broader central incisors. Thus, there is a tendency for increase in size—particularly breadth—in the maxillary incisors The central incisor is maximum for *H. neanderthalensis,* and the lateral maximum for *H. erectus* and not significantly smaller in *H. neanderthalensis.* There is a significant decrease in area and breadth of the maxillary incisors with the appearance of *H. sapiens.*

Both mandibular and maxillary incisors exhibit the same trends. The only statistically significant differences between *H. erectus* and *H. neanderthalensis* are found in the greater incisor breadths of the latter for all but the upper lateral incisor. Similarly, the only statistically significant differences between the australopithecines and *H. erectus* are increases for the latter. There is a general increase through *H. erectus,* and a particular increase in breadth with *H. neanderthalensis.* The subsequent decrease in *H. sapiens* is both statistically and morphologically significant.

b) Canines

There is statistical significance to the length, breadth, and area difference in the mandibular canine between *H. africanus* and *H. robustus.* Morphological significance is more difficult to ascertain. For instance, the length difference is only 6% greater than the maximum difference among extant groups. Differences between the australopithecines in breadth and area are less than the maximum differences among extant groups. There is only a 20% to 30% overlap between the taxa in these dimensions (Tables XXIII - XXV). Yet, Mayr recognizes as little as 10% overlap within the same species (1969:190). Neither taxon is significantly different from *H. erectus: H. africanus* is larger and *H. robustus* smaller. When the australopithecines are treated as a single taxon, they are not significantly different from *H. erectus* in length, breadth, or area of the lower canine.

There are no significant differences between *H. erectus* and *H. neanderthalensis* in any measure of size, but *H. sapiens* shows a significant decrease from the latter in all dimensions.

A comparison of the australopithecine maxillary canines indicates a lack of significant difference for length, breadth, and area. With respect to length, the measure of greatest difference, the range of *H. africanus* variation falls completely within the *H. robustus* range (Table XXVIII). Thus, the difference is not morphologically significant. When the australopithecines are compared as a single taxon with *H. erectus,* a non-significant breadth and area increase in the latter is disclosed. Indeed, about 20% of the *H. erectus* specimens exceed the range of australopithecine area (Table XXX).

There is a length and area decrease between *H. erectus* and *H. neanderthalensis.* In spite of this decrease, all *H. erectus* specimens fall completely within the *H. neanderthalensis* range of variation. Lastly, there is a significant decrease in breadth and area between the latter and *H. sapiens.*

The major problem with respect to trends in the canines stems from the australopithecines. If one treats the australopithecines as a single taxon, and there are a number of good reasons for doing so (Le Gros Clark 1967; Bielicki 1966; Brace 1963b, 1963c, 1967a; Dart 1954, 1955a; Garn, Lewis, and Walenga 1969; Simons 1967, 1968a; Simpson 1963; Day 1969; Day and Napier 1964; Davis 1964; Tobias 1969; Wolpoff 1968, 1969b, 1970b), then the apparent metric trend is approximately the same as for the incisors; that is, a slight increase through *H. erectus* is followed by a significant decrease (particularly in breadth) leading to *H. sapiens.* If, on the other hand, the australopithecines are to be separated, there is an apparent reduction and subsequent increase in lower canine size with *H. robustus.*

TABLE LXXXI. Liberian Chimpanzee Lower and Upper Central Incisor through Fourth Premolar Length and Breadth: Mean, Standard Error of the Mean (SE(M)), Range, Sample Size (N), and Coefficient of Variation (CV).

	LENGTH(M-D)					BREADTH(B-L)				
	MEAN	SE(M)	RANGE	N	CV	MEAN	SE(M)	RANGE	N	CV
LOWER I1										
LIBERIAN CHIMP	8.10	.07	7.10 - 9.50	53	6.5					
UPPER I1										
LIBERIAN CHIMP	12.00	.10	10.20 - 13.50	49	5.7					
LOWER I2										
LIBERIAN CHIMP	9.00	.07	7.90 - 10.00	46	5.1					
UPPER I2										
LIBERIAN CHIMP	9.50	.09	8.10 - 10.90	48	6.2					
LOWER C										
LIBERIAN CHIMP	10.10	.08	7.50 - 12.70	95	7.4	18.10	.23	13.50 - 25.00	62	9.9
UPPER C										
LIBERIAN CHIMP	13.10	.09	10.60 - 16.70	97	7.1	19.40	.32	13.80 - 27.10	54	11.9
LOWER P4										
LIBERIAN CHIMP	8.24	.05	7.00 - 10.00	128	6.6	9.04	.06	7.30 - 11.10	128	6.9
UPPER P4										
LIBERIAN CHIMP	7.50	.04	6.00 - 9.80	197	7.9	10.27	.04	7.30 - 12.20	194	5.6

TABLE LXXXII. Non-Human Primate Lower and Upper First Molar Length and Breadth: Mean, Standard Error of the Mean (SE(M)), Range, Sample Size (N), and Coefficient of Variation (CV).

	LENGTH(M-D)					BREADTH(B-L)				
LOWER M1	MEAN	SE(M)	RANGE	N	CV	MEAN	SE(M)	RANGE	N	CV
LIBERIAN CHIMP	11.24	.04	9.90 - 13.20	128	4.4	10.35	.05	9.20 - 12.00	128	5.0
MACACCA SPECIOSA	5.73	.14		26	12.6	3.66	.08		26	11.5
MACACCA MULATTA	6.22	.08		22	6.2	4.05	.11		24	13.1
CERCCP. ASCANIUD	5.32	.04	4.50 - 6.40	50	5.8	4.18	.04	3.00 - 4.90	50	6.2
CERCOCEBUS ALBIG.	6.70	.04	5.50 - 7.40	56	4.5	5.63	.04	4.50 - 6.40	55	5.9
UPPER M1										
LIBERIAN CHIMP	10.70	.04	9.00 - 12.60	226	5.0	11.57	.03	9.90 - 12.70	225	4.1
MACACCA SPECIOSA	5.35	.11		28	10.4	4.81	.09		28	10.2
MACACCA MULATTA	5.95	.09		22	6.8	5.03	.09		26	8.6
CERCCP. ASCANIUD	5.32	.03	4.50 - 5.90	50	4.1	4.99	.05	3.50 - 5.90	50	6.6
CERCOCEBUS ALBIG.	6.82	.03	6.00 - 7.40	56	3.5	6.60	.04	5.50 - 7.90	55	4.7

c) Premolars

The third lower premolars are an exception to the other 3 premolars in that there is no significant difference between the australopithecine taxa for length, breadth, or area. Otherwise, all of the premolars vary the same way. *H. robustus* is significantly larger than *H. africanus*. *H. erectus* is significantly smaller than either of the australopithecine taxa or both taken together as a single taxon. *H. neanderthalensis* is significantly smaller than *H. erectus,* but there is no significant difference between the former and *H. sapiens*.

In terms of morphological significance, the differences between the australopithecines are consistent for all of the premolars except the fourth upper one. In the other 3 premolars, the differences between the australopithecines in length, breadth, and area are less than the maxi-

TABLE LXXXIII. Non-Human Primate Lower and Upper Second Molar Length and Breadth: Mean, Standard Error of the Mean (SE(M)), Range, Sample Size (N), and Coefficient of Variation (CV).

LOWER M2	LENGTH(M-D)					BREADTH(B-L)				
	MEAN	SE(M)	RANGE	N	CV	MEAN	SE(M)	RANGE	N	CV
LIBERIAN CHIMP	11.11	.05	9.90 - 13.00	128	5.3	10.98	.05	9.50 - 12.60	126	4.6
MACACCA SPECIOSA	6.02	.12		26	10.4	4.53	.09		26	9.8
MACACCA MULATTA	6.61	.08		22	5.5	4.80	.10		24	9.6
CERCOP. ASCANIUD	5.72	.04	5.00 - 6.40	50	4.9	4.77	.05	4.00 - 5.40	49	6.7
CERCOCEBUS ALBIG.	7.47	.04	6.50 - 8.40	55	3.5	6.48	.04	5.50 - 7.40	54	4.8
UPPER M2										
LIBERIAN CHIMP	10.25	.04	8.70 - 11.90	229	5.8	11.62	.04	10.00 - 13.60	228	5.1
MACACCA SPECIOSA	5.92	.13		27	11.0	5.36	.09		28	8.4
MACACCA MULATTA	6.55	.06		22	4.4	5.68	.08		28	7.1
CERCOP. ASCANIUD	5.75	.05	5.00 - 6.40	49	5.6	5.61	.06	5.00 - 6.90	49	7.1
CERCOCEBUS ALBIG.	7.40	.05	6.00 - 8.40	53	4.5	7.20	.04	6.00 - 8.40	54	4.4

TABLE LXXXIV. Non-Human Primate Lower and Upper Third Molar Length and Breadth: Mean, Standard Error of the Mean (SE(M)), Range, Sample Size (N), and Coefficient of Variation (CV).

LOWER M3	LENGTH(M-D)					BREADTH(B-L)				
	MEAN	SE(M)	RANGE	N	CV	MEAN	SE(M)	RANGE	N	CV
LIBERIAN CHIMP	10.50	.06	9.20 - 12.40	117	6.0	10.38	.05	8.80 - 12.10	117	5.3
CERCOP. ASCANIUD	5.34	.06	4.00 - 6.40	45	7.7	4.45	.04	3.50 - 5.40	44	5.6
CERCOCEBUS ALBIG.	7.93	.08	6.00 - 9.40	47	6.6	6.26	.05	5.50 - 6.90	47	5.0
UPPER M3										
LIBERIAN CHIMP	9.34	.05	7.30 - 11.80	208	7.4	10.86	.04	9.20 - 13.20	209	5.4
CERCOP. ASCANIUD	4.58	.06	3.50 - 5.40	42	8.7	4.90	.06	4.50 - 5.90	41	7.6
CERCOCEBUS ALBIG.	6.75	.06	5.50 - 7.90	44	5.6	6.70	.05	5.50 - 7.90	45	4.9

mum differences among extant groups. In addition, there is extensive overlap between the 2 taxa. For the fourth upper premolar, the differences between the australopithecine length, breadth, and area measurements exceed the maximum difference among extant human groups. In addition, there is relatively little overlap between the frequency distributions. For instance, only 4% of the *H. robustus* specimens overlap with *H. africanus* in area (Table L).

In general, there is a consistent decrease over time in premolar size. A possible exception to this general trend is the fourth upper premolar in *H. robustus,* if it is to be recognized as a separate taxon. The general reduction trend, culminating with modern size teeth in *H. neanderthalensis,* is both statistically and morphologically significant.

d) Molars

Length, breadth, and area differences in the mandibular molars between the australopithecines are either not statistically significant, or are barely so. There is clearly no morphologically significant difference between the dimensions of these teeth. *H. erectus,* on the other hand, has significantly smaller mandibular molars than either of the australopithecine taxa separately, or both considered together as a single taxon. *H. neanderthalensis,* in turn, has teeth significantly smaller than *H. erectus,* but not significantly different from *H. sapiens.*

The maxillary molars show slightly greater differences. This can be seen particularly well in the comparison of the australopithecine taxa. The differences are statistically significant. Yet, the actual overlap is extensive; in no case does more than 20% of 1 taxon fall outside the range of variation of the other. In addition, the difference between them is inevitably less than the maximum difference among extant groups. Thus, there is no difference of morphological significance between the maxillary molars of the australopithecines.

Other differences in maxillary molars correspond to those in mandibular molars. The overall size decrease in hominid molars, resulting in modern size teeth by the time of *H. neanderthalensis,* is both statistically and morphologically significant.

SHAPE TRENDS OF INDIVIDUAL TEETH

With a few exceptions, the range of variation of tooth shape, as expressed by the dental index (100 L/B), is remarkably invariant when compared to the range of shape variation in extant groups. On the other hand, sexual differences in shape tend to be more distinct than such differences in length or breadth alone (Selmer-Olsen 1949; Garn, Lewis, and Kerewsky 1967a). When coupled with the fact that length-breadth correlations tend to be reasonably low (Selmer-Olsen 1949; Garn, Lewis, and Kerewsky 1968b), questions emerge with respect to the action of selection upon shape. Indeed, there are shape similarities throughout the dentition (Garn, Lewis, and Kerewsky 1967b). If selection is acting upon tooth shape, only a few taxonomically significant trends are disclosed by a perusal of the evidence.

The most consistent trend appears in incisor variation. With the exception of the lower lateral incisor, these teeth become relatively longer through *H. erectus.* Teeth of *H. neanderthalensis* are relatively broader, and teeth of *H. sapiens* again relatively longer. The lower lateral incisor differs in that the relative broadening begins with the australopithecines, rather than first appearing with *H. neanderthalensis.*

There is no statistically significant variation among any of the fossil taxa for any of the remaining teeth, with the exception of the lower third molar. The latter tooth is relatively longer in *H. robustus* than it is in any other hominid taxon. As could be expected, the second greatest length occurs in *H. africanus.* The difference between the australopithecines is statistically significant, although barely so. For the other teeth, the only statistically or morphologically significant differences in shape index occur with the relative decrease in broadness of *H. sapiens* compared with the corresponding shape in any of the fossil taxa. This is particularly apparent in the upper canine and fourth premolar, and in the lower third premolar. It is interesting to note that the relative buccolingual narrowing which the proposed taxon, "*Homo habilis,*" is supposed to exhibit (Leakey, Tobias, and Napier 1964; Leakey 1961c, 1966; Tobias 1966a) could only be used to argue for the inclusion of the specimens in *H. sapiens.* Robinson (1965b, 1966b, 1967) has already demonstrated that there is no narrowing trend for the lower third premolar in fossil hominids.

VARIABILITY

Dental variability was measured first by use of the coefficient of variation (Simpson, Roe, and Lewontin 1960:87-95; Mayr 1969:169-70). The advantage of the coefficient is that it presumably allows comparison of variabilities between samples with different means. This index must be approached with caution; there is really no reason why coefficients of variation of 5 in both mouse and elephant molars necessarily mean that the variability is the same. One could, perhaps, argue that when there is an allometric relation between 2 samples, the divisor of a coefficient comparing variation should be the allometric term, rather than the sample mean. The coefficient has its greatest value in the comparison of the same measurement in closely related samples.

Other indexes of relative variation have been proposed. Perhaps the most important of these is the variance of the logarithms of the sample values (Bader and Lehmann 1965; Lewontin 1966). This index has the advantage of invariance under multiplicative change. Thus, direct comparisons can be made between different samples, even when the units of measurement themselves are different. If the coefficient of variation of a sample is under 30, the variance of the natural logarithms can be approximated by the square of the coefficient of variation (Lewontin 1966:142). An additional property of this variation index is that it may be used in parametric statistical tests when sample sizes are too small to allow the coefficient of variation to be used (Wright 1952). The index was not used here for 2 reasons. The first is that the coefficients of variation can, after all, be compared statistically when sample sizes are large enough to allow *meaningful* comparisons to be made. The second reason stems from the fact that the index tends to underemphasize differences in variability when the coefficients of variation are very low, and overemphasize variability when the coefficients are relatively high.

Comparison of the coefficients of variation for length, breadth, and area in hominid species to non-human primate species indicates, with very few exceptions, that hominid dentitions tend to be more variable than non-human primate dentitions. Only in the case of the lower premolar are non-human primates clearly more variable than hominid species, corroborating a claim made by Schuman and Brace (1954:240). In the lower canine, and upper canine and premolars, non-human primate and hominid species variabilities are about equal. For most of these cases, variation in *H. sapiens* exceeds the non-human primates. Exceptions to the general trend shown by the canines and the lower third premolar are clearly due to differences in function and morphology. It is interesting that even with the great sexual dimorphism in non-human primate canines, they are not more variable than hominid canines in either the mandible or the maxilla. This data, then, supports the contention that hominids are the most dentally variable primate species.

An attempt was made to discern trends in the pattern of variation change among hominid species. With respect to length, no clear picture emerges. For instance, in the maxillary incisors, variability tends to increase through *H. erectus,* and then decrease or remain the same. For the mandibular incisors, however, *H. erectus* is more variable than *H. robustus,* but less variable than *H. africanus.* The latter, however, may be due to the very small sample size of *H. africanus* incisors. Canine variation follows no pattern at all, except that *H. erectus* is less variable than the australopithecines. In the posterior teeth, it is interesting that *H. neanderthalensis* is almost always more variable than *H. erectus,* and in turn, *H. sapiens* is always more variable than *H. neanderthalensis.* Australopithecine variation is less patterned. *H. robustus* is more variable than *H. africanus* about 2/3 of the time. *H. erectus* is more variable than *H. robustus* in the maxilla, and for almost all of the teeth in the mandible.

In breadth, clearer patterns of change in variability can be seen. In the mandible, the 3 anterior teeth change in the same way. The australopithecines are more variable than *H. erectus,* while *H. africanus* is more variable than *H. robustus. H. neanderthalensis* is about as variable as *H. erectus,* and *H. sapiens* shows a definite increase in variability. The maxillary incisors vary the same way, almost identically with the anterior maxillary teeth. The single exception is in the comparison of I^1 in *H. africanus* and *H. robustus.* The former is less variable. Variation in the maxillary canine is the same from *H. erectus* on. However, variation between the australopithecines themselves, and between the australopithecines and *H. erectus,* is almost exactly the opposite. In the posterior maxillary teeth, *H. africanus* tends to be less variable than *H. robustus.* On the other hand, *H. africanus* is either as variable or more variable in almost all of the mandibular posteriors. Similarly, *H. erectus* is equally or more variable than *H. robustus* in the mandibular posteriors, while it is almost always more variable in the maxillary posteriors. Comparing *H. erectus* to *H. neanderthalensis,* in both jaws the latter is equally or more variable in the premolars but equally or less variable in the molars. *H. sapiens* is equally or more variable than *H. neanderthalensis* in all the posteriors of both jaws. The lateral incisor, on the other hand, decreases in variability after *H. erectus,* and the canine decreases to *H. erectus,* but increases with *H. neanderthalensis.* The 2 maxillary premolars follow the same pattern as the maxillary canine. *H. robustus* is more variable than *H. africanus,* and *H. sapiens* is equally or more variable than *H. neanderthalensis.* In the mandible, the 2 premolars and the first molar have somewhat similar patterns of variability change. *H. robustus* is less variable than *H. africanus,* except for M_1, and *H. erectus* is equally or less variable than *H. robustus.* Variability increases in *H. neanderthalensis,* and decreases or remains the same in *H. sapiens.* The 2 other mandibular molars are more variable in *H. robustus* than they are in *H. africanus,* while variability decreases or remains the same in *H. erectus.* Variability in *H. neanderthalensis* increases for M_2 and decreases for M_3, while there is a consistent increase for *H. sapiens.* In the maxilla, the 3 molars act almost identically. *H. robustus* is more variable than *H. africanus* (except for M_3), while the former is exceeded by *H. erectus.* Variability decreases or remains the same in *H. neanderthalensis,* and increases or remains the same in *H. sapiens.*

Area variation for the 2 mandibular incisors was almost identical. *H. africanus* is more variable than *H. robustus.* However, while the australopithecines are equally or more variable than *H. erectus,* the latter is equally or more variable than *H. robustus. H. neanderthalensis* is more variable than *H. erectus,* and equally or less variable than *H. sapiens.* The mandibular canine varies in almost exactly the same manner, except that *H. neanderthalensis* is less variable than *H. erectus.* In the maxilla, variability increases for the central incisor through *H. erectus,* and then remains constant.

There is another approach to the analysis of variability changes. One can look at the range divided by n (sample size) times the standard deviation. In a sample with an approximately normal distribution, 98.76% of the sample should be within an interval of 2-1/2 standard deviations on either side of the mean. Variability may be, in this instance, thought of as the deviation of the sample from the normal approximation. Certainly this provides a means for making relative comparisons of the variabilities of different samples. By comparing the actual to the expected (if the distribution were normal) range, a measure of relative variation is established. Dividing the range by 5 times the standard deviation approximates such a measure. If the population were normal, the percentage index of 100 would indicate that all of the sample fell in an interval which would be expected to enclose 98.76% of the sample.

Tables LXXXV to LXXXIX examine this index for hominids, and Table XC examines it for length and breadth of non-human primates. Comparing the latter with the indexes of length and breadth variation in hominids (Tables LXXXV and LXXXVI) reveals the fact that *H. sapiens* is more variable for almost every tooth. The other hominid taxa are, by and large, less variable. Thus, conclusions reached by comparing coefficients of variation are corroborated. There is a definite trend for the hominids in length and breadth, as well as area (Table LXXXVII), dental index (Table LXXXVIII), and module (LXXXIX). Variability clearly increases over time, with the maximum value in *H. sapiens.*

Trends in dental variability are of particular importance with respect to questions concerning the mechanisms of dental reduction (Wolpoff 1969a). The general trend throughout the Pleistocene for dental reduction has been recognized by some (Keith 1915:453; Hooton 1938: 84-88, 1947:132-40; Dahlberg 1949, 1963a). Recently, however, 2 sets of hypotheses have emerged with respect to the actual mechanism of dental reduction. The first set deals with hypotheses of direct selection for tooth size reduction (Holloway 1967, 1968; Washburn 1968a; Mills 1963; Brues 1966). The second suggests that such reduction was the result of reduced or suspended selection (Brace 1963a, 1964b; Brace and Montagu 1965; Wolpoff 1969a).

The importance of trends in variability derives from the area of contradiction between reduction models based on selection and models based on relaxed selection. The reduced selection model suggests that random change in the genetic material, by changing parameters in a complex and interrelated developmental process, will tend to stop the process (Brace 1963a). Reduction of the size or complexity of the structure in question is the most likely effect, as changes leading to the increased size or complexity of the structure (for which selection has been reduced) would probably be disadvantageous (Wolpoff 1969a). Such random genetic changes come from 2 possible sources. The first is mutation accumulation for selectively neutral changes (Brace 1964b), and the second is shifts in selection acting on pleiotropic systems of genes when the selection for 1 of the structures is reduced (Wolpoff 1969a). The latter process might be termed the "probable pleiotropy effect." The accumulation of selectively neutral random genetic changes has been established for developmentally simple biochemical structures with relatively low levels of pleiotropy (Sarich 1968; Sarich and Wilson 1967a, 1967b; King and Jukes 1969). Selectively neutral changes in systems with higher developmental complexity and higher levels of pleiotropy would lead to structural reduction.

The reduced selection model, then, predicts an increase in variability in a structure in the process of reducing (Wolpoff 1969a). Reduction of a structure due to direct selection for smaller size would be accompanied by reduced variability (Simpson 1953). Indeed, of all the mechanisms which can orient the direction of evolutionary change (Holloway 1966; Prout 1964; Simpson 1953), only the reduction of selection is accompanied by an increase in variability.

The combined data for trends in variability changes show several things. There is clearly a trend for increased variability, tending to corroborate the reduced selection hypothesis. In some cases, the greatest variability is found in

TABLE LXXXV. Distribution of the Hominid Range divided by Five times the Standard Deviation for Length.

DISTRIBUTION OF RANGE/(5*SIGMA) FOR LENGTH(M-D)

	LOWER								UPPER							
	I1	I2	C	P3	P4	M1	M2	M3	I1	I2	C	P3	P4	M1	M2	M3
H. AFRICANUS	51	47	75	80	61	78	59	69	28	46	61	57	81	85	67	69
H. ROBUSTUS	60	50	64	90	106	82	63	68	73	59	82	73	72	79	74	82
H. ERECTUS	69	74	79	111	76	97	80	71	65	56	76	80	60	67	57	70
H. NEANDERTAL	75	97	123	121	102	110	93	105	83	68	92	78	73	112	91	83
H. SAPIENS	122	121	152	115	119	117	129	123	129	135	147	152	148	163	166	125
AUSTRALOPITHECINES	84	65	81	93	107	82	71	72	81	66	70	68	88	88	87	77
KRAPINA	53	66	74	62	65	60	72	68	65	65	76	51	65	69	68	46
NEANDERTAL	72	80	100	122	97	111	88	86	68	68	83	79	75	104	86	84
MT CARMEL	53	48	59	67	46	61	54	47	52	50	54	51	37	68	58	51
ALEUTS	145	114	114	117	111	91	77	83	106	75	100	89	119	95	111	109
AMERICAN NEGROS				51	53	77	74	74				57	74	74	75	94
AMERICAN WHITES(1)	105	115	135	118	147	126	98		116	126	120	119	129	111	120	
AMERICAN WHITES(2)				73	56	58	57	73				107	62	84	73	75
AUSTRALOID	63	55	58	80	78	72	86	67	56	44	59	81	72	65	74	62
CAUCASOID	72	86	90	102	109	77	100	104	76	77	73	96	109	111	86	77
DICKSON MOUND	117	111	104	113	149	96	98	101	86	112	97	108	96	103	106	102
E.GREENLAND ESKIMO					66	74	86	79			174	148	109	86	107	69
HARAPPA, INDIA						115	70	103						96	105	91
INDIAN	67	72	83	72	84	86	89	86	63	73	65	85	76	77	76	68
LAPPS	120	123	142	111	131	120	113	140	89	111	128	120	111	134	123	140
MALAY	39	38	64	65	70	77	86	59	46		36	69	52	71	75	43
NEW BRITAIN	92	85	95	79	95	101	96	105	100	78	76	103	109	93	97	107
PECOS PUEBLO	108	89	90	124	86	81	113	69	127	95	94	94	69	94	82	93
SUB SAHARAN	85	90	66	89	108	92	101	96	71	77	78	65	66	79	71	66

TABLE LXXXVI. Distribution of the Hominid Range divided by Five times the Standard Deviation for Breadth.

DISTRIBUTION OF RANGE/(5*SIGMA) FOR BREADTH(B-L)

	LOWER								UPPER							
	I1	I2	C	P3	P4	M1	M2	M3	I1	I2	C	P3	P4	M1	M2	M3
H. AFRICANUS	43	43	64	68	65	80	58	72	28	40	53	78	67	85	69	79
H. ROBUSTUS	62	56	65	67	79	83	68	63	61	66	70	70	84	81	77	88
H. ERECTUS	58	78	71	77	80	83	77	90	41	47	69	72	86	62	63	71
H. NEANDERTAL	71	89	86	106	104	101	86	99	88	98	79	90	84	138	93	96
H. SAPIENS	118	157	117	116	147	119	134	128	142	129	118	123	110	134	114	122
AUSTRALOPITHECINES	80	52	75	83	80	84	77	72	69	83	78	92	72	89	95	104
KRAPINA	34	58	58	63	82	67	82	79	52	83	61	48	52	84	65	44
NEANDERTAL	61	65	79	101	94	103	83	84	68	69	75	93	73	112	90	87
MT CARMEL	43	36	55	57	43	48	54	50	46	52	53	51	42	49	58	46
ALEUTS			109	109	109	116	89	89			119	108	109	101	89	114
AMERICAN NEGROS				68	60	75	58	83				74	66	66	80	70
AMERICAN WHITES(2)				62	58	58	75	84				107	72	84	67	80
AUSTRALOID	44	47	50	59	84	73	72	78	58	54	65	78	60	91	67	72
CAUCASOID	81	87	86	85	103	106	99	119	85	63	84	76	99	78	82	83
DICKSON MOUND	124	90	96	90	114	106	91	119	103	99	94	104	100	116	113	108
E.GREENLAND ESKIMO					85	84	107	82			177	117	92	92	75	122
HARAPPA, INDIA						90	83	86						87	93	93
INDIAN	59	66	67	75	68	67	81	82	74	72	58	72	75	83	64	66
LAPPS	104	110	98	126	134	144	119	118	112	133	115	167	131	120	109	137
MALAY	48	46	83	59	79	76	79	67	46		34	68	70	62	72	52
NEW BRITAIN	77	96	70	75	95	81	92	88	94	85	84	83	75	85	77	82
PECOS PUEBLO	109	92	87	80	101	104	94	82	132	109	97	80	83	113	85	113
SUB SAHARAN	88	106	71	96	118	100	96	94	78	78	71	83	82	66	75	70

TABLE LXXXVII. Distribution of the Hominid Range divided by Five times the Standard Deviation for Area.

DISTRIBUTION OF RANGE/(5*SIGMA) FOR L*B

	LOWER								UPPER							
	I1	I2	C	P3	P4	M1	M2	M3	I1	I2	C	P3	P4	M1	M2	M3
H. AFRICANUS	44	45	70	67	58	70	62	74	27	44	43	71	87	75	69	64
H. ROBUSTUS	70	56	66	84	88	83	66	65	57	65	72	76	75	77	78	70
H. ERECTUS	65	73	74	103	69	81	83	86	53	55	54	81	76	72	61	68
H. NEANDERTAL	72	92	107	131	116	98	89	90	82	82	99	82	69	105	91	77
H. SAPIENS	124	148	104	137	158	118	144	123	111	143	147	111	111	146	134	123
AUSTRALOPITHECINES	80	68	79	85	92	79	75	71	66	78	76	81	78	88	94	77
KRAPINA	35	59	61	58	59	63	73	77	59	86	74	52	53	69	67	47
NEANDERTAL	69	67	105	124	108	106	91	79	69	63	93	81	70	108	89	70
MT CARMEL	40	37	50	58	38	54	54	45	47	48	54	44	46	63	54	48
CAUCASOID	77	83	87	87	113	94	101	99	71	77	84	86	98	89	88	67
INDIAN	60	68	77	81	81	68	76	83	59	67	66	78	76	63	78	70
AUSTRALOID	43	48	54	69	78	69	87	78	47	44	69	65	62	78	67	63
DICKSON MOUND	128	102	103	91	126	106	100	107	92	96	104	101	94	108	107	115
HARAPPA, INDIA						103	78	85						90	92	103
SUB SAHARAN	85	96	71	94	104	100	99	94	78	73	75	74	74	72	73	69
MALAY	37	36	75	55	61	74	65	58	45		35	69	61	75	68	51
NEW BRITAIN	90	105	76	86	107	98	96	102	104	68	78	85	78	97	84	86

TABLE LXXXVIII. Distribution of the Hominid Range divided by Five times the Standard Deviation for Dental Index.

DISTRIBUTION OF RANGE/(5*SIGMA) FOR (100*L)/B

	LOWER								UPPER							
	I1	I2	C	P3	P4	M1	M2	M3	I1	I2	C	P3	P4	M1	M2	M3
H. AFRICANUS	47	42	69	57	58	71	83	67	28	47	58	70	71	76	56	79
H. ROBUSTUS	60	51	65	77	84	79	75	65	62	59	72	65	73	90	76	93
H. ERECTUS	64	64	62	88	88	98	81	88	59	48	66	71	62	67	78	80
H. NEANDERTAL	71	74	121	97	95	112	86	90	100	96	106	88	91	144	100	116
H. SAPIENS	127	114	123	133	120	167	151	174	120	133	122	126	122	177	142	144
AUSTRALOPITHECINES	76	62	66	79	91	105	92	86	70	69	76	91	104	100	83	97
KRAPINA	36	56	63	81	65	71	86	66	57	75	62	41	61	72	61	46
NEANDERTAL	69	68	75	70	89	95	74	78	73	82	86	79	77	128	100	105
MT CARMEL	47	37	55	55	44	46	49	53	42	47	47	55	43	69	57	55
CAUCASOID	78	97	79	145	112	102	123	136	74	84	105	90	103	108	113	90
INDIAN	65	59	85	79	76	117	100	84	63	55	62	70	85	76	85	67
AUSTRALOID	39	45	54	67	81	83	101	84	53	55	72	95	70	77	74	81
DICKSON MOUND	98	96	105	121	143	120	121	123	99	99	119	93	103	99	136	117
HARAPPA, INDIA						102	94	84						111	98	78
SUB SAHARAN	71	98	89	90	88	96	77	102	63	94	81	88	73	71	77	86
MALAY	36	39	63	63	66	62	78	63	49		36	67	62	73	70	49
NEW BRITAIN	104	103	92	91	91	89	102	128	62	68	90	95	103	94	105	87

the teeth of *H. neanderthalensis,* and in others *H. sapiens* has the maximum amount of variability. This should not be surprising, as many teeth of the earlier taxon have already reduced to modern size. There are 3 possible terminations for a reduction trend due to reduced selection. The structure can reduce until selection for its maintenance in reduced form is operative; the structure can reduce until selection acting on the pleiotropic effects of some of its genetic background allows no further change (such a structure is described as vestigial); or reduction can lead to the eventual disappearance of the structure. In the case of the second possibility, the reduced structure will be maintained with a relatively great amount of variability as a vestigial structure (Simpson 1953:75). It appears that the size of the dentition in living man is being maintained in reduced dimensions by direct selection. Thus, after reduction is complete, variability again decreases. If some teeth of *H. neanderthalensis* are as reduced as selection will allow,

TABLE LXXXIX. Distribution of the Hominid Range divided by Five times the Standard Deviation for Module.

DISTRIBUTION OF RANGE/(5*SIGMA) FOR (L+B)/2

	LOWER								UPPER							
	I1	I2	C	P3	P4	M1	M2	M3	I1	I2	C	P3	P4	M1	M2	M3
H. AFRICANUS	43	46	69	65	60	67	61	74		42	43	73	87	74	69	64
H. ROBUSTUS	65	56	65	81	85	82	67	65	57	64	70	75	78	77	78	72
H. ERECTUS	57	71	74	104	68	84	83	83	53	55	54	80	78	71	61	69
H. NEANDERTAL	72	91	108	131	116	99	86	92	79	81	99	84	68	103	89	77
H. SAPIENS	128	154	103	135	148	119	140	122	109	146	147	112	110	157	135	125
AUSTRALOPITHECINES	76	69	77	81	88	79	76	70	66	77	75	83	76	87	94	78
KRAPINA	33	59	60	56	60	63	73	76	59	85	74	49	54	70	67	47
NEANDERTAL	63	65	104	124	107	105	90	80	66	63	93	84	66	102	88	69
MT CARMEL	41	36	49	55	35	55	54	44	47	50	53	45	45	59	56	47
CAUCASOID	78	81	85	86	110	93	102	103	71	77	84	86	100	89	88	68
INDIAN	59	66	77	81	78	66	75	83	62	66	65	75	76	62	75	69
AUSTRALOID	43	48	52	65	79	69	84	78	46	43	68	68	61	78	66	61
DICKSON MOUND	130	101	99	92	124	107	97	109	90	99	105	104	94	109	106	114
HARAPPA, INDIA						104	80	84						92	94	104
SUB SAHARAN	87	97	69	96	105	101	97	91	75	70	77	77	75	71	73	68
MALAY	37	35	75	52	61	71	65	57	42		33	69	62	73	68	46
NEW BRITAIN	88	100	74	86	101	96	95	103	103	64	77	80	77	96	83	80

TABLE XC. Distribution of the Non-Human Primates Ranges divided by Five times the Standard Deviations for Length and Breadth.

DISTRIBUTION OF RANGE/(5*SIGMA) FOR LENGTH(M-D)

	LOWER								UPPER							
	I1	I2	C	P3	P4	M1	M2	M3	I1	I2	C	P3	P4	M1	M2	M3
LIBERIAN CHIMP	90	91	138		111	131	105	101	95	94	131	117	128	133	108	130
CERCOP. ASCANIUD						122	99	117						127	87	94
CERCOCEBUS ALBIG.						126	146	130						116	145	126

DISTRIBUTION OF RANGE/(5*SIGMA) FOR BREADTH(B-L)

	LOWER								UPPER							
	I1	I2	C	P3	P4	M1	M2	M3	I1	I2	C	P3	P4	M1	M2	M3
LIBERIAN CHIMP			127		122	107	121	119			115	118	168	116	122	135
CERCOP. ASCANIUD						146	87	151						145	94	75
CERCOCEBUS ALBIG.						115	122	90						154	149	145

one would expect the variability of these teeth to be reduced in *H. sapiens.*

The observed trends for increased variability are more apparent in posterior teeth than in anteriors. Posterior teeth have undergone relatively greater reduction, as has been demonstrated both here and in other studies (Garn, Lewis, and Walenga 1969).

There is no consistent relationship between *H. africanus* and *H. robustus* with respect to dental variation, a point already noted by several authors (Tobias 1965b; Wolpoff 1968). If anything, *H. robustus* is the taxon with greater dental variability, contrary to claims based on smaller sample sizes (Robinson 1956).

It may thus be concluded that the trends in variability, although not as distinctive and unequivocable as the trends in individual tooth size, are consistent with the latter when interpreted by a model of reduction due to the relaxation of selection. The evolution of human culture, through changes in diet and technology, ultimately replaced the dentition in many of its functions. Subsequently, selection was relaxed.

DENTAL CORRELATIONS

Many authors have attempted dental correlations between corresponding teeth in the same jaw as well as in opposite jaws. Ritter (1933) correlated the mesiodistal length of both incisors of both jaws in all combinations. Every correlation coefficient was in excess of .5. Even higher correlations were found for *H. sapiens* for each incisor (Tables XCI and XCII). Bolton (1958) established a positive correlation between all teeth of the maxilla and the corresponding mandibular teeth, as did Selmer-Olsen (1949) and Gabriel (1955). Correlations have been used to study both mesiodistal (Garn, Lewis, and Kerewsky 1966c) and buccolingual (Garn, Lewis, and Kerewsky 1967c) asymmetry. Lastly, there are a number of correlation analyses of the relation of teeth in the same jaw (Gabriel 1955; Ritter 1933; Garn, Lewis, and Kerewsky 1965b; Lundstrom 1943; Ono 1960; Seipel 1946). The results of 2 such studies (Moorrees and Reed 1964; Selmer-Olsen 1949) have been reproduced here (Tables IC and C).

A graphical method of correlation has been recently proposed (Brabrant and Twiesselman 1964a, 1964b; Twiesselman and Brabrant 1960) but was not utilized.

Tables XCI through C are concerned with dental correlations. Tables XCI through XCVIII show the correlation of each tooth with its corresponding number on the opposite side and the opposite jaw in all (6) combinations. Table IC gives correlations for mesiodistal crown diameters of a North American sample ranging from 131 to 171. This table was adapted from Table 3 in Moorrees and Reed (1964:689). Table XC gives the inter-dental length and breadth correlations for a large Lapp sample. The data was taken from Table 25 in Selmer-Olsen (1949:95).

Many authors measure only 1 side of each jaw. Others, feeling that 1 side does not adequately represent the individual, use the average of both sides for each measurement. Still others measure every tooth. The final procedure was employed in this work. The first 2 tactics are used in order to eliminate bias in small samples when remains of some individuals are relatively complete, and others are not. However, whether this procedure eliminates bias is questionable. Unless skeletal material is relatively complete, the difficulties of recognizing tooth pairs from the same jaw are legion (Mann 1968). For this reason, it is best to consider all fossil teeth in a sample separately. Then, however, it is necessary to treat all teeth in any sample the same way, so that comparisons are made between samples collected in equivalent ways. This procedure is supported by the distribution of correlations.

The correlation tables consistently show a high correlation between each tooth and its opposite number for both lower (LL/LR) and upper (UL/UR) jaws in the species *H. sapiens.* However, there is a good deal of variation among extant populations, not all of which is accounted for by sample size. The correlations between opposite teeth in the same jaw are almost always higher than are those for either opposing or opposite teeth in opposite jaws. In addition, the correlations between opposite teeth in the same jaw are inevitably higher than correlations between the same tooth and any other tooth in the jaw. However, the correlations are only high enough to justify elimination in a sample of 1 side of the jaw for the most proximal tooth in each morphological class. In the more distal teeth, the amount of variation in each tooth increases (Garn and Lewis 1962; Garn, Lewis, and Vicinus 1962; Grahen 1962; Garn, Lewis, and Kerewsky 1965b). Thus, it is no surprise that the correlation between opposite tooth pairs decreases distally in each morphological group. It has long been recognized that bilateral asymmetry increases distally within each morphological group for measures of size (Garn, Lewis, and Kerewsky 1966c, 1967c), as well as cusp number and crown morphology (Garn, Lewis, and Kerewsky 1966b).

Looking again at the correlations for *H. sapiens,* it is interesting to note that the correlation of opposites in the mandible is usually greater than or the same as correlations for the maxilla in anterior teeth, while the opposite tends to be the case in the posterior teeth.

Lastly, these correlations relate to a contention about the selective importance of crown area made several years ago (See Brace 1967b:810, footnote). If crown area is the trait upon which selection most directly acts, one would expect the correlations between tooth pair areas to be higher than between either lengths or breadths. This is almost always the case for the samples considered here.

TABLE XCI. Correlations for the Central Incisor. The following abbreviations are used: LL (lower left), LR (lower right), UL (upper left), UR (upper right).

CORRELATIONS FOR I1	LL/LR	LL/UL	LL/UR	LR/UL	LR/UR	UL/UR
			LENGTH(M-D)			
H. NEANDERTHALENSIS	.88	.86	.77	.63	.44	.97
H. SAPIENS	.90	.76	.74	.78	.68	.93
CAUCASOID	.95	.83	.84	.89	.88	.95
INDIAN	.91	.99	.80	.43	.94	.93
DICKSON MOUND	.91	.61	.51	.59	.51	.90
NEW BRITAIN	.59	.03	.85	.57	.26	.37
SUB SAHARAN	.93	-.87	.89	-.62	.86	.83
			BREADTH(B-L)			
H. NEANDERTHALENSIS	.80	.80	.32			
H. SAPIENS	.91	.75	.69	.75	.74	.93
CAUCASOID	.94	.90	.80	.97	.78	.89
INDIAN	.99	.05	-.52	-.05	-.60	.74
DICKSON MOUND	.90	.73	.70	.70	.70	.89
NEW BRITAIN	.50	.57	.81	.22	.56	.86
SUB SAHARAN	.97	.87	.81	.70	.97	.99
			AREA(L*B)			
H. NEANDERTHALENSIS	.85		.81			
H. SAPIENS	.88	.77	.77	.76	.75	.94
CAUCASOID	.97	.94	.94	.95	.92	.95
INDIAN	.75	.28	.22	-.06	-.12	.87
DICKSON MOUND	.89	.70	.68	.65	.66	.90
NEW BRITAIN	.39	.13	.77	-.30	-.09	.55
SUB SAHARAN	.97			.06	.98	.98

TABLE XCII. Correlations for the Lateral Incisor. The following abbreviations are used: LL (lower left), LR (lower right), UL (upper left), UR (upper right).

CORRELATIONS FOR I2	LL/LR	LL/UL	LL/UR	LR/UL	LR/UR	UL/UR
			LENGTH(M-D)			
H. NEANDERTHALENSIS	.50	.72	-.37	.88	.36	.96
H. SAPIENS	.82	.72	.67	.72	.72	.90
CAUCASOID	.83	.82	.69	.91	.87	.93
NEW BRITAIN	.45	.62	.71	.44	.43	.59
DICKSON MOUND	.90	.34	.36	.45	.46	.87
			BREADTH(B-L)			
H. NEANDERTHALENSIS	.96			.77		.92
H. SAPIENS	.76	.67	.60	.62	.57	.84
CAUCASOID	.75	.77	.82	.77	.70	.91
NEW BRITAIN	.51	-.04	-.10	.06	.49	.73
DICKSON MOUND	.82	.52	.44	.56	.45	.73
			AREA(L*B)			
H. NEANDERTHALENSIS	.91			.84		.94
H. SAPIENS	.79	.79	.73	.73	.68	.91
CAUCASOID	.84	.89	.86	.90	.87	.96
NEW BRITAIN	.45	.83	.15	.49	.29	.70
DICKSON MOUND	.87	.55	.52	.58	.52	.84

TABLE XCIII. Correlations for the Canine. The following abbreviations are used: LL (lower left), LR (lower right), UL (upper left), UR (upper right).

CORRELATIONS FOR C	LL/LR	LL/UL	LL/UR	LR/UL	LR/UR	UL/UR
			LENGTH(M-D)			
H. NEANDERTHALENSIS	.70	.76	.73	.87	.75	.89
H. SAPIENS	.88	.74	.72	.74	.77	.88
CAUCASOID	.93	.55	.28	.70	.72	.91
INDIAN	.91					.77
NEW BRITAIN	.46	.68	.54	.33	.54	.67
DICKSON MOUND	.93	.77	.79	.79	.83	.89
			BREADTH(B-L)			
H. NEANDERTHALENSIS	.82	.85	.86	-.28	.93	.89
H. SAPIENS	.88	.75	.75	.77	.83	.94
CAUCASOID	.82	.50	.64	.68	.82	.84
INDIAN	.98					.97
NEW BRITAIN	.89	.85	.77	.74	.84	.96
DICKSON MOUND	.86	.82	.79	.79	.78	.93
			AREA(L*B)			
H. NEANDERTHALENSIS	.80	.92	.90	.65	.77	.86
H. SAPIENS	.91	.79	.78	.79	.85	.94
CAUCASOID	.96	.51	.63	.67	.76	.93
INDIAN	.98					.97
NEW BRITAIN	.69	.80	.57	.60	.74	.90
DICKSON MOUND	.92	.87	.83	.85	.85	.93

TABLE XCIV. Correlations for the Third Premolar. The following abbreviations are used: LL (lower left), LR (lower right), UL (upper left), UR (upper right).

CORRELATIONS FOR PM3	LL/LR	LL/UL	LL/UR	LR/UL	LR/UR	UL/UR
			LENGTH(M-D)			
H. AFRICANUS	.66					
H. ROBUSTUS	.77					
H. ERECTUS	.86					
H. NEANDERTHALENSIS	.62	.59	.81	.32	.39	.82
H. SAPIENS	.87	.70	.70	.70	.72	.87
CAUCASOID	.95	.83	.87	.86	.83	.92
INDIAN	.74	.48	.42	.53	.63	.92
NEW BRITAIN	.66	.40	.13	.10	-.07	.86
DICKSON MOUND	.88	.54	.72	.55	.74	.74
			BREADTH(B-L)			
H. ROBUSTUS	.84					
H. ERECTUS	.72					
H. NEANDERTHALENSIS	.77	.66	.90	.59	.46	.89
H. SAPIENS	.81	.69	.59	.65	.64	.87
CAUCASOID	.36	.51	.33	.45	.34	.67
INDIAN	.69	.62	.58	.38	.47	.97
NEW BRITAIN	.74	.48	-.04	.34	.09	.90
DICKSON MOUND	.92	.69	.66	.66	.70	.86
			AREA(L*B)			
H. ROBUSTUS	.60					
H. ERECTUS	.95					
H. NEANDERTHALENSIS	.67	.76	.91	.65	.50	.89
H. SAPIENS	.93	.77	.73	.74	.74	.91
CAUCASOID	.85	.81	.84	.82	.86	.91
INDIAN	.87	.73	.82	.46	.63	.96
NEW BRITAIN	.90	.46	-.19	.13	-.04	.88
DICKSON MOUND	.93	.70	.74	.71	.79	.82

TABLE XCV. Correlations for the Fourth Premolar. The following abbreviations are used: LL (lower left), LR (lower right), UL (upper left), UR (upper right).

CORRELATIONS FOR PM4	LL/LR	LL/UL	LL/UR	LR/UL	LR/UR	UL/UR
			LENGTH(M-D)			
H.AFRICANUS						.98
H.ROBUSTUS	.88					.88
H.ERECTUS	.39				.61	1.00
H.NEANDERTHALENSIS	.90	.61	.77	.92	.83	.75
H.SAPIENS	.90	.48	.60	.49	.66	.86
CAUCASOID	.92	.22	.54	.44	.79	.79
INDIAN	.86	.97	.91	.91	.76	.98
NEW BRITAIN	.98	.13	.55	.10	.53	.94
DICKSON MOUND	.84	.75	.63	.68	.65	.86
SUB SAHARAN						
			BREADTH(B-L)			
H.AFRICANUS						.63
H.ROBUSTUS	.89					.99
H.ERECTUS	.92				.82	1.00
H.NEANDERTHALENSIS	.80	-.42	.53	.58	.76	.90
H.SAPIENS	.84	.68	.65	.61	.64	.90
CAUCASOID	.66	.49	.46	.13	.37	.85
INDIAN	.67	.59	.83	.79	.87	.93
NEW BRITAIN	.86	.04	.01	.15	.23	.85
DICKSON MOUND	.83	.83	.76	.69	.63	.92
SUB SAHARAN	.82					
			AREA(L*B)			
H.AFRICANUS						.86
H.ROBUSTUS	.89					.95
H.ERECTUS	.94				.89	1.00
H.NEANDERTHALENSIS	.81	.45	.90	.75	.95	.82
H.SAPIENS	.91	.56	.58	.59	.64	.93
CAUCASOID	.91	.49	.53	.55	.77	.92
INDIAN	.86	.85	.99	.93	.91	.98
NEW BRITAIN	.96	-.00	.01	.06	.16	.95
DICKSON MOUND	.86	.84	.77	.78	.77	.91
SUB SAHARAN	.94					

TABLE XCVI. Correlations for the First Molar. The following abbreviations are used: LL (lower left), LR (lower right), UL (upper left), UR (upper right).

CORRELATIONS FOR M1	LL/LR	LL/UL	LL/UR	LR/UL	LR/UR	UL/UR
			LENGTH(M-D)			
H.AFRICANUS						.95
H.ROBUSTUS	.97					.96
H.ERECTUS					.90	
H.NEANDERTHALENSIS	.95	.49	.60	.44	.44	.98
H.SAPIENS	.90	.70	.54	.68	.55	.84
CAUCASOID	.93	.82	.66	.85	.77	.72
INDIAN	.78	.73	.39	.62	.48	.88
NEW BRITAIN	.89	.29	.06	.32	.18	.79
DICKSON MOUND	.84	.81	.70	.71	.67	.78
HARAPPA, INDIA	.57	.52	.31	.22	.20	.81
SUB SAHARAN	.96	.98			.56	.98
AUSTRALOID						.93
			BREADTH(B-L)			
H.AFRICANUS						.92
H.ROBUSTUS	.93					
H.NEANDERTHALENSIS	.61	.91	.58	.87	.77	.58
H.SAPIENS	.88	.65	.52	.61	.55	.92
CAUCASOID	.90	.41	.33	.41	.37	.90
INDIAN	.94	.88	.35	.82	.35	.63
NEW BRITAIN	.91	.43	.33	.45	.36	.97
DICKSON MOUND	.76	.76	.70	.78	.79	.94
HARAPPA, INDIA	.83	.32	-.06	.03	-.15	.88
SUB SAHARAN	.84				.76	
AUSTRALOID						.86
			AREA(L*B)			
H.AFRICANUS						.99
H.ROBUSTUS	.99					.98
H.NEANDERTHALENSIS	.86	.83	.85	.75	.50	.94
H.SAPIENS	.93	.76	.63	.75	.63	.91
CAUCASOID	.95	.74	.58	.72	.62	.81
INDIAN	.90	.94	.41	.91	.49	.67
NEW BRITAIN	.95	.39	.13	.43	.22	.90
DICKSON MOUND	.87	.89	.82	.85	.80	.93
HARAPPA, INDIA	.77	.54	.27	.33	.17	.84
SUB SAHARAN	.96				.72	
AUSTRALOID	.98					.97

TABLE XCVII. Correlations for the Second Molar. The following abbreviations are used: LL (lower left), LR (lower right), UL (upper left), UR (upper right).

CORRELATIONS FOR M2	LL/LR	LL/UL	LL/UR	LR/UL	LR/UR	UL/UR
			LENGTH(M-D)			
H.AFRICANUS						.97
H.ROBUSTUS	.99					.98
H.ERECTUS	.10				.93	.99
H.NEANDERTHALENSIS	.81	.91	.87	.75	.75	.91
H.SAPIENS	.89	.68	.71	.69	.73	.78
CAUCASOID	.91	.80	.87	.80	.90	.86
INDIAN	.94	.77	.80	.93	.85	.84
NEW BRITAIN	.83	.32	.30	.54	.45	.75
DICKSON MOUND	.79	.68	.66	.63	.67	.87
HARAPPA, INDIA	.66	.25	.34	.18	.30	.34
SUB SAHARAN	.95			.99	.97	.99
AUSTRALOID	.99					.94
			BREADTH(B-L)			
H.AFRICANUS	.86					.99
H.ROBUSTUS	.99					.99
H.ERECTUS	.93				.88	.99
H.NEANDERTHALENSIS	.68	.59	.74	.61	.74	.58
H.SAPIENS	.92	.65	.65	.69	.68	.91
CAUCASOID	.83	.10	.52	.31	.35	.80
INDIAN	.95	.85	.80	.90	.89	.94
NEW BRITAIN	.93	.27	.23	.36	.28	.94
DICKSON MOUND	.89	.79	.86	.81	.90	.91
HARAPPA, INDIA	.92	.23	.51	.08	.38	.82
SUB SAHARAN	.86			.96	.89	.99
AUSTRALOID	.86					.90
			AREA(L*B)			
H.AFRICANUS	.98					.96
H.ROBUSTUS	.99					1.00
H.ERECTUS	.76				.97	1.00
H.NEANDERTHALENSIS	.82	.90	.90	.83	.82	.87
H.SAPIENS	.95	.76	.77	.79	.79	.91
CAUCASOID	.88	.60	.80	.73	.88	.85
INDIAN	.94	.96	.92	.90	.86	.92
NEW BRITAIN	.94	.33	.28	.48	.38	.90
DICKSON MOUND	.90	.80	.85	.79	.87	.94
HARAPPA, INDIA	.92	.09	.54	-.14	.42	.69
SUB SAHARAN	.97			.97	.95	1.00
AUSTRALOID	.95					.92

TABLE XCVIII. Correlations for the Third Molar. The following abbreviations are used: LL (lower left), LR (lower right), UL (upper left), UR (upper right).

CORRELATIONS FOR M3	LL/LR	LL/UL	LL/UR	LR/UL	LR/UR	UL/UR
			LENGTH(M-D)			
H.ROBUSTUS	.91					.93
H.ERECTUS	.87					
H.NEANDERTHALENSIS	.74	.40	.70	.12	.32	.72
H.SAPIENS	.82	.64	.60	.65	.62	.79
CAUCASOID	.87	.69	.64	.74	.85	.79
INDIAN	.89	.41	.62	.47	.72	.84
NEW BRITAIN	.66	.53	.48	.57	.44	.73
DICKSON MOUND	.76	.67	.51	.73	.62	.76
HARAPPA, INDIA	.75	.28	.62	.60	.60	.56
AUSTRALOID	.91					.47
SUB SAHARAN	.85		.99		.90	
			BREADTH(B-L)			
H.ROBUSTUS	.92					.92
H.ERECTUS	.43					
H.NEANDERTHALENSIS	.85	.85	.73	.49	.73	.63
H.SAPIENS	.82	.75	.65	.61	.50	.85
CAUCASOID	.73	.56	.53	.37	.29	.92
INDIAN	.81	.85	.94	.75	.54	.82
NEW BRITAIN	.89	.38	.35	-.02	.05	.83
DICKSON MOUND	.75	.53	.44	.66	.50	.86
HARAPPA, INDIA	.90	.94	.83	.74	.71	.69
AUSTRALOID	-.15					.97
SUB SAHARAN	.75				.94	
			AREA(L*B)			
H.ROBUSTUS	.92					.99
H.ERECTUS	.91					
H.NEANDERTHALENSIS	.82	.59	.78	.25	.64	.70
H.SAPIENS	.89	.75	.71	.71	.68	.89
CAUCASOID	.84	.73	.72	.64	.81	.92
INDIAN	.96	.57	.84	.57	.86	.84
NEW BRITAIN	.83	.57	.47	.35	.33	.78
DICKSON MOUND	.84	.67	.52	.76	.66	.86
HARAPPA, INDIA	.87	.88	.86	.86	.68	.77
AUSTRALOID	.29					.90
SUB SAHARAN	.90				.96	

TABLE IC. North American Mesiodistal Crown Diameter Correlations.

MAXILLA

	I1	I2	C	PM3	PM4	M1
I2	.52					
C	.48	.50				
PM3	.44	.36	.49			
PM4	.44	.28	.42	.67		
M1	.38	.30	.37	.35	.44	
M2	.32	.26	.21	.36	.51	.50

MANDIBLE

	I1	I2	C	PM3	PM4	M1
I2	.73					
C	.54	.62				
PM3	.41	.41	.53			
PM4	.49	.46	.53	.76		
M1	.37	.38	.44	.40	.40	
M2	.38	.39	.40	.44	.44	.45

TABLE C. Lapp Interdental Length and Breadth Correlations. n is the Sample Size, and r the Correlation.

LAPP INTER-DENTAL LENGTH CORRELATIONS

	MAXILLA		MANDIBLE	
	n	r	n	r
I1 - I2	177	.62		
I2 - C	248	.60		
C - PM3	401	.68	429	.57
PM3-PM4	439	.74	434	.70
PM4- M1	474	.53	438	.46
M1 - M2	526	.58	486	.70
M2 - M3	346	.38	312	.39

LAPP INTER-DENTAL BREADTH CORRELATIONS

	MAXILLA n	MAXILLA r	MANDIBLE n	MANDIBLE r
C - PM3	374	.59	410	.63
PM3- PM4	391	.77	426	.73
PM4- M1	408	.55	443	.53
M1 - M2	463	.80	512	.76
M2 - M3	317	.48	314	.62

5. Summations Along the Tooth Row and Dental Ratios

SUMMED DIMENSIONS

Some consideration was given to combinations of summed dimensions for anterior and posterior groups (Tables CI to CX). Averages were taken of summed values. Thus, sample sizes were reduced in all cases: only a relatively small proportion of individuals have dentitions complete enough to sum.

One way to prevent the reduction of sample size is to use the sums of the averages for each tooth, rather than the averages of the sums. These, however, are not necessarily the same. I have compared the sum of the averages to the average of the sums for length and area of the anterior tooth row (I1 to C) for the 5 taxa considered here. Examination of the percentage differences is of some interest. The minimum difference is .5% for maxillary area in *H. sapiens,* and the maximum is 7.2% for maxillary area in *H. erectus.* Maxillary differences were almost always greater than mandibular ones, and the differences were greater in area most of the time. In 8 out of the 20 possibilities, the average of the sums was less than the sum of the averages. Lastly, the average error of all the comparisons was 2.1%.

a) Anterior Sums

Tables CI and CVI examine the mandibular and maxillary sums of I1 and I2. In the mandible, length and breadth differences between the australopithecines and *H. erectus* are not statistically significant, while the area difference is barely so. Comparing *H. africanus* to *H. robustus,* the only significant difference is the very slight one in breadth. Differences between the remaining taxa are only sometimes significant: the *H. erectus-H. neanderthalensis* length and breadth differences are barely so, and there is no significance to the area difference (as well as to the *H. neanderthalensis-H. sapiens* length difference). In general, there is extensive overlap among all the hominid taxa. This is not true for the extant groups: the American Indians fall completely outside the range of variation for the Australian aborigines in both length and area. The first really significant reduction in incisor size occurs with anatomically modern *H. sapiens.* This taxon has mandibular incisor sets significantly narrower (less breadth) and with less area than is the case for *H. neanderthalensis.* These differences alone are greater than the maximum corresponding difference among extant groups.

For the maxillary incisor sums (Table CVI), this pattern emerges even more strongly. Here, there is no statistical difference in any of the comparisons of summed incisors between adjacent taxa, with the exception of the length, breadth, and area reduction from *H. neanderthalensis* to *H. sapiens.* The breadth and area differences appear to have morphological significance while the length difference probably does not. Thus, the length for *H. neanderthalensis* falls within the range of variation in extant groups while the breadth and area do not. The breadth and area evince more difference between the taxa than the maximum difference among extant groups.

Mandibular anterior sums from I1 to C are given in Table CIII. When considering these 3 teeth, differences with no statistical significance occur, in all dimensions, between the australopithecines and *H. erectus,* and in length between *H. africanus* and *H. robustus.* However, there is not great statistical significance to the length differences among the other taxa. The differences between *H. africanus* and *H. robustus* border on morphological significance. Thus, the difference in length is less than the extant maximum; the difference in breadth is greater than the extant maximum; and the area difference is about the same. If the australopithecines are borderline, then differences between *H. erectus* and either *H. robustus* or *H. neanderthalensis* are not morphologically significant. In contrast, the breadth rereduction between *H. neanderthalensis* and *H. sapiens* is morphologically significant. The latter difference exceeds the maximum difference among extant groups.

Maxillary sums from I1 to C are presented in Table CVII. There is a clear pattern of variation, in that no difference between any of the fossil taxa is statistically significant, except again the reduction in breadth and area from *H. neanderthalensis* to *H. sapiens.* The *H. neanderthalensis* breadth and area means fall outside the range of variation for extant groups. The subsequent reduction is greater than the maximum difference among extant groups. Thus, the reduction in breadth and area has morphological significance.

In conclusion, there is great consistency to the trends in length, breadth, and area for the summed anterior teeth of the mandible and maxilla. There do not appear to be any trends of morphological significance, with the exception of the significant reduction in breadth and area between *H. neanderthalensis* and *H. sapiens.*

b) Posterior Sums

Tables CIII and CIV give the sums for the posterior mandibular teeth. Values for sums from P3 - M3 and from C - M3 are given respectively. Both sets of sums show no statistically significant differences between *H. neanderthalensis* and *H. sapiens* in any of the 3 dimensions. Differences among the other taxa are statistically significant. The question of morphological significance is more difficult to ascertain. Differences between *H. africanus* and *H. robustus* are greater than the corresponding maximum differences among the extant groups considered here. Morphological significance would seem to be indicated on this basis. On the other hand, a similar comparison between the hominid taxa and extant groups using the sums of individual tooth averages in each group (Table CXLVII) suggests otherwise. The percentage difference between 2 groups may be expressed with respect to the mean of the 2 groups. Calculated this way, the summed mandibular area difference for the australopithecines is 11%. The greatest percentage difference between extant groups is 32%. This posterior area estimate shows more overlap than the estimate based on the average of posterior sums because the sample size is much greater. For the same reason, the former estimate is a far more likely representation of the actual group parameters. Thus, the variation between extant groups was found to be 3 times as great as the difference between *H. africanus* and *H. robustus.* The difference between *H. erectus* and *H. africanus* was 28% and thus bordered on morphological significance, while the difference between *H. robustus* and *H. erectus* was clearly morphologically significant. In comparison, *H. erectus* and *H. neanderthalensis* differed by 18% (greatly exceeding the percentage difference between the australopithecines), and *H. neanderthalensis* and *H. sapiens* differed by 9%. Even given the maximum estimated 5% error arising from the utilization of summed averages, the great similarity existing between the 2 australopithecine taxa is clear. There has been a consistent and morphologically significant trend throughout the Pleistocene for reduction of the posterior mandibular dentition.

Tables CVIII and CIX give the data for the maxillary sums P3-M3 and C-M3, respectively. The maxillary posterior sums vary identically, and much as the mandibular with a few exceptions. There is no statistical significance to the length differences between *H. neanderthalensis* and both *H. erectus* and *H. sapiens.* In addition, there is no statistical significance to the area difference between *H. neanderthalensis* and *H. sapiens.* With respect to morphological significance, it is again best to use the data derived

TABLE CI. Summed Length (L), Breadth (B), and Area (L*B) from Mandibular I1 and I2: Mean, Range, Sample Size (N), and Coefficient of Variation (CV).

LOWER I1-I2	L(M-D)				B(B-L)				L*B			
	MEAN	RANGE	N	CV	MEAN	RANGE	N	CV	MEAN	RANGE	N	CV
H. AFRICANUS	12.5	9.2 - 14.5	6	15.6	14.3	12.9 - 16.2	5	7.5	87	67.8 - 105.3	5	16.6
H. ROBUSTUS	11.9	11.4 - 12.3	6	2.9	13.0	12.5 - 14.2	6	5.0	78	71.0 - 86.0	6	6.2
H. ERECTUS	13.0	10.5 - 14.7	14	9.3	14.3	13.2 - 17.1	13	8.1	92	81.8 - 114.9	13	10.9
H. NEANDERTAL	12.0	10.3 - 13.8	30	8.1	15.1	13.2 - 17.5	28	6.8	91	71.9 - 107.7	28	10.2
H. SAPIENS	11.9	8.1 - 14.3	195	8.9	12.5	8.5 - 16.5	185	8.9	75	41.0 - 113.0	181	14.2
AUSTRALOP.	12.2	9.2 - 14.5	12	12.1	13.6	12.5 - 16.2	11	8.7	80	68.8 - 105.3	11	10.8
KRAPINA	11.9	11.4 - 12.9	5	11.9	16.2	14.7 - 17.5	5	6.3	97	86.8 - 107.4	5	8.6
NEANDERTAL	12.2	10.3 - 13.8	19	8.0	15.1	13.3 - 16.2	18	4.5	92	83.6 - 104.7	18	6.7
MT CARMEL	11.5	10.5 - 13.7	6	9.2	14.0	13.2 - 15.7	5	6.8	82	71.9 - 107.7	5	15.5
AUSTRALOID	13.3	12.8 - 14.3	6	3.9	13.6	12.8 - 14.8	4	6.6	89	84.0 - 96.0	4	6.4
SUB SAHARAN	12.4	9.7 - 14.2	28	8.3	13.2	8.5 - 16.5	24	12.7	83	41.0 - 102.0	24	18.3
DICKSON MD	12.1	10.5 - 14.1	93	5.7	12.1	10.3 - 13.9	91	6.9	73	58.0 - 92.0	91	9.6
INDIAN	12.1	11.0 - 12.5	10	4.0	12.5	11.2 - 13.8	10	7.0	75	70.0 - 81.0	9	5.8
NEW BRITAIN	12.0	10.6 - 13.4	28	6.8	12.6	11.3 - 14.6	27	5.8	75	62.0 - 86.0	26	8.7
CAUCASOID	10.7	8.1 - 14.0	29	13.4	12.9	11.2 - 16.0	26	9.5	69	51.0 - 113.0	26	22.2

TABLE CII. Summed Length (L), Breadth (B), and Area (L*B) from Mandibular I1 to C: Mean, Range, Sample Size (N), and Coefficient of Variation (CV).

LOWER I1-C	L(M-D)				B(B-L)				L*B			
	MEAN	RANGE	N	CV	MEAN	RANGE	N	CV	MEAN	RANGE	N	CV
H. AFRICANUS	21.3	18.2 - 23.7	5	9.8	24.6	22.8 - 26.2	4	5.2	178	164.1- 196.3	4	7.4
H. ROBUSTUS	19.7	18.7 - 20.3	5	3.5	21.0	20.4 - 22.2	5	3.3	140	130.0- 153.0	5	6.1
H. ERECTUS	21.1	18.2 - 23.6	12	7.6	23.8	21.4 - 27.8	12	7.5	170	145.6- 204.4	12	10.0
H. NEANDERTAL	19.9	17.5 - 22.8	30	6.6	24.1	21.4 - 27.8	28	6.5	162	130.3- 194.9	28	9.0
H. SAPIENS	19.2	14.2 - 22.4	180	7.8	20.4	14.5 - 25.0	170	7.8	133	82.0- 178.0	167	12.9
AUSTRALOP.	20.5	18.2 - 23.6	10	8.9	22.4	20.4 - 26.2	9	10.3	154	130.0- 196.0	9	14.0
KRAPINA	20.1	19.2 - 21.2	5	3.8	25.3	22.6 - 27.8	5	7.1	171	151.6- 194.9	5	9.3
NEANDERTAL	20.0	17.5 - 21.9	19	6.2	24.4	21.4 - 25.9	18	5.0	164	150.1- 192.4	18	6.7
MT CARMEL	19.4	17.7 - 22.8	6	8.9	22.3	21.6 - 22.8	5	2.0	148	130.3- 171.4	5	9.6
AUSTRALOID	21.1	20.0 - 21.8	6	3.0	22.3	21.0 - 24.3	4	6.8	160	148.0- 176.0	4	7.7
SUB SAHARAN	19.9	16.5 - 22.4	25	7.5	20.9	14.5 - 24.2	21	11.3	141	82.0- 172.0	21	17.4
INDIAN	19.5	18.6 - 20.5	10	2.5	20.4	18.9 - 22.7	9	7.0	134	124.0- 149.0	9	6.6
DICKSON MD	19.4	17.4 - 22.2	85	5.2	20.0	17.1 - 23.0	84	6.6	132	101.0- 158.0	84	9.7
NEW BRITAIN	19.4	17.8 - 21.2	25	4.6	20.6	18.8 - 23.9	24	6.0	134	114.0- 153.0	23	7.8
CAUCASOID	17.4	14.2 - 21.3	28	11.4	21.0	18.4 - 25.0	25	7.8	124	94.0- 178.0	25	18.3

TABLE CIII. Summed Length (L), Breadth (B), and Area (L*B) from Mandibular P3 to M3: Mean, Range, Sample Size (N), and Coefficient of Variation (CV).

LOWER P3-M3	L(M-D)				B(B-L)				L*B			
	MEAN	RANGE	N	CV	MEAN	RANGE	N	CV	MEAN	RANGE	N	CV
H.AFRICANUS	62.3	58.8 - 71.6	8	6.4	65.0	59.7 - 69.7	6	4.9	834	754.6 - 1014.2	6	10.1
H.ROBUSTUS	69.8	65.9 - 76.3	11	4.8	70.6	65.9 - 76.5	11	4.9	1007	882.8 - 1183.8	11	9.9
H.ERECTUS	57.3	52.1 - 68.7	15	4.7	57.1	50.4 - 61.1	14	5.8	656	557.2 - 731.0	14	8.4
H.NEANDERTAL	49.0	40.5 - 55.2	25	6.5	50.8	41.5 - 56.6	25	6.7	510	351.0 - 615.0	25	12.0
H.SAPIENS	48.8	41.4 - 61.4	225	6.6	49.5	39.0 - 56.5	219	5.6	496	353.0 - 649.0	216	11.0
AUSTRALOP	66.7	58.8 - 76.3	19	7.8	68.7	59.7 - 76.5	17	6.3	946	754.6 - 1183.8	17	13.3
KRAPINA	50.2	50.0 - 50.5	2	.7	50.9	50.8 - 51.0	2	.3	522	520.0 - 525.0	2	.7
NEANDERTAL	48.8	40.5 - 55.2	21	7.0	50.8	41.5 - 56.6	21	7.2	509	351.0 - 615.0	21	12.9
MT CARMEL	49.6	47.4 - 51.8	2	6.3	50.2	48.1 - 52.3	2	5.9	510	467.0 - 553.0	2	11.9
SUB SAHARAN	50.0	43.4 - 61.4	37	7.9	49.9	39.0 - 54.5	34	6.2	505	353.0 - 588.0	34	11.2
NEW BRITAIN	49.7	44.2 - 56.4	31	5.3	51.0	47.5 - 55.2	30	4.1	520	433.0 - 640.0	30	8.5
AUSTRALOID	49.7	46.3 - 55.3	19	6.3	51.4	47.6 - 56.5	20	4.9	524	450.0 - 649.0	19	11.1
DICKSON MOUND	49.0	41.9 - 55.0	69	5.4	49.1	42.8 - 55.2	68	5.3	495	380.0 - 626.0	68	10.0
INDIAN	48.8	43.7 - 55.4	25	6.1	49.4	45.0 - 53.3	22	5.3	499	401.0 - 604.0	22	11.7
CAUCASOID	46.5	41.4 - 53.0	39	6.4	47.9	41.1 - 53.0	38	5.5	457	353.0 - 542.0	38	10.3

TABLE CIV. Summed Length (L), Breadth (B), and Area (L*B) from Mandibular C to M3: Mean, Range, Sample Size (N), and Coefficient of Variation (CV).

LOWER C-M3	L(M-D)				B(B-L)				L*B			
	MEAN	RANGE	N	CV	MEAN	RANGE	N	CV	MEAN	RANGE	N	CV
H. AFRICANUS	70.2	67.8 - 74.1	6	2.9	74.1	68.8 - 77.3	5	4.3	887	845.6- 920.4	5	3.0
H. ROBUSTUS	78.8	73.7 - 83.6	5	5.3	80.8	75.8 - 84.6	5	5.3	1112	967.0-1243.0	5	6.1
H. ERECTUS	64.4	59.6 - 67.6	11	3.8	66.1	58.6 - 71.1	12	5.7	722	621.0- 803.4	11	7.9
H. NEANDERTAL	56.9	52.5 - 63.3	22	5.2	59.6	54.8 - 65.5	21	4.9	580	512.0- 691.0	21	9.0
H. SAPIENS	56.2	46.4 - 69.4	158	6.7	57.4	45.0 - 65.2	157	5.7	553	389.0- 700.0	151	11.3
AUSTRALOP.	74.1	67.8 - 83.6	11	7.1	77.5	68.8 - 84.6	10	6.3	1000	845.6-1243.0	10	13.8
KRAPINA	58.3	58.2 - 58.5	2		59.2	58.9 - 59.5	2		590	585.0- 595.0	2	
NEANDERTAL	56.6	52.5 - 63.3	18	5.5	59.8	54.8 - 65.5	17	5.2	579	512.0- 691.0	17	9.6
MT CARMEL	57.4	54.7 - 60.1	2		58.6	56.1 - 61.2	2		576	525.0- 627.0	2	
AUSTRALOID	61.5	59.7 - 63.3	4	2.6	62.3	59.2 - 65.2	4	4.2	658	605.0- 686.0	4	5.6
SUB SAHARAN	57.4	50.2 - 69.4	24	8.7	57.2	45.0 - 62.3	22	7.4	555	394.0- 655.0	22	12.7
NEW BRITAIN	57.0	51.2 - 61.7	25	4.1	58.9	55.0 - 62.9	27	4.0	576	487.0- 653.0	25	7.5
INDIAN	56.9	51.8 - 63.7	11	6.7	58.5	54.0 - 62.9	8	5.9	579	483.0- 685.0	8	13.6
DICKSON MD	56.4	48.2 - 63.4	63	5.4	57.1	49.9 - 64.0	65	5.3	554	427.0- 700.0	63	10.1
CAUCASOID	53.2	46.4 - 60.5	26	7.2	55.8	48.5 - 61.0	24	5.1	509	389.0- 606.0	24	10.8

TABLE CV. Summed Length (L), Breadth (B), and Area (L*B) from Mandibular I1 to M3: Mean, Range, Sample Size (N), and Coefficient of Variation (CV).

LOWER I1-M3	L(M-D)				B(B-L)				L*B			
	MEAN	RANGE	N	CV	MEAN	RANGE	N	CV	MEAN	RANGE	N	CV
H. AFRICANUS	80.1	78.3 - 82.0	2		89.7	88.6 - 90.9	2		955	951.0- 960.0	2	
H. ROBUSTUS	90.5	86.0 - 95.0	5	4.3	93.6	88.4 - 97.1	5	4.6	1187	1000.0-1314.0	5	1.6
H. ERECTUS	76.3	69.9 - 82.3	7	5.8	81.8	77.2 - 86.7	7	3.9	817	708.2- 916.8	7	7.8
H. NEANDERTAL	68.8	63.1 - 76.7	22	4.9	74.4	68.7 - 82.6	22	4.8	665	562.6- 785.4	22	7.3
H. SAPIENS	68.2	56.3 - 82.4	114	6.9	69.4	53.5 - 77.0	103	5.5	623	435.0- 779.0	101	10.7
AUSTRALOP.	87.6	78.3 - 95.0	7	6.9	92.5	88.4 - 97.1	7	4.4	1121	951.0-1314.0	7	4.4
KRAPINA	70.0	69.9 - 70.0	2		74.3	73.6 - 74.9	2		677	671.6- 682.4	2	
NEANDERTAL	68.9	63.5 - 76.7	16	7.9	75.2	68.9 - 82.6	16	4.8	672	596.8- 785.4	16	7.2
MT CARMEL	67.5	63.1 - 71.7	4	3.9	71.7	68.7 - 74.4	4	3.8	636	562.6- 703.4	4	7.6
AUSTRALOID	74.9	72.5 - 76.7	4	2.7	73.1	72.2 - 74.1	2		719	689.0- 749.0	2	
SUB SAHARAN	69.9	59.9 - 82.4	17	8.6	69.0	53.5 - 75.6	12	9.2	617	435.0- 720.0	12	13.9
NEW BRITAIN	69.5	65.3 - 75.1	20	3.7	71.0	66.5 - 73.7	18	3.4	650	575.0- 733.0	18	6.3
DICKSON MD	68.8	60.6 - 75.6	43	4.7	69.5	64.1 - 77.0	43	4.8	634	517.0- 779.0	43	9.0
INDIAN	68.5	64.2 - 75.9	9	6.1	69.5	65.3 - 74.6	6	5.7	629	554.0- 726.0	6	12.4
CAUCASOID	63.6	56.3 - 74.2	21	8.1	68.7	60.6 - 74.0	20	5.3	576	449.0- 708.0	20	11.7

TABLE CVI. Summed Length (L), Breadth (B), and Area (L*B) from Maxillary I1 to I2: Mean, Range, Sample Size (N), and Coefficient of Variation (CV).

UPPER I1-I2	L(M-D)				B(B-L)				L*B			
	MEAN	RANGE	N	CV	MEAN	RANGE	N	CV	MEAN	RANGE	N	CV
H. AFRICANUS	16.4	16.1 - 16.8	2		14.8	14.4 - 15.2	2		124	119.0- 129.0	2	
H. ROBUSTUS	17.4	16.5 - 19.0	4	5.5	15.5	15.2 - 15.7	3	1.4	137	129.5- 149.3	3	6.3
H. ERECTUS	18.5	15.3 - 20.0	4	10.1	17.8	16.2 - 20.9	3	12.5	162	124.1- 209.0	3	21.7
H. NEANDERTAL	17.6	14.8 - 21.0	19	11.4	17.0	14.7 - 20.5	15	9.7	151	112.0- 207.0	15	18.6
H. SAPIENS	16.2	11.2 - 20.9	182	8.8	14.4	11.7 - 19.4	179	8.7	118	75.0- 184.0	177	15.0
AUSTRALOP.	17.1	16.1 - 19.0	6	8.5	15.2	14.4 - 15.7	5	9.7	132	119.0- 149.3	5	13.2
KRAPINA	18.3	17.9 - 18.5	3	1.9	17.7	16.5 - 18.8	3	6.6	162	153.0- 173.0	3	6.1
NEANDERTAL	18.0	15.0 - 21.0	11	11.8	17.5	16.1 - 20.5	8	9.1	160	124.0- 207.0	8	19.2
MT CARMEL	16.3	14.8 - 19.7	5	11.8	15.2	14.7 - 16.2	4	4.4	126	112.0- 149.0	4	13.7
SUB SAHARAN	17.5	15.0 - 20.9	18	9.4	15.1	12.0 - 18.9	18	11.4	134	90.0- 184.0	18	18.1
DICKSON MD	16.5	14.7 - 18.6	95	5.4	14.1	11.7 - 16.2	94	6.1	116	87.0- 142.0	94	10.0
NEW BRITAIN	16.4	14.9 - 18.2	23	5.3	14.3	13.2 - 15.9	23	4.5	118	101.0- 136.0	21	6.9
AUSTRALOID	16.2	13.5 - 18.9	8	12.3	15.7	12.4 - 19.4	8	17.1	130	87.0- 165.0	8	25.9
INDIAN	16.0	12.9 - 16.9	9	7.6	13.9	11.9 - 14.6	9	5.8	112	82.0- 122.0	9	10.7
CAUCASOID	14.7	11.2 - 18.4	28	12.9	14.6	12.8 - 17.8	26	10.1	110	75.0- 161.0	26	21.4

TABLE CVII. Summed Length (L), Breadth (B), and Area (L*B) from Maxillary I1 to C: Mean, Range, Sample Size (N), and Coefficient of Variation (CV).

UPPER I1-C	L(M-D)				B(B-L)				L*B			
	MEAN	RANGE	N	CV	MEAN	RANGE	N	CV	MEAN	RANGE	N	CV
H. AFRICANUS	26.3	26.0 - 26.6	2		24.6	24.1 - 25.1	2		220	215.0- 226.0	2	
H. ROBUSTUS	26.1	24.8 - 28.0	4	4.5	25.6	24.3 - 26.1	4	3.8	225	216.6- 242.9	3	5.4
H. ERECTUS	28.3	24.2 - 29.9	4	8.3	28.3	25.7 - 32.6	3	10.8	264	208.7- 320.2	3	17.3
H. NEANDERTAL	25.7	22.7 - 30.0	10	9.4	26.3	24.2 - 27.5	9	4.2	229	197.0- 267.0	9	10.7
H. SAPIENS	24.5	18.7 - 29.4	164	7.5	23.0	18.8 - 30.3	160	7.7	190	131.0- 258.0	160	13.0
AUSTRALOP	26.2	24.8 - 28.0	6	6.2	25.3	24.1 - 26.1	6	5.9	223	215.0- 242.9	5	12.1
KRAPINA	27.8	27.8 - 27.8	1	.0	25.8	25.8 - 25.8	1	.0	239	239.0- 239.0	1	.0
NEANDERTAL	25.9	22.7 - 30.0	7	10.3	26.9	26.0 - 27.5	6	2.4	237	211.0- 267.0	6	9.8
MT CARMEL	24.1	24.0 - 24.2	2	.6	24.7	24.2 - 25.2	2	2.9	201	197.0- 204.0	2	2.6
SUB SAHARAN	25.8	21.0 - 29.4	14	9.7	23.8	18.8 - 26.7	14	10.3	207	131.0- 250.0	14	17.7
DICKSON MD	24.9	21.9 - 27.6	85	4.8	22.7	19.1 - 25.7	85	5.4	190	140.0- 227.0	85	8.9
NEW BRITAIN	24.8	23.2 - 26.5	22	4.3	23.0	21.6 - 25.9	20	4.5	192	168.0- 228.0	20	7.1
AUSTRALOID	24.4	21.8 - 26.9	8	8.0	25.2	19.8 - 30.3	8	15.2	208	145.0- 258.0	8	20.1
INDIAN	24.2	20.9 - 25.2	8	5.9	22.4	20.0 - 23.8	8	5.5	182	146.0- 195.0	8	9.0
CAUCASOID	22.7	18.7 - 27.4	27	10.7	23.3	20.8 - 28.2	25	8.7	178	131.0- 258.0	25	18.7

TABLE CVIII. Summed Length (L), Breadth (B), and Area (L*B) from Maxillary P3 to M3: Mean, Range, Sample Size (N), and Coefficient of Variation (CV).

UPPER P3-M3	L(M-D)				B(B-L)				L*B			
	MEAN	RANGE	N	CV	MEAN	RANGE	N	CV	MEAN	RANGE	N	CV
H. AFRICANUS	57.0	55.3 - 59.5	5	2.0	69.4	68.3 - 70.0	5	2.9	802	786.8 - 830.7	5	2.2
H. ROBUSTUS	64.5	58.8 - 71.6	9	6.5	80.8	71.8 - 95.1	9	9.5	1060	858.2 - 1363.9	9	16.0
H. ERECTUS	49.6	45.1 - 60.5	8	10.7	62.5	57.7 - 75.2	8	9.0	631	528.6 - 923.0	8	20.7
H. NEANDERTAL	45.5	37.7 - 52.6	16	8.7	57.5	52.3 - 62.3	17	5.2	530	416.0 - 668.0	16	12.5
H. SAPIENS	45.2	35.0 - 56.9	169	7.5	54.9	43.0 - 65.9	165	7.3	504	307.0 - 710.0	164	13.5
AUSTRALOP.	61.8	55.3 - 71.6	14	8.1	76.7	68.3 - 95.1	14	10.7	968	786.8 - 1363.9	14	19.0
NEANDERTAL	45.0	37.7 - 52.6	13	9.1	57.6	52.3 - 62.3	14	5.6	523	416.0 - 668.0	13	13.2
MT CARMEL	47.3	43.6 - 49.4	3	6.8	57.0	54.6 - 58.4	3	3.7	547	485.0 - 583.0	3	9.9
AUSTRALOID	48.1	43.9 - 53.5	19	6.1	58.7	49.8 - 65.9	17	9.1	576	446.0 - 710.0	17	14.3
NEW BRITAIN	46.5	42.7 - 50.8	32	4.0	56.9	52.3 - 63.0	32	4.9	537	455.0 - 653.0	31	8.1
SUB SAHARAN	46.2	39.4 - 56.9	11	11.3	53.9	44.3 - 61.0	10	9.5	498	362.0 - 619.0	10	17.0
INDIAN	45.1	42.9 - 48.4	12	4.5	53.3	49.9 - 57.8	12	5.1	490	434.0 - 550.0	12	7.8
DICKSON MD	44.8	38.0 - 49.4	64	5.5	54.2	48.5 - 62.8	64	5.2	495	391.0 - 633.0	64	10.2
CAUCASOID	42.6	35.0 - 51.4	29	10.2	53.2	43.0 - 60.5	28	8.6	466	307.0 - 617.0	28	17.2

TABLE CIX. Summed Length (L), Breadth (B), and Area (L*B) from Maxillary C to M3: Mean, Range, Sample Size (N), and Coefficient of Variation (CV).

UPPER C-M3	L(M-D)				B(B-L)				L*B			
	MEAN	RANGE	N	CV	MEAN	RANGE	N	CV	MEAN	RANGE	N	CV
H. AFRICANUS	66.6	65.6 - 68.3	3	1.9	79.3	78.4 - 79.8	3	1.8	895	883.8- 913.4	3	1.5
H. ROBUSTUS	74.9	67.5 - 80.4	4	7.9	94.6	80.6 - 104.8	4	10.4	1234	930.4-1448.3	4	18.1
H. ERECTUS	60.6	54.1 - 70.8	4	11.2	75.5	68.7 - 84.2	4	8.5	782	620.6-1016.0	4	20.2
H. NEANDERTAL	53.7	44.2 - 62.6	15	9.3	67.6	60.6 - 73.2	15	5.2	625	484.3- 778.0	14	11.7
H. SAPIENS	53.4	42.0 - 66.0	145	6.9	63.2	51.0 - 77.4	144	7.0	572	363.0- 829.0	142	12.8
AUSTRALOP.	71.3	65.6 - 80.4	7	8.2	88.0	78.4 - 104.8	7	12.1	1088	883.8-1448.3	7	21.9
NEANDERTAL	53.8	44.2 - 62.6	12	9.4	67.5	60.6 - 73.2	12	5.7	612	500.0- 778.0	11	12.3
MT CARMEL	56.0	52.5 - 58.7	3	6.1	65.1	63.1 - 68.5	3	4.9	632	484.3- 582.9	3	7.8
AUSTRALOID	57.0	52.6 - 63.7	13	6.7	68.6	58.4 - 77.4	12	9.1	666	561.0- 829.0	12	14.4
NEW BRITAIN	54.6	50.8 - 59.0	23	3.6	65.0	62.5 - 72.3	23	4.2	600	541.0- 687.0	22	6.8
SUB SAHARAN	53.7	45.4 - 66.0	10	11.0	61.8	51.1 - 70.5	9	9.4	553	403.0- 657.0	9	16.1
INDIAN	53.6	50.9 - 56.6	11	3.8	62.1	58.2 - 67.2	11	5.1	566	502.0- 632.0	11	7.2
DICKSON MD	53.1	46.1 - 58.4	61	5.2	62.8	56.5 - 72.6	61	5.2	566	463.0- 722.0	61	9.9
CAUCASOID	51.1	42.0 - 60.7	24	9.4	61.6	51.0 - 71.0	25	8.4	537	363.0- 715.0	24	17.0

TABLE CX. Summed Length (L), Breadth (B), and Area (L*B) from Maxillary I1 to M3: Mean, Range, Sample Size (N), and Coefficient of Variation (CV).

UPPER I1-M3	L(M-D)				B(B-L)				L*B			
	MEAN	RANGE	N	CV	MEAN	RANGE	N	CV	MEAN	RANGE	N	CV
H. AFRICANUS	82.6	81.9 - 83.5	3		93.8	92.3 - 94.9	3		1014	1005.2-1023.9	3	
H. ROBUSTUS	97.0	96.5 - 97.4	2		119.3	118.1 - 120.4	2		1580	1577.5-1581.5	2	
H. ERECTUS	81.1	70.5 - 90.4	3		93.4	86.7 - 100.0	2		912	778.5-1044.7	2	
H. NEANDERTAL	72.8	66.8 - 80.5	10	6.3	83.9	77.5 - 89.7	10	4.5	779	667.0- 919.0	10	10.0
H. SAPIENS	69.3	56.6 - 84.2	110	6.2	77.3	63.1 - 88.2	104	5.9	686	493.0- 876.0	104	10.7
AUSTRALOP.	88.3	81.9 - 97.4	5	8.0	91.4	92.3 - 120.4	5	10.2	1240	1005.2-1581.5	5	22.3
NEANDERTAL	73.2	66.8 - 80.5	7	7.1	84.9	77.5 - 89.7	7	4.6	792	667.0- 919.0	7	10.7
MT CARMEL	71.8	68.7 - 73.5	3	3.0	81.5	78.5 - 83.7	3	2.7	748	687.6- 787.2	3	5.8
AUSTRALOID	70.8	66.4 - 74.4	8	3.7	80.3	71.3 - 85.9	7	7.8	722	653.0- 777.0	7	6.6
NEW BRITAIN	70.8	67.2 - 77.2	16	3.8	79.7	76.0 - 87.3	14	3.9	727	678.0- 814.0	14	6.0
SUB SAHARAN	70.7	60.4 - 84.2	9	10.7	75.4	63.1 - 86.7	8	9.8	666	493.0- 801.0	8	1.7
DICKSON MD	69.6	61.6 - 74.7	51	4.7	77.0	69.4 - 86.9	51	4.9	686	571.0- 838.0	51	9.3
INDIAN	69.2	64.1 - 73.3	8	4.1	76.1	71.0 - 80.2	8	4.3	673	600.0- 715.0	8	6.9
CAUCASOID	66.7	56.6 - 78.8	18	9.2	77.4	69.6 - 88.2	16	6.9	668	525.0- 876.0	16	.6

from the comparison of summed averages because of the greater number of extant groups represented, as well as the greater sample size available for each group. Table CXLVII shows a 24% difference between the australopithecine groups. This can be compared with the 40% maximum difference among the extant groups—almost *twice* as great. The difference between *H. africanus* and *H. robustus* exceeds the difference between the former and *H. erectus.*

Two conclusions emerge: (1) the difference between the australopithecines is not morphologically significant; (2) there is a clearly significant trend to the reduction of the posterior teeth throughout the Pleistocene. The presence of such a trend for both the summed mandibular and maxillary posterior dentitions makes the great similarity between the australopithecines, when compared to subsequent taxa, all the most significant.

The extent of posterior reduction shown for *H. sapiens* is somewhat misleading. Third molar agenesis is a phenomena of increasing frequency in extant groups (Banks 1934; Nanda 1954; Hunt 1959; Brothwell, Carbonell, and Goose 1963; Goldstein 1932; Hellman 1936; Garn, Lewis, and Vicinus 1963). It seems to have a definite relationship to the size of the jaw: some authors have suggested that smaller jaws select for fewer teeth (Hellman 1936; Keith 1925). No case of third molar agenesis is known in a hominid species other than *H. sapiens.* However, factors of use, and resulting stress on the bone, are known to influence mandible size developmentally (Campbell 1966:182; Oppenheimer 1964, 1966, 1967; J. Howell 1917; Baker 1941; Hunt 1959; Watt and Williams 1951), so that the dental reduction more likely results from the same factors which act to reduce mandible size (Hunt 1959): mainly, the relaxation of selection maintaining large teeth for mastication, gripping, and holding functions (Brose and Wolpoff 1971; Wolpoff 1969a). Indeed, third molar agenesis is closely related to the reduction of the number of other teeth (Garn and Lewis 1962; Garn, Lewis, and Vicinus 1962), as well as to cusp reduction (Davies 1968), and size reduction (Garn, Lewis, and Kerewsky 1964c) in the remaining teeth. As such, the increasing frequency of missing third molars represents an extension of the general trend: reduction in the grinding area of the posterior teeth. Finding no significant difference between *H. sapiens* and *H. neanderthalensis* in the posterior summed teeth is an artifact of the way in which the sample was collected; only those dentitions were summed in which the third molar was present. In actuality, taking third molar agenesis into account leaves *H. sapiens* with a posterior dentition significantly reduced.

c) Entire Tooth-Row Sums

Tables CV and CX give summed parameters for the entire tooth row. The length difference, both mandibular and maxillary, between *H. sapiens* and *H. neanderthalensis* is not statistically significant. All other differences between adjacent taxa are statistically significant. In the mandibular dentition, it is interesting to note that while almost no 2 temporally adjacent taxa (excepting *H. robustus* and *H. erectus*) have morphologically significant differences, the total size reduction in the Pleistocene is clearly of morphological significance. This includes the comparison of *H. erectus* with all australopithecines. By way of contrast, almost all of the maxillary comparisons are of morphological significance. This is surely an artifact of the very small sample sizes for *H. africanus* (3 from 2 individuals), *H. robustus* (2 from 1 individual), and *H. erectus* (2 from 2 individuals). With sample sizes this small, it is specimens, and not the taxa from which they were sampled, which are being compared.

DENTAL RATIOS OF INDIVIDUAL TEETH

There has been only limited use of tooth-to-tooth ratios, the so-called "step ratios" (Goose 1963:132), in the literature (Selmer-Olsen 1949; Weidenreich 1943; Robinson 1956; Tobias 1967a; Senyurek 1953; Dahlberg 1962, 1963a; Frisch 1965; von Koenigswald 1962b; Garn, Lewis, and Kerewsky 1964a). Dental ratios for length, breadth, and area have been calculated here, comparing a number of different teeth (Tables CXI to CXLII). The species and extant group values for the ratios were calculated from the sum of the available ratios, rather than the ratio of the sums.

a) Anterior to Anterior Ratios

Table CXI considers the ratio of the mandibular I1 to C, and Table CXII considers the corresponding maxillary ratio. Length, breadth, and area ratios for the mandible show all of the fossil hominid taxa either almost or completely within the range of variation for extant groups of *H. sapiens*, with the single exception of *H. africanus*. The smaller ratio in *H. africanus* (30% smaller in area ratio) thus has apparent morphological significance. That is, the canines are relatively larger with respect to the central incisors in *H. africanus*, but reduced in all other hominid taxa.

The maxillary ratios have exactly the same pattern of variation for length. Breadth and area ratios place the *H. africanus* range of variation within the modern extant group range. Possible morphological significance appears with respect to the relatively longer maxillary canines (compared with central incisors) in the *H. africanus* maxilla (there are 2 ratios calculated for 1 individual—STS 52). One individual cannot, by itself, characterize the taxon.

Examination of both the mandibular (Table CXIII) and maxillary (Table CXIV) I2/C ratios demonstrates the same pattern; all fossil hominid taxa are morphologically similar with the exception of a relatively larger canine for *H. africanus*. The only apparent exception is the slightly enlarged canine area, corresponding to a reduced ratio, for the *H. robustus* maxillae.

TABLE CXI. Ratio of Mandibular I1 to C for Length (L), Breadth (B), and Area (L*B): Mean, Range, Sample Size (N), and Coefficient of Variation (CV).

LOWER I1/C	L(M-D)				B(B-L)				L*B			
	MEAN	RANGE	N	CV	MEAN	RANGE	N	CV	MEAN	RANGE	N	CV
H. AFRICANUS	62.1	44.4 - 73.2	5	17.6	67.3	58.3 - 81.0	4	12.6	40.4	28.2 - 52.3	4	15.5
H. ROBUSTUS	71.9	64.7 - 75.7	6	6.0	78.0	73.0 - 92.0	6	9.1	56.2	47.3 - 68.7	6	12.4
H. ERECTUS	73.8	64.9 - 85.4	9	7.8	75.0	66.7 - 83.3	9	7.2	56.5	47.1 - 71.1	9	11.2
H. NEANDERTAL	69.0	52.9 - 86.2	24	9.9	80.7	68.6 - 110.0	16	12.5	56.2	43.3 - 78.6	16	16.5
H. SAPIENS	76.0	59.2 - 101.5	186	9.9	75.7	62.8 - 93.3	176	7.8	57.4	40.5 - 85.2	172	13.7
AUSTRALOP.	67.5	44.4 - 75.7	11	14.4	74.6	58.3 - 92.0	10	13.0	50.0	28.2 - 68.7	10	13.1
KRAPINA	67.7	65.9 - 71.1	3	4.3								
NEANDERTAL	71.1	52.9 - 86.2	15	10.3	79.0	68.6 - 90.9	13	8.5	55.6	48.1 - 68.1	13	12.8
MT CARMEL	64.3	60.2 - 71.4	6	6.7	88.4	71.9 - 110.0	3	22.1	58.7	43.3 - 78.6	3	30.7
AUSTRALOID	82.8	73.8 - 95.6	6	10.7	76.3	75.0 - 77.8	4	1.5	59.1	55.9 - 62.1	4	5.9
SUB SAHARAN	79.2	65.9 - 100.0	25	12.1	80.7	70.0 - 93.3	21	8.4	64.3	46.3 - 85.2	21	16.0
NEW BRITAIN	77.8	62.0 - 101.5	26	10.3	77.1	62.8 - 87.7	26	8.6	59.6	46.8 - 78.8	24	13.3
DICKSON MOUND	75.2	62.2 - 87.0	87	7.6	73.3	62.8 - 82.4	85	5.8	55.1	40.5 - 70.9	85	11.1
INDIAN	73.7	59.2 - 87.1	10	13.2	76.7	67.2 - 83.6	9	7.1	57.2	47.2 - 63.2	9	10.8
CAUCASOID	73.0	59.7 - 88.0	29	10.2	76.8	66.7 - 88.2	26	8.0	56.1	46.9 - 75.1	26	13.3

TABLE CXLVII. Summed Posterior Areas from Individual Tooth Averages.

AREAS OF THE POSTERIOR MAXILLARY DENTITION

	"AFRICANUS"	"ROBUSTUS"	"ERECTUS"	"NEANDERTAL"	"SAPIENS"	AUSTRALOID	INDIAN	CAUCASOID	JAPANESE	LAPP
PM3	111	142	103	81	73	84	73	64	69	57
PM4	112	169	92	76	70	81	68	63	63	55
M1	170	205	151	137	126	150	128	122	115	102
M2	211	244	154	133	118	142	122	113	110	97
M3	200	261	130	116	103	124	102	100	92	77
Sum	804	1021	630	543	490	581	493	464	449	388

AREAS OF THE POSTERIOR MANDIBULAR DENTITION

	"AFRICANUS"	"ROBUSTUS"	"ERECTUS"	"NEANDERTAL"	"SAPIENS"	AUSTRALOID	INDIAN	CAUCASOID	JAPANESE	LAPP
PM3	112	116	85	71	59	63	58	55	56	48
PM4	121	148	89	70	65	70	65	60	61	51
M1	182	202	154	131	127	140	130	121	120	110
M2	219	233	161	132	120	134	125	116	112	101
M3	211	242	149	129	116	132	120	112	100	81
Sum	845	941	638	533	487	539	498	464	449	391

TABLE CXII. Ratio of Maxillary I1 to C for Length (L), Breadth (B), and Area (L*B): Mean, Range, Sample Size (N), and Coefficient of Variation (CV).

UPPER I1/C	L(M-D)				B(B-L)				L*B			
	MEAN	RANGE	N	CV	MEAN	RANGE	N	CV	MEAN	RANGE	N	CV
H. AFRICANUS	95.4	93.9 - 96.9	2	2.2	84.2	82.8 - 85.6	2	2.3	80.3	80.3 - 80.4	2	.1
H. ROBUSTUS	110.9	108.9 - 116.9	5	6.6	79.0	77.8 - 82.5	4	2.5	90.0	84.8 - 94.8	4	4.0
H. ERECTUS	102.4	84.7 - 114.6	6	13.0	80.2	70.8 - 89.7	5	9.7	80.4	64.8 - 94.5	5	10.9
H. NEANDERTAL	110.5	80.0 - 133.3	13	13.3	83.7	75.0 - 96.5	12	7.9	91.9	61.8 - 108.4	12	16.7
H. SAPIENS	106.3	78.5 - 137.5	180	8.7	86.3	71.4 - 103.2	177	6.6	91.9	59.5 - 127.5	176	11.4
AUSTRALOP.	106.5	93.9 - 116.9	7	9.1	80.7	77.8 - 82.5	6	5.4	86.8	80.3 - 94.8	6	6.2
KRAPINA	109.3	107.5 - 111.1	2	2.3	88.4	88.2 - 88.6	2	.4	96.6	94.8 - 98.5	2	2.7
NEANDERTAL	114.5	80.0 - 133.3	8	14.5	82.5	77.3 - 93.2	7	6.4	93.6	61.8 - 106.7	7	16.7
MT CARMEL	100.5	91.3 - 112.4	3	10.7	83.5	75.0 - 96.5	3	13.7	84.7	68.5 - 108.4	3	24.8
AUSTRALOID	111.6	83.3 - 137.5	9	13.7	86.6	71.4 - 97.8	9	11.4	97.0	59.5 - 122.1	9	18.8
SUB SAHARAN	111.2	93.7 - 133.3	15	8.8	85.7	73.7 - 102.4	15	7.4	95.4	69.1 - 117.6	15	13.0
NEW BRITAIN	106.3	93.3 - 120.5	23	6.8	87.1	77.7 - 98.7	22	6.6	92.7	77.4 - 107.1	21	8.9
DICKSON MOUND	105.9	91.0 - 126.7	90	5.4	85.5	77.3 - 102.1	90	5.2	90.6	75.1 - 116.3	90	8.1
INDIAN	103.5	94.7 - 111.2	10	5.2	87.3	78.0 - 103.2	10	8.9	90.4	79.0 - 110.4	10	10.5
CAUCASOID	103.1	78.5 - 132.1	30	14.3	88.0	75.6 - 101.9	28	7.5	91.6	64.5 - 127.5	28	17.0

TABLE CXIII. Ratio of Mandibular I2 to C for Length (L), Breadth (B), and Area (L*B): Mean, Range, Sample Size (N), and Coefficient of Variation (CV).

LOWER I2/C	L(M-D)				B(B-L)				L*B			
	MEAN	RANGE	N	CV	MEAN	RANGE	N	CV	MEAN	RANGE	N	CV
H.AFRICANUS	73.2	57.8 - 85.2	5	17.6	77.2	72.9 - 81.0	3	5.3	50.9	42.1 - 63.2	3	21.5
H.ROBUSTUS	80.7	71.8 - 85.9	5	6.7	80.7	76.4 - 85.9	5	4.9	65.3	54.8 - 73.8	5	10.6
H.ERECTUS	81.8	77.8 - 86.4	6	3.8	81.8	72.3 - 89.0	7	8.3	66.9	56.2 - 74.8	5	10.4
H.NEANDERTAL	82.8	68.2 - 97.2	31	7.3	87.2	77.8 - 114.3	19	11.6	72.2	62.2 - 106.7	19	14.8
H.SAPIENS	87.2	70.5 - 110.0	205	7.4	81.5	64.9 - 127.3	194	8.1	71.1	47.6 - 117.9	189	12.1
AUSTRALOP.	77.0	57.8 - 85.9	10	13.2	79.4	72.9 - 85.9	8	5.2	59.9	42.1 - 73.8	8	18.0
KRAPINA	80.6	76.2 - 84.3	6	3.8	88.3	88.3 - 88.3	2	.1	73.6	72.8 - 74.5	2	1.6
NEANDERTAL	84.3	68.2 - 97.2	20	8.2	85.7	77.8 - 109.8	14	10.2	71.4	63.0 - 106.7	14	15.6
MT CARMEL	79.4	75.9 - 82.2	5	2.8	93.6	77.8 - 114.3	3	20.0	75.2	62.2 - 90.4	3	18.9
AUSTRALOID	89.6	81.0 - 98.5	6	8.0	79.0	74.1 - 87.5	4	7.9	67.3	63.9 - 74.4	4	7.2
INDIAN	89.5	84.3 - 97.6	11	4.9	81.7	77.4 - 88.6	10	4.6	73.5	67.9 - 83.9	10	6.5
DICKSON MOUND	88.3	76.7 - 97.6	92	4.8	80.2	71.6 - 95.9	91	6.3	70.8	58.2 - 85.6	91	8.3
SUB SAHARAN	86.3	71.8 - 100.0	29	7.2	84.8	71.7 - 127.3	23	13.3	73.3	51.8 - 117.9	23	18.1
NEW BRITAIN	85.3	72.2 - 98.6	30	7.8	81.1	64.9 - 100.0	30	7.8	68.5	58.2 - 83.2	27	10.4
CAUCASOID	85.1	70.5 - 110.0	34	12.2	82.7	66.7 - 94.1	31	7.3	70.7	47.6 - 99.3	31	17.0

TABLE CXIV. Ratio of Maxillary I2 to C for Length (L), Breadth (B), and Area (L*B): Mean, Range, Sample Size (N), and Coefficient of Variation (CV).

UPPER I2/C	L(M-D)				B(B-L)				L*B			
	MEAN	RANGE	N	CV	MEAN	RANGE	N	CV	MEAN	RANGE	N	CV
H.AFRICANUS	69.9	65.9 - 74.5	4	5.2	66.0	59.6 - 70.7	4	8.5	46.3	39.3 - 52.7	4	13.3
H.ROBUSTUS	81.1	71.1 - 101.1	6	13.1	71.6	65.0 - 75.8	5	5.7	58.2	46.2 - 71.7	5	16.1
H.ERECTUS	89.2	78.1 - 105.3	3	16.0	83.9	77.9 - 88.9	3	6.7	75.3	60.8 - 93.6	3	22.2
H.NEANDERTAL	87.0	69.6 - 100.0	13	12.9	85.7	72.7 - 100.0	11	10.0	75.6	50.9 - 100.0	11	22.0
H.SAPIENS	88.4	61.2 - 121.2	187	9.6	78.6	54.3 - 98.7	185	8.2	69.8	33.3 - 102.9	183	14.3
AUSTRALOP.	76.6	65.9 - 101.1	10	13.1	69.1	59.6 - 75.2	9	7.8	52.9	39.3 - 71.7	9	18.7
KRAPINA	91.9	91.9 - 91.9	1	.0	89.2	89.2 - 89.2	1	.0	82.0	82.0 - 82.0	1	.0
NEANDERTAL	88.9	70.0 - 100.0	10	12.4	87.5	72.7 - 100.0	8	9.9	79.3	50.9 - 100.0	8	20.9
MT CARMEL	75.0	69.6 - 80.5	2	10.3	76.4	75.8 - 77.0	2	1.1	57.3	53.6 - 61.0	2	9.1
SUB SAHARAN	95.2	82.4 - 121.2	15	11.6	80.5	69.5 - 91.5	15	7.6	77.0	57.2 - 102.9	15	16.6
INDIAN	89.7	61.2 - 101.2	9	12.6	75.6	54.3 - 85.5	10	11.2	68.4	33.3 - 83.1	9	20.9
DICKSON MOUND	89.2	71.8 - 103.4	95	7.2	78.1	60.6 - 94.8	95	7.7	69.8	43.9 - 87.2	95	12.3
AUSTRALOID	87.6	66.7 - 110.0	9	16.8	77.9	57.1 - 89.3	10	13.0	69.2	38.1 - 95.8	9	25.9
NEW BRITAIN	87.0	68.5 - 100.0	29	8.0	78.9	72.5 - 86.4	27	4.6	68.6	53.0 - 82.5	27	9.7
CAUCASOID	83.2	67.5 - 103.8	28	10.7	80.6	66.7 - 98.7	26	9.6	67.7	47.6 - 83.9	26	15.2

TABLE CXV. Ratio of Mandibular P3 to P4 for Length (L), Breadth (B), and Area (L*B): Mean, Range, Sample Size (N), and Coefficient of Variation (CV).

LOWER P3/P4	L(M-D)				B(B-L)				L*B			
	MEAN	RANGE	N	CV	MEAN	RANGE	N	CV	MEAN	RANGE	N	CV
H.AFRICANUS	98.5	89.2 - 111.1	8	9.2	96.7	78.6 - 108.3	7	9.8	93.6	78.6 - 115.7	7	14.9
H.ROBUSTUS	87.5	63.4 - 103.1	13	11.7	91.6	80.9 - 107.0	13	7.9	80.3	56.4 - 101.3	13	16.0
H.ERECTUS	99.7	88.9 - 112.6	18	6.1	99.3	90.1 - 113.7	18	6.3	98.8	87.4 - 105.7	18	6.0
H.NEANDERTAL	106.2	80.6 - 135.6	36	10.8	99.8	87.3 - 122.2	36	8.1	106.2	72.1 - 150.7	36	15.5
H.SAPIENS	96.8	57.1 - 123.3	325	8.1	94.8	68.4 - 115.4	322	6.9	92.0	48.1 - 132.9	319	12.1
AUSTRALOPITH	91.7	63.4 - 111.1	21	12.0	93.4	78.6 - 108.3	20	8.8	85.0	56.4 - 115.7	20	17.0
KRAPINA	100.8	96.1 - 103.7	4	3.6	97.7	90.7 - 102.2	4	5.1	98.4	94.0 - 106.0	4	5.3
NEANDERTAL	108.2	90.0 - 135.6	29	10.4	100.5	87.3 - 122.2	29	8.5	108.9	89.0 - 150.7	29	15.1
MT CARMEL	93.3	80.6 - 104.5	3	12.9	96.0	89.5 - 102.2	3	6.6	90.1	72.1 - 106.8	3	19.3
INDIAN	100.2	76.8 - 123.3	30	11.6	92.8	73.1 - 107.8	26	9.6	93.7	56.2 - 132.9	26	19.2
CAUCASOID	99.0	85.7 - 114.9	70	6.8	93.7	68.4 - 112.6	69	6.5	93.0	58.6 - 119.9	69	9.8
SUB SAHARAN	98.0	75.6 - 111.9	45	7.6	96.3	68.9 - 112.5	44	8.6	94.8	52.1 - 125.6	44	13.7
DICKSON MD	95.6	83.5 - 111.9	114	5.2	94.6	84.7 - 113.3	114	4.9	90.5	74.3 - 113.3	114	8.3
AUSTRALOID	95.1	78.5 - 114.3	20	9.1	96.9	84.2 - 113.3	21	8.4	92.6	76.0 - 115.7	20	14.6
NEW BRITAIN	95.1	67.9 - 109.0	39	9.1	96.1	83.5 - 115.4	39	6.7	91.6	56.7 - 111.6	39	12.6

TABLE CXVI. Ratio of Maxillary P3 to P4 for Length (L), Breadth (B), and Area (L*B): Mean, Range, Sample Size (N), and Coefficient of Variation (CV).

UPPER P3/P4	L(M-D)				B(B-L)				L*B			
	MEAN	RANGE	N	CV	MEAN	RANGE	N	CV	MEAN	RANGE	N	CV
H.AFRICANUS	97.3	88.9 - 109.0	10	7.1	96.4	92.9 - 99.2	10	2.5	93.9	82.5 - 103.5	10	7.8
H.ROBUSTUS	90.7	75.2 - 97.1	12	5.8	91.0	83.2 - 96.6	12	4.1	82.7	62.6 - 89.0	12	8.4
H.ERECTUS	106.1	95.4 - 121.4	10	7.0	101.9	95.7 - 110.9	11	4.6	108.6	94.6 - 134.7	10	10.5
H.NEANDERTAL	105.1	77.8 - 123.3	24	9.5	101.2	92.8 - 122.6	23	6.5	106.1	77.8 - 129.2	23	11.1
H.SAPIENS	104.1	79.6 - 134.8	253	7.4	100.8	79.4 - 116.1	249	5.2	105.2	71.5 - 138.1	249	10.6
AUSTRALOPITH	93.7	75.2 - 109.0	22	7.2	93.5	83.2 - 99.2	22	4.5	87.8	62.6 - 103.5	22	10.3
KRAPINA	105.3	98.8 - 111.8	2	8.8	101.7	96.2 - 107.1	2	7.6	107.4	95.0 - 119.8	2	16.4
NEANDERTAL	105.5	77.8 - 123.3	19	8.8	99.8	92.8 - 108.7	18	4.9	105.3	77.8 - 129.2	18	11.6
MT CARMEL	102.6	82.7 - 117.1	3	17.4	108.9	100.0 - 122.6	3	11.0	110.3	101.4 - 117.1	3	7.3
INDIAN	106.1	89.9 - 119.7	20	8.7	101.0	91.4 - 109.7	20	5.1	107.4	89.2 - 130.6	20	12.2
NEW BRITAIN	105.3	79.6 - 121.6	46	7.4	100.7	89.4 - 114.1	45	4.6	106.8	87.1 - 138.1	45	9.9
DICKSON MD	104.8	88.8 - 121.8	99	6.0	102.0	93.8 - 116.1	98	4.2	107.2	85.8 - 136.9	98	8.8
AUSTRALOID	103.4	84.5 - 118.4	21	7.4	98.8	81.6 - 111.8	20	7.0	102.4	77.2 - 118.7	20	10.6
SUB SAHARAN	103.3	91.4 - 117.1	20	6.1	100.7	93.9 - 110.4	20	4.4	104.2	88.9 - 122.9	20	8.9
CAUCASOID	101.8	79.7 - 134.8	42	9.5	98.9	79.4 - 114.3	41	7.0	100.6	71.5 - 136.2	41	13.5

Thus, there is a progressive pattern of canine reduction relative to the incisors. This pattern is somewhat clearer in the mandible than it is in the maxilla, although it exists in both jaws. This trend seems to place *H. africanus* apart from the other hominid taxa.

The last possible anterior to anterior ratio is I2/I1. This ratio was not calculated here. Tobias (1967a:152), Senyurek (1953), and Selmer-Olsen (1949:61-62) have calculated the ratio for area, module, and breadth in extinct and extant hominids. Apparently, all fossil taxa can be included in the range of variation of extant groups.

b) Posterior to Posterior Ratios

Tables CXV to CXXXVIII present data for the ratios of posterior to posterior teeth in both the mandible and the maxilla.

Table CXV is concerned with the ratio of the third to the fourth lower premolars. According to von Koenigswald (1962b:125), hominid evolution is characterized by a progressive "deterioration" of the anterior premolar in comparison to the posterior premolar. If this were the case, *H. robustus* would have to be considered an "ultra hominid" (as von Koenigswald indeed suggests), and *H. neanderthalensis* would have to be the most primitive of all hominids with larger anterior than posterior premolars, on the average. For length, American Indians also exhibit this "archaic" condition. In actuality, while the fossil species are both outside of the range of variation for extant groups in length and area, this distribution only emphasizes the lack of any consistent trends in the ratio. Considering the australopithecines as 1 point on a line, and *H. sapiens* as another, there has been no relative reduction of the anterior mandibular premolar, although there have been morphologically significant changes (both reductions and increases) in the intervening taxa.

Again according to von Koenigswald (1962b: 122-23), the maxillary premolars of all the australopithecines stand in exception to both hominids and pongids. Here, his conclusions rest on a firmer base. Table CXVI examines the ratio of the anterior to the posterior maxillary premolars. In both *H. africanus* and *H. robustus*, the ratio is less than 100; the anterior tooth is relatively reduced when compared with the posterior for length, breadth, and area. For all other hominid taxa, and for all extant groups, the posterior tooth is relatively smaller. In *H. robustus* not 1 individual specimen has a smaller posterior premolar. On the other hand, larger posterior premolars appear with some frequency in all hominid taxa. Thus, the average reduction of the posterior premolar is a species characteristic for *H. erectus, H. neanderthalensis,* and *H. sapiens,* but not an individual level distinguishing characteristic for any of these. The confusion between characteristics which distinguish species (but not necessarily all the individuals in the species) with those that distinguish individuals has suggested both nonexistent differences when sample sizes were small, and individual traits used to characterize species (Simons and Pilbeam 1965), and has hidden real differences when overlap in ranges was taken to mean identity (Garn, Lewis, and Kerewsky 1964a). While no apparent trends exist in the ratio of the mandibular premolars, the ratio of the maxillary premolars has undergone a significant change with the relative reduction of the posterior tooth from *H. erectus* on.

Some attention has been given to the relative proportions of the molars. For instance, in comparing the size of the first and second molars in both jaws, Garn, Lewis, and Kerewsky (1964a:590) conclude that the ratio between them which was "claimed to distinguish fossil man from modern man does nothing of the sort." They found that in 43% of the Ohio "Whites" of both sexes studied, and in 43% of the Pima Indians of both sexes, the maxillary M1 was the same size as, or smaller than, M2. The corresponding percentages for the mandibular molars are 14% and 25%. However, overlap is not synonymous with identity. The average molar size ratio for these teeth (M1/M2) is over 100 for both jaws in both groups. Selmer-Olsen (1949:64) gives the inverse of this ratio for 24 extant groups. In every case, for both length and breadth, the average ratio M1/M2 is over 100.

Table CXXIII gives the distribution of mandibular M1/M2. Of all the hominid taxa, only *H. sapiens* has a ratio of over 100. No extant group is under 100. Indeed, there is a continuous increase in this ratio for length, breadth, and area from *H. africanus,* with the largest second molars relative to the first, to *H. sapiens,* with the second molars so relatively reduced that they are, on the average, smaller than the first molars.

TABLE CXVII. Ratio of Mandibular P3 to M1 for Length (L), Breadth (B), and Area (L*B): Mean, Range, Sample Size (N), and Coefficient of Variation (CV).

LOWER P3/M1	L(M-D)				B(B-L)				L*B			
	MEAN	RANGE	N	CV	MEAN	RANGE	N	CV	MEAN	RANGE	N	CV
H.AFRICANUS	73.0	67.1 - 86.2	9	8.5	91.3	81.5 - 101.4	9	6.7	66.7	56.4 - 83.6	9	12.6
H.ROBUSTUS	66.1	56.1 - 72.9	12	7.8	84.4	73.0 - 92.4	12	6.8	55.9	47.0 - 67.1	12	11.6
H.ERECTUS	68.7	62.6 - 79.6	16	7.1	81.4	69.0 - 90.9	14	6.7	55.8	44.1 - 62.9	13	10.1
H.NEANDERTAL	68.5	52.6 - 96.2	33	11.0	81.2	71.4 - 92.4	33	5.9	55.7	40.9 - 81.1	33	13.9
H.SAPIENS	62.8	48.0 - 79.0	315	7.4	73.3	57.6 - 80.0	314	7.3	46.1	30.3 - 67.1	309	12.0
AUSTRALOP	69.1	56.1 - 86.2	21	9.4	87.4	73.0 - 101.4	21	7.7	60.5	47.0 - 83.6	21	14.9
KRAPINA	68.5	63.5 - 78.2	4	9.6	80.2	76.0 - 83.0	4	3.8	55.0	50.1 - 64.9	4	12.2
NEANDERTAL	68.6	52.6 - 96.2	27	11.6	81.7	71.8 - 92.4	27	5.9	56.2	40.9 - 81.1	27	14.1
MT CARMEL	67.1	62.6 - 71.6	2	9.5	75.7	71.4 - 80.0	2	8.0	51.0	44.7 - 57.3	2	17.4
SUB SAHARAN	65.0	53.1 - 75.9	48	7.3	75.9	63.2 - 86.4	46	6.8	49.3	33.5 - 61.7	46	12.3
CAUCASOID	62.9	50.0 - 75.0	65	7.3	74.4	61.8 - 89.5	65	6.6	46.9	31.8 - 67.1	65	11.1
DICKSON MOUND	62.7	56.2 - 71.4	105	5.9	71.4	61.7 - 82.4	105	5.7	44.8	36.3 - 55.0	105	9.5
AUSTRALOID	62.3	52.6 - 72.7	20	7.3	72.7	64.9 - 81.8	21	7.2	45.4	35.2 - 59.5	20	12.7
NEW BRITAIN	62.1	53.5 - 71.8	41	7.0	75.5	65.6 - 88.5	43	7.3	47.2	39.1 - 62.2	41	11.5
INDIAN	61.8	52.5 - 79.0	29	10.4	69.9	57.6 - 84.1	25	9.5	43.1	30.3 - 56.9	25	15.7

TABLE CXVIII. Ratio of Maxillary P3 to M1 for Length (L), Breadth (B), and Area (L*B): Mean, Range, Sample Size (N), and Coefficient of Variation (CV).

UPPER P3/M1	L(M-D)				B(B-L)				L*B			
	MEAN	RANGE	N	CV	MEAN	RANGE	N	CV	MEAN	RANGE	N	CV
H.AFRICANUS	72.3	68.0 - 75.2	7	3.7	92.7	87.5 - 98.5	7	3.9	67.1	62.2 - 72.0	7	6.0
H.ROBUSTUS	70.3	64.4 - 73.1	10	4.6	92.7	86.8 - 101.5	10	4.8	65.1	59.6 - 68.9	10	5.9
H.ERECTUS	72.3	66.4 - 81.0	10	5.8	92.8	88.5 - 101.7	11	4.7	67.3	60.1 - 82.3	10	9.5
H.NEANDERTAL	71.4	54.9 - 87.5	23	10.6	85.7	74.8 - 97.6	24	7.0	61.5	45.9 - 72.5	23	12.1
H.SAPIENS	67.7	53.6 - 82.0	255	7.5	81.7	62.8 - 100.9	255	6.5	55.4	36.7 - 76.2	252	11.2
AUSTRALOP.	71.1	64.4 - 75.2	17	4.4	92.7	86.8 - 101.5	17	4.3	65.9	59.6 - 72.0	17	5.9
KRAPINA	73.3	73.3 - 73.3	1	.0	97.6	97.6 - 97.6	1	.0	71.5	71.5 - 71.5	1	.0
NEANDERTAL	72.1	59.1 - 87.5	17	10.6	85.3	74.8 - 96.0	18	7.2	61.9	49.2 - 72.5	17	11.4
MT CARMEL	68.3	54.9 - 74.5	5	11.7	84.9	80.0 - 90.3	5	4.5	58.1	45.9 - 65.3	5	14.0
SUB SAHARAN	69.2	63.3 - 75.0	19	4.1	83.0	64.8 - 100.0	17	9.9	57.7	44.6 - 68.4	17	10.5
DICKSON MOUND	69.0	59.4 - 81.1	97	6.2	81.4	73.9 - 90.6	97	4.3	56.2	44.1 - 67.3	97	8.6
AUSTRALOID	68.4	53.6 - 80.4	20	10.4	80.8	65.6 - 93.9	20	9.3	55.7	37.1 - 72.2	19	15.9
INDIAN	67.6	58.5 - 82.0	21	9.5	81.2	71.3 - 100.0	21	8.7	55.0	42.0 - 73.8	21	15.3
CAUCASOID	66.3	55.0 - 78.0	40	8.5	80.6	62.8 - 100.9	41	8.4	53.5	36.7 - 76.2	40	14.1
NEW BRITAIN	66.1	55.6 - 76.9	53	6.7	83.4	73.0 - 92.1	54	4.4	55.1	42.2 - 67.9	53	9.6

TABLE CXIX. Ratio of Mandibular P3 to M2 for Length (L), Breadth (B), and Area (L*B): Mean, Range, Sample Size (N), and Coefficient of Variation (CV).

LOWER P3/M2	L(M-D)				B(B-L)				L*B			
	MEAN	RANGE	N	CV	MEAN	RANGE	N	CV	MEAN	RANGE	N	CV
H.AFRICANUS	64.2	55.6 - 69.4	8	7.6	84.1	76.3 - 93.3	8	6.6	53.9	45.7 - 59.5	8	10.1
H.ROBUSTUS	60.5	52.9 - 65.1	10	7.5	80.2	68.9 - 91.7	10	8.3	48.5	41.5 - 59.3	10	11.5
H.ERECTUS	67.5	56.6 - 77.8	16	7.8	79.8	68.5 - 88.5	15	6.4	54.4	44.1 - 63.7	15	10.3
H.NEANDERTAL	64.6	47.6 - 73.2	33	8.7	78.8	67.5 - 91.7	34	6.1	51.0	33.3 - 66.0	33	11.9
H.SAPIENS	64.1	50.0 - 79.3	310	7.8	75.7	61.8 - 88.6	311	6.7	48.7	33.0 - 64.7	304	12.2
AUSTRALOP	62.1	52.9 - 69.4	18	7.9	81.9	68.9 - 93.3	18	7.8	50.9	41.5 - 59.5	18	11.8
KRAPINA	63.9	62.5 - 66.4	3	3.3	78.0	75.7 - 80.0	3	2.8	49.9	47.3 - 53.1	3	6.0
NEANDERTAL	65.0	47.6 - 73.2	27	8.6	79.1	67.5 - 91.7	28	6.6	51.5	33.3 - 66.0	27	12.2
MT CARMEL	61.7	51.3 - 68.6	3	14.8	76.9	74.8 - 79.0	3	2.7	47.4	39.5 - 51.4	3	14.4
CAUCASOID	65.4	50.0 - 76.1	68	8.6	75.9	63.6 - 84.8	68	5.7	49.7	33.2 - 60.9	68	11.5
NEW BRITAIN	65.2	55.6 - 75.5	37	7.8	78.8	67.2 - 88.5	38	6.7	51.7	42.0 - 64.6	36	11.5
SUB SAHARAN	65.0	56.0 - 75.0	46	5.9	77.2	65.5 - 88.5	46	7.1	50.2	38.6 - 64.1	45	11.5
INDIAN	64.8	53.4 - 79.3	25	10.8	72.9	61.8 - 87.4	23	8.3	47.2	33.0 - 64.7	22	16.6
AUSTRALOID	63.4	50.0 - 72.6	21	9.5	76.4	66.0 - 88.6	22	7.3	48.6	34.0 - 63.0	21	14.9
DICKSON MOUND	62.8	54.4 - 75.2	106	6.2	74.2	63.6 - 84.7	105	5.7	46.6	37.0 - 63.7	105	10.3

TABLE CXX. Ratio of Maxillary P3 to M2 for Length (L), Breadth (B), and Area (L*B): Mean, Range, Sample Size (N), and Coefficient of Variation (CV).

UPPER P3/M2	L(M-D)				B(B-L)				L*B			
	MEAN	RANGE	N	CV	MEAN	RANGE	N	CV	MEAN	RANGE	N	CV
H.AFRICANUS	64.9	62.0 - 70.7	6	4.9	83.8	79.1 - 94.4	6	6.7	54.6	49.2 - 66.7	6	11.8
H.ROBUSTUS	64.4	57.6 - 73.9	9	8.6	83.0	78.1 - 94.4	8	6.2	52.6	45.0 - 62.4	8	11.5
H.ERECTUS	74.0	60.3 - 87.0	8	12.2	86.8	81.6 - 102.5	9	8.0	64.3	49.2 - 87.1	8	18.4
H.NEANDERTAL	72.6	57.7 - 90.0	23	9.9	85.3	72.0 - 113.2	23	9.9	62.1	45.3 - 93.4	23	16.5
H.SAPIENS	72.2	46.9 - 90.0	248	8.6	82.2	61.8 - 105.6	247	6.8	59.6	30.6 - 89.2	245	12.9
AUSTRALOP.	64.6	57.6 - 73.9	15	7.1	83.4	78.1 - 94.4	14	6.2	53.4	45.0 - 66.7	14	11.3
KRAPINA	82.5	82.5 - 82.5	1	.0	113.2	113.2 - 113.2	1	.0	93.4	93.4 - 93.4	1	.0
NEANDERTAL	72.1	57.7 - 90.0	17	10.8	82.5	72.0 - 96.0	17	6.6	59.6	45.3 - 75.9	17	14.2
MT CARMEL	72.2	66.7 - 75.9	5	5.0	89.3	82.0 - 95.7	5	5.9	64.4	61.3 - 69.5	5	5.7
INDIAN	73.9	61.9 - 87.1	21	9.4	82.4	75.3 - 91.7	21	6.4	61.1	48.1 - 79.3	21	14.2
NEW BRITAIN	72.9	63.6 - 90.0	49	8.1	83.3	68.3 - 95.5	49	6.1	60.9	48.1 - 77.8	48	12.3
AUSTRALOID	72.8	60.5 - 84.9	21	8.7	80.3	66.2 - 97.1	22	9.5	58.6	45.7 - 69.3	21	11.3
DICKSON MOUND	72.6	61.9 - 87.0	95	6.6	82.4	72.4 - 93.0	94	4.7	60.0	48.1 - 78.4	94	9.4
CAUCASOID	70.5	46.9 - 85.9	38	12.5	82.3	65.3 - 105.6	38	9.4	58.3	30.6 - 85.0	38	18.6
SUB SAHARAN	69.2	61.7 - 77.7	19	6.5	81.0	61.8 - 89.2	18	8.6	56.2	38.3 - 67.9	18	13.6

TABLE CXXI. Ratio of Mandibular P4 to M1 for Length (L), Breadth (B), and Area (L*B): Mean, Range, Sample Size (N), and Coefficient of Variation (CV).

LOWER P4/M1	L(M-D)				B(B-L)				L*B			
	MEAN	RANGE	N	CV	MEAN	RANGE	N	CV	MEAN	RANGE	N	CV
H.AFRICANUS	76.5	72.0 - 79.2	7	3.2	93.9	86.3 - 113.8	7	10.6	71.9	63.2 - 88.9	7	12.6
H.ROBUSTUS	75.0	60.7 - 88.4	15	10.1	93.5	81.6 - 100.8	13	6.1	72.1	56.1 - 87.8	13	12.4
H.ERECTUS	67.2	57.1 - 83.2	15	8.8	82.3	72.1 - 92.5	16	6.1	54.9	47.7 - 60.0	14	7.7
H.NEANDERTAL	64.7	54.2 - 89.3	37	10.7	81.9	68.8 - 96.6	37	8.1	53.1	39.7 - 76.5	37	15.7
H.SAPIENS	65.2	49.6 - 104.6	330	9.3	77.3	64.2 - 111.2	328	7.3	50.3	32.6 - 90.1	325	13.4
AUSTRALOPITH	75.5	60.7 - 88.4	22	8.4	93.6	81.6 - 113.8	20	7.7	72.0	56.1 - 88.9	20	12.2
KRAPINA	66.1	58.5 - 75.5	6	8.3	81.6	74.4 - 91.5	6	7.1	54.2	45.4 - 69.0	6	15.4
NEANDERTAL	64.1	54.2 - 89.3	28	11.7	82.4	68.8 - 96.6	28	8.6	53.0	39.7 - 76.5	28	16.7
MT CARMEL	67.6	66.1 - 68.6	3	2.0	77.2	74.1 - 79.1	3	3.5	52.2	49.0 - 53.9	3	5.3
NEW BRITAIN	67.2	56.2 - 104.6	51	14.3	79.6	69.3 - 92.7	50	7.1	53.1	40.8 - 90.1	50	17.1
SUB SAHARAN	66.2	54.0 - 78.9	51	8.0	79.2	68.4 - 111.2	49	8.0	52.2	36.9 - 87.8	49	13.5
AUSTRALOID	65.6	58.4 - 78.1	23	7.9	75.8	67.0 - 86.0	23	7.4	49.8	39.2 - 67.1	23	12.6
DICKSON MD	65.5	56.8 - 75.9	100	6.1	75.7	66.1 - 84.9	100	5.9	49.7	38.3 - 63.4	100	10.0
CAUCASOID	63.8	54.6 - 85.0	64	7.6	78.6	66.1 - 93.6	64	6.9	50.0	40.4 - 63.6	63	10.0
INDIAN	61.5	49.6 - 81.0	33	9.7	74.2	64.2 - 84.5	32	7.0	45.7	32.6 - 59.6	32	14.5

TABLE CXXII. Ratio of Maxillary P4 to M1 for Length (L), Breadth (B), and Area (L*B): Mean, Range, Sample Size (N), and Coefficient of Variation (CV).

UPPER P4/M1	L(M-D)				B(B-L)				L*B			
	MEAN	RANGE	N	CV	MEAN	RANGE	N	CV	MEAN	RANGE	N	CV
H.AFRICANUS	70.3	61.5 - 76.2	9	6.7	95.2	91.2 - 100.0	8	3.2	67.2	57.1 - 74.0	8	8.6
H.ROBUSTUS	79.8	75.2 - 88.4	10	5.1	101.6	94.3 - 112.1	10	5.2	82.1	74.9 - 95.9	9	9.4
H.ERECTUS	68.4	65.3 - 73.0	11	3.8	91.4	88.3 - 93.9	11	1.7	62.5	59.9 - 67.4	11	3.7
H.NEANDERTAL	66.5	54.0 - 83.3	25	10.1	85.7	68.3 - 94.0	25	7.4	57.0	41.6 - 71.5	25	12.6
H.SAPIENS	65.2	46.5 - 86.8	262	8.6	81.1	65.9 - 100.0	261	6.6	53.0	33.7 - 73.0	257	12.6
AUSTRALOPITH	75.3	61.5 - 88.4	19	8.6	98.7	91.2 - 112.1	18	5.5	75.1	57.1 - 95.9	17	13.5
KRAPINA	65.5	65.5 - 65.5	1	.0	91.1	91.1 - 91.1	1	.0	59.7	59.7 - 59.7	1	.0
NEANDERTAL	66.4	54.0 - 83.3	20	11.2	85.8	75.4 - 93.7	20	6.3	57.0	41.6 - 71.5	20	12.8
MT CARMEL	66.9	63.6 - 70.7	4	4.3	83.9	68.3 - 94.0	4	13.1	56.2	45.3 - 66.5	4	15.5
SUB SAHARAN	66.7	55.6 - 77.0	20	8.0	81.7	66.7 - 98.1	19	9.6	54.5	41.9 - 69.4	19	14.8
DICKSON MD	66.1	51.9 - 75.7	101	6.8	79.9	66.4 - 89.7	102	5.3	52.9	37.8 - 64.9	101	10.4
AUSTRALOID	66.1	59.8 - 72.7	20	4.7	82.0	72.2 - 91.7	19	5.7	54.2	44.8 - 66.7	19	9.4
CAUCASOID	65.5	46.5 - 86.8	41	11.6	81.8	70.0 - 95.9	41	7.7	54.1	33.7 - 73.0	39	15.8
INDIAN	64.2	55.0 - 85.7	20	12.4	80.5	65.9 - 100.0	20	10.4	52.1	37.6 - 72.5	20	20.3
NEW BRITAIN	62.9	52.0 - 83.0	56	7.7	82.9	75.4 - 91.2	55	4.4	52.0	39.6 - 59.1	55	9.5

TABLE CXXIII. Ratio of Mandibular M1 to M2 for Length (L), Breadth (B), and Area (L*B): Mean, Range, Sample Size (N), and Coefficient of Variation (CV).

LOWER M1/M2	L(M-D)				B(B-L)				L*B			
	MEAN	RANGE	N	CV	MEAN	RANGE	N	CV	MEAN	RANGE	N	CV
H.AFRICANUS	87.4	78.4 - 91.7	9	5.6	90.6	86.0 - 96.3	8	3.7	78.9	68.2 - 86.9	8	8.8
H.ROBUSTUS	92.1	86.2 - 98.0	16	4.3	94.8	87.8 - 100.0	16	4.1	87.3	77.2 - 96.7	16	7.2
H.ERECTUS	98.7	86.0 - 111.2	20	6.3	97.2	88.5 - 104.0	19	4.0	96.7	83.8 - 115.6	19	8.0
H.NEANDERTAL	95.9	77.7 - 109.5	46	7.2	97.8	84.7 - 114.9	47	5.6	93.8	68.0 - 121.7	45	10.9
H.SAPIENS	103.1	84.6 - 127.8	435	6.5	103.4	86.4 - 128.6	429	5.2	106.7	75.1 - 146.7	425	9.7
AUSTRALOPITH	90.4	78.4 - 98.0	25	5.3	93.4	86.0 - 100.0	24	4.5	84.5	68.2 - 96.7	24	8.9
KRAPINA	97.4	93.3 - 100.8	7	3.1	98.2	89.6 - 105.3	7	5.8	95.7	85.8 - 106.1	7	8.4
NEANDERTAL	95.1	77.7 - 105.9	35	7.5	97.4	84.7 - 114.9	37	5.7	92.9	68.0 - 121.7	35	11.2
MT CARMEL	100.7	90.9 - 109.5	4	8.2	101.4	98.7 - 104.7	3	3.0	100.9	89.7 - 114.6	3	12.6
HARAPPA	107.6	90.9 - 127.8	47	7.8	108.2	95.0 - 128.6	44	7.0	116.9	90.9 - 146.7	44	11.2
INDIAN	104.7	90.1 - 120.0	31	5.6	103.5	87.0 - 110.8	31	5.0	108.1	91.3 - 123.4	30	7.8
NEW BRITAIN	104.2	89.3 - 118.2	65	5.7	103.7	98.2 - 115.2	63	3.5	108.5	87.7 - 136.1	62	7.8
CAUCASOID	103.0	84.6 - 117.0	98	6.2	101.5	86.4 - 116.0	97	4.7	104.6	75.1 - 123.3	97	8.5
AUSTRALOID	101.4	87.1 - 118.1	29	8.1	104.3	91.5 - 114.4	29	4.9	106.1	85.6 - 133.1	29	12.1
DICKSON MD	101.0	90.2 - 117.7	101	5.3	103.3	89.2 - 115.9	100	4.4	104.5	86.0 - 127.6	100	8.3
SUB SAHARAN	101.0	88.8 - 117.1	55	6.0	102.2	89.8 - 120.0	54	5.7	103.5	83.3 - 130.3	54	9.3

TABLE CXXIV. Ratio of Maxillary M1 to M2 for Length (L), Breadth (B), and Area (L*B): Mean, Range, Sample Size (N), and Coefficient of Variation (CV).

UPPER M1/M2	L(M-D)				B(B-L)				L*B			
	MEAN	RANGE	N	CV	MEAN	RANGE	N	CV	MEAN	RANGE	N	CV
H.AFRICANUS	91.2	83.2 - 97.9	13	4.9	90.3	83.3 - 98.6	13	5.4	82.4	73.1 - 94.9	13	9.3
H.ROBUSTUS	90.3	81.1 - 99.3	12	6.5	90.2	84.3 - 96.6	11	4.0	82.3	73.7 - 93.0	11	8.5
H.ERECTUS	101.7	89.0 - 118.0	11	7.1	93.8	90.1 - 100.8	11	3.5	95.4	80.2 - 110.4	11	9.1
H.NEANDERTAL	105.7	75.8 - 125.0	32	9.5	99.1	87.7 - 116.0	32	6.9	104.8	72.8 - 134.6	32	11.9
H.SAPIENS	106.4	66.7 - 155.7	381	9.0	101.2	82.4 - 122.2	381	5.8	107.9	54.9 - 175.2	375	12.2
AUSTRALOPITH	90.8	81.1 - 99.3	25	5.6	90.2	83.3 - 98.6	24	4.7	82.4	73.1 - 94.9	24	8.7
KRAPINA	115.1	112.6 - 117.5	2	3.0	107.6	99.2 - 116.0	2	11.0	123.7	116.7 - 130.7	2	8.0
NEANDERTAL	104.0	75.8 - 125.0	23	9.4	97.1	87.7 - 115.0	23	6.2	101.0	72.8 - 125.2	23	10.7
MT CARMEL	108.7	98.4 - 124.4	7	9.7	103.0	93.3 - 110.8	7	5.1	111.8	102.5 - 134.6	7	10.1
NEW BRITAIN	109.9	93.5 - 133.3	68	7.6	100.0	90.6 - 110.9	68	3.9	110.0	92.7 - 143.0	67	9.6
INDIAN	108.5	96.4 - 118.3	24	5.2	101.4	84.7 - 109.9	24	5.3	110.0	95.3 - 123.0	24	6.8
CAUCASOID	106.6	79.1 - 128.6	43	10.3	102.0	89.1 - 118.9	43	5.4	108.8	79.8 - 150.8	43	13.2
AUSTRALOID	105.9	95.7 - 113.6	22	5.0	98.9	90.1 - 115.1	24	6.2	105.4	92.1 - 123.2	21	7.7
DICKSON MD	105.4	86.7 - 121.5	113	6.7	101.0	89.3 - 116.0	113	4.4	106.7	78.2 - 136.5	113	9.9
HARAPPA	105.0	66.7 - 155.7	83	13.1	103.0	82.4 - 122.2	82	8.0	108.4	54.9 - 175.2	81	17.4
SUB SAHARAN	102.3	90.0 - 113.6	21	5.9	98.4	86.1 - 110.3	19	5.1	100.5	84.1 - 118.1	19	8.6

TABLE CXXV. Ratio of Mandibular M1 to M3 for Length (L), Breadth (B), and Area (L*B): Mean, Range, Sample Size (N), and Coefficient of Variation (CV).

LOWER M1/M3	L(M-D)				B(B-L)				L*B			
	MEAN	RANGE	N	CV	MEAN	RANGE	N	CV	MEAN	RANGE	N	CV
H.AFRICANUS	88.3	77.9 - 99.3	5	9.8	92.3	87.9 - 101.6	4	6.9	79.3	68.7 - 96.4	4	15.1
H.ROBUSTUS	86.6	80.6 - 92.5	13	4.4	96.1	86.8 - 113.1	13	7.6	83.3	70.3 - 104.6	13	11.1
H.ERECTUS	103.3	87.0 - 118.0	15	8.2	102.9	92.8 - 116.1	14	6.2	106.9	80.7 - 132.2	14	11.7
H.NEANDERTAL	98.8	70.0 - 144.6	38	12.4	101.9	88.5 - 136.2	37	9.7	101.4	65.0 - 178.6	37	21.6
H.SAPIENS	104.2	79.4 - 135.1	358	8.1	105.8	78.5 - 138.5	355	7.1	110.7	76.4 - 187.0	350	12.9
AUSTRALOPITH	87.1	77.9 - 99.3	18	6.1	95.2	86.8 - 113.1	17	7.4	82.4	68.7 - 104.6	17	11.8
KRAPINA	99.7	92.6 - 106.0	4	6.5	104.9	100.9 - 110.1	4	3.7	104.6	93.5 - 114.8	4	9.1
NEANDERTAL	98.2	70.0 - 144.6	30	13.8	100.8	88.5 - 136.2	30	10.5	99.9	65.0 - 178.6	30	23.8
MT CARMEL	101.9	97.9 - 108.5	4	4.7	109.2	105.0 - 113.1	3	3.7	111.4	102.8 - 122.7	3	9.2
HARAPPA	109.3	85.7 - 133.3	38	10.2	112.7	100.0 - 137.5	37	7.5	123.5	91.3 - 183.3	37	14.8
SUB SAHARAN	105.3	87.4 - 128.1	48	8.1	104.4	87.2 - 131.7	46	7.2	110.1	86.2 - 168.7	46	13.6
CAUCASOID	104.3	90.9 - 135.1	59	7.5	105.5	78.5 - 138.5	59	8.6	110.4	78.5 - 187.0	59	14.8
INDIAN	104.1	79.4 - 116.1	31	6.8	104.9	95.1 - 114.0	30	4.5	109.3	76.4 - 124.6	30	9.1
AUSTRALOID	103.2	87.7 - 114.2	29	7.6	104.4	89.8 - 117.8	29	7.0	107.9	78.8 - 129.2	29	11.6
DICKSON MD	102.8	82.6 - 132.6	85	7.8	106.7	86.0 - 125.9	85	6.1	109.8	84.9 - 146.5	85	11.5
NEW BRITAIN	102.7	88.1 - 122.5	61	7.0	104.3	90.3 - 115.5	58	5.3	107.4	89.9 - 141.6	57	9.5

TABLE CXXVI. Ratio of Maxillary M1 to M3 for Length (L), Breadth (B), and Area (L*B): Mean, Range, Sample Size (N), and Coefficient of Variation (CV).

UPPER M1/M3	L(M-D)				B(B-L)				L*B			
	MEAN	RANGE	N	CV	MEAN	RANGE	N	CV	MEAN	RANGE	N	CV
H.AFRICANUS	93.7	86.9 - 97.6	3	6.4	89.4	85.1 - 96.6	3	7.0	83.9	75.1 - 94.3	3	11.5
H.ROBUSTUS	89.4	76.9 - 107.8	10	10.6	86.6	82.4 - 90.3	9	3.4	78.5	69.1 - 88.9	9	8.5
H.ERECTUS	106.1	98.1 - 117.4	9	5.9	96.6	86.7 - 103.4	9	6.6	102.3	90.5 - 113.1	9	7.3
H.NEANDERTAL	112.5	82.8 - 136.7	25	12.9	104.2	89.3 - 127.1	26	8.5	118.4	90.3 - 168.9	25	18.7
H.SAPIENS	117.5	70.0 - 155.7	266	10.4	107.1	82.4 - 137.5	270	8.0	126.3	60.7 - 186.9	261	14.9
AUSTRALOPITH	89.8	76.9 - 107.8	14	9.8	87.3	82.4 - 96.6	12	4.4	79.8	69.1 - 94.3	12	9.4
NEANDERTAL	113.0	82.8 - 136.7	20	13.5	104.4	89.3 - 127.1	21	9.1	119.5	90.3 - 168.9	20	20.1
MT CARMEL	110.6	92.4 - 121.5	5	11.2	103.0	98.2 - 112.6	5	6.0	113.8	97.9 - 131.8	5	11.9
NEW BRITAIN	121.9	93.3 - 144.9	49	8.2	105.6	90.3 - 116.0	52	5.1	128.6	94.1 - 163.0	49	10.8
DICKSON MD	117.9	80.4 - 140.7	81	9.0	108.2	90.1 - 126.9	82	6.8	127.6	83.2 - 168.5	81	13.4
INDIAN	117.2	100.0 - 150.0	14	11.7	108.3	89.7 - 131.9	14	8.7	127.2	103.2 - 177.4	14	16.8
CAUCASOID	116.9	85.6 - 138.9	32	11.3	104.4	90.6 - 113.9	33	5.5	122.0	84.7 - 157.9	32	13.9
SUB SAHARAN	116.0	99.0 - 134.5	15	8.8	107.3	95.2 - 125.0	13	8.4	125.6	104.0 - 149.7	13	10.7
AUSTRALOID	115.2	104.5 - 140.9	20	9.7	105.1	94.9 - 123.5	20	7.8	121.7	100.8 - 150.0	18	12.6
HARAPPA	114.7	70.0 - 155.7	50	13.9	110.0	82.4 - 137.5	49	11.8	127.1	60.7 - 186.9	49	21.4

TABLE CXXVII. Ratio of Mandibular M2 to M3 for Length (L), Breadth (B), and Area (L*B): Mean, Range, Sample Size (N), and Coefficient of Variation (CV).

LOWER M2/M3	L(M-D)				B(B-L)				L*B			
	MEAN	RANGE	N	CV	MEAN	RANGE	N	CV	MEAN	RANGE	N	CV
H.AFRICANUS	101.2	89.5 - 109.6	8	5.8	100.7	89.8 - 105.5	8	4.9	102.1	80.4 - 113.0	8	9.9
H.ROBUSTUS	94.6	86.7 - 101.3	14	4.1	102.0	88.1 - 113.8	14	5.9	96.5	82.4 - 108.2	14	7.2
H.ERECTUS	104.2	89.3 - 119.0	19	8.1	104.8	97.6 - 114.0	18	4.6	108.7	92.3 - 135.7	18	9.9
H.NEANDERTAL	103.0	88.8 - 155.4	40	11.8	103.9	92.3 - 143.7	41	9.0	107.9	88.5 - 197.5	40	21.3
H.SAPIENS	101.5	77.6 - 139.0	369	8.2	102.6	77.0 - 151.3	363	6.9	104.4	77.8 - 210.2	361	13.2
AUSTRALOPITH	97.0	86.7 - 109.6	22	5.8	101.5	88.1 - 113.8	22	5.5	98.5	80.4 - 113.0	22	8.5
KRAPINA	101.8	96.7 - 108.6	4	5.3	106.1	103.6 - 109.5	4	2.5	107.8	104.7 - 112.6	4	3.2
NEANDERTAL	103.8	90.0 - 155.4	31	12.9	103.1	92.3 - 143.7	32	10.2	108.1	88.5 - 197.5	31	24.0
MT CARMEL	98.9	88.8 - 107.7	5	7.0	107.2	104.0 - 108.9	5	1.9	106.0	92.3 - 114.6	5	7.9
SUB SAHARAN	104.1	88.0 - 128.3	50	7.4	102.0	82.9 - 129.3	48	7.0	105.9	82.9 - 141.4	48	11.5
DICKSON MD	102.9	82.7 - 132.6	91	8.0	103.5	82.9 - 124.7	90	6.3	106.7	83.7 - 158.3	90	12.1
HARAPPA	102.4	81.8 - 131.2	41	8.9	105.3	94.4 - 131.2	40	6.9	107.9	86.6 - 157.5	40	13.1
CAUCASOID	101.7	82.6 - 139.0	61	8.4	104.0	77.0 - 151.3	60	8.3	106.3	79.3 - 210.2	60	16.7
AUSTRALOID	101.6	86.9 - 120.0	32	8.1	100.4	80.5 - 115.3	32	7.5	102.3	77.8 - 132.0	32	13.4
INDIAN	98.8	86.5 - 118.3	28	7.1	101.2	89.8 - 117.1	28	5.5	100.2	81.7 - 125.5	28	10.8
NEW BRITAIN	98.2	77.6 - 121.0	58	7.8	100.7	84.1 - 112.9	55	5.7	99.0	80.1 - 136.6	55	11.0

TABLE CXXVIII. Ratio of Maxillary M2 to M3 for Length (L), Breadth (B), and Area (L*B): Mean, Range, Sample Size (N), and Coefficient of Variation (CV).

UPPER M2/M3	L(M-D)				B(B-L)				L*B			
	MEAN	RANGE	N	CV	MEAN	RANGE	N	CV	MEAN	RANGE	N	CV
H.AFRICANUS	104.0	99.3 - 106.6	6	2.5	99.2	95.5 - 104.1	6	3.2	103.3	94.9 - 110.8	6	5.2
H.ROBUSTUS	98.8	92.4 - 114.1	14	6.5	97.2	90.1 - 102.5	14	4.1	95.9	87.7 - 108.1	14	6.7
H.ERECTUS	105.0	88.5 - 125.9	10	10.0	102.7	92.7 - 108.6	10	5.0	108.0	82.0 - 136.7	10	12.6
H.NEANDERTAL	109.0	90.8 - 144.4	28	11.4	105.8	88.8 - 121.9	28	7.2	115.7	88.8 - 168.5	27	17.3
H.SAPIENS	110.3	77.5 - 137.5	282	9.3	105.8	85.7 - 132.9	286	7.3	116.9	77.1 - 177.2	277	14.0
AUSTRALOPITH	100.1	92.4 - 114.1	21	5.9	97.8	90.1 - 104.1	20	3.8	98.1	87.7 - 110.8	20	7.0
NEANDERTAL	111.5	95.5 - 144.4	22	11.4	106.7	99.2 - 121.9	22	6.6	119.5	98.3 - 168.5	21	17.1
MT CARMEL	99.8	90.8 - 105.3	6	5.7	102.3	88.8 - 111.8	6	8.8	102.2	88.8 - 117.0	6	11.4
SUB SAHARAN	111.8	96.2 - 125.0	19	7.9	106.9	96.0 - 125.0	16	7.8	120.1	98.3 - 152.8	16	11.4
DICKSON MD	111.6	89.0 - 133.8	83	8.0	107.2	90.0 - 132.9	84	6.7	119.8	82.8 - 177.2	83	12.7
NEW BRITAIN	111.1	77.5 - 134.5	50	9.5	105.6	88.1 - 120.7	52	5.9	117.7	78.1 - 153.9	49	13.5
CAUCASOID	110.1	89.1 - 135.0	33	10.4	101.7	85.7 - 114.7	33	7.1	112.2	77.1 - 143.7	33	14.0
AUSTRALOID	109.7	100.0 - 137.5	22	9.5	105.0	95.4 - 115.1	24	4.7	115.0	97.8 - 150.0	21	11.3
HARAPPA	108.4	88.2 - 133.3	56	10.4	106.5	87.5 - 131.2	57	9.3	116.1	84.4 - 164.1	56	16.9
INDIAN	108.3	89.8 - 132.4	14	10.5	105.8	93.3 - 121.5	14	7.6	114.9	87.8 - 153.8	14	15.6

Indeed, although the range of variation in *H. sapiens* overlaps almost every fossil *individual,* the prominent trend of relative reduction between hominid *species* should not be overlooked. The ratio of mandibular M1/M3 (Table CXXV) shows a similar, but not identical pattern. In this case, the hominid species fall into 2 contrasting groups with respect to length, breadth, and area. The first group, *H. africanus* and *H. robustus,* has ratios well under 100, and the second group made up of the remaining taxa has ratios over 100. Again, there is a clear trend of reduction in the third mandibular molar relative to the first. Interestingly, comparison of the mandibular second to third molars (Table CXXVII) establishes no particular pattern of variation. Extant groups within *H. sapiens* disclose a range of differences in this ratio (M2/M3) from under 100 to over it, a range large enough to include almost all the fossil taxa. *H. robustus* is the exception, with a ratio slightly less than the minimum for an extant group. Thus, there is no trend, or for that matter significant change, in the ratio M2/M3. That is, there is no morphologically significant reduction of M_3 relative to M_2.

Variation in the patterns of change in the maxillary molar relative proportions is similar to that of the mandible. Here, however, there are 3 rather than 2 distinct types of patterns. In the first type of pattern, the taxa *H. africanus* and *H. robustus* form a contrasting group to the other 3 taxa; the former have significantly lower ratios. The second pattern differs from the first only in that *H. erectus* forms an intermediate between 2 australopithecine taxa and the group consisting of *H. neanderthalensis* and *H. sapiens.* In the third pattern, there is no significant change between any of the hominid taxa when compared with the range of variation in extant groups. The first pattern holds for the length ratio of M1/M2 (Table CXXIV). The second pattern holds for the breadth and area ratios of M1/M2 as well as for M1/M3 ratios of all 3 measures (Table CXXVI). The third pattern holds for M2/M3 ratios of all 3 measures (Table CXXVIII) as it did for the mandibular ratio. Thus, as was the case with the mandible, there is a clear trend for the reduction of M^2 and M^3 relative to M^1, but no reduction of M^3 relative to M^2. The only real difference is that in the maxilla, the trend is more prolonged and more extreme. Thus, there are greater differences between the beginning and end points of the trend. *H. erectus* holds an intermediate rather than a completely modernized position for the maxillary ratios.

Another ratio which has received some attention in the literature is the relative breadths of the premolars and the first molar (Dahlberg 1962). In particular, the ratio of P4/M1 breadths has been considered (Dahlberg 1963a). Howell (personal communication) has stated that this ratio is distinctively high for *H. robustus*; that is, the ratio has taxonomic significance. Indeed, Table 1 in Dahlberg's study (1963a) shows Swartkrans as the only hominid sample with a P4/M1 mandibular breadth ratio of over 100. It is therefore crucial to look at the relations of the premolars to the first molar in hominid taxa, rather than in samples representing groups of lower taxonomic status, or representing sites.

Table CXXI gives the P4/M1 ratio for mandibular teeth. For length, breadth, and area, the 2 australopithecine taxa are indistinguishable from each other and significantly different from the subsequent hominid taxa. Thus, there is clear evidence for a trend in relative P_4 reduction when compared with M_1. The ratio does not exceed 100 in breadth for any hominid taxon. The pattern of variation in the maxillary P4/M1 ratio is almost identical (Table CXXII). In the maxilla, however, *H. robustus* has a ratio for length, breadth, and area which is greater than the *H. africanus* ratio. The *H. africanus* ratio is significantly greater than that of *H. erectus* in breadth and area. The breadth and area ratios for *H. erectus,* in turn, are intermediate between the australopithecines and *H. neanderthalensis* (as well as *H. sapiens*). Similar to molar ratio variation, changes in the maxilla are both more prolonged and more extreme than they are in the mandible.

An examination of the mandibular P3/M1 ratio (Table CXVII) indicates relatively larger anterior premolars in length, breadth, and area for *H. africanus.* The ratio is significantly smaller for all other hominid taxa. Relative to M_1, P_3 reduced first in hominid evolution. In the maxillary dentition, a significant reduction in the P3/M1 ratio (Table CXVIII) does not occur until *H. sapiens* with respect to length, and first occurs in *H. neanderthalensis* for breadth and area. Relative P_3 reduction occurs, then, after P_4 reduction, in contradistinction to the mandible.

Tables CXIX and CXX examine the mandibular and maxillary P3/M2 ratios. For the mandible, there is no significant change in the ratio for length and area. The breadth ratio, however, shows a consistent decrease from *H. africanus* to *H. sapiens.* In the maxilla, on the other hand, there is no significant change in breadth or area, but a morphologically significant *increase* in the ratio for length. This ratio is somewhat complicated by the relative reduction of M2 compared with M1, so that it is difficult and perhaps not meaningful to discern trends.

In sum, these posterior to posterior ratios clearly show a pattern of dental reduction throughout the dentition. In most cases, the 2 australopithecine taxa stand in contrast to the remaining hominid taxa, with *H. erectus* sometimes intermediate and otherwise with the recent taxa. Comparisons with M1 are of particular interest. In general, these ratios show more gradual but ultimately more extensive change in the maxilla than in the mandible. There seems to be no real difference between the relative reduction of the second and third molars in either jaw. The trend of relative reduction in the third molar of hominids has already been established (Frisch 1965:72-78). The order of premolar reduction relative to M1 is reversed in the 2 jaws, with the posterior tooth reducing first in the maxilla, and the anterior tooth first in the mandible.

c) Anterior to Posterior Ratios

Tables CXXIX to CXLII are concerned with the ratios of anterior to posterior teeth. The interpretation of these ratios is usually somewhat difficult because unlike ratios within anterior or posterior groups, differences in selection acting upon the numerator and denominator leave the selective importance of the fraction (ratio) less clear.

Table CXXIX is concerned with the ratio of mandibular I1/M1. Weidenreich has utilized this ratio in his discussion of the evolutionary position of "*Sinanthropus*" (1943). Taking the ratio of the areas, he gives 81 as the value in chimpanzees and 27 as the value in gorillas (p. 264). This extensive variation between 2 closely related primate species with relatively similar diets and feeding habits (Goodall 1963; Schaller 1963:149-69) makes differences in the morphological significance of the ratio hard to establish. It is interesting to note that on the basis of root size, Weidenreich estimated an area index of 22.4 for "*Plesianthropus*," and 11.6 for "*Paranthropus*" (1943:268). The corresponding indexes calculated for *H. africanus* and *H. robustus* are 22.9 and 16.0. With respect to the distribution of the index, both australopithecine taxa are significantly smaller than subsequent hominid taxa in length and area. In breadth, however, the *H. africanus* value falls within the range of variation in extant hominid groups. In all cases, *H. robustus* is significantly smaller than *H. africanus.* In both breadth and area, the ratio is significantly greater in *H. neanderthalensis* than it is in either *H. sapiens* or *H. erectus.* While there are no unambiguous trends, it is evident that compared with M_1, the australopithecine central incisors are relatively smaller (particularly in length) than other taxa, while they are relatively broader and larger in *H. neanderthalensis.* The ratio is significantly decreased in *H. sapiens.*

Comparison of mandibular I2/M1 (Table CXXXIII) gives an almost identical picture. The only exceptions are that values for *H. africanus* are almost indistinguishable from those of *H. erectus,* while the breadth and area reductions of *H. sapiens* from the *H. neanderthalensis* condition are even more extensive than in I1/M1 ratios.

Table CXLI compares mandibular C to M_1. Yet another variation of the initial pattern is evident. *H. robustus* still represents a minimum value for the ratio, and *H. neanderthalensis* a maximum. However, while the ratio for *H. africanus* was significantly less than that of *H. erectus* for I1/M1, and the same for I2/M2, it is significantly greater for C/M1.

Relative to the first molar, the pattern of variation for the 3 anterior teeth remains constant for all taxa: *H. robustus* is minimum, *H. erectus* larger, *H. neanderthalensis* maximum, and *H. sapiens* significantly reduced. *H. africanus* ratios gradually increase distally so that while the central incisor ratio is small, as in *H. robustus,* the canine ratio is large, as in *H. neanderthalensis.*

Weidenreich also discusses the maxillary I1/M1 ratio (1943:264), giving values of 102 for chimpanzee and 52 for gorilla ratios. As with the mandibular ratios, the variability is extensive.

TABLE CXXIX. Ratio of Mandibular I1 to M1 for Length (L), Breadth (B), and Area (L*B): Mean, Range, Sample Size (N), and Coefficient of Variation (CV).

LOWER I1/M1	L(M-D)				B(B-L)				L*B			
	MEAN	RANGE	N	CV	MEAN	RANGE	N	CV	MEAN	RANGE	N	CV
H. AFRICANUS	43.9	34.5 - 47.4	7	9.2	52.3	46.2 - 62.8	6	10.2	22.9	18.0 - 28.5	6	13.1
H. ROBUSTUS	36.6	33.5 - 38.1	7	4.9	43.6	39.4 - 51.1	7	9.8	16.0	13.4 - 19.2	7	12.9
H. ERECTUS	48.3	38.4 - 47.4	10	11.2	57.5	49.6 - 64.8	9	7.6	28.3	24.1 - 33.5	9	9.6
H. NEANDERTAL	50.1	38.5 - 68.7	22	15.4	67.0	55.7 - 73.4	15	7.0	34.1	24.3 - 45.2	15	17.4
H. SAPIENS	47.2	37.4 - 65.0	186	9.2	53.8	43.7 - 70.2	169	9.3	25.4	17.6 - 36.8	166	13.3
AUSTRALOP.	40.3	33.5 - 47.4	14	12.2	47.6	39.4 - 62.8	13	14.1	19.2	13.4 - 28.5	13	16.1
KRAPINA	46.5	45.7 - 47.0	3	1.5								
NEANDERTAL	52.2	38.5 - 68.7	15	16.1	67.7	61.0 - 73.4	13	5.6	34.8	28.2 - 45.2	13	16.4
MT CARMEL	44.9	39.1 - 50.0	4	10.4	62.2	55.7 - 68.7	2	14.9	29.3	24.3 - 34.4	2	24.3
AUSTRALOID	49.8	45.3 - 52.2	6	5.3	55.9	54.5 - 57.6	3	2.8	27.5	26.1 - 28.5	3	4.6
SUB SAHARAN	48.8	39.8 - 65.0	24	14.7	57.2	44.2 - 64.7	19	8.6	28.1	17.6 - 36.8	19	19.1
NEW BRITAIN	48.0	41.9 - 54.3	30	6.6	54.3	46.6 - 61.5	27	7.6	26.0	22.5 - 32.5	26	9.1
DICKSON MOUND	47.0	39.7 - 53.8	81	6.8	51.2	43.7 - 63.2	79	6.9	24.1	19.0 - 29.9	79	9.3
INDIAN	46.3	39.1 - 56.5	10	12.2	52.3	47.3 - 59.4	8	6.5	25.0	23.4 - 28.8	8	6.7
CAUCASOID	45.4	37.4 - 53.9	32	9.8	58.1	49.5 - 70.2	28	10.4	26.3	19.7 - 35.0	28	16.1

TABLE CXXX. Ratio of Maxillary I1 to M1 for Length (L), Breadth (B), and Area (L*B): Mean, Range, Sample Size (N), and Coefficient of Variation (CV).

UPPER I1/M1	L(M-D)				B(B-L)				L*B			
	MEAN	RANGE	N	CV	MEAN	RANGE	N	CV	MEAN	RANGE	N	CV
H. AFRICANUS	76.7	76.2 - 77.2	2	.9	58.7	58.6 - 58.9	2	.4	45.1	44.9 - 45.2	2	.6
H. ROBUSTUS	66.4	65.8 - 66.9	3	0.7	44.3	43.5 - 45.2	2	1.9	29.3	28.9 - 29.7	2	1.4
H. ERECTUS	81.9	72.0 - 89.3	5	7.0	64.9	56.0 - 76.6	4	11.8	52.3	43.0 - 63.3	4	13.8
H. NEANDERTAL	85.6	57.1 - 100.0	18	12.0	70.2	60.0 - 83.5	14	11.6	60.2	36.0 - 74.4	14	18.3
H. SAPIENS	80.8	62.0 - 104.8	192	8.4	62.9	48.1 - 93.8	190	9.0	50.8	35.8 - 78.2	185	13.6
AUSTRALOP.	70.5	65.8 - 77.2	5	8.4	51.5	43.5 - 58.9	4	14.2	37.2	28.9 - 45.2	4	16.8
KRAPINA	80.7	80.6 - 80.8	2	.1	77.3	76.7 - 77.9	2	1.1	62.4	61.9 - 62.8	2	1.0
NEANDERTAL	87.7	57.1 - 100.0	11	13.7	70.7	63.0 - 83.5	8	11.9	62.5	36.0 - 74.4	8	19.5
MT CARMEL	82.8	74.0 - 90.9	5	8.6	65.8	60.0 - 77.0	4	12.0	54.6	44.8 - 67.7	4	20.1
SUB SAHARAN	82.1	65.9 - 95.2	17	9.8	67.2	56.0 - 77.2	17	10.6	55.6	38.2 - 64.3	17	13.3
DICKSON MOUND	82.5	71.8 - 101.1	97	6.6	61.5	55.1 - 72.0	94	5.4	50.7	42.8 - 66.8	94	9.9
AUSTRALOID	81.6	67.0 - 104.8	9	14.4	67.1	50.8 - 93.8	9	20.6	55.3	35.8 - 78.2	9	27.6
CAUCASOID	77.9	62.0 - 90.0	28	10.9	65.3	48.1 - 80.1	27	11.0	51.0	36.2 - 71.3	26	19.0
INDIAN	77.5	72.4 - 85.6	11	5.0	63.2	57.7 - 72.9	11	8.7	48.9	44.2 - 54.5	11	7.7
NEW BRITAIN	77.3	64.5 - 84.5	28	5.4	61.4	57.5 - 67.2	30	4.0	47.4	38.2 - 52.1	26	6.8

TABLE CXXXI. Ratio of Mandibular I1 to P3 for Length (L), Breadth (B), and Area (L*B): Mean, Range, Sample Size (N), and Coefficient of Variation (CV).

LOWER I1/P3	L(M-D)				B(B-L)				L*B			
	MEAN	RANGE	N	CV	MEAN	RANGE	N	CV	MEAN	RANGE	N	CV
H.AFRICANUS	59.7	40.0 - 69.8	6	19.9	58.7	47.6 - 69.2	4	15.2	33.2	23.1 - 45.4	4	34.5
H.ROBUSTUS	58.8	56.5 - 61.8	6	3.5	51.8	45.2 - 63.2	6	13.0	30.4	25.6 - 35.7	6	12.0
H.ERECTUS	70.3	65.1 - 77.7	10	5.9	68.4	61.4 - 78.9	6	9.0	48.1	43.3 - 53.6	6	7.5
H.NEANDERTAL	70.4	57.7 - 79.3	20	8.5	82.1	69.6 - 92.0	15	7.9	58.0	42.4 - 70.5	15	14.1
H.SAPIENS	76.0	59.7 - 101.7	184	10.0	73.7	60.2 - 93.7	173	8.4	56.3	41.2 - 83.7	170	13.6
AUSTRALOP.	59.2	40.0 - 69.8	12	13.8	54.6	45.2 - 69.2	10	14.7	31.5	23.1 - 45.4	10	23.1
KRAPINA	71.4	69.4 - 74.0	3	3.3	.0	.0 - .0	0	.0	.0	.0 - .0	0	.0
NEANDERTAL	71.6	57.7 - 79.3	13	8.1	83.2	77.8 - 92.0	12	5.6	59.2	51.9 - 67.2	12	9.6
MT CARMEL	66.1	61.0 - 77.6	4	11.7	77.6	69.6 - 90.9	3	15.0	52.9	42.4 - 70.5	3	29.1
AUSTRALOID	83.3	72.9 - 91.5	5	8.2	73.2	66.7 - 80.0	3	9.1	58.3	57.1 - 59.3	3	1.9
NEW BRITAIN	78.9	64.6 - 101.5	24	10.1	72.2	60.2 - 82.1	23	8.1	57.1	41.9 - 70.7	22	13.0
SUB SAHARAN	77.1	61.5 - 100.0	26	13.3	74.9	63.7 - 93.1	22	10.7	58.6	42.7 - 83.7	22	21.9
INDIAN	76.7	62.9 - 101.7	11	15.6	76.5	65.0 - 90.9	8	10.2	61.2	50.0 - 69.1	8	10.9
DICKSON MOUND	75.4	66.2 - 86.8	86	6.8	72.4	61.2 - 83.7	84	6.2	54.7	43.0 - 70.4	84	9.4
CAUCASOID	72.3	59.7 - 83.8	29	9.8	77.5	66.7 - 93.7	28	9.6	56.2	41.2 - 78.3	28	14.8

TABLE CXXXII. Ratio of Maxillary I1 to P3 for Length (L), Breadth (B), and Area (L*B): Mean, Range, Sample Size (N), and Coefficient of Variation (CV).

UPPER I1/P3	L(M-D)				B(B-L)				L*B			
	MEAN	RANGE	N	CV	MEAN	RANGE	N	CV	MEAN	RANGE	N	CV
H. AFRICANUS	108.7	108.1 - 109.2	2	.7	64.5	64.1 - 64.8	2	.9	70.0	70.0 - 70.1	2	.2
H. ROBUSTUS	98.9	91.7 - 107.8	5	6.1	49.4	45.3 - 55.7	3	9.2	48.4	42.0 - 60.0	3	12.3
H. ERECTUS	114.4	97.3 - 124.1	6	8.4	69.9	59.5 - 84.7	5	12.3	79.1	69.5 - 103.3	5	14.5
H. NEANDERTAL	125.3	100.0 - 153.2	14	14.8	79.9	67.0 - 110.9	12	13.6	95.0	68.6 - 114.3	11	17.5
H. SAPIENS	119.6	95.4 - 150.0	176	8.1	77.2	63.8 - 103.9	175	8.5	92.7	69.3 - 131.0	72	13.7
AUSTRALOP.	101.7	91.7 - 109.2	7	7.5	55.4	45.3 - 64.8	5	12.6	57.1	42.0 - 70.1	5	14.6
KRAPINA	125.0	125.0 - 125.0	1		81.2	81.2 - 81.2	1		101.5	101.5 - 101.5	1	
NEANDERTAL	126.1	100.0 - 150.0	9	14.2	82.4	76.2 - 110.9	8	14.3	98.8	77.3 - 114.3	7	14.0
MT CARMEL	123.6	102.4 - 153.2	4	20.1	72.8	67.0 - 82.0	3	11.1	83.8	68.6 - 110.8	3	28.0
AUSTRALOID	126.2	114.3 - 146.7	9	7.0	83.7	68.1 - 103.9	9	17.0	105.7	77.8 - 131.0	9	17.6
SUB SAHARAN	120.4	101.2 - 137.5	17	7.8	79.2	69.2 - 94.4	17	9.2	95.5	72.6 - 121.9	17	13.8
DICKSON MOUND	119.9	101.9 - 147.5	81	6.6	75.7	66.3 - 86.4	81	6.0	90.9	74.3 - 127.3	81	10.8
CAUCASOID	118.5	95.4 - 150.0	30	11.2	80.7	69.2 - 95.2	28	8.0	96.4	74.3 - 125.0	28	16.0
NEW BRITAIN	117.8	101.1 - 137.2	26	7.5	73.9	63.8 - 84.0	27	6.4	87.2	69.3 - 111.2	24	11.3
INDIAN	114.5	98.8 - 124.7	11	7.3	78.5	72.4 - 87.5	11	8.1	90.2	72.4 - 107.5	11	14.0

TABLE CXXXIII. Ratio of Mandibular I2 to M1 for Length (L). Breadth (B), and Area (L*B): Mean, Range, Sample Size (N), and Coefficient of Variation (CV).

LOWER I2/M1	L(M-D)				B(B-L)				L*B			
	MEAN	RANGE	N	CV	MEAN	RANGE	N	CV	MEAN	RANGE	N	CV
H. AFRICANUS	52.8	47.4 - 54.9	5	6.0	61.9	60.2 - 63.1	4	1.9	32.7	29.2 - 34.4	4	6.5
H. ROBUSTUS	41.7	36.0 - 45.3	6	8.9	45.7	41.8 - 51.7	6	8.1	19.1	15.0 - 22.4	6	15.0
H. ERECTUS	53.5	40.7 - 59.0	12	10.0	64.5	58.4 - 72.0	10	6.1	33.7	29.1 - 38.4	9	9.2
H. NEANDERTAL	59.3	45.8 - 86.2	31	13.9	72.0	60.9 - 81.8	20	7.3	42.7	33.1 - 62.3	20	19.3
H. SAPIENS	54.3	41.7 - 65.0	203	7.0	58.1	44.2 - 87.1	189	9.6	31.6	20.8 - 46.3	184	12.5
AUSTRALOP.	46.7	36.0 - 54.9	11	14.3	52.2	41.8 - 63.1	10	16.6	24.5	15.0 - 34.4	10	17.8
KRAPINA	56.5	54.0 - 60.0	6	4.2	72.2	68.6 - 75.8	2	7.1	40.2	37.2 - 43.2	2	10.4
NEANDERTAL	60.9	45.8 - 86.2	21	15.8	73.3	66.1 - 81.8	15	6.1	44.5	33.6 - 62.3	15	19.4
MT CARMEL	55.5	52.2 - 57.6	4	4.3	65.2	60.9 - 71.4	3	8.5	35.7	33.1 - 39.6	3	9.6
INDIAN	56.[illegible]	51.2 - 62.0	11	6.5	55.8	53.7 - 61.6	9	4.6	31.5	27.5 - 34.4	9	8.8
DICKSON MOUND	55.5	46.9 - 63.2	85	5.0	56.1	48.3 - 64.5	84	6.3	31.2	26.8 - 38.1	84	8.5
SUB SAHARAN	53.5	46.0 - 65.0	28	7.1	60.5	45.3 - 87.1	21	13.5	32.3	20.8 - 46.2	21	15.6
AUSTRALOID	53.3	49.6 - 59.1	5	7.4	59.4	53.8 - 63.6	3	8.5	32.2	28.8 - 37.6	3	14.8
NEW BRITAIN	53.3	48.3 - 59.3	33	6.3	57.4	44.2 - 76.5	32	9.8	30.4	25.5 - 39.3	29	11.0
CAUCASOID	52.7	41.7 - 63.3	38	9.6	61.9	50.0 - 73.2	35	9.8	32.7	20.8 - 46.3	35	17.7

TABLE CXXXIV. Ratio of Maxillary I2 to M1 for Length (L), Breadth (B), and Area (L*B): Mean, Range, Sample Size (N), and Coefficient of Variation (CV).

UPPER I2/M1	L(M-D)				B(B-L)				L*B			
	MEAN	RANGE	N	CV	MEAN	RANGE	N	CV	MEAN	RANGE	N	CV
H.AFRICANUS	54.5	48.3 - 59.3	3	10.3	44.8	41.2 - 50.0	3	10.3	24.6	19.9 - 29.7	3	19.9
H.ROBUSTUS	48.0	45.4 - 55.7	5	9.1	46.2	41.0 - 57.6	4	16.6	22.7	18.8 - 32.1	4	27.9
H.ERECTUS	68.6	56.6 - 82.6	3	19.1	70.4	64.5 - 75.9	3	8.1	48.8	36.5 - 62.7	3	27.0
H.NEANDERTAL	68.6	54.9 - 81.0	17	9.5	69.1	54.9 - 80.0	15	11.0	47.7	32.1 - 56.6	15	17.3
H.SAPIENS	67.2	46.7 - 91.2	193	10.3	57.1	34.9 - 77.9	192	10.0	38.5	16.3 - 60.2	188	16.5
AUSTRALOP.	50.4	45.4 - 59.3	8	11.1	45.6	41.0 - 57.6	7	13.4	23.5	18.8 - 32.1	7	22.9
KRAPINA	66.4	66.4 - 66.4	1	.0	80.0	80.0 - 80.0	1	.0	53.1	53.1 - 53.1	1	.0
NEANDERTAL	71.2	64.3 - 81.0	12	6.3	72.4	67.0 - 78.3	10	4.3	52.0	45.3 - 56.6	10	7.6
MT CARMEL	61.5	54.9 - 71.0	4	12.0	58.3	54.9 - 62.1	4	5.1	35.7	32.1 - 38.9	4	8.0
SUB SAHARAN	70.7	55.6 - 91.2	16	10.9	61.1	54.5 - 76.4	16	10.4	43.3	30.6 - 55.6	16	15.1
DICKSON MOUND	69.2	54.1 - 83.2	97	8.0	55.9	44.5 - 63.4	96	6.6	38.7	24.0 - 49.1	96	12.0
INDIAN	68.5	46.7 - 81.6	10	14.2	55.2	34.9 - 64.8	11	13.3	38.2	16.3 - 45.4	10	21.3
CAUCASOID	63.4	50.0 - 77.7	26	10.4	60.8	48.9 - 77.8	25	14.4	39.0	25.0 - 60.2	24	23.7
NEW BRITAIN	63.4	51.7 - 73.2	34	8.2	55.8	49.6 - 60.0	33	4.8	35.3	28.4 - 41.9	32	9.8
AUSTRALOID	62.9	49.2 - 74.9	8	17.6	59.9	45.5 - 77.9	9	17.1	38.6	24.4 - 57.0	8	33.9

TABLE CXXXV. Ratio of Mandibular I2 to P3 for Length (L), Breadth (B), and Area (L*B): Mean, Range, Sample size (N), and Coefficient of Variation (CV).

LOWER I2/P3	L(M-D)				B(B-L)				L*B			
	MEAN	RANGE	N	CV	MEAN	RANGE	N	CV	MEAN	RANGE	N	CV
H.AFRICANUS	70.1	52.0 - 81.2	6	18.6	66.5	63.5 - 69.2	4	3.6	44.0	34.4 - 54.6	4	24.8
H.ROBUSTUS	67.1	62.6 - 71.3	5	5.3	53.1	47.4 - 58.8	5	10.1	35.8	30.2 - 41.9	5	15.1
H.ERECTUS	82.9	74.1 - 95.7	10	9.0	75.8	68.2 - 86.7	7	8.4	59.9	52.5 - 69.2	7	9.5
H.NEANDERTAL	83.2	73.3 - 97.2	25	8.0	91.1	82.8 - 113.9	16	9.1	76.5	60.7 - 110.7	16	16.3
H.SAPIENS	87.3	69.5 - 106.1	200	8.0	79.5	65.3 - 115.3	191	8.8	69.7	49.4 - 103.6	185	13.2
AUSTRALOP.	68.7	52.0 - 81.2	11	14.0	59.1	47.4 - 69.2	9	13.8	39.5	30.2 - 54.6	9	22.4
KRAPINA	81.6	76.7 - 87.7	5	4.9	90.2	90.2 - 90.2	1	.0	74.3	74.3 - 74.3	1	.0
NEANDERTAL	84.0	73.3 - 97.2	17	9.2	91.4	82.8 - 113.9	14	9.7	76.8	60.7 - 110.7	14	17.4
MT CARMEL	80.9	78.9 - 83.3	3	2.8	88.7	88.7 - 88.7	1	.0	74.0	74.0 - 74.0	1	.0
INDIAN	93.5	79.3 - 105.5	11	9.0	82.7	75.0 - 97.0	9	8.4	76.0	64.6 - 92.1	8	11.0
AUSTRALOID	89.8	80.0 - 97.1	5	7.6	77.7	70.8 - 84.4	3	8.8	68.1	61.1 - 75.6	3	10.7
DICKSON MOUND	88.8	78.0 - 101.3	89	5.9	79.0	65.3 - 92.3	88	5.7	70.3	58.1 - 83.6	88	8.1
NEW BRITAIN	86.0	73.4 - 97.1	26	7.2	77.2	67.8 - 96.3	27	8.7	66.5	52.9 - 81.9	24	12.4
CAUCASOID	84.4	71.4 - 106.1	36	10.1	82.5	66.7 - 100.0	35	10.1	70.0	49.8 - 103.6	35	17.9
SUB SAHARAN	84.0	69.5 - 94.3	30	8.2	78.6	65.9 - 115.3	24	14.0	66.6	49.4 - 103.3	24	19.7

TABLE CXXXVI. Ratio of Maxillary I2 to P3 for Length (L), Breadth (B), and Area (L*B): Mean, Range, Sample Size (N), and Coefficient of Variation (CV).

UPPER I2/P3	L(M-D)				B(B-L)				L*B			
	MEAN	RANGE	N	CV	MEAN	RANGE	N	CV	MEAN	RANGE	N	CV
H.AFRICANUS	76.3	65.2 - 83.9	4	10.4	51.6	47.1 - 56.9	4	9.6	39.5	30.7 - 45.9	4	17.3
H.ROBUSTUS	68.3	62.9 - 82.1	6	11.0	48.0	44.1 - 56.7	5	10.6	33.5	27.9 - 46.6	5	23.2
H.ERECTUS	95.0	75.0 - 122.0	4	20.7	71.7	63.3 - 83.9	4	12.1	69.3	51.7 - 102.3	4	33.0
H.NEANDERTAL	96.7	78.0 - 112.5	14	9.3	79.6	66.7 - 99.5	13	11.0	76.1	53.7 - 96.4	12	17.2
H.SAPIENS	99.6	69.0 - 125.6	176	8.9	70.0	48.9 - 92.7	175	10.0	70.0	33.7 - 102.8	172	15.8
AUSTRALOP.	71.5	62.9 - 83.9	10	11.6	49.6	44.1 - 56.9	9	10.2	36.2	27.9 - 46.6	9	21.0
KRAPINA	106.9	106.9 - 106.9	1	.0	82.2	82.2 - 82.2	1	.0	87.8	87.8 - 87.8	1	.0
NEANDERTAL	98.3	88.7 - 112.5	10	7.1	83.1	72.7 - 99.5	9	8.8	80.6	67.9 - 96.4	8	12.1
MT CARMEL	87.8	78.0 - 100.0	3	12.7	68.4	66.7 - 69.9	3	2.4	60.2	53.7 - 69.9	3	14.3
SUB SAHARAN	103.6	85.4 - 125.6	17	8.9	73.6	62.3 - 88.7	17	11.1	76.6	53.2 - 99.6	17	17.3
DICKSON MOUND	101.1	82.6 - 121.1	82	8.1	68.4	53.5 - 77.4	82	7.0	69.3	44.2 - 87.8	82	12.4
INDIAN	99.3	69.0 - 107.5	10	11.1	67.7	48.9 - 81.6	11	11.5	67.6	33.7 - 85.0	10	19.9
AUSTRALOID	98.8	80.0 - 113.5	9	11.8	75.3	57.1 - 90.5	10	15.3	75.5	51.9 - 102.8	9	24.4
CAUCASOID	96.5	83.3 - 112.7	28	8.4	74.6	62.0 - 92.7	26	11.3	72.6	54.8 - 100.4	26	17.6
NEW BRITAIN	95.9	81.2 - 111.3	28	8.5	66.6	60.6 - 73.2	27	5.4	63.6	52.0 - 80.3	26	11.1

TABLE CXXXVII. Ratio of Mandibular C to P3 for Length (L), Breadth (B), and Area (L*B): Mean, Range, Sample Size (N), and Coefficient of Variation (CV).

LOWER C/P3	L(M-D)				B(B-L)				L*B			
	MEAN	RANGE	N	CV	MEAN	RANGE	N	CV	MEAN	RANGE	N	CV
H. AFRICANUS	93.8	83.0 - 108.2	8	7.7	86.0	78.0 - 91.7	7	5.2	81.2	71.7 - 99.2	7	11.3
H. ROBUSTUS	79.4	68.3 - 86.7	6	7.9	66.2	61.5 - 69.6	5	5.6	53.9	46.0 - 60.3	5	11.0
H. ERECTUS	92.2	77.8 - 105.5	17	8.0	92.7	72.9 - 105.0	17	8.6	85.3	65.8 - 99.2	14	11.5
H. NEANDERTAL	100.9	71.4 - 119.0	36	7.9	99.9	83.3 - 111.1	31	6.5	101.4	59.5 - 129.8	31	12.0
H. SAPIENS	100.6	75.8 - 133.3	242	7.7	98.1	77.8 - 118.5	243	7.2	99.0	71.3 - 152.4	233	12.2
AUSTRALOPITH.	87.6	68.3 - 108.2	14	12.3	77.8	61.5 - 91.7	12	12.8	69.8	46.0 - 99.2	12	18.9
KRAPINA	101.9	93.0 - 112.3	5	7.5	96.4	87.8 - 102.2	4	6.6	98.5	88.8 - 106.7	4	7.5
NEANDERTAL	99.9	71.4 - 115.4	27	7.9	100.3	83.3 - 111.1	24	6.6	100.8	59.5 - 128.2	24	12.1
MT CARMEL	106.4	101.2 - 119.0	4	8.0	101.9	96.7 - 109.1	3	6.3	109.7	97.9 - 129.8	3	15.9
INDIAN	102.9	89.9 - 116.7	15	7.3	99.9	92.1 - 110.2	11	5.2	102.1	86.1 - 115.9	11	9.5
DICKSON MOUND	101.8	83.9 - 119.1	113	6.3	99.2	85.9 - 118.5	114	6.5	101.6	82.0 - 132.1	111	11.2
AUSTRALOID	100.4	93.2 - 114.3	5	8.2	101.8	88.9 - 110.0	5	9.0	101.6	95.5 - 104.3	5	3.6
NEW BRITAIN	99.8	88.5 - 115.4	30	7.0	95.4	83.3 - 117.5	34	7.5	94.5	79.3 - 113.1	29	9.3
CAUCASOID	99.4	75.8 - 133.3	37	9.7	100.1	77.8 - 114.3	36	7.8	99.7	71.3 - 152.4	36	14.2
SUB SAHARAN	96.8	83.3 - 113.3	35	8.8	94.3	84.4 - 107.3	34	6.4	91.6	71.7 - 115.6	34	13.1

TABLE CXXXVIII. Ratio of Maxillary C to P3 for Length (L), Breadth (B), and Area (L*B): Mean, Range, Sample Size (N), and Coefficient of Variation (CV).

UPPER C/P3	L(M-D)				B(B-L)				L*B			
	MEAN	RANGE	N	CV	MEAN	RANGE	N	CV	MEAN	RANGE	N	CV
H.AFRICANUS	108.9	98.9 - 115.1	4	6.6	78.2	75.8 - 80.5	4	2.6	85.0	78.1 - 87.6	4	5.4
H.ROBUSTUS	91.5	79.8 - 111.6	8	12.3	66.8	57.1 - 77.6	8	10.9	61.8	45.5 - 86.6	8	23.1
H.ERECTUS	110.7	95.9 - 115.9	7	6.1	85.5	67.4 - 96.0	7	11.8	95.1	64.7 - 109.3	7	16.3
H.NEANDERTAL	110.4	92.8 - 133.3	24	8.5	93.0	81.6 - 112.0	22	7.9	102.8	81.6 - 133.3	22	12.1
H.SAPIENS	113.2	89.7 - 150.0	222	7.4	89.5	75.0 - 112.9	223	7.2	101.5	74.5 - 150.0	221	11.9
AUSTRALOPITH	97.3	79.8 - 115.1	12	13.3	70.6	57.1 - 80.5	12	11.5	69.5	45.5 - 87.6	12	23.5
KRAPINA	116.2	116.2 - 116.2	1	.0	92.1	92.1 - 92.1	1	.0	107.0	107.0 - 107.0	1	.0
NEANDERTAL	109.7	92.8 - 133.3	20	9.0	94.0	81.6 - 112.0	18	8.2	103.2	81.6 - 133.3	18	13.1
MT CARMEL	112.9	106.1 - 120.3	3	6.3	87.4	85.0 - 89.3	3	2.5	98.6	93.3 - 102.2	3	4.7
CAUCASOID	115.7	89.7 - 133.9	36	8.7	92.1	77.3 - 112.9	37	7.5	106.9	77.3 - 145.0	36	13.2
INDIAN	114.0	98.2 - 136.2	18	8.0	89.8	80.0 - 97.7	18	6.5	102.5	80.4 - 123.5	18	12.0
AUSTRALOID	113.9	103.2 - 150.0	15	9.9	96.7	78.7 - 106.9	15	7.5	110.2	87.7 - 150.0	15	13.4
DICKSON MD	113.5	98.7 - 138.3	93	6.7	88.2	75.0 - 101.1	92	5.9	100.1	74.5 - 138.8	92	10.4
NEW BRITAIN	111.5	94.0 - 127.1	37	7.0	86.0	76.9 - 105.6	38	7.4	96.3	77.3 - 124.8	37	11.6
SUB SAHARAN	108.7	96.8 - 124.6	17	6.6	91.0	82.1 - 100.0	17	5.1	99.0	85.7 - 121.8	17	9.5

TABLE CXXXIX. Ratio of Mandibular C to P4 for Length (L), Breadth (B), and Area (L*B): Mean, Range, Sample Size (N), and Coefficient of Variation (CV).

LOWER C/P4	L(M-D)				B(B-L)				L*B			
	MEAN	RANGE	N	CV	MEAN	RANGE	N	CV	MEAN	RANGE	N	CV
H.AFRICANUS	91.7	80.6 - 100.0	7	8.6	82.1	67.9 - 87.3	5	9.8	76.1	56.3 - 85.1	5	15.5
H.ROBUSTUS	65.9	50.3 - 75.7	5	16.8	57.1	53.3 - 61.4	5	5.7	37.8	26.8 - 44.9	5	20.5
H.ERECTUS	91.6	73.7 - 105.9	11	10.4	92.6	74.3 - 112.2	13	11.6	87.1	68.4 - 104.4	9	14.7
H.NEANDERTAL	107.3	90.9 - 142.1	37	10.1	98.8	86.6 - 125.0	34	8.6	106.4	83.5 - 156.2	34	15.3
H.SAPIENS	96.4	61.3 - 116.4	236	8.4	93.2	73.9 - 116.8	240	8.2	90.2	45.3 - 122.7	232	13.0
AUSTRALOPITH	81.0	50.3 - 100.0	12	19.7	69.6	53.3 - 87.3	10	20.7	56.9	26.8 - 85.1	10	39.1
KRAPINA	105.7	96.4 - 118.1	6	6.9	97.9	86.6 - 110.8	6	9.6	103.8	83.5 - 130.7	6	15.1
NEANDERTAL	108.7	90.9 - 142.1	27	10.9	99.1	90.0 - 125.0	24	9.2	108.3	85.2 - 156.2	24	16.2
MT CARMEL	100.4	95.8 - 105.7	4	5.2	98.0	96.4 - 98.9	4	1.2	98.4	92.6 - 104.6	4	6.3
INDIAN	101.4	90.0 - 116.4	15	8.1	96.5	82.4 - 114.9	14	10.1	97.9	83.6 - 122.7	14	14.0
CAUCASOID	97.6	76.9 - 114.3	35	8.7	95.1	77.8 - 116.8	33	8.5	93.1	71.3 - 114.3	33	11.2
DICKSON MD	97.3	84.2 - 112.9	110	5.8	93.6	81.4 - 108.3	113	6.6	91.2	70.9 - 122.2	110	10.8
AUSTRALOID	94.9	82.9 - 105.0	6	8.0	98.9	86.7 - 113.1	6	12.1	93.9	78.8 - 118.7	6	15.6
SUB SAHARAN	94.1	76.2 - 111.5	29	9.5	91.2	73.9 - 105.9	29	8.5	85.9	60.0 - 104.1	29	13.3
NEW BRITAIN	93.4	61.3 - 108.2	34	11.8	90.3	74.0 - 110.6	36	10.0	84.8	45.3 - 113.6	33	15.8

TABLE CXL. Ratio of Maxillary C to P4 for Length (L), Breadth (B), and Area (L*B): Mean, Range, Sample Size (N), and Coefficient of Variation (CV).

UPPER C/P4	L(M-D)				B(B-L)				L*B			
	MEAN	RANGE	N	CV	MEAN	RANGE	N	CV	MEAN	RANGE	N	CV
H.AFRICANUS	106.1	104.2 - 107.7	3	1.7	75.7	72.9 - 79.2	3	4.2	80.3	77.6 - 82.5	3	3.1
H.ROBUSTUS	77.2	73.3 - 83.0	4	5.9	59.2	53.9 - 64.9	4	8.5	45.9	39.7 - 53.9	4	14.4
H.ERECTUS	115.1	106.2 - 121.5	7	4.3	87.2	64.5 - 96.7	7	12.7	100.6	68.5 - 112.0	7	14.6
H.NEANDERTAL	114.9	100.0 - 127.0	23	6.9	92.8	81.6 - 117.9	21	8.4	106.5	87.7 - 133.6	21	11.6
H.SAPIENS	117.6	90.3 - 156.5	224	8.6	90.3	75.5 - 115.4	224	8.0	106.6	70.2 - 155.5	223	13.6
AUSTRALOPITH	89.6	73.3 - 107.7	7	17.7	66.3	53.9 - 79.2	7	14.6	60.6	39.7 - 82.5	7	31.4
KRAPINA	114.8	114.8 - 114.8	1	.0	88.6	88.6 - 88.6	1	.0	101.7	101.7 - 101.7	1	.0
NEANDERTAL	114.5	100.0 - 127.0	19	7.1	93.9	81.6 - 117.9	17	8.6	107.4	90.7 - 133.6	17	11.9
MT CARMEL	117.5	107.1 - 124.3	3	7.8	87.6	81.8 - 93.0	3	6.4	103.2	87.7 - 112.6	3	13.1
INDIAN	121.7	94.7 - 147.5	17	10.9	91.0	79.6 - 105.4	17	9.2	111.4	75.9 - 155.5	17	18.8
DICKSON MD	118.6	98.7 - 145.5	97	7.4	89.8	76.9 - 108.7	97	6.2	106.8	81.9 - 155.1	97	12.2
CAUCASOID	118.1	93.3 - 156.5	36	11.1	91.8	75.5 - 115.4	37	9.6	108.8	81.1 - 149.3	36	16.0
NEW BRITAIN	116.8	90.3 - 138.1	37	7.5	86.8	75.5 - 107.1	36	7.6	102.1	81.2 - 127.3	36	11.1
AUSTRALOID	115.8	102.6 - 127.6	15	5.9	96.2	76.5 - 111.2	15	9.8	111.7	79.9 - 127.6	15	12.9
SUB SAHARAN	112.6	96.8 - 129.0	16	8.1	90.8	82.6 - 100.0	16	5.1	102.3	84.7 - 129.0	16	11.0

TABLE CXLI. Ratio of Mandibular C to M1 for Length (L), Breadth (B), and Area (L*B): Mean, Range, Sample Size (N), and Coefficient of Variation (CV).

LOWER C/M1	L(M-D)				B(B-L)				L*B			
	MEAN	RANGE	N	CV	MEAN	RANGE	N	CV	MEAN	RANGE	N	CV
H.AFRICANUS	69.3	62.6 - 77.6	6	9.5	79.0	74.2 - 86.6	5	5.9	55.9	47.5 - 66.4	5	14.1
H.ROBUSTUS	51.2	44.5 - 58.6	6	10.5	55.3	52.9 - 61.8	6	6.1	28.4	23.6 - 36.2	6	16.0
H.ERECTUS	65.1	50.0 - 85.9	13	13.9	78.7	67.7 - 91.7	13	8.4	51.1	38.5 - 74.0	12	19.9
H.NEANDERTAL	71.0	58.3 - 100.0	36	11.3	81.8	62.5 - 95.2	34	8.6	58.4	43.7 - 90.7	34	17.2
H.SAPIENS	62.7	49.5 - 75.9	234	6.1	72.0	60.2 - 94.7	236	8.1	45.2	36.0 - 66.3	226	10.8
AUSTRALOPITH	60.2	44.5 - 77.6	12	18.3	66.0	52.9 - 86.6	11	19.6	40.9	23.6 - 66.4	11	38.0
KRAPINA	69.6	64.3 - 72.7	6	4.2	79.6	71.8 - 85.8	6	6.0	55.3	50.0 - 59.3	6	6.9
NEANDERTAL	71.6	58.3 - 100.0	26	12.8	83.9	72.7 - 95.2	24	7.4	60.6	46.8 - 90.7	24	17.9
MT CARMEL	69.2	63.5 - 72.5	4	5.7	72.4	62.5 - 78.3	4	10.0	50.1	43.7 - 56.1	4	13.0
DICKSON MD	63.4	54.6 - 71.3	100	5.0	71.1	60.8 - 87.9	101	7.2	45.0	36.9 - 61.2	98	9.8
NEW BRITAIN	62.7	51.9 - 68.9	40	5.9	71.3	62.4 - 83.0	44	7.8	44.4	36.0 - 52.8	39	8.7
SUB SAHARAN	62.6	57.0 - 75.9	31	7.1	71.7	63.2 - 82.7	29	7.7	45.1	37.2 - 58.9	29	11.7
INDIAN	62.2	55.8 - 67.3	15	6.5	71.1	60.2 - 87.9	13	11.7	44.1	37.2 - 57.1	13	13.7
CAUCASOID	62.1	49.5 - 71.1	36	7.4	75.8	63.6 - 94.7	35	8.6	47.1	38.4 - 66.3	35	12.8
AUSTRALOID	59.8	50.4 - 69.6	5	12.1	75.2	72.6 - 78.6	5	3.3	44.8	38.3 - 50.6	5	10.0

TABLE CXLII. Ratio of Maxillary C to M1 for Length (L), Breadth (B), and Area (L*B): Mean, Range, Sample Size (N), and Coefficient of Variation (CV).

UPPER C/M1	L(M-D)				B(B-L)				L*B			
	MEAN	RANGE	N	CV	MEAN	RANGE	N	CV	MEAN	RANGE	N	CV
H.AFRICANUS	78.1	73.3 - 81.1	3	5.3	69.5	68.8 - 70.7	3	1.5	54.3	50.7 - 56.3	3	5.8
H.ROBUSTUS	63.1	57.2 - 75.7	5	13.1	63.7	54.8 - 78.8	5	15.9	40.8	31.4 - 59.7	5	29.8
H.ERECTUS	79.1	69.6 - 85.0	8	5.8	80.2	60.5 - 87.5	8	10.6	63.7	42.2 - 71.2	8	14.3
H.NEANDERTAL	77.4	63.6 - 90.3	22	9.2	80.4	68.0 - 89.3	21	7.1	61.7	52.9 - 76.2	21	11.2
H.SAPIENS	76.2	64.3 - 92.0	226	6.3	72.9	61.2 - 96.5	228	7.9	55.5	40.3 - 83.6	225	11.2
AUSTRALOPITH	68.7	57.2 - 81.1	8	14.8	65.9	54.8 - 78.8	8	12.5	45.9	31.4 - 59.7	8	25.4
KRAPINA	72.6	72.6 - 72.6	1	.0	87.9	87.9 - 87.9	1	.0	63.8	63.8 - 63.8	1	.0
NEANDERTAL	77.2	63.6 - 90.3	17	10.3	81.1	70.8 - 89.3	16	6.3	62.0	52.9 - 76.2	16	12.4
MT CARMEL	79.2	75.8 - 81.1	4	3.1	75.4	68.0 - 80.6	4	7.1	59.7	55.0 - 65.4	4	7.3
DICKSON MD	77.6	68.3 - 91.7	98	5.4	71.6	61.4 - 83.0	98	5.2	55.6	47.2 - 68.6	98	8.5
CAUCASOID	76.9	66.3 - 92.0	33	7.4	74.8	62.4 - 95.5	35	9.4	57.8	45.5 - 83.6	33	14.1
INDIAN	76.2	65.0 - 83.4	18	6.2	72.2	64.3 - 89.5	19	8.0	54.9	45.5 - 65.4	18	10.0
AUSTRALOID	75.8	65.6 - 81.9	15	7.2	77.9	61.2 - 96.5	14	11.6	59.3	40.3 - 75.9	14	16.8
SUB SAHARAN	74.7	66.7 - 81.8	14	6.6	75.1	64.8 - 91.4	14	9.3	56.2	43.2 - 70.3	14	12.0
NEW BRITAIN	73.1	64.3 - 81.1	43	5.6	71.7	61.8 - 90.9	43	7.8	52.5	40.9 - 70.8	43	10.3

Measured again from tooth roots, the estimated ratio for "*Plesianthropus*" was 41.4 and for "*Paranthropus*" 45.5 (1943:268). A comparison with the area ratios calculated here (Table CXXX) indicates less correspondence with the mandibular ratio estimates. The *H. africanus* value is 45.1, and the *H. robustus* value is 29.3 (representing 2 teeth from 1 individual–with the largest molar size of all specimens). The pattern of maxillary I1/M1 ratio variation is similar to the mandibular pattern. *H. robustus* has the minimum value, significantly smaller than *H. africanus. H. neanderthalensis* ratios are maximum, significantly greater than *H. erectus* and *H. sapiens.* However, it should be pointed out that all the ratios for *H. africanus* are calculated for 1 individual, as are 2 of the 3 *H. robustus* ratios.

The maxillary I2/M1 ratio (Table CXXXIV) distribution is somewhat different. In this case, *H. africanus* and *H. robustus* are not significantly different. Both are significantly smaller than subsequent hominid taxa. The maximum for the ratio is in *H. erectus.* Subsequent values decrease, and the reduction of the ratio in *H. sapiens* is quite significant.

An examination of the C/M1 maxillary ratio (Table CXLII) shows a pattern intermediate between the previous 2. *H. robustus* is minimum, significantly smaller than *H. africanus* in length and area, although not in breadth where the australopithecines are indistinguishable and much smaller than subsequent taxa. The values of the ratio are maximum for *H. erectus,* and decrease significantly with *H. sapiens.*

The maxillary ratios, then, show patterns of change similar, but not identical to the mandibular patterns. *H. sapiens* has reduced maxillary anteriors, when compared with M^1. However, the difference between *H. sapiens* and the earlier taxa is not as great as was true for the mandible. Indeed, the maxilla in general shows less variation than does the mandible with respect to comparisons of anterior teeth to M1 Again unlike the mandible, the values of the ratio for *H. africanus* in both breadth and area tend to be more similar to *H. robustus* than they are to *H. erectus.*

Table CXXXI gives the mandibular I1/P3 ratios. There is a clear trend to the variation of this ratio. In all 3 dimensions, the australopithecines are indistinguishable from each other, but stand in contrast to the other 3 hominid taxa with relatively greater ratios. In length, *H. erectus* stands with the recent taxa, while in breadth and area this species is intermediate between the australopithecines and the recent taxa.

The mandibular I2/P3 ratios are presented in Table CXXXV. There is exactly the same pattern of variation. There is no more difference between the australopithecine taxa than there is among extant groups. The australopithecines are, on the other hand, quite different from the recent hominid taxa. As in the I1/P3 ratio, *H. erectus* is intermediate for breadth and area. Also, *H. sapiens,* when compared with *H. neanderthalensis,* has a smaller ratio for breadth and area. This was also the case for the I1/P3 ratio.

Table CXXXVII gives the distribution of the mandibular C/P3 ratio. This ratio for both jaws has been used by several other authors to separate the australopithecine taxa from each other (Robinson 1956:148; Tobias 1967a:156), and to align *H. africanus* with *H. erectus* (Robinson 1963a:598). Both of these authors used a smaller sample size than is now available for the respective australopithecine taxa, and neither made comparisons with other hominid taxa or the ranges of individuals or extant groups. Thus, the comparisons and conclusions of this study may not agree with those mentioned here. For length and area, the *H. africanus* and *H. erectus* values are not significantly different. In the breadth ratio, the difference between these taxa is about the same as the maximum difference among extant groups. For all 3 measurements, *H. robustus* has the minimum ratios for all taxa, and is significantly smaller than *H. africanus.*

The mandibular C/P4 comparison (Table CXXXIX) shows the same pattern of relationships. The major difference is that for breadth and area, the *H. africanus* value is significantly smaller than *H. erectus.* The australopithecine taxa are different enough in this ratio so that the actual ranges of variation do not overlap. This was also true for the C/P3 breadth and area ratios. In the C/P4 ratio, the *H. sapiens* value is smaller than the value for *H. neanderthalensis.* The difference is about the same as the maximum difference among extant groups.

The ratios of the anterior teeth with the premolars all show a significant increase. In addition, all the ratios except C/P3 clearly differentiate the 2 australopithecine taxa from the more recent taxa, although not necessarily from each other.

Table CXXXII gives the maxillary I1/P3 ratios. *H. africanus* and *H. erectus* have values which are not significantly different and which are intermediate between *H. robustus* and *H. neanderthalensis* and *H. sapiens.* The length value for the *H. robustus* ratio is not significantly different from the *H. africanus* value, although the breadth and area ratios are. It should be remembered that *H. africanus* is represented by 2 values from 1 individual. Thus, of the australopithecines, only *H. robustus* can properly be compared with other taxa.

The sample sizes of the I2/P3 maxillary ratio (Table CXXXVI) allow a better comparison to be made with *H. africanus. H. africanus* is not significantly different from *H. robustus* in this ratio, and the 2 are significantly smaller than the more recent taxa.

The distributions of the maxillary C/P3 (Table CXXXVIII) and C/P4 (Table CXL) ratios are almost identical. *H. robustus* is minimum, and is significantly smaller than *H. africanus. H. erectus* falls with the more recent taxa. The only difference is that in the C/P3 ratio, *H. africanus* and *H. erectus* were not significantly different, while for the C/P4 ratios they were. The same difference existed in the comparison of the mandibular ratios.

For the ratios of the maxillary anterior teeth with the premolars, the pattern of variation is not dissimilar to the mandibular comparisons. Sample size was too small to make comparisons with *H. africanus* for I1. The I2/P3 and C/P4 comparisons placed the australopithecine taxa apart from subsequent hominids, although only the I2/P3 ratio placed them with each other. The C/P3 ratio only separated out *H. robustus.*

There are 3 different patterns running through the anterior-posterior comparisons. In the first, both australopithecine taxa have ratios significantly smaller than the subsequent taxa, but similar to each other. In the second, the australopithecines have ratios significantly smaller than subsequent taxa, and *H. robustus* has a significantly smaller ratio than *H. africanus.* In the third pattern, *H. robustus* alone has a ratio significantly smaller than the other taxa. These patterns have been listed in order of relative frequency.

DENTAL RATIOS OF SUMMED TOOTH SETS

The only author who has utilized ratios of summed tooth sets, to my knowledge, is Selmer-Olsen (1949:67-69). He compares the summed lengths from I1 to C with the summed lengths of the first 2 molars for both jaws. The ratios calculated here are not comparable with these.

The advantage of comparing tooth sets is that one can be definitive about the relation of the anterior to the posterior teeth, without letting 1 ratio act as an estimate of that comparison, as so many authors do. In Table CXLIII to CXLVI, mandibular and maxillary ratios are calculated for the incisors compared with the remaining teeth, and for the incisors and the canine compared with the remaining teeth. Morphologically, one would expect the canine to fit best with the incisors, rather than with the premolars and molars. However, there is no significant difference in the variability of either the mandibular or maxillary tooth sums I1 - I2 compared with I1 - C, or C - M3 compared with P3 - M3 (Tables CI to CIV and CVI to CIX). In calculating ratios for summed tooth sets, an index was calculated comparing length to length, area to area, and length to area.

Comparing the anterior to the posterior tooth sets in this way reveals a very consistent pattern. There is a significant increase in this ratio through the Pleistocene. *H. robustus* has the minimum ratio, and is significantly smaller than *H. africanus* with the exception of the length to length comparison in both jaws for the ratio of incisors to remaining teeth. In the comparison of length to area, *H. erectus* stands intermediate between earlier and later taxa. This is not true for the other 2 ratios. For these, *H. erectus* stands with the recent taxa. Lastly, *H. africanus* is not significantly smaller than *H. erectus* in the maxillary length to length and length to area comparisons. It is significantly smaller in all other instances. There is no significant difference between *H. sapiens* and *H. neanderthalensis.*

TABLE CXLIII. Ratio of summed dental dimensions from Mandibular I1 to I2, compared to the summed dimensions from C to M3: Mean, Range, Sample Size (N), and Coefficient of Variation (CV). The Ratios considered are Length to Length (L/L), Length to Area (L/Area), and Area to Area (Area/Area).

LOWER I/CM3	L/L				L/AREA				AREA/AREA			
	MEAN	RANGE	N	CV	MEAN	RANGE	N	CV	MEAN	RANGE	N	CV
H. AFRICANUS	16.8	13.3 - 19.6	4	14.2	14.6	11.9 - 16.6	3	13.8	10.8	8.4 - 12.5	3	16.3
H. ROBUSTUS	15.1	13.6 - 16.7	5	8.4	10.8	9.2 - 12.7	5	14.4	6.9	5.7 - 8.1	5	15.1
H. ERECTUS	19.9	17.4 - 21.7	7	5.8	18.2	15.3 - 20.9	8	7.8	13.5	12.1 - 15.2	7	7.3
H. NEANDERTAL	21.2	17.9 - 23.9	22	8.2	20.9	17.0 - 25.4	21	10.6	15.5	12.3 - 18.7	21	10.5
H. SAPIENS	21.0	16.2 - 24.5	116	7.1	21.5	16.1 - 26.1	111	9.9	13.5	10.1 - 19.0	103	11.9
AUSTRALOP	15.9	13.3 - 19.6	9	11.0	12.2	9.2 - 15.4	8	16.3	8.4	5.7 - 12.5	8	17.2
KRAPINA	19.9	19.5 - 20.3	2		19.7	19.2 - 20.2	2		14.8	14.8 - 14.8	2	
NEANDERTAL	21.7	17.9 - 23.9	16	8.1	21.3	17.0 - 25.4	15	11.4	16.1	13.5 - 18.7	15	8.7
MT CARMEL	19.8	19.2 - 20.7	4	3.1	20.1	18.5 - 22.3	4	6.9	13.8	12.3 - 16.1	4	10.5
AUSTRALOID	21.8	21.2 - 23.0	4	3.7	20.4	19.2 - 21.1	4	4.4	13.4	12.9 - 13.8	2	
INDIAN	21.5	19.2 - 23.9	9	7.4	21.9	17.8 - 25.6	7	14.0	13.6	12.5 - 14.5	6	6.2
SUB SAHARAN	21.3	18.7 - 24.5	17	9.2	22.4	18.6 - 26.1	15	10.6	14.7	10.5 - 17.1	12	14.9
NEW BRITAIN	21.2	19.0 - 23.1	20	5.8	21.0	18.5 - 23.8	20	7.6	13.2	11.3 - 15.6	18	10.2
DICKSON MD	21.0	19.1 - 23.2	43	5.0	21.4	17.3 - 24.6	43	7.9	13.0	11.0 - 15.0	43	7.4
CAUCASOID	20.1	16.2 - 23.3	21	9.4	21.2	16.1 - 25.4	20	12.8	13.8	10.1 - 19.0	20	16.4

TABLE CXLIV. Ratio of summed dental dimensions from Mandibular I1 to C, compared to the summed dimensions from P3 to M3: Mean, Range, Sample Size (N), and Coefficient of Variation (CV). The Ratios considered are Length to Length (L/L), Length to Area (L/Area), and Area to Area (Area/Area).

LOWER IC/PM3	L/L				L/AREA				AREA/AREA			
	MEAN	RANGE	N	CV	MEAN	RANGE	N	CV	MEAN	RANGE	N	CV
H. AFRICANUS	34.2	30.3 - 36.9	4	7.8	27.9	24.6 - 29.9	3	8.5	23.4	21.0 - 26.0	3	8.8
H. ROBUSTUS	27.9	24.5 - 30.5	5	9.6	19.1	15.8 - 22.2	5	14.9	13.6	11.0 - 15.4	5	14.9
H. ERECTUS	37.8	34.1 - 40.9	7	6.3	33.5	28.9 - 37.6	8	8.1	27.8	23.5 - 30.8	7	7.3
H. NEANDERTAL	40.5	35.0 - 45.0	22	6.3	39.4	31.8 - 46.3	21	9.4	31.6	27.3 - 36.4	21	8.4
H. SAPIENS	38.8	32.3 - 43.4	121	5.6	38.7	31.3 - 46.7	116	11.9	27.1	21.4 - 38.7	116	7.6

TABLE CXLV. Ratio of summed dental dimensions from Maxillary I1 to I2, compared to the summed dimensions from C to M3: Mean, Range, Sample Size (N), and Coefficient of Variation (CV). The Ratios considered are Length to Length (L/L), Length to Area (L/Area), and Area to Area (Area/Area).

UPPER I/CM3	L/L				L/AREA				AREA/AREA			
	MEAN	RANGE	N	CV	MEAN	RANGE	N	CV	MEAN	RANGE	N	CV
H. AFRICANUS	25.0	24.5 - 25.6	2		18.6	18.2 - 19.0	2		14.0	13.4 - 14.6	2	
H. ROBUSTUS	21.3	21.1 - 21.4	2		11.7	11.7 - 11.7	2		9.1	8.9 - 9.2	2	
H. ERECTUS	29.2	27.7 - 32.1	3	7.0	22.2	19.3 - 23.9	3	9.3	22.0	19.0 - 25.0	2	
H. NEANDERTAL	30.0	24.0 - 35.3	9	12.6	29.9	24.0 - 35.3	9	13.9	21.3	15.9 - 25.5	9	11.7
H. SAPIENS	30.2	24.2 - 36.4	110	7.5	28.4	21.6 - 37.2	108	10.4	20.3	14.7 - 29.4	104	13.0
AUSTRALOP.	23.2	21.1 - 25.6	4	8.2	15.2	11.7 - 19.0	4	22.7	11.5	8.9 - 14.6	4	21.7
NEANDERTAL	31.3	24.0 - 35.3	6	12.2	31.1	24.0 - 35.3	6	12.2	22.6	15.9 - 25.5	6	14.7
MT CARMEL	27.7	25.2 - 30.9	3	8.5	27.7	25.2 - 30.9	3	8.6	18.9	16.6 - 22.6	3	14.0
SUB SAHARAN	31.6	26.4 - 36.0	9	9.6	31.1	23.3 - 37.2	8	13.6	21.7	16.7 - 26.2	8	12.8
DICKSON MD	30.6	27.3 - 36.4	51	5.5	28.7	22.1 - 36.6	51	8.9	20.2	16.0 - 25.1	51	8.6
INDIAN	29.9	25.2 - 32.2	8	7.1	28.4	24.9 - 31.4	8	7.1	19.9	15.7 - 22.6	8	9.7
NEW BRITAIN	29.9	26.8 - 32.3	16	5.5	27.2	23.3 - 30.3	16	7.7	19.3	17.1 - 21.6	14	6.3
AUSTRALOID	29.7	25.0 - 34.5	8	12.6	26.7	21.6 - 30.8	7	11.9	21.2	14.7 - 29.4	7	28.4
CAUCASOID	28.6	24.2 - 32.0	18	8.0	27.3	23.4 - 35.4	18	11.4	20.4	15.7 - 27.4	16	18.5

TABLE CXLVI. Ratio of summed dental dimensions from Maxillary I1 to C, compared to the summed dimensions from P3 to M3: Mean, Range, Sample Size (N), and Coefficient of Variation (CV). The Ratios considered are Length to Length (L/L), Length to Area (L/Area), and Area to Area (Area/Area).

UPPER IC/PM3	L/L				L/AREA				AREA/AREA			
	MEAN	RANGE	N	CV	MEAN	RANGE	N	CV	MEAN	RANGE	N	CV
H. AFRICANUS	47.1	46.5 - 47.7	2		33.4	32.9 - 33.8	2		27.9	27.2 - 28.7	2	
H. ROBUSTUS	36.2	36.0 - 36.3	2		18.9	18.8 - 19.0	2		15.9	15.9 - 16.0	2	
H. ERECTUS	52.5	49.4 - 55.8	3	4.9	38.5	32.4 - 42.5	3	11.4	40.4	36.6 - 44.2	2	
H. NEANDERTAL	54.0	47.5 - 59.8	9	8.2	54.3	47.5 - 59.8	9	8.1	39.6	34.3 - 45.3	9	10.3
H. SAPIENS	54.6	45.2 - 63.6	115	10.2	49.9	39.4 - 64.7	113	9.7	37.9	28.5 - 55.0	113	13.1
AUSTRALOP.	41.6	36.0 - 47.7	4	13.2	26.1	18.8 - 33.8	4	27.7	21.9	15.9 - 28.7	4	27.5
NEANDERTAL	55.1	47.5 - 59.8	6	7.6	55.5	47.5 - 59.8	6	7.3	40.8	35.0 - 45.3	6	9.2
MT CARMEL	51.8	48.5 - 57.6	3	7.8	51.9	48.5 - 57.6	3	7.8	37.0	34.3 - 41.8	3	9.1
DICKSON MD	55.1	50.3 - 63.6	51	4.8	50.0	39.4 - 61.7	51	8.8	37.9	32.4 - 46.9	51	7.5
SUB SAHARAN	55.0	48.0 - 60.7	9	8.3	52.3	41.4 - 58.0	8	11.0	39.1	33.0 - 46.8	8	11.0
INDIAN	53.8	48.4 - 57.0	8	5.1	49.3	46.1 - 53.8	8	5.5	37.0	32.3 - 39.8	8	5.9
AUSTRALOID	52.7	45.2 - 57.5	8	9.0	46.6	42.4 - 54.2	7	9.2	39.8	28.5 - 55.0	7	24.2

6. Conclusions

SUMMARY OF THE MAJOR POINTS

1) There are no significant trends to mandibular incisor size variation in *fossil* hominid taxa. There is, however, a general tendency of breadth increase through *H. neanderthalensis.* There is a morphologically significant trend to the increase in maxillary incisor breadth. The maximum breadth values are reached in *H. neanderthalensis.* The reduction of mandibular and maxillary incisor size in *H. sapiens* is morphologically significant for length, breadth, and area.

2) Both mandibular and maxillary canine size are maximum in *H. africanus.* There is a significant decrease in the size of the *H. robustus* mandibular canines, while the maxillary canines are not significantly changed. Compared with *H. robustus,* mandibular canines increase significantly in the Mid-Pleistocene, according to the data used here. However, using a larger canine sample size, both a "*t*" test and a Mann-Whitney *U* test demonstrate no significant differences on the 1% level between either mandibular or maxillary canine areas of *H. africanus* and *H. erectus,* and of *H. robustus* and *H. erectus* (Wolpoff 1970b). If the australopithecines are treated as a single taxon, there is no significant trend to canine size variation in the Lower and Middle Pleistocene. In fact, the sizes of australopithecine and *H. erectus* canines are almost identical. While large canines are maintained in *H. neanderthalensis*—almost of *H. erectus* size—the *H. sapiens* decrease is both statistically and morphologically significant.

3) The premolars show a consistent and significant decrease over time. The 1 exception is P^4 in *H. robustus,* a tooth significantly greater in this taxon than in *H. africanus.* If the australopithecines are treated as a single taxon, there are no exceptions to this general reduction trend. *H. neanderthalensis* has modern-sized premolars.

4) The molars show a consistent and significant decrease throughout the Pleistocene, culminating in *H. neanderthalensis* with modern-sized teeth.

5) In comparing *H. africanus* with *H. robustus,* only 2 teeth show differences with morphological significance. The mandibular canine of *H. robustus* is significantly smaller, while the maxillary fourth premolar of this taxon is significantly larger. The differences between them among all of the other teeth are not morphologically significant; that is, the differences are less than those which regulary occur within extant groups of men.

6) In comparing the australopithecines with *H. erectus,* all of the significant differences appear in the posterior teeth; the premolars and molars are significantly smaller. There is no significant difference in the anterior teeth, although they tend to be slightly larger in *H. erectus.*

7) In comparing *H. erectus* with *H. neanderthalensis,* the latter has smaller posterior teeth. The anterior teeth are not significantly different, except for the increase in *H. neanderthalensis* maxillary incisor breadth.

8) In comparing *H. neanderthalensis* with *H. sapiens,* there is no significant difference in the posterior teeth. On the other hand, the anterior

teeth of *H. sapiens* exhibit a consistent and significant reduction.

9) With 2 exceptions, there are no significant trends, and only a few significant differences, in tooth shape as expressed by the dental index. The first exception is in incisor shape. The teeth become relatively longer through *H. erectus,* broader in *H. neanderthalensis,* and longer again in *H. sapiens.* The second exception is in M_3. This tooth has an exceptionally high index in *H. robustus.*

10) Variability in hominids, as measured by the coefficient of variation, is greater than or equal to that in the non-human primates. The only exception is P_3. When measured by the range-standard deviation index, *H. sapiens* is more variable in all teeth than the non-human primates, while the other hominid taxa are equally or less variable.

11) Using the coefficient of variation as a measure, some trends occurred in the evolution of variability. For length, the posterior teeth increase in variability from *H. erectus* on. For the anteriors, *H. sapiens* tends to be the most variable taxon. In breadth and area, there is a definite tendency, although not a uniform trend, for variability to increase through time among the recent hominid taxa. When the range-standard deviation index is used to measure variability, there is a uniform and significant increase in variability throughout the Pleistocene in length, breadth, area, dental index, and module.

12) There is no consistent pattern of relationship in variability between *H. africanus* and *H. robustus.* If anything, *H. robustus* is somewhat more variable.

13) Correlations of individual teeth with their opposites are high, but not high enough to justify using 1 side to represent the jaw. Mandibular correlations are higher in the anteriors, while maxillary correlations are higher in the posteriors.

14) There is a decrease in correlations distally in each tooth group. Correlations between pairs of teeth are higher than correlations between adjacent teeth.

15) Area correlations are higher than length or breadth correlations.

16) There is a great consistency to the trends in length, breadth, and area sums for the anterior teeth of the mandible and maxilla. There do not seem to be any trends of morphological significance with the exception of the significant reduction of breadth and area between *H. neanderthalensis* and *H. sapiens.* There is a tendency for size increase through the Middle Pleistocene.

17) For both mandibular and maxillary summed posterior teeth, there is a significant and consistent trend of reduction from the australopithecines through *H. neanderthalensis.* The difference between the australopithecine taxa is not morphologically significant. There is no difference between *H. neanderthalensis* and *H. sapiens.*

18) The lack of metric difference in the summed posteriors between *H. neanderthalensis* and *H. sapiens* is a somewhat misleading artifact of the sampling procedure. While third molar agenesis is relatively common in extant groups, it is unknown in fossil man. In summing the posteriors, only those jaws with all 3 molars were used. In actuality, there is a significant decrease in summed posterior teeth as the result of missing third molars, rather than because of reduced tooth size.

19) In sums taken for the entire tooth row, all differences between adjacent taxa are significant, with the exception of the differences between *H. sapiens* and *H. neanderthalensis.* The sample size allowing this summation was prohibitively small.

20) In the examination of anterior tooth ratios, there is a progressive pattern of canine reduction relative to both incisors. This pattern is somewhat clearer in the mandible than in the maxilla. The trend places *H. africanus* apart from the other taxa. There were no significant differences in the ratio of the incisors to each other.

21) The posterior to posterior ratios show a tendency for relative reduction distally in each tooth group. In M1 comparisons, the 2 australopithecine taxa stand in contradistinction to the remaining taxa. *H. erectus* is either intermediate or completely modern.

22) Comparisons with M1 show more gradual but ultimately more extensive change in the maxilla than in the mandible. There is no real difference between the relative reduction of the second and third molars in either jaw. The order of relative premolar reduction is reversed in the 2 jaws: the posterior tooth reduces first in the maxilla, and the anterior tooth first in the mandible.

23) The ratio of the anterior to posterior premolars shows no consistent pattern of change in

the mandible. In the maxilla, this ratio is significantly smaller (less than 100) in the australopithecine taxa, compared with other hominid taxa.

24) There are 3 different patterns which characterize the anterior to posterior tooth comparisons. In the first, both australopithecine taxa have ratios significantly smaller than those of other hominid taxa, but similar to each other. The second is like the first except that in addition, *H. robustus* has a significantly smaller ratio than *H. africanus.* In the third pattern, *H. robustus* has a significantly smaller ratio than the other hominid taxa. The first pattern, tending to characterize incisor comparisons, is the most frequent.

25) Comparison of the ratios of anterior to posterior summed tooth sets reveals a consistent trend: the ratio increases significantly through *H. neanderthalensis.* A relative decrease in the posterior dentition is thus indicated.

APPLICATION OF THE SELECTION MODEL

I believe that the metric data unambiguously supports the model of selection discussed earlier. The australopithecine dentition exhibits a maximization of posterior grinding area. The highest incidence of vegetable foods in any hominid taxon is thus suggested. In this respect, *H. africanus* and *H. robustus,* if they are separate species, cannot be distinguished. The canines and incisors of most australopithecines are reduced to the early hominid condition: they are large, but not ape-like or baboon-like in any sense. There is some evidence for the presence of slightly projecting canines in both the australopithecines and in *H. erectus.* This condition is not rare in modern man (Adloff 1908, 1927; Remane 1927; Taylor 1969b). The australopithecines may represent the very end of the trend for canine reduction resulting from the substitution of weapons for teeth as a means of defense. This is indicated by the fact that there is a reduction of the canines, relative to incisor size, following the australopithecines. Mid-Pleistocene hominids have relatively reduced canines, as do all subsequent hominid taxa. There is a general tendency for the size increase of the anterior teeth through the Middle Plestocene. Breadth is affected more extensively by this increase than length. I suggest that these teeth were used in manipulation of the environment as is characteristic of a culture-bearing hominid, rather than primarily in feeding and defense, from the australopithecines on. The tendency for increasing size follows direct evidence for extensive environmental manipulation seen in the record of non-perishable artifacts (Bordes 1968; Chard 1969). This tendency continues until the development of large numbers of efficient, special purpose tools in the Levalloiso-Mousterian industries of the Middle Paleolithic (Brose and Wolpoff 1971). Relevant behavioral changes follow from these changes in technology. A single purpose tool is generally more effective in the specific task it was designed for than any general purpose tool. With respect to the action of selection upon hominid morphology, the major implication of changes from general to specific tools concerns the use of the jaws as a vise. The importance of this usage is indicated by the maintenance of large anterior teeth (actually increasing in breadth for *early* Neandertals) throughout the Lower and Middle Pleistocene, while the posterior dentition progressively reduces. To put a hole in a piece of wood with a knife requires more use of a vise than if one were using a drill. That is, the development of special purpose tools reduces selection for both *force* and *power* (force over time) in the anterior dentition, through a combination of less strenuous use, and use over shorter periods of time (Brose and Wolpoff 1971). Indeed, the reduction of the anterior dentition is part of a general trend reducing skeletal and muscular rugosity, replacing them with more efficient technology. With the relaxation of selection, the anterior dentition and supporting structures decreased in size. The increased variability in the anterior teeth of both *H. neanderthalensis* and *H. sapiens* indicates that it was the reduction of selection for large size, rather than the substitution of selection for smaller size, which led to the subsequent size decrease.

The reduction of the posterior dentition clearly follows the archaeological evidence of increasing hominid meat-gathering activities, first as scavengers (Dart 1957; M. Leakey 1967; Chard 1969; Clark 1964; Washburn and Howell 1960; Tobias 1967d), and later as hunters (Washburn and Hamburg 1965; M. Leakey 1966; Leakey 1965; Washburn and Lancaster 1968). Both the extensive hunting of megafauna, and the specialized and intensive hunting of particular species, occurred with regularity by 1/2 million years ago, in the Middle Paleolithic (Howell 1960, 1961, 1965b). The evidence for these dietary shifts depends on assuming a graminivorous diet (Jolly 1970) for early hominids (Wolpoff 1970a).

Reduction of selection for extensive posterior grinding area comes within the australopithecines themselves. The progressive shift to increasing amounts of meat in the diet is evidenced by the sequence of living sites in Bed I at Olduvai Gorge. While the earliest sites contain scavenged material and the remains of very slow game, later sites contain remains of whole juvenile and eventually adult specimens brought back to the living area and butchered (Leakey 1964, 1965; M. Leakey 1967; Bordes 1968). The shift to an efficient hunting hominid economy has been documented in East Africa in the period of time from roughly 2 million to 1 million years ago. By the time of *H. erectus,* hunting habits are both extensive and intensive (Brose and Wolpoff 1971; Washburn and Lancaster 1968). The appearance of fire in temperate areas about 400,000 years ago (Oakley 1966) results in the suspension of the remaining selection for relatively large posterior teeth. By the time of *H. neanderthalensis,* the posteriors are reduced to modern size. Subsequent reduction of the mandible and maxilla following the relaxation of selection acting on large size in the anterior dentition and supporting structures results in the reduction of the jaws themselves, the crowding of the entire dentition, and is leading to the eventual loss of the last tooth to erupt—the third molar. The increasing variability in the posterior dentition indicates that it was relaxation of selection for large size, rather than substitution of selection for small size, which oriented the reduction of the posterior teeth. The increasing frequency of third molar agenesis, on the other hand, may well be due to a shift in selection following from the general decrease in jaw size which began in the Neolithic (Dahlberg 1945, 1960, 1962), or to the lack of mesio-distal dimension loss because of decreasing interstitial wear (Begg 1954; Wolpoff 1970a).

The one factor common to all of the hominid metric dental evolution, orienting in one way or another all of the trends which have been described, is culture. Culture is both man's major adaptive mechanism and the most important influence acting upon his morphological adaptation (Brace and Montagu 1965; Wolpoff 1968; Washburn 1960; Bartholomew and Birdsell 1953; Mayr 1950). The use of culture as man's major adaptive mechanism can be seen in the eventual reduction of the anterior dentition, resulting from the relaxation of selection for robust teeth by the development of efficient tools. The morphological adaptation to culture can be seen in the increasing frequency of third molar agenesis, in the trend of increasing anterior tooth size through the Middle Pleistocene, and of greatest importance, in the evolution of brain size and complexity (Washburn 1960; Wolpoff 1969b). Culture has been, and continues to be, the major factor orienting the direction of hominid dental evolution.

Bibliography

ABEL, W.
1930 "Kritische Untersuchungen über *Australopithecus africanus* Dart," *Morphologisches Jahrbuch von Gegenbaurs,* 65:539-640.
1933 "Zähne und Kiefer in ihren Wechselbeziehungen bei Suschmannern, Hottentotten, Negern, und deren Bastarden," *Zeitschrift für Morphologie und Anthropologie,* 31:314-61.

ADAM, K. D.
1954 "Die zeitliche Stellung der Urmenschen-Fundschicht von Steinheim an der Murr innerhalb des Pleistozäns," *Eiszeitalter und Gegenwart,* 4/5:18-21.
1961 "Die Bedeutung der pleistozänen Säugetierfaunen Mitteleuropas für die Geschichte des Eiszeitalters," *Stuttgarter Beiträge zur Naturkunde,* 78:1-34.

ADAM, W.
1943 "The Keilor Fossil Skull: Palate and Upper Dental Arch," *Memoir of the Natural History Museum of Victoria,* 13:71-77.

ADLOFF, P.
1907 "Die Zähne des *Homo primigenisus* von Krapina," *Anatomischer Anzeiger,* 31:273-82.
1908 *Das Gebiss des Menschen und der Anthropomorphen.* Springer, Berlin.
1909 "Zur Frage der Systematischen Stellung des Menschen von Krapina," *Anatomischer Anzeiger,* 34:105-10.
1927 "Das Gebiss des Menschen und der Anthropoiden und das Abstammungsproblem," *Zeitschrift für Morphologie und Anthropologie,* 26:431-49.
1931a "Das Gebiss von *Australopithecus africanus* Dart. Einige erganzende Bemerkungen zum Eckzahnproblem," *Zeitschrift für Anatomie und Entwicklungsgeschichte,* 97:145-56.
1931b "Der Eckzahn des Menschen und das Abstammungsproblem," *Zeitschrift für Anatomie und Entwicklungsgeschichte,* 94:94-116.
1932 "Uber die Bedeutung des Gebiss für die Beurteilung der zum Menschen in Beziehung stehenden fossilen Reste," *Anatomischer Anzeiger,* 75:542-49.
1938 "Das Gebiss von *Sinanthropus Pekinensis,*" *Zeitschrift für Morphologie und Anthropologie,* 37:490-537.
1939 "Die Südafrikanischen Fossilen Menschenaffen und der Ursprung des Menschen Gebiss," *Anthropologischer Anzeiger,* 16:72-76.
1949 "Bemerkungen über das Gebiss der Südafrikanischen Fossilen Anthropoiden *Paranthropus* und *Plesianthropus,*" *Zeitschrift für Morphologie und Anthropologie,* 41:259-67.

AMPOULANGE, A.
1959 "La Sépulture Néolithique de 'Pas Estret,'" *Annales de Paléontologie,* 44:47-84.

ANDERSON, J. E.
1965 "Human Skeleton of Tehuacan," *Science,* 148:496-97.

ARAMBOURG, C.
1954 "L'Hominien Fossile de Ternifine,"

Comptes Rendus de l'Académie des Sciences, Série D, 239:893-95.

1955a "Une Découverte Récente en Paléontologie Humaine, l'Atlanthropus de Ternifine," *Quaternaria,* 2:5-13.

1955b "Une Nouvelle Mandibule d'Atlanthropus du Gisement de Ternifine," *Comptes Rendus de l'Académie des Sciences, Série D,* 241:895-97.

1955c "A Recent Discovery in Human Paleontology, Atlanthropus of Ternifine," *American Journal of Physical Anthropology,* 13:191-202.

1956 Une 3eme Mandibule d'Atlanthropus Découverte à Ternifine," *Quaternaria,* 3:1-4.

1957 "Récentes Découvertes de Paléontologie Humaine Réalisées en Afrique du Nord Française," *Proceedings of the Third Pan African Congress on Prehistory,* pp. 186-94.

1958 "Les Stades Évolutifs de l'Humanité," *The Leech,* 28:106-11.

1963 "Le Gisement de Ternifine," *Archives de l'Institute de Paléontologie Humaine,* 32.

1965 "Le Gisement Mousterien et l'Homme du Jebel Irhound (Maroc)," *Quaternaria,* 7:1-8.

ARAMBOURG, C., and P. BIBERSON

1956 "Fossil Human Remains from the Paleolithic Site of Sidi Abderrahman (Morocco)," *American Journal of Physical Anthropology,* 14:267-90.

ARAMBOURG, C., J. CHAVAILLON, and Y. COPPENS

1967 "Premiers Résultats de la Nouvelle Mission de l'Omo (1967)," *Comptes Rendus de l'Académie des Sciences, Série D,* 265:1891-96.

ARAMBOURG, C., and Y. COPPENS

1967 "Sur la Découverte, dans le Pleistocene Inférieur de la Vallée de l'Omo, d'une Mandibule d'Australopithecien," *Comptes Rendus de l'Académie des Sciences, Série D,* 265:689-90.

1968 "Découverte d'un Australopithecien Nouveau dans les Gisements de l'Omo (Ethiopie)," *South African Journal of Science,* 64:58-59.

ASHTON. E. H., and S. ZUCKERMAN

1950a Some Quantitative Dental Characteristics of the Chimpanzee, Gorilla, and Orangoutan," *Philosophical Transactions of the Royal Society of London,* Series B, 234:471-84.

1950b "The Influence of Geographic Isolation on the Skulls of the Green Monkey (*Cercopithecus aethiops*)," *Proceedings of the Royal Society, Series B,* 137:212-38.

BADER, R. S., and W. H. LEHMANN

1965 "Phenotypic and Genotypic Variation in Odontometric Traits of the House Mouse," *American Midland Naturalist,* 74:28-38.

BAILIT, H. L., S. J. DEWITT, and R. A. LEIGH

1968 "The Size and Morphology of the Nasioi Dentition," *American Journal of Physical Anthropology,* 28:271-88.

BAILIT, H. L., and J. S. FRIEDLAENDER

1966 "Tooth Size Reduction: A Hominid Trend," *American Anthropologist,* 68:665-72.

BAKER, L. W.

1941 "The Influence of the Formative Dental Organs on the Growth of the Bones of the Face," *American Journal of Orthodontics,* 27:489-506.

BANKS, H. V.

1934 "Incidence of Third Molar Development," *Angle Orthodontist,* 4:223-33.

BARNES, D. S.

1969 "Tooth Morphology and Other Aspects of the Teso Dentition," *American Journal of Physical Anthropology,* 30:183-94.

BARRETT, M. J., T. BROWN, and M. R. MACDONALD

1963 "Dental Observations on Australian Aborigines: Mesiodistal Crown Diameters of Permanent Teeth," *Australian Dental Journal,* 8:150-56.

BARRETT, M. J., T. BROWN, and I. V. OZOIS

1964 "Dental Observations on Australian Aborigines: Buccolingual Crown Diameters of Deciduous and Permanent Teeth," *Australian Dental Journal,* 9:280-85.

BARTHOLOMEW, G. A., and J. B. BIRDSELL

1953 "Ecology and the Protohominids," *American Anthropologist,* 55:481-98.

BAY, R.

1958 "Das Gebiss des Neandertalers," *Hun-*

dert Jahre Neanderthaler (ed. G.H.R. von Koenigswald), pp. 123-40. Kemik en Zoon N. V., Utrecht.

BAYLAC, P., R. CAMMAS *et al.*

1950 "Découverte Récentes dans les Grottes de Montmaurin, Haute-Garonne," *L'Anthropologie,* 54:262-71.

BEGG, P. R.

1954 "Stone Age Man's Dentition," *American Journal of Orthodontics,* 40:298-312, 373-83, 462-75, 517-31.

BEHM-BLANCKE, G.

1958 "Umwelt, Kultur, und Morphologie des eem-interglazialen Menschen von Ehringsdorf bei Weimar," *Hundert Jahre Neanderthaler* (ed. G. H. R. von Koenigswald), pp. 141-50. Kemik en Zoon N. V., Utrecht.

BERCKHEMER, F.

1933 "Ein Menschen-Schädel aus den diluvailen Schottern von Steinheim," *Anthropologischer Anzeiger,* 10:318-21.

1937 "Bemerkungen zu H. Weinert's Abhandlung 'Der Urmenschen-Schädel von Steinheim,'" *Verhandlungen der Gesellschaft für Physische Anthropologie,* 8:49-58.

BERLIN, V.

1956 "Odontologische Befunde am 'Svaerdborg–Individuum,'" *Zeitschrift für Morphologie und Anthropologie,* 47:382-406.

BIBERSON, P.

1963 "Human Evolution in Morocco in the Framework of the Paleoclimatic Variations of the Atlantic Pleistocene," *African Ecology and Human Evolution* (eds. F. C. Howell and F. Bourlière), pp. 417-47. Aldine, Chicago.

1964 "La Place des Hommes du Paleolithique Marocain dans la Chronologie du Pleistocene Atlantique," *L'Anthropologie,* 68:475-526.

BIELICKI, T.

1966 "On 'Homo habilis,'" *Current Anthropology,* 7:576-78.

BIGGERSTAFF, R. H.

1966 "Metric and Taxonomic Variation in the Dentitions of Two Asian Cercopithecoid Species of Macaca," *American Journal of Physical Anthropology,* 24:231-38.

1967 "The Anterior Migration of Dentitions and Anterior Crowding: A Review," *Angle Orthodontist,* 37:227-40.

BISHOP, W. W., and J. D. CLARK, eds.

1967 *Background to Evolution in Africa.* University of Chicago, Chicago.

BLACK, G. V.

1895 "An Investigation of the Physical Characters of Human Teeth," *Dental Cosmos,* 37:469-84.

1902 *Descriptive Anatomy of the Human Teeth.* White Dental Manufacturing Company, Philadelphia.

1908 *Operative Dentistry.* Medicodental, Chicago.

BLACKWELDER, R. E.

1967 *Taxonomy, a Text and Reference Book.* Wiley, New York.

BLANC, A. C.

1954 "Reperti Fossili Neandertalaini Grotta del Fossellone al Monte Circeo: Circeo IV," *Quaternaria,* 1:171-75.

1958a "Il Primo Reperto Fossile Neandertaliano del Selento," *Quaternaria,* 5:271-79.

1958b "Torre in Pietra, Saccopastore, Monte Circeo. On the Position of the Mousterian Culture in the Pleistocene Sequence of the Rome Area," *Hundert Jahre Neanderthaler* (ed. G. H. R. von Koenigswald), pp. 167-74. Kemink en Zoon H. V., Utrecht.

1960 "Leura I: Der Erste fossile Funde eines Neandertalers von Salento," *Anthropologischer Anzeiger,* 24:292-98.

BOBOC, G.

1965 "Studiu Statistic si Citeva Consideratii Asupra Latimii Dintilor Temporari si Definitivi," *Stomatologia,* 12:345-54.

BOLTON, W. A.

1958 "Disharmony in Tooth Size and Its Relation to the Analysis and Treatment of Malocclusion," *Angle Orthodontist,* 28:113-28.

BONE, E. L.

1955 "Une Clavicule et un Nouveau Fragment Mandibulaire *d'Australopithecus prometheus,*" *Palaeontologia Africana,* 3:87-101.

1957 "Les Fouilles 1955 au Terril de Makapansgat," *Proceedings of the Third Pan African Congress on Prehistory,* pp.

149-54.

VON BONIN, G.

1935 "The Magdalenian Skeleton from Cap-Blanc in the Field Museum of Natural History," *Illinois Medical and Dental Monographs,* 1:1-76.

BORDES, F.

1968 *The Old Stone Age.* McGraw-Hill, New York.

BOSTANCI, E.

1964 "An Examination of a Neandertal Type Fossil Skull Found in the Chalcidique Peninsula," *Turk Tarih Kurumu Belleten,* 28:373-81.

BOULE, M.

1913 *L'Homme Fossile de la Chapelle aux Saints.* Masson, Paris.

BOULE, M., and H. V. VALLOIS

1932 "L'Homme Fossile d'Asselar, Sahara," *Archives de l'Institute de Paléontologie Humaine,* 9.

1957 *Fossil Men.* Dryden, New York.

BRABRANT, H.

1963a "Observations sur la Denture Humaine en France et en Belgique à l'Époque Gallo-Romaine et au Moyen Age," *Bulletin du Groupement Internationale pour la Recherche Scientifique en Stomatologie,* 6:169-296.

1963b "Observations Anthropologique et Odontologique sur Dents les Hutu du Rwanda," *Annales de Musée Royal Afrique Centrale, Série in-8, Sciences humaines,* 47:1-30.

1965 "Observations sur la Denture des Pygmées de l'Afrique Centrale," *Bulletin du Groupement Internationale pour la Recherche Scientifique en Stomatologie,* 8:27-49.

BRABRANT, H., A. SAHLY, and M. BOUYSSOU

1961 "Étude des Dents Préhistorique les Station Archéologique des Matelles (Département de l'Herault, France)," *Bulletin du Groupement Internationale pour la Recherche Scientifique en Stomatologie,* 4:382-448.

BRABRANT, H. and F. TWIESSELMAN

1964a "L'Évolution de la Denture Humaine en Europe Occidentale," *Archives de Biologie,*75:709-44.

1964b "Observations sur l'Évolution de la Denture Permanente Humaine en Europe Occidentale," *Bulletin du Groupement Internationale pour la Recherche Scientifique en Stomatologie,* 7:11-84.

BRACE, C. L.

1962a "Cultural Factors in the Evolution of the Human Dentition," *Culture and the Evolution of Man* (ed. M. F. A. Montagu), pp. 343-54. Oxford, New York.

1962b "Refocusing on the Neandertal Problem," *American Anthropologist,* 64:729-41.

1963a "Structural Reduction in Evolution," *American Naturalist,* 97:39-49.

1963b "Review of 'Evolution and Hominisation' (ed. G. Kurth)," *American Journal of Physical Anthropology,* 21:87-91.

1963c "Review of 'Ideas on Human Evolution' (ed. W. W. Howells)," *Human Biology,* 35:545-48.

1964a "The Fate of the 'Classic' Neandertals: A Consideration of Hominid Catastrophism," *Current Anthropology,* 5:3-43.

1964b "The Probable Mutation Effect," *American Naturalist,* 97:453-55.

1967a *The Stages of Human Evolution.* Prentice Hall, Englewood Cliffs.

1967b "Environment, Tooth Form, and Size in the Pleistocene," *Journal of Dental Research,* 46:809-16.

1967c "More on the Fate of the 'Classic' Neandertals," *Current Anthropology,* 7:204-14.

BRACE, C. L., and S. MOLNAR

1967 "Experimental Studies in Human Tooth Wear," *American Journal of Physical Anthropology,* 27:213-22.

BRACE, C. L., and M. F. A. MONTAGU

1965 *Man's Evolution.* Macmillan, New York.

BRAIN, C. K.

1958 "The Transvaal Ape-Man Bearing Cave Deposits," *Transvaal Museum Memoir,* 11.

1967 "The Transvaal Museum's Fossil Project at Swartkrans," *South African Journal of Science,* 63:378-84.

BRAMBLETT, C. A.

1967 "Pathology in the Darajani Baboon," *American Journal of Physical Anthropology,* 26:331-40.

BREDER, C. M.
1944 "Ocular Anatomy and Light Sensitivity Studies on the Blind Fish from Cueva de los Sabinos, Mexico," *Zoologica,* 94:131-43.

BREKHUS, P. J., W. D. ARMSTRONG, and W. J SIMON
1937 "Biting Force of Athletes at University of Minnesota," *Journal of Dental Research,* 16:309.

BRESCIA, H.
1961 *Applied Dental Anatomy.* Mosby, St. Louis.

BRIGGS, L. C.
1948 "Les Hommes Paleolithique de Rabat et Tangier: Etude Comparative," *Bulletin de la Société d'Historie Naturelle de l'Afrique du Nord,* 39:105-14.
1955 "Stone Age Races of North Africa," *Bulletin of the American School of Prehistoric Research,* 18.
1968 "Hominid Evolution in Northwest Africa and the Question of the North African 'Neanderthaloids,'" *American Journal of Physical Anthropology,* 29:377-86.

BRONOWSKI, J., and W. M. LONG
1951 "Statistical Methods in Anthropology," *Nature,* 168:794-95.
1952 "Statistics of Discrimination in Anthropology," *American Journal of Physical Anthropology,* 10:385-94.
1953 "The Australopithecine Milk Canines," *Nature,* 172:251.

BROOM, R.
1925 "Some Notes on the Taungs Skull," *Nature,* 115:569-71.
1929 "Note on the Milk Dentition of *Australopithecus,*" *Proceedings of the Zoological Society of London,* 99:85-88.
1939a "Les Singes Anthropoides Fossiles de l'Afrique Sud et Leurs Relations à l'Homme," *Revue Scientifique,* 77:172-75.
1939b "The Dentition of *Plesianthropus* and *Paranthropus,*" *Annals of the Transvaal Museum,* 19:303-14.
1950 "The Genera and Species of the South African Fossil Ape Men," *American Journal of Physical Anthropology,* 8:1-13.

BROOM, R., and J. T. ROBINSON
1950 "Man Contemporaneous with the Swartkrans Ape-Man," *American Journal of Physical Anthropology,* 8:151-55.
1952 "Swartkrans Ape-Man," *Transvaal Museum Memoir,* 6.

BROOM, R., J. T. ROBINSON, and G. W. SCHEPERS
1950 "Sterkfontein Ape-Man, *Plesianthropus transvaalensis,*" *Transvaal Museum Memoir,* 4.

BROOM, R., and G. W. H. SCHEPERS
1946 "The South African Fossil Ape-Men, the Australopithecinae," *Transvaal Museum Memoir,* 2.

BROSE, D. S., and M. H. WOLPOFF
1971 "Early Upper Paleolithic Man and Late Middle Paleolithic Tools," *American Anthropologist* 73 (in press).

BRÖSTE, K., K. FISCHER-MULLER, and P. O. PEDERSEN
1944 "The Mediaeval Norsemen at Gardar," Anthropological Investigations, *Meddelelser om Grønland,* 89:1-62.

BROTHWELL, D. R.
1958 "Teeth in Earlier Human Populations," *Proceedings of the Nutrition Society,* 18:54-64.
1959 "Upper Pleistocene Human Skull from Niah Caves," *Sarawak Museum Journal,* 9:323-49.
1967 "Some Problems and Objectives Related to the Study of Dental Variation in Human Populations," *Journal of Dental Research,* 46:938-41.

BROTHWELL, D. R., ed.
1963 *Dental Anthropology.* Pergamon, New York.

BROTHWELL, D. R., V. M. CARBONELL, and D. H. GOOSE
1963 "Congenital Absence of Teeth in Human Populations," *Dental Anthropology* (ed. D. R. Brothwell), pp. 179-90. Pergamon, New York.

BRUES, A.
1966 "'Probable Mutation Effect' and the Evolution of Hominid Teeth and Jaws," *American Journal of Physical Anthropology,* 25:169-70.

BUETTNER-JANUSCH, J.
1966 *The Origins of Man.* Wiley, New York.

1968 "Man's Place in Nature," *Journal of Investigative Dermatology,* 51:309-23.

BURKITT, A. N.

1928 "Neanderthal Man and the Natives of New Caledonia," *Nature,* 122:474-75.

BUTLER, P. M.

1939 "Studies of the Mammalian Dentition. Differentiation of the Post-Canine Dentition," *Proceedings of the Zoological Society of London,* B, 109:1-36.

1963 "Tooth Morphology and Primate Evolution," *Dental Anthropology* (ed. D. R. Brothwell), pp. 1-14. Pergamon, New York.

BUXTON, L. H. D.

1928 "Excavation of a Mousterian Rock-Shelter at Devil's Tower, Gibraltar: Human Remains," *Journal of the Royal Anthropological Institute,* 58:57-85.

CALDWELL, J. R.

1959 "The Mississippian Period," *Illinois Archaeological Survey,* 1:33-39.

CAMPBELL, B.

1966 *Human Evolution.* Aldine, Chicago.

CAMPBELL, T. D.

1925 *Dentition and Palate of the Australian Aboriginal.* Hassell Press, Adelaide.

1939 "Food and Food Habits of the Australian Aborigines in Relation to Their Dental Conditions," *Australian Journal of Dentistry,* 43:1-15, 45-55, 73-87, 141-56, 177-98.

1941 "A Suggested Reconstruction of the Missing Anterior Teeth of the Cohuna Specimen," *Records of the South Australian Museum,* 7:235-36.

CARTER, J.

1928 "The Teeth of the Rhodesian Man," *Rhodesian Man and Associated Remains* (W. P. Pycraft *et al.*), pp. 64-65. British Museum, London.

CHANG, KWANG-CHIH

1962 "New Evidence on Fossil Man in China," *Science,* 136:749-60.

CHARD, C. S.

1969 *Man in Prehistory.* McGraw-Hill, New York.

CHIA, L. P.

1957 "Notes on the Human and some other Mammalian Remains from Changyang, Hupei," *Vertebrata Palasiatica,* 3:247-52.

CHIARELLI, B., ed.

1969 *Taxonomy and Phylogeny of the Old World Primates with Special Reference to the Origin of Man.* Rosenberg and Sellier, Torino.

CHOQUET, J.

1908 "Étude Comparative des Dents Humaines dans les différentes Races," *L'Odontologic,* 39:49-56, 107-21, 145-74.

CLARK, J. D.

1964 "Comment on: 'The Human Revolution,' (C. F. Hockett and R. Ascher)," *Current Anthropology,* 5:155-56.

CLARK, J. D., ed.

1957 *Proceedings of the 3rd Pan-African Congress on Prehistory.* Chatto and Windus, London.

CLARK, J. D., K. P. OAKLEY, L. H. WELLS, and J. MCCLELLAND

1947 "New Studies on the Rhodesian Man," *Journal of the Royal Anthropological Institute,* 77:7-32.

CLINCH, L. A.

1963 "A Longitudinal Study of the Mesiodistal Crown Diameters of the Deciduous Teeth and Their Permanent Successors," *European Orthodontic Society,* Report 39:202-15.

COLE, FAY-COOPER, and T. DEUEL

1937 *Rediscovering Illinois.* University of Chicago, Chicago.

COOKE, H. B. S.

1963 "Pleistocene Mammal Faunas of Africa, with Particular Reference to Southern Africa," *African Ecology and Human Evolution* (eds. F. C. Howell and F. Bourlière), pp. 65-116. Aldine, Chicago.

COON, C. S.

1957 *The Seven Caves.* Knopf, New York.

1963 *The Origin of Races.* Knopf, New York.

CROOK, J. H., and P. ALDRICH-BLAKE

1968 "Ecological and Behavioral Contrasts between Sympatric Ground Dwelling Primates," *Folia Primatologia,* 8:192-227.

CROOK, J. H., and J. S. GARTLAN

1966 "Evolution of Primate Societies," *Nature,* 210:1200-1203.

CURTIS, G. H.

1967 "Notes on some Miocene to Pleistocene Potassium/Argon Results," *Background to Evolution in Africa* (eds. W. W.

Bishop and J. D. Clark), pp. 365-70. University of Chicago, Chicago.

DAHLBERG, A. A.

1945 "The Changing Dentition of Man," *Journal of the American Dental Association,* 32:676-90.

1949 "The Dentition of the American Indian," *The Physical Anthropology of the American Indian* (ed. W. S. Laughlin), pp. 138-76. Viking Fund, New York.

1960a "The Giant Olduvai Hominid Tooth," *Nature,* 188:962.

1960b "The Dentition of the First Agriculturalists (Jarmo, Iraq)," *American Journal of Physical Anthropology,* 18:243-56.

1961 "Relationship of Tooth Size to Cusp Number and Groove Formation of Occlusal Surface Patterns of Lower Molar Teeth," *Journal of Dental Research,* 40:34-38.

1962 "On the Teeth of Early Sapiens," *Evolution and Hominisation* (ed. A. Kurth), pp. 205-211. Fischer, Stuttgart.

1963a "Dental Evolution and Culture," *Human Biology,* 35:237-49.

1963b "Analysis of the American Indian Dentition," *Dental Anthropology* (ed. D. R. Brothwell), pp. 149-78. Pergamon, New York.

1963c "Genetic Aspects of the Evolution of the Human Dentition," *Genetics and Dental Health* (ed. C. J. Witkop), pp. 113-20.

1965 "Evolutionary Background of Dental and Facial Growth," *Journal of Dental Research,* 44:151-60.

DAHLBERG, A. A., ed.

1963 "Conference on the Genetic Aspects of Oral Structures," *Journal of Dental Research,* 43.

DART, R. A.

1925 "*Australopithecus africanus:* The Man-Ape of South Africa," *Nature,* 115:195-99.

1934 "The Dentition of *Australopithecus africanus,*" *Folia Anatomica Japonica,* 12:207-22.

1948a "The First Human Mandible from the Cave of Hearths, Makapansgat," *South African Archaeological Bulletin,* 3:96-98.

1948b "The Makapansgat Proto-Human, *Australopithecus prometheus,*" *American Journal of Physical Anthropology,* 6:259-64.

1948c "The Adolescent Mandible of *Australopithecus prometheus,*" *American Journal of Physical Anthropology,* 6:391-412.

1949a "The Cranio-Facial Fragment of *Australopithecus prometheus,*" *American Journal of Physical Anthropology,* 7:187-214.

1949b "The Second Adult Palate of *Australopithecus prometheus,*" *American Journal of Physical Anthropology,* 7:335-38.

1954 "The Second Adult Female Mandible of *Australopithecus prometheus,*" *American Journal of Physical Anthropology,* 12:313-43.

1955a "*Australopithecus prometheus* and *Telanthropus capensis,*" *American Journal of Physical Anthropology,* 13:67-96.

1955b "The First Australopithecine Fragment from the Makapansgat Pebble Culture Stratum," *Nature,* 176:170-71.

1957 "The Osteodontokeratic Culture of *Australopithecus prometheus,*" *Transvaal Museum Memoir,* 10.

1960a "The Status of Gigantopithecus," *Anthropologischer Anzeiger,* 24:139-45.

1960b "*Pithecanthropus* and *Australopithecus,*" *Zeitschrift für Morphologie und Anthropologie,* 50:261-74.

1962a "The Makapansgat Pink Breccia Australopithecine Skull," *American Journal of Physical Anthropology,* 20:119-26.

1962b "A Cleft Adult Mandible and Nine other Lower Jaw Fragments from Makapansgat," *American Journal of Physical Anthropology,* 20:267-86.

1963 "The Carnivorous Propensity of Baboons," *Symposia of the Zoological Society of London* (eds. J. Napier and N. A. Barnicot), Number 10:49-56.

DARWIN, C.

1859 *On the Origin of Species by Means of Natural Selection, or Preservation of Favoured Races in the Struggle for Life.* Murray, London.

1874 *The Descent of Man, and Selection in Relation to Sex,* Revised edition. Murray, London.

DAVID, P.

1960 "Étude des Deux Dents Neanderthaliennes découvertes à La Chaise (Charente), Grotte Saurd," *Bulletin de la Société Préhistorique Française,* 57:424-27.

DAVID, P., and F. BORDES

1950 "Découverte d'une Calotte Cranienne Fragmentaire et des Dents Humaines dans un Niveau Mousterien Ancien de La Chaise (Charente)," *Comptes Rendus de l'Académie des Sciences, Série D,* 230: 779-80.

DAVIES, P. L.

1968 "Relationship of Cusp Reduction in the Permanent Mandibular First Molar to Agenesis of Teeth," *Journal of Dental Research,* 47:499.

DAVIES, T. G. H., and P. O. PEDERSEN

1938 "The Degree of Attrition of the Deciduous Teeth and First Permanent Molars of Primitive and Urbanized Greenland Natives," *British Dental Journal,* 99:35-43.

DAVIS, P. R.

1964 "Fossil Hominids from Bed I, Olduvai Gorge, Tanganyika: A Tibia and a Fibula," *Nature,* 201:967-69.

DAY, M.

1965 *Guide to Fossil Man.* World, Cleveland.

1969 "Femoral Fragment from a Robust Australopithecine from Olduvai Gorge, Tanzania," *Nature,* 221:230-33.

DAY, M. H., and J. R. NAPIER

1964 "Hominid Fossils from Bed I, Olduvai Gorge, Tanganyika: Fossil Foot Bones," *Nature,* 201:969-71.

DE BEER, G. R.

1958 *Embryos and Ancestors.* Clarendon, Oxford.

DE TERRA, M.

1903 "Mitteilungen zum Krapina-Fund unter besonderer Berücksichtigung der Zähne," *Schweizerische Vierteljahrsschrift für Zahnheilkunde,* 13.

1905 *Beitrage zu einer Odontographie der Menschenrassen.* Freise, Zurich.

DEVORE, I.

1963 "Comparative Ecology and Behavior of Monkeys and Apes," *Classification and Human Evolution* (ed. S. L. Washburn), pp. 301-19. Aldine, Chicago.

1964 "The Evolution of Social Life," *Horizons in Anthropology* (ed. S. Tax), pp. 25-36. Aldine, Chicago.

DEVORE, I., and S. L. WASHBURN

1963 "Baboon Ecology and Human Evolution," *African Ecology and Human Evolution* (eds. F. C. Howell and F. Bourlière), pp. 335-67. Aldine, Chicago.

DIECK, W.

1923 "Das Gebiss des *Homo mousteriensis* Hauseri und seine Rekonstruktion," *Odontologisk Tidskrift,* 3.

1925 "Das Gebiss des *Homo mousteriensis* Hauseri," *Urgeschichte auf Grundlage praktischer Ausgrabungen und Forschungen* (O. Hauser), pp. 125-33. Thüringer, Jena.

DOBZHANSKY, T., M. K. HECHT, and W. C. STEERE, eds.

1967 *Evolutionary Biology,* Volume 1. Meredith, New York.

DOCKRELL, R. B.

1956 "Tooth Size in Irish (Aran Island) Families," *European Orthodontic Society,* Report 32:200-216.

DOLAMORE, W. H.

1908 "The Relation of the Deciduous to the Permanent Teeth," *Royal Dental Hospital* (Britain) *Gazette for 1908:*144-56.

DRENNAN, M. R.

1929a "The Dentition of a Bushman Tribe," *Annals of the South African Museum,* 24:61-88.

1929b "An Australoid Skull from Cape Flats," *Journal of the Royal Anthropological Institute,* 59:417-21.

DREYER, J. F.

1935 "A Human Skull from Florisbad, Orange Free State," *Koninklijke Akademie Wetenschappen te Amsterdam,* 35:119-28.

DUBOIS, E.

1922 "The Proto-Australian Fossil Man of Wadjak, Java," *Koninklijke Akademie Wetenschappen te Amsterdam,* 23:1013-51.

1924 "On the Principle Characters of the Cranium and the Femur, the Mandible and the Teeth of *Pithecanthropus erectus*," *Koninklijke Akademie Wetenschappen te Amsterdam*, 27:265-78.

ELSNER, F. W.
1913 "Die Zähne von La Rochette," *Archiv für Anthropologie*, 41:127-29.
1917 "Die Unterkiefer der Spätdiluvailen Fundstätte 'Hohlerfels' bei Nürnberg und ihre Rassenmorphologische Bedeutung," *Archiv für Anthropologie*, 43:313-36.

EMERSON, A. E.
1961 "Vestigial Characters of Termites, and Processes of Regressive Evolution," *Evolution*, 15:115-31.

EMILIANI, C.
1968 "The Pleistocene Epoch and the Evolution of Man," *Current Anthropology*, 9:27-47.

ENNOUCHI, E.
1953 "Découverte d'un Homme de Mechta, à Rabat," *L'Anthropologie*, 57:272-83.
1962 "Un Néanderthalien: l'Homme de Jebel Irhound," *L'Anthropologie*, 66:279-99.
1963 "Les Néanderthaliens du Jebel Irhound (Maroc)," *Comptes Rendus de l'Académie des Sciences, Série D*, 256:2459-60
1968 "Le Deuxieme Crane de l'Homme d'Irhoud," *Annales de Paléontologie Vertèbres*, 54:117-28.

ERDBRINK, D. P.
1965 "A Quantification of the *Dryopithecus* and other Lower Molar Patterns in Man and some of the Apes," *Zeitschrift für Morphologie und Anthropologie*, 57:70-108.
1967 "A Quantification of Lower Molar Patterns in Deutero-Malayans," *Zeitschrift für Morphologie und Anthropologie*, 59:40-56.

ERGARTNER, W.
1949 "Zur Stammengeschichtlichen Einstufung von *Australopithecus africanus* Dart," *Mitteilungen der Anthropologischen Gesellschaft in Wien*, 78/79:2-14.
1950 "Fossile Menschenaffen aus Südafrika," *Mitteilungen der Anthropologischen Gesellschaft in Wien*, 80:157-212.

ETKIN, W.
1954 "Social Behavior and the Evolution of Man's Mental Faculties," *American Naturalist*, 88:129-42.
1963 "Social Factors in the Emergence of Man," *Human Biology*, 35:299-310.

EWING, J. F.
1963 "A Probable Neandertal from Ksar Akil, Lebanon," *American Journal of Physical Anthropology*, 21:101-4.

FALCONER, D. S.
1960 *Introduction to Quantitative Genetics.* Ronald, New York.

FEREMBACH, D.
1954 "Note sur une Mandibule Presumée de Magdelanien III," *Société d'Anthropologie de Paris, Bulletin et Memoires, Série 10*, 5:25-34.
1957 "Les Restes Humains de L'Abri Lachaud," *Société d'Anthropologie de Paris, Bulletin et Memoires, Série 10*, 8:61-80.
1958 "Note sur la Dent Aurignacienne Trouvée dans L'Abri Blanchard," *Société d'Anthropologie de Paris, Bulletin et Memoires, Série 10*, 9:199-202.
1964 "Les Australopithecines," *Société Études et Recherches Préhistorique*, 13.
1965a "Les Ossements Humains de Salemas (Portugal)," *Comunicacoes dos Servicos Geologicos de Portugal*, 48:165-84.
1965b "La Molaire Humaine Inférieur Mousterienne de Bombarral (Portugal)," *Comunicacoes dos Servicos Geologicos de Portugal*, 48:185-90.

FILIPSSON, R., and L. GOLDSON
1963 "Correlation between Tooth Width, Width of the Head, Length of the Head, and Stature," *Acta Odontologica Scandanavia*, 21:359-65.

FOUCHE, L., ed.
1937 *Mapungubwe. Ancient Bantu Civilization on the Limpopo*, Volume II. Cambridge University Press, London.

FRAIPONT, J., and M. LOHEST
1887 "La Race Humaine de Néanderthal ou de Canstadt en Belgique," *Archives de Biologie*, 7:587-758.

FREEDMAN, L.
1957 "The Fossil Cercopithecoidea of South

Africa," *Annals of the Transvaal Museum,* 43:121-262.

1960 "Some New Cercopithecoid Specimens from Makapansgat, South Africa," *Palaeontologia Africana,* 7:7-45.

1961 "New Cercopithecoid Fossils, Including a New Species from Taung, Cape Provence, South Africa," *Annals of the South African Museum,* 46:1-14.

FRISCH, J. E.

1963 "Dental Variability in a Population of Gibbons," *Dental Anthropology* (ed. D. R. Brothwell), pp. 15-28. Pergamon, New York.

1965 "Trends in the Evolution of the Hominoid Dentition," *Bibliotheca Primatologica,* Fasc. 3.

GABRIEL, A.

1955 "The Correlation of the Size of Human Teeth with One Another and with Certain Jaw Measurements," *Dental Journal of Australia,* 27:174-86.

GALLOWAY, A.

1937 "The Skeletal Remains of Mapungubwe," *Mapungubwe,* Volume II (ed. L. Fouche), pp. 127-74. Cambridge University Press, London.

1959 *The Skeletal Remains of Bambandyanalo.* Witwatersrand University Press, Johannesburg.

GARN, S. M.

1964 "Culture and the Direction of Human Evolution," *Culture and the Direction of Human Evolution* (ed. S. M. Garn), pp. 3-18. Wayne State University Press, Detroit.

1966 "Nutrition in Physical Anthropology," *American Journal of Physical Anthropology,* 24:289-92.

GARN, S. M., A. A. DAHLBERG, A. B. LEWIS, and R. KEREWSKY

1966 "Groove Pattern, Cusp Size, and Tooth Size," *Journal of Dental Research,* 45:970.

GARN, S. M., and A. B. LEWIS

1958 "Tooth Size, Body Size, and 'Giant' Fossil Man," *American Anthropologist,* 60:874-80.

1962 "The Relationship Between Third Molar Agenesis and Reduction in Tooth Number," *Angle Orthodontist,* 32:14-18.

1963 "Phylogenetic and Intra-Specific Variations in Tooth Sequence Polymorphism," *Dental Anthropology* (ed. D. R. Brothwell), pp. 29-52. Pergamon, New York.

GARN, S. M., A. B. LEWIS, A. A. DAHLBERG, and R. KEREWSKY

1966 "Interaction Between Relative Molar Size and Relative Number of Cusps," *Journal of Dental Research,* 45:1240.

GARN, S. M., A. B. LEWIS, and R. KEREWSKY

1964a "Relative Molar Size and Fossil Taxonomy," *American Anthropologist,* 66:587-92.

1964b "Sex Difference in Tooth Size," *Journal of Dental Research,* 43:306.

1964c "Third Molar Agenesis and Variation in the Size of the Remaining Teeth," *Nature,* 201:839.

1965a "Genetic, Nutritional, and Maturational Correlates of Dental Development," *Journal of Dental Research,* 44:228-42.

1965b "Size Interrelationships of the Mesial and Distal Teeth," *Journal of Dental Research,* 44:350-54.

1965c "X-Linked Inheritance of Tooth Size," *Journal of Dental Research,* 44:439-41.

1966a "Sexual Dimorphism in the Buccolingual Tooth Diameter," *Journal of Dental Research,* 45:1819.

1966b "Bilateral Asymmetry and Concordance in Cusp Number and Crown Morphology of the Mandibular First Molar," *Journal of Dental Research,* 45:1820.

1966c "The Meaning of Bilateral Asymmetry in the Permanent Dentition," *Angle Orthodontist,* 36:55-62.

1966d "Relationship between Sexual Dimorphism in Tooth-Size and Body-Size as Studied within Families," *Archives of Oral Biology,* 12:299-301.

1967a "Sex Differences in Tooth Shape," *Journal of Dental Research,* 46:1470.

1967b "Shape Similarities Throughout the Dentition," *Journal of Dental Research,* 46:1481.

1967c "Buccolingual Size Asymmetry and Its Developmental Meaning," *Angle Orthodontist,* 37:186-93.

1967d "Communalities in the Size Differences in Teeth of Brothers and Sisters," *Archives of Oral Biology,* 12:575-81.

1968a "The Magnitude and Implications of the

Relationship between Tooth Size and Body Size," *Archives of Oral Biology*, 13:129-31.

1968b "Relationship between Buccolingual and Mesiodistal Tooth Diameters," *Journal of Dental Research*, 47:495.

GARN, S. M., A. B. LEWIS, R. KEREWSKY, and K. JEGART

1965 "Sex Differences in Intraindividual Tooth Size Communalities," *Journal of Dental Research*, 44:476-79.

GARN, S. M., A. B. LEWIS, D. R. SWINDLER, and R. KEREWSKY

1967 "Genetic Control of Sexual Dimorphism in Tooth Size," *Journal of Dental Research*, 46:963-72.

GARN, S. M., A. B. LEWIS, and J. H. VICINUS

1962 "Third Molar Agenesis and Reduction in the Number of Other Teeth," *Journal of Dental Research*, 41:717.

1963 "Third Molar Polymorphism and Its Significance to Dental Genetics," *Journal of Dental Research*, 42:1344-63.

GARN, S. M., A. B. LEWIS, and A. WALENGA

1968a "Evidence for a Secular Trend in Tooth Size over Two Generations," *Journal of Dental Research*, 47:503.

1968b "The Genetic Basis of Crown-Size Profile Pattern," *Journal of Dental Research*, 47:1289-91.

1968c "Maximum Confidence Values for Permanent Tooth Size," *Archives of Oral Biology*, 13:841-44.

1968d "Crown-Size Profile Pattern Comparisons of 14 Populations," *Archives of Oral Biology*, 13:1235-42.

1969 "Crown-Size Profile Patterns and Presumed Evolutionary Trends," *American Anthropologist*, 71:79-84.

GARN, S. M., and C. G. ROHMANN

1962 "X-Linked Inheritance of Developmental Timing in Man," *Nature*, 196:695-96.

GARN, S. M., and Z. SHAMIR

1958 *Methods for Research in Human Growth*. Thomas, Springfield.

GENET-VARCIN, E.

1962 "Évolution de la Couronne de la Seconde Prémolaire," *Annales de Paléontologie*, 48:59-82.

1966 "Étude des Dents Permanentes Prouvenant du Gisement Mousterien de la Croze del Dua," *Annales de Paléontologie Vertèbres*, 52:89-114.

GENET-VARCIN, E. and M. MIQUEL

1967 "Contribution à l'Étude du Squelette Magdalenian de L'Abri Lafaye, a Bruniquel," *L'Anthropologie*, 71:467-78.

GENET-VARCIN, E. and R. VILAIN

1963 "Un Seconde Sepultare Mesolithique à Culoz," *Annales de Paléontologie*, 49:305-34.

GESSAIN, P.

1959 "Le Dentition des Eskimo d'Angmassalik, Génétique Croissance et Pathologie," *Société d'Anthropologie de Paris, Bulletin et Memories*, Série 10:364-96.

GIESELER, W.

1957 "Die Fossilgeschichte des Menschen," *Die Evolution der Organismen* (ed. G. Heberer), pp. 951-1109. Fischer, Stuttgart.

GILES, E.

1956 "Cranial Allometry in the Great Apes," *Human Biology*, 28:43-58.

GIVENS, D.

1968 "On the Peopling of America," *Current Anthropology*, 9:219.

GOAZ, P. W., and M. C. MILLER

1966 "A Preliminary Description of the Dental Morphology of the Peruvian Indian," *Journal of Dental Research*, 45:106-19.

GOLDSTEIN, M. S.

1932 "Congenital Absence and Impactation of the Third Molar in the Eskimo Mandible," *American Journal of Physical Anthropology*, 16:381-88.

GONDA, K.

1959 "On the Sexual Difference in the Dimensions of Human Teeth," *Journal of the Anthropological Society of Nippon*, 67:151-63.

GOODALL, J.

1963 "Feeding Behavior of Wild Chimpanzees," *Symposia of the Zoological Society of London* (eds. J. Napier and N. A. Barnicot), Number 10:39-48.

GOOSE, D. H.

1963 "Dental Measurement: An Assessment of Its Value in Anthropological Studies," *Dental Anthropology* (ed. D. R. Brothwell), pp. 125-48. Pergamon,

New York.
1967 "Preliminary Study of Tooth Size in Families," *Journal of Dental Research,* 46:959-62.

GORJANOVIC-KRAMBERGER, K.
1901 "Der Paläolische Mensch und sein Zeitgnossen aus dem Diluvium von Krapina in Kroatien I," *Mitteilungen der Anthropologischen Gesellschaft in Wien,* 31:164-97.
1902 "Der Paläolische Mensch und sein Zeitgnossen aus dem Diluvium von Krapina in Kroatien II," *Mitteilungen der Anthropologischen Gesellschaft in Wien,* 32:189-216.
1904 "Der Paläolische Mensch und sein Zeitgnossen aus dem Diluvium von Krapina in Kroatien III," *Mitteilungen der Anthropologischen Gesellschaft in Wien,* 34:187-99.
1905 "Der Paläolische Mensch und sein Zeitgnossen aus dem Diluvium von Krapina in Kroatien IV," *Mitteilunger der Anthropologischen Gesellschaft in Wien,* 35:197-229.
1906 *Der diluvaile Mensch von Krapina in Kroatia. Ein Beitrag zur Paläonthropologie.* Kreidels, Wiesbaden. Volume II of *Studien über die Entwicklungs-Mechanik des Primatenskelletes* (ed. O. Walkhoff), pp. 59-277.
1907 "Die Kronen und Wurzeln der Mahlzähne des *Homo primigenisus* und ihre genetische Bedeutung," *Anatomischer Anzeiger,* 31:97-134.
1908 "Die Zähne des *Homo primigenisus* von Krapina," *Anatomischer Anzeiger,* 32:145-56.
1910 "Die Verwandschaftlichen Beziehungen zwischen dem *Homo Heidelbergensis* aus Mauer und dem *Homo primigenisus* aus Krapina in Kroatien," *Anatomischer Anzeiger,* 35:359-64.

GRAHNEN, H.
1962 "Hereditary Factors in Relation to Dental Caries and Congenitally Missing Teeth," *Genetics and Dental Health* (ed. C. J. Witkop, Jr.), pp. 194-204. McGraw-Hill, New York.

GREENE, D. L., G. H. EWING, and G. J. ARMELAGOS
1967 "Dentition of a Mesolithic Population from Wadi Halfa, Sudan," *American Journal of Physical Anthropology,* 27:41-56.

GREGORY, W. K.
1922 *The Origin and Evolution of the Human Dentition.* Williams and Williams, Baltimore.
1951 *Evolution Emerging: A Survey of Changing Patterns from Primeval Life to Man.* 2 volumes. Macmillan, New York.

GREGORY, W. K., and M. HELLMAN
1926a "The Dentition of *Dryopithecus* and the Origin of Man," *Anthropological Papers of the American Museum of Natural History,* 28:1-123.
1926b "Crown Patterns in Fossil and Recent Human Molar Teeth and their Meaning," *Natural History,* 26:300-309.
1939 "Dentition of the Extinct South African Ape-Man, *Plesianthropus,*" *Annals of the Transvaal Museum,* 19:339-73.

GRIFFIN, J. B., ed.
1952 *Archaeology of the Eastern United States.* University of Chicago, Chicago.

GUENTHER, E. W.
1964 "Zur Altersdatierung der "Homo" Fundschicht von Ehringsdorf bei Weimar," *Zeitschrift für Morphologie und Anthropologie,* 56:23-32.

GUPTA, P., P. C. DUTTA, and A. BASU
1962 "Human Remains from Harappa," *Anthropological Survey of India,* Memoir 9:3-186.

HALL, R. L.
1966 "Current Research: Northern Mississippi Valley," *American Antiquity,* 31:604.
1967a "Current Research: Northern Mississippi Valley," *American Antiquity,* 32:268.
1967b "Current Research: Northern Mississippi Valley," *American Antiquity,* 32:570-71.
1968 "Current Research: Northern Mississippi Valley," *American Antiquity,* 33:537.

HARRISSON, T.
1959 "Radio-Carbon Dates from Niah," *Sarawak Museum Journal,* 9:136-38.

HEBERER, G.
1956 "Die Fossilgeschichte der Hominoidea," *Primatologia,* 1:379-561.
1965 "Uber der Systematischen Ort und den Physisch-Phychischen Status der Australopithecinen," *Menschliche Abstammungslehre* (ed. G. Heberer), pp.

310-56. Fischer, Stuttgart.
1966 "Uber die Osteodontokeratische 'Kultur' der Australopithecinen," *Quartär,* 17:21-50.

HEIM, JEAN-LOUIS
1968 "Les Restes Néandertaliens de La Ferrassie. Nouvelles Données sur la Stratigraphy et Inventaire des Squelettes," *Comptes Rendus de l'Académie des Sciences, Série D,* 266:576-78.

HEINZ, N.
1966 "L'Arcade Alvéolare de la Mandibule des Hominides Croissance, Variabilitié, Évolution," *Annales de Paléontologie Vertèbres,* 52:67-86.

HELLMAN, M.
1919 "Dimensions Versus Form in Teeth and Their Bearing on the Morphology of the Dental Arch," *International Journal of Orthodontia and Oral Surgery,* 5, Number 11.
1928 "Racial Characters in the Human Dentition," *Proceedings of the American Philosophical Society,* 67:157-74.
1936 "Our Third Molar Teeth: Their Eruption, Presence, and Absence," *Dental Cosmos,* 78:750-62.

HENNIG, E.
1948 "Quatärfaunen und Urgeschichte Ostafrikas," *Naturwissenschaftliche Rundschau,* 1:212-17.

HENRI-MARTIN, G.
1923 "L'Homme Fossile de La Quina," *Archives de Morphologie Générale et Experimentale,* 15:1-253.
1926 *Recherches sur l'Évolution au Mousterien dans le Gisement de La Quina (Charente): L'Enfant Fossile de La Quina,* 4. Paris.

HIGGS, E. S.
1961a "North Africa and Mount Carmel: Recent Developments," *Man,* 61:138-39.
1961b "Some Pleistocene Faunas of the Mediterranean Coastal Areas," *Proceedings of the Prehistoric Society,* 27:144-54.

HILLEBRAND, E.
1909 "Beiträge zur Morphologie der Menschlichen Zähne," *Pester Medizinisch-chirurgische Presse* (Budapest), 45.

HJELMMAN, G.
1928 "Morphologische Beobachtungen an den Zähnen der Finnen," *Acta Societatis Medicorum Fennicae Duodecim,* 11:1-132.

HOCKETT, C. F., and R. ASCHER
1964 "The Human Revolution," *Current Anthropology,* 5:135-68.

HOLLOWAY, R. L., Jr.
1966 "'Structural Reduction' through the Probable Mutation Effect," *American Journal of Physical Anthropology,* 25:7-11.
1967 "Tools and Teeth: Some Speculations Regarding Canine Reduction," *American Anthropologist,* 69:63-67.
1968 "Reply to Professor Washburn," *American Anthropologist,* 70:101-6.

HOOIJER, D. A.
1962 "The Middle Pleistocene Fauna of the Near East," *Evolution und Hominisation* (ed. G. Kurth), pp. 81-83. Fischer, Stuttgart.

HOOTON, E. A.
1938 *Apes, Men, and Morons.* Allen and Unwin, London.
1947 *Up From The Ape,* Revised edition. Macmillan, New York.

HOSAKA, T.
1936 "Statistiche Untersuchungen über die Zähne bei Chinesen mit besonderer Berucksichtigung der Rassenunterschiede," *Journal of Oriental Medicine,* 24:1065-90, 1230-51; 25: 348-68.

HOWELL, A. H., and R. S. MANLY
1948 "An Electronic Gauge for Measuring Oral Forces," *Journal of Dental Research,* 27:705-12.

HOWELL, F. C.
1958 "Upper Pleistocene Men of the Southwest Asian Mousterian," *Hundert Jahre Neanderthaler* (ed. G. H. R. von Koenigswald), pp. 185-98. Kemik en Zoon N. V., Utrecht.
1960 "European and Northwest African Middle Pleistocene Hominids," *Current Anthropology,* 1:195-232.
1961 "More on Mid-Pleistocene Hominids," *Current Anthropology,* 2:117-20.
1963 "Transcript of Discussions on African

Ecology and Human Evolution," (eds. F. C. Howell and F. Bourlière), pp. 547-654. Aldine, Chicago.
1965a "Comment on: 'New Discoveries in Tanganyika,' (P. V. Tobias)," *Current Anthropology*, 6:399-401.
1965b *Early Man.* Life Nature Library, Time, New York.
1967 "Review of *'Man Apes or Ape Men,'* (W. E. LeGros Clark)," *American Journal of Physical Anthropology*, 27:95-101.
1968a "Review of *'Olduvai Gorge. Volume II: The Cranium and Maxillary Dentition of* Australopithecus (*Zinjanthropus*) boisei' (by P. V. Tobias)," *American Anthropologist*, 70:1028-30.
1968b "Omo Research Expedition," *Nature*, 219:567-72.
1968c "Recent Advances in Human Evolutionary Studies," *Quarterly Review of Biology*, 42:471-513.
1969 "Remains of Hominidae from Pliocene/Pleistocene Formations in the Lower Omo Basin, Ethiopia," *Nature*, 223:1234-39.

HOWELL, F. C., and F. BOURLIÈRE, eds.
1963 *African Ecology and Human Evolution.* Aldine, Chicago.

HOWELL, J. A.
1917 "An Experimental Study of the Effect of Stress and Strain on Bone Development," *Anatomical Record*, 13:233-52.

HOWELLS, W. W.
1966 "Homo Erectus," *Scientific American*, 215:46-53.
1967 *Mankind in the Making*, Revised edition. Doubleday, Garden City.

HRDLICKA, A.
1911 "Human Dentition and Teeth from the Evolutionary and Racial Standpoint," *The Dominion Dental Journal* (Ontario), 21:1-15.
1916 "Physical Anthropology of the Lenape or Delawares and of the Eastern Indians in General," *Smithsonian Institution Bureau of American Ethnology, Bulletin 62.*
1923a "Dimensions of the First and Second Lower Molars with their Bearing on the Piltdown Problem and on Man's Phylogeny," *American Journal of Physical Anthropology*, 6:195-216.
1923b "Variations in the Dimensions of the Lower Molars in Man and Anthropoid Apes," *American Journal of Physical Anthropology*, 6:423-38.
1924 "New Data on the Teeth of Early Man and Certain European Fossil Apes," *American Journal of Physical Anthropology*, 7:109-37.
1927 "The Neandertal Phase of Man," *Journal of the Royal Anthropological Institute*, 57:249-74.
1930 "The Skeletal Remains of Early Man," *Smithsonian Miscellaneous Collections*, 83.
1952 *Practical Anthropometry* (ed. T. D. Steward). Wistar, Philadelphia.

HUNT, E. E., Jr.
1959 "The Continuing Evolution of Modern Man," *Cold Spring Harbor Symposium on Quantitative Biology*, 24:245-54.
1960 "Malocclusion and Civilization," *American Journal of Orthodontics*, 47:406-21.

HUNTER, W. S., and W. R. PRIEST
1960 "Errors and Discrepancies in Measurement of Tooth Size," *Journal of Dental Research*, 39:405-8.

HUXLEY, J. S.
1932 *Problems of Relative Growth.* Methuen, London.
1942 *Evolution, The Modern Synthesis.* Allen, London.

ISAAC, G.
1965 "The Peninj Beds—An Early Middle Pleistocene Formation West of Lake Natron, *Quaternaria*, 7:101-30.
1967 "The Stratigraphy of the Peninj Group—Early Middle Pleistocene Formations West of Lake Natron," *Background to Evolution in Africa* (eds. W. W. Bishop and J. D. Clark), pp. 229-58. University of Chicago, Chicago.

JACOB, T.
1967a "Recent Pithecanthropus Finds in Indonesia," *Current Anthropology*, 8:501-4.
1967b "Racial Identification of the Bronze Age Human Dentitions from Bali, Indonesia," *Journal of Dental Research* 46:903-10.

JACOBSHAGEN, E.
1957 "Der Schädelrest der Frau von

Rhünda," *Antomischer Anzeiger,* 104:64-87.

JAMES, W. W.
1960 *The Jaws and Teeth of Primates.* Pitman Medical Publishing, London.

JANZER, O.
1927 "Die Zähne der Neu-Pommern," *Vierteiljahrschrift für Zahnheilkunde,* 43:289-319, 401-34.

JELINEK, J.
1953 "The Fossil Man of Dolni Vestonice III," *Anthropozoikum,* 3:37-92.
1962 "Der Unterkiefer von Ochoz: Ein Beitrag zu seiner Phylogenetischen Stellung," *Anthropos (Studie z Oboru Anthropologie, Paleoetnologie, Paleontologie, a Kvarterni . Geologie),* 5:261-85.
1964 "Betrachtungen über die Verwandschaft der Anthropologischen Funde Dolni Vestonice, Abri Pataud, und Markina Gora," *Zeitschrift für Morphologie und Anthropologie,* 56:18-23.
1966 "Jaw of an Intermediate Type of Neandertal Man from *Czechoslovakia,*" *Nature,* 212:701-2.
1969 "Neanderthal Man and *Homo sapiens* in Central and Eastern Europe," *Current Anthropology,* 10:475-503.

JENKS, A. E.
1936 *Pleistocene Man In Minnesota.* University of Minnesota Press, Minneapolis.

JOHNSTON, F. E., and C. E. SNOW
1961 "The Re-Assessment of the Age and Sex of the Indian Knoll Skeletal Population," *American Journal of Physical Anthropology,* 19:237-44.

JOLLY, C. J.
1970 "The Seed-Eaters: a New Model of Hominid Differentiation Based on a Baboon Analogy," *Man,* 5:1-26.

JORGENSEN, K. D.
1955 "The Dryopithecus Pattern in Recent Danes and Dutchmen," *Journal of Dental Research,* 34:195-208.

JULLIEN, R.
1965 *Les Hommes Fossiles de La Pierre Taillée.* Boubée, Paris.

KAHLKE, H. D.
1962 "Zur relativen Chronologie ostasiatischer Mittelpleistozän-Faunen und Hominoidea-Funde," *Evolution und Hominisation* (ed. G. Kurth), pp. 84-107. Fischer, Stuttgart.

KAJAVA, Y.
1912 "Die Zähne der Lappen, Anthropologische Zahnstudien," Sumoen Hammas Laakariseuran Toimituksia. *Finska Tadlakarsallskapets Forhandlingar,* 10:1-64.

KALLAY, J.
1949 "Einige Besonderheiten der Premolaren bei *Homo diluvialis* e Krapina," *Folia Stomatologia,* 2:25-36.
1955 "Krapina Unterkiefer I und Paradentose im Pleistozän," *Osterreich Zeitschrift für Stomatologie,* 2:57-63.

KANTOROWICZ, A.
1931 "Morphologie der Zähne," *Handwörterbuch des Gesamten Zahnheilkunde,* 4:3266-67.

KEENE, H. J.
1967 "Australopithecine Dental Dimensions in a Contemporary Population," *American Journal of Physical Anthropology,* 27:379-84.

KEITH, A.
1912 "Description of the Teeth of the Paleolithic Man from Jersey," *Journal of Anatomy and Physiology,* 46:12-27.
1913 "Problems Relating to the Teeth of Earlier Forms of Prehistoric Man," *Proceedings of the Royal Society of Medicine,* 6:103-19.
1915 *The Antiquity of Man.* Williams and Norgate, London.
1924 "Neandertal Man in Malta," *Journal of the Royal Anthropological Institute,* 54:251-75.
1925 *The Antiquity of Man,* Revised edition. 2 volumes. Lippincott, Philadelphia.
1931 *New Discoveries Relating to the Antiquity of Man.* Williams and Norgate, London.
1948 *A New Theory of Human Evolution.* Watts, London.

KING, J. L., and T. H. JUKES
1969 "Non-Darwinian Evolution," *Science,* 164:788-98.

KLAATSCH, H.
1903 "Bericht über einen Anthropologischen Streifzug nach London und auf das Plateau von Süd-England," *Zeitschrift*

für Ethnologie, 35:875-920.

1909a "Die Neuesten Ergebnisse der Paläontologie des Menschen und ihre Bedeutung für das Abstammungsproblem," *Zeitschrift für Ethnologie,* 41:537-84.

1909b "Die Fortschritte der Lehre von der Neanderthalrasse," *Ergebnisse der Anatomie und Entwickelungsgeschichte,* 17:431-62.

KLAATSCH, H., and O. HAUSER

1909a "*Homo mousterensis* Hauseri," *Archiv für Anthropologie,* 7:287-97.

1909b "*Homo aurignacensis* Hauseri," *Prähistorische Zeitschrift,* 1:273-369.

KLATSKY, M., and R. L. FISCHER

1953 *The Human Mascatory Apparatus.* Dental Items of Interest, New York.

KINZEY, W. G.

1970 "Rates of Evolutionary Change in Hominid Canine Teeth," *Nature,* 225:296.

KOBY, F., ed.

1956 "Une Incisive Néanderthalienne Trouvée en Suisse," *Verhandlungen der Natur Gesellschaft Basel,* 67:1-15.

VON KOENIGSWALD, G. H. R.

1937 "Ein Unterkiefer Fragment von *Pithecanthropus* aus den Trinilschichten Mitteljavas," *Koninklijke Akademie Wetenschappen te Amsterdam,* 40:883-93.

1940 "Neue *Pithecanthropus*-Funde 1936-1938. Ein Beitrag zur Kenntnis der Praehominiden," *Dienst van den Mijnbouw in Nederlandsch-Indie, Wetenschappen Mededeelingen,* 28.

1942 "The South African Man-Apes and *Pithecanthropus,*" *Carnegie Institute of Washington, Contributions to Paleontology,* 530:205-18.

1950 "Fossil Hominids from the Lower Pleistocene of Java," *International Geological Congress, Great Britain (1948),* Part 9:59-61.

1952 "*Gigantopithecus blacki* von Koenigswald, A Giant Fossil Hominid from the Pleistocene of Southern China," *Anthropological Papers of the American Museum of Natural History,* 43:295-325.

1953a "The Australopithecinae and Pithecanthropus I," *Koninklijke Akademie Wetenschappen te Amsterdam, Series B,* 56:403-13.

1953b "The Australopithecinae and Pithecanthropus II," *Koninklijke Akademie Wetenschappen te Amsterdam, Series B,* 56:427-38.

1954a "*Pithecanthropus, Meganthropus,* and the Australopithecinae," *Nature,* 173:795-97.

1954b "The Australopithecinae and Pithecanthropus III," *Koninklijke Akademie Wetenschappen te Amsterdam, Series B,* 57:85-91.

1955 "Remarks on the Correlation of Mammalian Faunas of Java, India, and the Plio-Pleistocene Boundary," *Koninklijke Akademie Wetenschappen te Amsterdam, Series B,* 59:204-10.

1956 *Meeting Prehistoric Man.* Thames and Hudson, London.

1957a "Bemerkungen zum Gebiss der Australopithecinen," *Anthropologischer Anzeiger,* 21:54-61.

1957b "*Meganthropus* and the Australopithecinae," *Proceedings of the Third Pan African Congress on Prehistory,* pp. 158-60.

1957c "Remarks on Gigantopithecus and other Hominid Remains from Southern China," *Koninklijke Akademie Wetenschappen te Amsterdam, Series B,* 60:153-59.

1958a "The Hominisation of the Masticatory Apparatus, and Modifications of Diet," *Les Processus de l'Hominisation.* Colloque Internationale du Centre Nationale de la Recherche Scientifique, pp. 59-78, Paris.

1958b "*Gigantopithecus* and *Australopithecus,*" *The Leech (Johannesburg),* 28:101-5.

1960 "Remarks on a Fossil Human Molar from Olduvai, Bed II," *Koninklijke Akademie Wetenschappen te Amsterdam, Series B,* 63:20-25.

1962a *The Evolution of Man.* University of Michigan Press, Ann Arbor.

1962b "General Remarks on the Absolute Length and Relations in Size of the Premolars in Early and Modern

Hominids," *Bibliotheca Primatologica,* 1:120-30.
1962c "Das absolute Alter des *Pithecanthropus erectus* Dubois," *Evolution and Hominisation* (ed. G. Kurth), pp.112-19. Fischer, Stuttgart.
1963 "Zur Systematic der Hominiden," *Zeitschrift für Morphologie und Anthropologie,* 53:124-38.
1965a "Die Phylogenetische Stellung der Australopithecinen," *Anthropologischer Anzeiger,* 27:273-77.
1965b "Der Alter der Hominiden," *Anthropologischer Anzeiger,* 29:163-70.
1967 "Evolutionary Trends in the Deciduous Molars of the Hominoidea," *Journal of Dental Research,* 46:779-86.

VON KOENIGSWALD, G. H. R., ed.
1958 *Hundert Jahre Neanderthaler.* Kemik en Zoon N. V., Utrecht.

VON KOENIGSWALD, G. H. R., and F. WEIDENREICH
1939 "The Relationship Between *Pithecanthropus* and *Sinanthropus,*" *Nature,* 144:926-29.

KOKKOROS, M. M., and A. KAMELLIS
1960 "Découverte d'un Crane d'Homme Paléolithique dans la Péninsule Chalcidique (Petralona)," *L'Anthropologie,* 64:438-46.

KORENHOF, C. A. W.
1960 *Morphogenetical Aspects of the Human Upper Molar.* Uitgeversmaatschappij Neerlandia, Utrecht.

KORKHAUS, G.
1930 "Die Verebung der Kornenform und Grosse menschlicher Zähne," *Zeitschrift für Anatomie und Entwicklungsgeschichte,* 91:594-617.

KRAUS, B. S., and S. W. OKA
1967 "Wrinkling of Molar Crowns: New Evidence," *Science,* 157:328-29.

KRETZOI, M., and L. VERTES
1965 "Upper Biharian (Intermindel) Pebble-Industry Occupation Site in Western Hungary," *Current Anthropology,* 6:74-87.

KRIZ, M.
1903 *Beiträge zur Kenntnis der Quartärzeit in Mähren.* Steinitz.

KRUG, R.
1952 "*Australopithecus prometheus* Dart," *Zeitschrift für Morphologie und Anthropologie,* 43:276-87.

KURTEN, B.
1959 "New Evidence on the Age of Pekin Man," *Vertebrata Palasiatica,* 3:173-75.
1962 "The Relative Ages of the Australopithecines of Transvaal and the Pithecanthropines of Java," *Evolution und Hominisation* (ed. G. Kurth), pp. 74-80. Fischer, Stuttgart.
1967 "Some Quantitative Approaches to Dental Microevolution," *Journal of Dental Research,* 46:817-28.

KURTH, G.
1965 "Die (Eu)Homininen," *Menschliche Abstammungslehre* (ed. G. Heberer), pp. 337-425. Fischer, Stuttgart.

KURTH, G., ed.
1962 *Evolution and Hominisation.* Fischer, Stuttgart.

KUSTALOGLU, O. A.
1961 "*Australopithecus* and *Paranthropus* Dentitions," *Southwest Journal of Anthropology,* 17:226-38.

LAMPEL, G.
1963 "Variationsstatistische und Morphologische Untersuchungen am Gebiss der Cercopithecinen," *Acta Anatomica,* Supplementum 45, Volume 49:1-122.

LANCASTER, J. B.
1968 "On the Evolution of Tool-Using Behavior," *American Anthropologist,* 70:56-66.

LAVELLE, C. L. B.
1968 "Anglo-Saxon and Modern British Teeth," *Journal of Dental Research,* 47:811-15.

VAN LAWICK-GOODALL, J.
1967 *My Friends the Wild Chimpanzees.* National Geographic Society, Washington, D. C.

LEAKEY, L. S. B.
1935 *Stone Age Races of Kenya.* Oxford, London.
1953 *Adam's Ancestors: The Evolution of Man and His Culture,* Fourth edition. Methuen, London.
1958 "Recent Discoveries at Olduvai Gorge, Tanganyika," *Nature,* 181:1099-1103.
1959 "A New Fossil Skull from Olduvai," *Nature,* 184:491-93.
1960a "An Alternative Explanation of the

Supposed Giant Hominid Deciduous Tooth from Olduvai," *Nature,* 185:408.

1960b "Recent Discoveries at Olduvai Gorge," *Nature,* 188:1050-52.

1961a "A New Lower Pliocene Fossil Primate from Kenya," *Annals and Magazine of Natural History, Series 13,* 4:689-96.

1961b "New Finds at Olduvai Gorge," *Nature,* 189:649-50.

1961c "The Juvenile Mandible from Olduvai," *Nature,* 191:417-18.

1963a "East African Hominoidea and the Classification within this Superfamily," *Classification and Human Evolution* (ed S. L. Washburn), pp. 32-49. Aldine, Chicago.

1963b "Very Early East African Hominidae and their Ecological Setting," *African Ecology and Human Evolution* (eds. F. C. Howell and F. Bourlière), pp. 448-57. Aldine, Chicago.

1964 "The New Olduvai Hominid Discoveries and their Geologic and Faunal Setting," *Proceedings of the Geological Society of London,* 1617:104-9.

1965 *Olduvai Gorge, Volume I: A Preliminary Report on the Geology and Fauna.* Cambridge University Press, London.

1966 "*Homo habilis, Homo erectus,* and the Australopithecines," *Nature,* 209:1279-81.

1967 "An Early Miocene Member of Hominidae," *Nature,* 213:155-63.

1968a "The Lower Dentition of *Kenyapithecus africanus,*" *Nature,* 217:827-30.

1968b "Upper Miocene Primates from Kenya," *Nature,* 218:527-28.

1968c "Bone Smashing by Late Miocene Hominidae," *Nature,* 218:528-30.

LEAKEY, L. S. B., and M. D. LEAKEY

1964 "Recent Discoveries of Fossil Hominids in Tanganyika: At Olduvai and Near Lake Natron," *Nature,* 202:5-7.

LEAKEY, L. S. B., P. V. TOBIAS, and J. R. NAPIER

1964 "A New Species of the Genus *Homo* from Olduvai Gorge," *Nature,* 202:7-9.

LEAKEY, M. D.

1966 "Review of the Oldowan Culture from Olduvai Gorge," *Nature,* 210:462-66.

1967 "Preliminary Survey of the Cultural Materials from Beds I and II, Olduvai Gorge," *Background to Evolution in Africa* (eds. W. W. Bishop and J. D. Clark), pp. 417-46. University of Chicago, Chicago.

LEE, R. B.

1968 "What Hunters do for a Living, or, How to Make Out on Scarce Resources," *Man the Hunter* (eds. R. B. Lee and I. DeVore), pp. 30-48. Aldine, Chicago.

LEE, R. B., and I. DEVORE, eds.

1968 *Man the Hunter.* Aldine, Chicago.

LEGOUX, P.

1966 *Détermination de l'Age Dentaire de Fossiles de la Lignée Humaine.* Maloine, Paris.

LEGROS CLARK, W. E.

1947 "Observations on the Anatomy of the Fossil Australopithecinae," *Journal of Anatomy,* 81:300-333.

1949 "New Paleontological Evidence Bearing on the Evolution of the Hominoidea," *Quarterly Journal of the Geological Society,* 105:7-51.

1950 "Hominid Characters of the Australopithecine Dentition," *Journal of the Royal Anthropological Institute,* 80:37-54.

1951a "Comments on the Dentition of the Fossil Australopithecinae," *Man,* 51:18-20.

1951b "The Dentition of the Australopithecinae," *Man,* 51:32.

1964 *The Fossil Evidence for Human Evolution,* Second edition. University of Chicago, Chicago.

1967 *Man-Apes or Ape-Men?* Holt, Rinehart, and Winston, New York.

LEIGH, R. W.

1928 "Dental Pathology of Aboriginal California," *University of California Publications in American Archaeology and Ethnology,* 23:399-440.

1937 "Dental Morphology and Pathology of Pre-Spanish Peru," *American Journal of Physical Anthropology,* 22:267-95.

LEROI-GOURHAN, A.

1958 "Étude des Restes Humains Fossiles Prouvenant des Grottes d'Arcy-sur-Cure," *Annales de Paléontologie,* 44:87-148.

LEWIS, D. W., and R. M. GRAINGER

1967 "Sex-Linked Inheritance of Tooth Size:

A Family Study," *Archives of Oral Biology,* 12:539-44.

LEWONTIN, R. C.
1966 "On the Measurement of Relative Variability," *Systematic Zoology,* 15:141-42.

LINDGREN, B. W., and G. W. MCELRATH
1959 *Introduction to Probability and Statistics.* Macmillan, New York.

LIVINGSTONE, F.
1961 "More on Middle Pleistocene Hominids," *Current Anthropology,* 2:117-18.
1964 "Comment on: 'The Human Revolution,' (C. F. Hockett and R. Ascher)," *Current Anthropology,* 5:150-51.

LUNDSTROM, A.
1943 "Intermaxillara Tandbreddsforhallanden och Tandstallningen," *Svensk Tandlakare-Tidskrift* (Stockholm), 36:575-624.
1948 *Tooth Size and Occlusion in Twins.* Karger, New York.
1952 "On the Correlation Between Tooth Size and the Irregularities of the Teeth (Crowding, Spacing)," *Archives of Orthodontics,* 1:29-33.

LYSELL, L.
1957 "Correlation of the Mesiodistal Width of the Deciduous and Permanent Incisors," *Sartryck ur Odontologism Tidskrift,* 65:571-78.
1958 "Quantitative and Qualitative Determination of Attrition and Ensuing Tooth Migration," *Acta Odontologia Scandanavia,* 16:267-93.

MCALESTER, A. L.
1962 "Some Comments on the Species Problem," *Journal of Paleontology,* 36:1377-81.

MCBURNEY, C. B. M.
1967 *The Haua Fteah (Cyrenaica) and the Stone Age of the South-East Mediterranean.* Cambridge University Press, London.

MCBURNEY, C. B. M., J. C. TREVOR, and L. H. WELLS
1953 "The Haua Fteah Fossil Jaw," *Journal of the Royal Anthropological Institute,* 83:73-85.

MCCOWN, T., and A. KEITH
1939 *The Stone Age of Mount Carmel,* Volume II. *The Fossil Human Remains from the Levalloiso-Mousterian.* Claredon, Oxford.

MACCURDY, G. G.
1924 *Human Origins.* Appleton, New York.

MACINTOSH, N. W. G., and B. C. W. BARKER
1965 "The Osteology of Aboriginal Man in Tasmania," *The Oceania Monographs,* 12.

MCKINLEY, K. R.
1971 "Survivorship in Gracile and Robust australopithecines: A Demographic Comparison and a Proposed Birth Model," *American Journal of Physical Anthropology* (in press).

MAGLIO, V. J.
1970 "Early Elephantidae of Africa and a Tenative Correlation of African Plio-Pleistocene Deposits," *Nature,* 225:328-32.

MALY, J.
1939 "Les Cranes de l'Homme Fossile de Dolni Vestonice," *L'Anthropologie,* 17:71-192.

MANN, A. E.
1968 *The Paleodemography of Australopithecus.* Ph.D. thesis, University of California, Berkeley.

MARCIAS, J.
1934 "Découverte de Restes Humains Fossiles dans les Grès Quaternaires de Rabat," *L'Anthropologie,* 44:579-83.

MARGENAU, H., and G. M. MURPHY
1956 *The Mathematics of Physics and Chemistry.* Van Nostrand, New York.

MARKS, P.
1953 "Preliminary Note on the Discovery of a New Jaw of *Meganthropus* von Koenigswald in the Lower Middle Pleistocene of Sangiran, Central Java," *Madjalah Ilmu Alam Untuk Indonesia (Indonesian Journal of Natural Science),* 109:26-33.

MARSEILLIER, E.
1945 *Les Dents Humaines Morphologie.* Gauthier-Villars, Paris.

MARTIN, R.
1928 *Lehrbuch der Anthropologie,* Volume II. Fischer, Jena.

MARTYN, J. S.
1967 "Pleistocene Deposits and New Fossil Localities in Kenya," *Nature,* 215:476-79.

MASKA, K. J.
1886 *Der diluvaile Mensch in Mähren.* Landes-Oberschule, Neutitschein.

MASON, R. J.
1962 "Australopithecines and Artifacts at Sterkfontein. Part II, The Sterkfontein Stone Artifacts and Their Maker," *South African Archaeological Bulletin,* 17:109-26.
1966 *The Cave of Hearths in Prehistory.* University of Witwatersrand, Johannesburg.

MATIEGKA, J.
1929 "The Skull of the Fossil Man Brno III and the Cast of Its Interior," *L'Anthropologie,* 7:90-107.
1938 Home predmostensis *Fosilni clovek z Predmosti na Morave.* Czechoslovakian Academy of Science and Art Publication, Prague.

MAYR, E.
1950 "Taxonomic Categories in Fossil Hominids," *Cold Spring Harbor Symposium on Quantitative Biology,* 15:109-18.
1969 *Principles of Systematic Zoology.* McGraw-Hill, New York.

MEGGITT, M. J.
1957 "Notes on the Vegetable Foods of the Walbiri of Central Australia," *Oceania,* 28:141-45.

MERBS, C. F.
1968 "Anterior Tooth Loss in Arctic Populations," *Southwest Journal of Anthropology,* 24:20-32.

MIJSBERG, W. A.
1931 "On Sexual Differences in the Teeth of the Javanese," *Koninklijke Akademie Wetenschappen te Amsterdam, Series B,* 34:1111-15.

MILES, A. E. W.
1963 "The Dentition in the Assessment of the Individual Age in Skeletal Material," *Dental Anthropology* (ed. D. R. Brothwell), pp. 191-209. Pergamon, New York.

MILLS, J. R. E.
1963 "Occlusion and Malocclusion in Primates," *Dental Anthropology* (ed. D. R. Brothwell), pp. 29-52. Pergamon, New York.

MIYABARA, T.
1916 "An Anthropological Study of the Masticatory System in the Japanese (1): The Teeth," *Dental Cosmos,* 16:739-49.

MOLLESON, T. I., and K. P. OAKLEY
1966 "The Relative Antiquity of the Ubeidiya Hominid," *Nature,* 209:1268-69.

MOLNAR, S.
1968 "Experimental Studies in Human Tooth Wear," *American Journal of Physical Anthropology,* 28:361-68.

MONTANDON, G.
1936 "Les Cranes Cromagoides de la Biscordine," *Revue Anthropologie,* 46:105-39.
1938 "Perspectives de Phylogenie Humaine Suggérées par la Morphologie Auriculaire et Dentaire du Sinanthrope," *Revue Scientifique,* 76:561-68.
1939 "Les Dents des Paranthropiens," *Revue Scientifique,* 77:635-49.

MOORREES, C. F. A.
1957 *The Aleut Dentition. A Correlative Study of Dental Characteristics in an Eskimoid People.* Harvard University, Cambridge.
1959 *The Dentition of the Growing Child.* Harvard University, Cambridge.
1962 "Genetic Considerations in Dental Anthropology," *Genetics and Dental Health* (ed. C. J. Witkop), pp. 101-12. McGraw-Hill, New York.

MOORREES, C. F. A., and J. M. CHADHA
1962 "Crown Diameters of Corresponding Tooth Groups in the Deciduous and Permanent Dentition," *Journal of Dental Research,* 41:466-70.

MOORREES, C. F. A., and R. B. REED
1964 "Correlations Among Crown Diameters of Human Teeth," *Archives of Oral Biology,* 9:685-97.

MOORREES, C. F. A., S. Ø. THOMSEN, E. JENSEN, and P. K. YEN
1957 "Mesiodistal Crown Diameters of the Deciduous and Permanent Teeth in Individuals," *Journal of Dental Research,* 36:39-47.

MOSS, M. L., P. S. CHASE, and R. I. HOWES, Jr.
1967 "Comparative Odontometry of the Permanent Post-Canine Dentition of American Whites and Negroes," *Ameri-*

can Journal of Physical Anthropology, 27:125-42.

MOVIUS, H. L.
1956 "New Paleolithic Sites Near Ting Ts'un in the Fen River, Shansi Provence, North China," *Quaternaria,* 3:13-26.

MOVIUS, H. L., and H. V. VALLOIS
1959 "Crane Proto-Magdalenian et Venus du Periogordien Final Trouvés dans L'Abri Pataud, les Eyzies (Dordogne)," *L'Anthropologie,* 63:213-32.

MÜHLREITER, E., and TH. E. DE JONGE-COHEN
1928 *Anatomie des Menschlichen Gebiss.* Felix, Leipzig.

MÜLLER-BECK, R.
1967 *Urgeschichte der Menschheit,* Revised edition. Kohlhammer, Stuttgart.

NAGER, G.
1960 "Der Vergleich zwischen dem Raumlichen Verhalten des Dentinkronenreliefs und dem Schmelzreleif der Zähnkrone," *Acta Anatomica,* 42:226-50.

NANDA, R. S.
1954 "Agenesis of the Third Molar in Man," *American Journal of Orthodontics,* 40:698-706.

NARR, K. J.
1962 "Menschenfunde an der Grenze von Mittel - und Jungpälolithikum in Europa (einige chronologische Aspekte)," *Evolution und Hominisation* (ed. G. Kurth), pp. 221-28. Fischer, Stuttgart.

NEHRING, A.
1895 "Uber ein Menschlichen Molar aus dem Diluvium von Taubach bei Weimar," *Zeitschrift für Ethnologie,* 1885:573-77.

NELSON, C. T.
1938 "The Teeth of the Indians of Pecos Pueblo," *American Journal of Physical Anthropology,* 23:261-93.

NEUMANN, G. K.
1937 "Preliminary Notes on the Crania from Fulton County, Illinois," *Rediscovering Illinois* (eds. F. Cole and T. Deuel), pp. 227-64. University of Chicago, Chicago.

NICHOLLS, B.
1914 "A Contribution to the Study of the Teeth of the Australian and Tasmanian Aboriginals," *Transactions of the VIth International Dental Congress,* 67-102.

NOBEL, H. E.
1926 "The Teeth of the Richmond River Blacks," *Australian Journal of Dentistry,* 30:4-12.

OAKLEY, K. A.
1966 *Frameworks for Dating Fossil Man,* Second edition. Aldine, Chicago.

OAKLEY, K. P., and B. G. CAMPBELL
1967 *Catalogue of Fossil Hominids.* Part I: Africa. British Museum, London.

OKLADNIKOV, A. P. *et al.*
1949 *Teshik-Tash: Paleoliticheskii Chelovek.* Trudy Nauchno-Issledovatelskogo Instituta Anthropologii, Moscow.

OLIVIER, G.
1960 *Pratique Anthropologique.* Freres, Paris.

ONO, H.
1960 "Mesiodistal Diameters of Primary and Permanent Teeth and their Correlation in the Arch," *Journal of Japanese Stomatological Society,* 27:221-34.

OPPENHEIMER, A. M.
1964 "Tool Use and Crowded Teeth in Australopithecinae," *Current Anthropology,* 5:419-21.
1966 "Reply to Criticisms," *Current Anthropology,* 7:357-59.
1967 "In Re 'Tooth Size Reduction: A Hominid Trend,'" *American Anthropologist,* 69:514-15.

OSBORN, H. F.
1907 *Evolution of the Mammalian Molar Teeth.* Macmillan, New York.

OSBORNE, R. H.
1963 "The Respective Role of Twin, Sibling, Family, and Population Methods in Dentistry and Medicine," *Journal of Dental Research,* 43:1276-87.
1967 "Some Genetic Problems in Interpreting the Evolution of the Human Dentition," *Journal of Dental Research,* 46:945-48.

OSBORNE, R. H., and F. V. DE GEORGE
1959 *Genetic Basis of Morphological Variation.* Harvard, Cambridge.

OSBORNE, R. H., S. L. HOROWITZ, and F. V. DE GEORGE
1958 "Genetic Variation of Tooth Dimensions: A Twin Study of the Permanent Anterior Teeth," *American Journal of Human Genetics,* 10:350-56.

OZEGOVIC, F.
1958 "Die Bedeutung der Endeckung des Diluvialen Menschen von Krapina in Kroatien," *Hundert Jahre Neanderthaler* (ed. G. H. R. von Koenigswald), pp. 27-31. Kemik en Zoon N. V., Utrecht.

PALMA DI CESNOLA, A., and P. MESSERI
1967 "Quatre Dents Humains Paléolithiques Trouvées dans des Cavernes de l'Italie Meriodonale," *L'Anthropologie,* 71:249-61.

PARRATT, L. G.
1961 *Probability and Experimental Errors in Science.* Wiley and Sons, New York.

PATTE, E.
1957 *L'Enfant Néanderthalien du Pêch de l'Aze.* Masson, Paris.
1959 "La Dentition des Néanderthaliens I," *Annales de Paléontologie,* 45:223-38.
1960a "La Dentition des Néanderthaliens II," *Annales de Paléontologie,* 46:197-288.
1960b "Découverte d'un Néanderthalien dans La Vienne," *L'Anthropologie,* 64:512-17.
1961 "La Dentition des Néanderthaliens III," *Annales de Paléontologie,* 47:253-304.

PATTERSON, B., and W. W. HOWELLS
1967 "Hominid Humeral Fragment from the Early Pleistocene of Northwestern Kenya," *Science,* 156:64-66.

PEDERSEN, P. O.
1938 "Investigation into Dental Conditions of about 3000 Ancient and Modern Greenlanders," *Dental Record,* 58:191-98.
1949 "The East Greenland Eskimo Dentition. Numerical Variations and Anatomy," *Meddelelser om Grønland,* 142:1-244.

PEI, WEN-CHUNG
1954 "New Light on Peking Man," *China Reconstructs,* 3:33-36.
1957a "Discovery of *Gigantopithecus* Mandible and other Material in Liu-Cheng District of Central Kwangsi in South China," *Vertebrata Palasiatica,* 1:65-72.
1957b "Giant Ape's Jaw Bone Discovered in Southern China," *American Anthropologist,* 59:834-38.
1957c "Le Gigantopitheque," *Melanges Pittard* (ed. Mme. de Saint-Perier), pp. 265-71. Chastrusse, Brive.

PEI, WEN-CHUNG, and Y. H. LI
1958 "Discovery of a Third Mandible of Gigantopithecus in Liu-Cheng, Kwangsi, South China," *Vertebrata Palasiatica,* 2:198-200.

PEI, WEN-CHUNG, and JU-KANG WOO
1956 "New Materials of *Gigantopithecus* Teeth from South China," *Acta Palaeontologia Sinica,* 4:489-90.

PENROSE, L. S.
1954 "Some Recent Trends in Human Genetics," *Proceedings of the 9th International Congress of Genetics (Bellagio),* 1:521-30.

PERRET, G.
1943 "Jungsteinzeitliche und Frühbronzeitliche Skelettrests Alt-Preussens," *Zeitschrift für Morphologie und Anthropologie,* 40:334-66.

PILBEAM, D. R.
1966 "Notes on *Ramapithecus,* the Earliest Known Hominid, and *Dryopithecus,*" *American Journal of Physical Anthropology,* 25:1-5.
1967 "Man's Earliest Ancestors," *Science Journal,* February:47-53.
1968 "The Earliest Hominids," *Nature,* 219:1335-38.
1970 "*Gigantopithecus* and the Origins of Hominidae," *Nature,* 225:516-19.

PILBEAM, D. R., and E. L. SIMONS
1965 "Some Problems in Hominid Classification," *American Scientist,* 53:237-59.

PIVETEAU, J.
1951 "Restes Humains de la Grotte de la Verrerie à Macassargues (Gard)," *Annales de Paléontologie,* 37:175-83.
1957 *Traité de Paléontologie VII. Vers la Forme Humaine le Problem Biologique de l'Homme les Époques de l'Intelligence.* Masson, Paris.
1963 "La Grotte de Regourdou I," *Annales de Paléontologie,* 49:285-304.
1964 "La Grotte de Regourdou II," *Annales de Paléontologie Vertèbres,* 50:23-62.
1966 "La Grotte de Regourdou III," *Annales de Paléontologie Vertèbres,* 52:63-94.
1967 "Un Pariétal Humain de la Grotte du Lazaret (Alpes-Maritimes)," *Annales de Paléontologie Vertèbres,* 53:166-99.

PIVETEAU, J., H. DE LUMLEY, and M. DE LUMLEY
1963 "Découverte de Restes Néanderthaliens dans la Grotte de l'Hortus," *Comptes*

Rendus de l'Academie des Sciences, Série D, 256:40-44.

PLUMMER, H. C.

1940 *Probability and Frequency.* Macmillan, London.

DE PONCINS, G.

1941 *Kabloona.* Reynal and Hitchcock, New York.

POST, R. H.

1962a "Population Differences in Red and Green Color Vision: A Review and a Query on Relaxed Selection," *Eugenics Quarterly,* 9:131-46.

1962b "Population Differences in Visual Acuity: A Review with Speculative Notes on Selection Relaxation," *Eugenics Quarterly,* 9:189-212.

1963 "Colorblindness in Britain, France, and Japan: A Review with Notes on Relaxed Selection," *Eugenics Quarterly,* 10:110-18.

1964 "Hearing Acuity among Negroes and Whites," *Eugenics Quarterly,* 11:65-81.

1966a "Breast Cancer, Lactation, and Genetics," *Eugenics Quarterly,* 13:1-29.

1966b "Deformed Nasal Septa and Relaxed Selection," *Eugenics Quarterly,* 13:101-12.

PROUT, T.

1964 "Observations on Structural Reduction in Evolution," *American Naturalist,* 98:239-49.

PYCRAFT, W. P. *et al.*

1928 *Rhodesian Man and Associated Remains.* British Museum, London.

RECHE, O.

1928 "Die Schädel aus der Ancyluszeit von Pritzeber See," *Archiv für Anthropologie,* 21:122-90.

REMANE, A.

1927 "Studieren über die Phylogenie des Menschlichen Eckzahns," *Zeitschrift für Anatomie und Entwicklungsgeschichte,* 82:391-481.

1930 "Zur Mesztechnik der Primatenzähne," *Handbuch der biologischen Arbeitsmethoden* (ed. E. Abderhanden), Volume 7, pp. 609-35. Urban and Schwarzenberg, Berlin.

1951 "Die Zähne des Meganthropus africanus," *Zeitschrift für Morphologie und Anthropologie,* 42:311-29.

1952a "Der Vordere Prämolar von *Australopithecus prometheus* und die morphologische Stellung des Australopithecinengebissen," *Zeitschrift für Morphologie und Anthropologie,* 43:288-310.

1952b "Methodische Probleme der Hominiden-Phylogenie I," *Zeitschrift für Morphologie und Anthropologie,* 44:188-200.

1954a "Structure and Relationships of *Meganthropus africanus,*" *American Journal of Physical Anthropology,* 12:123-26.

1954b "Methodische Probleme der Hominiden-Phylogenie II," *Zeitschrift für Morphologie und Anthropologie,* 46:225-68.

1957 "Methodische Probleme der Hominiden-Phylogenie III," *Zeitschrift für Morphologie und Anthropologie,* 48:28-54.

1960 "Die Stellung von Gigantopithecus," *Anthropologischer Anzeiger,* 24:146-59.

1961 "Zähne und Gebiss," *Primatologia,* 3:637-846.

RENSCH, B.

1959 *Evolution Above the Species Level.* Wiley, New York.

RICHARDSON, M. E., C. P. ADAMS, and T. P. G. MCCARTNEY

1963 "Analysis of Tooth Measuring Methods on Dental Casts," *Transactions of the European Orthodontics Society,* 39:285-301.

RITCHIE, S. G.

1923 "The Dentition of the Western and Central Eskimos," *Report of the Canadian Arctic Expedition 1913-1918,* 12.

RITTER, R.

1933 "Untersuchungen über die mesiodistalen Grossenverhältnisse der Zähne des Oberkeifers zu danen des Unterkeifers," *Fortschritte der Orthodontik,* 3.

ROBINSON, J. T.

1952 "Some Hominid Features of the Ape-Man Dentition," *Official Journal of the Dental Association of South Africa,* 7:102-13.

1953a "The Nature of *Telanthropus capensis,*"

Nature, 171:33.
1953b "*Telanthropus* and Its Phylogenetic Significance," *American Journal of Physical Anthropology*, 11:445-501.
1953c "*Meganthropus*, Australopithecines, and Hominids," *American Journal of Physical Anthropology*, 11:1-38.
1954a "Phyletic Lines in the Prehominids," *Zeitschrift für Morphologie und Anthropologie* 46:269-73.
1954b "Prehominid Dentition and Hominid Evolution," *Evolution*, 8:324-34.
1954c "The Genera and Species of the Australopithecinae," *American Journal of Physical Anthropology*, 12:181-200.
1955 "Further Remarks on the Relationship between *Meganthropus* and the Australopithecines," *American Journal of Physical Anthropology*, 13:429-45.
1956 "The Dentition of the Australopithecinae," *Transvaal Museum Memoir*, 9.
1960a "An Alternative Interpretation of the Supposed Giant Hominid Deciduous Tooth from Olduvai," *Nature*, 185:407-8.
1960b "The Affinities of the New Olduvai Australopithecine," *Nature*, 186:456-57.
1961a "The Australopithecines and Their Bearing on the Origin of Man and of Stone Toolmaking," *South African Journal of Science*, 57:3-16.
1961b "The Origin and Adaptive Radiation of the Australopithecines," *Evolution and Hominisation* (ed. G. Kurth), pp. 120-40. Fischer, Stuttgart.
1961c "Australopithecines and the Origin of Man," *Annual Report of the Smithsonian Institution for 1961*, pp. 479-500.
1962 "Australopithecines and Artifacts at Sterkfontein. Part I, Sterkfontein Stratigraphy and the Significance of the Extension Site," *South African Archaeological Bulletin*, 17:87-107.
1963a "Australopithecines, Culture, and Phylogeny," *American Journal of Physical Anthropology*, 21:595-605.
1963b "Adaptive Radiation in the Australopithecines and the Origin of Man," *Classification and Human Evolution* (ed. S. L. Washburn), pp. 385-416. Aldine, Chicago.
1964 "Some Critical Phases in the Evolution of Man," *South African Archaeological Bulletin*, 19:3-12.
1965a "Comment on 'New Discoveries in Tanganyika' by P. V. Tobias," *Current Anthropology*, 6:403-6.
1965b "*Homo 'habilis'* and the Australopithecines," *Nature*, 205:121-24.
1965c "Relationships and Trends in Hominid Evolution," *Time and Stratigraphy in the Evolution of Man* (eds. C. B. Hunt, W. L. Straus, Jr., and M. G. Wolman), pp. 22-29. National Academy of Sciences National Research Council (Publication 1469), Washington, D. C.
1966a "The Emergence of Man," Read at Peabody Museum Centennial Meetings (Xerox version made available by the author).
1966b "The Distinctiveness of *Homo habilis*," *Nature*, 209:957-60.
1967 "Variation and the Taxonomy of the Early Hominids," *Evolutionary Biology I* (eds. T. Dobzhansky, M. K. Hecht, and W. C. Steere), pp. 69-100. Meredith, New York.
1968 "Skull of Early Hominid," *Nature*, 219:981-82.

ROBINSON, J. T., and E. F. ALLIN
1966 "On the Y of the Dryopithecus Pattern of Mandibular Molar Teeth," *American Journal of Physical Anthropology*, 25:323-24.

ROGINSKII, J. J.
1954 "Morphological Characteristics of the Child's Skull from the Late Mousterian Layer of the Starosel'je Cave," *Sovietskaia Etnografiia*, 1:27-39.

ROMER, A. S.
1966 *Vertebrate Paleontology*, Third edition. University of Chicago, Chicago.

ROSENZWEIG, K. A., and Y. ZILBERMAN
1967 "Dental Morphology of the Jews from Yemen and Cochin," *American Journal of Physical Anthropology*, 26:15-22.

SAHLY, A., H. BRABRANT, and M. BOUYSSOU
1962 "Observations sur les Dents et les Maxillaires du Mesolithique et de l'Age du Fer, Trouvés dans la Grotte de Rouffignac, Départment de la Dordogne, France," *Bulletin du Groupe-*

ment Internationale pour la Recherche Scientifique en Stomatologie, 5:252-85.

DE SAINT-PERIER, MME.
1957 *Melanges Pittard.* Chastrusse, Brive.

DE SAINT-PERIER, R.
1950 "La Grotte d'Isturitz III," *Archives de l'Institute de Paléontologie Humaine,* Memoire, 25.

SARICH, V.
1968 "The Origin of the Hominids: An Immunological Approach," *Perspectives on Human Evolution* (eds. S. L. Washburn and P. C. Jay), pp. 94-121. Holt, Rinehart, and Winston, New York.

SARICH, V., and A. C. WILSON
1967a "Immunological Time Scale for Hominid Evolution," *Science,* 158:1200-1202.
1967b "Rates of Albumin Evolution in Primates," *Proceedings of the National Academy of Science,* 58:142-48.

SARTONO, S.
1961 "Notes on a New Find of a *Pithecanthropus* Mandible," *Publikasi Teknik Seri Paleontologi,* 2.

SAUTER, M.
1956 "La Squelette Préhistorique de la Grotte du Bichon," *Archives des Sciences Physiques et Naturelles, Geneva,* 9:330-35.
1957 "Étude des Vestiges Osseux Humains des Grottes Préhistoriques de Fraincourt," *Archives Suisses d'Anthropologie Générale,* 22:6-37.

SAXE, A. A.
1966 "Social Dimensions of Mortuary Practices in a Mesolithic Population from Wadi Halfa, Sudan." Paper read at American Anthropological Association meeting (Pittsburgh).

SCHALLER, G. G.
1963 *The Mountain Gorilla: Ecology and Behavior.* University of Chicago, Chicago.

SCHLAGINHAUFEN, O.
1925 *Die Menschlichen Skeletreste aus der Steinzeit des Wauwilersees (Luzern).* Rentsch, Leipzig.

SCHOETENSACK, O.
1908 *Der Unterkiefer des* Homo heidelbergensis *aus den Sanden von Maur bei Heidelberg. Ein Beitrag zur Paläontologie des Menschen.* Leipzig.

SCHROETER, C.
1966 *The Dentition of Man: An Atlas of Tooth Morphology.* University of Washington, Seattle.

SCHUMAN, E. L., and C. L. BRACE
1954 "Metric and Morphologic Variations in the Dentition of the Liberian Chimpanzee," *Human Biology,* 26:239-68.

SCHWALBE, G.
1913 "Kritische Besprechung von Boule's Werk: 'L'homme fossile de La Chapelle-aux-Saints' mit eigenen Untersuchungen," *Zeitschrift für Morphologie und Anthropologie,* 16:527-610.
1914 "Uber einen bei Ehringsdorf in der Nähe von Weimar gefunden Unterkiefer des *Homo primigenisus,*" *Anatomischer Anzeiger,* 47:337-45.

SCHWERTZ, F.
1914 "Zwei Schädel von Buggisen aus Celebes," *Archiv für Anthropologie,* 42:89-97.
1917 "Morphologische Untersuchungen an Zähnen von Alamannen aus dem V bis X Jahrhundert," *Archiv für Anthropologie,* 43:1-43.

SCOTT, J. H., and N. B. SYMONS
1961 *Introduction to Dental Anatomy.* Livingstone, Edinburgh.

SEGAL, A. H.
1963 *Morphology and Anatomy of the Human Dentition.* Year Book Medical, Chicago.

SEIPEL, C. M.
1946 "Variations of Tooth Position: A Metric Study of Variation and Adaptation in the Deciduous and Permanent Dentitions," *Svensk Tandläkare-Tidskrift,* 39:Supplementum.

SELMER-OLSEN, R.
1949 "An Odontometrical Study of the Norwegian Lapps," *Skrifter Det Norske Videnskaps-Akademi I Oslo, Mathematisk-Naturvidenskapelig Klasse,* 65(3):1-168.

SENYUREK, M. S.
1940 "Fossil Man in Tangier," *Papers of the Peabody Museum of American Archaeology and Ethnology,* 16(3):1-27.
1941 "The Dentition of *Plesianthropus* and *Paranthropus,*" *Annals of the Transvaal*

Museum, 20:293-302.

1946 "A Study of the Skulls from Masat Nayuk," *Turk Tarih Kurumu Belleten,* 10:243-54.

1950 "A Note on Three Skulls from Alaca Hoyuk," *Turk Tarih Kurumu Belleten,* 14:71-84.

1952 "A Study of the Dentition of the Ancient Inhabitants of Alara Hoyuk," *Turk Tarih Kurumu Belleten,* 16:153-224.

1953 "The Relative Size of the Permanent Incisors in the Suborder Anthropoidea," *Anatolia,* 2:47-85.

1955 "A Note on the Teeth of *Meganthropus africanus* Weinert from Tanganyika Territory," *Turk Tarih Kurumu Belleten,* 19:1-54.

1957a "The Skeleton of the Fossil Infant Found in Shanidar Cave, Northern Iraq. Preliminary Report," *Revue Annuelle de l'Institute d'Archaeologie de l'Université d'Ankara,* 2:49-55.

1957b "A Further Note on the Paleolithic Shanidar Infant," *Revue annuelle de l'Institute d'Archaeologie de l'Université d'Ankara,* 2:111-21.

1958 "A Study of a Human Skeleton Found in Okuxini in the Provence of Antalya," *Turk Tarih Kurumu Belleten,* 22:491-516.

1959 *A Study of the Deciduous Teeth of the Fossil Shanidar Infant.* Publication of the Faculty of Languages, History, and Geography, Number 128, University of Ankara.

SERGI, S.

1944 "Craniometria e Craniografia del primo Paleanthropo di Saccopastore," *Richerche di Morfologia,* 21:733-91.

1948 "Il Cranio del Secondo Paleanthropo di Saccopastore," *Palaeontographia Italica,* 42:25-164.

1954 "La Mandibola Neandertaliana Circeo II," *Rivista di Anthropologia,* 41:305-44.

1958 "Die Neandertalischen Palaeanthropen in Italien," *Hundert Jahre Neanderthaler* (ed. G. H. R. von Koenigswald), pp. 38-51. Kemink en Zoon N. V., Utrecht.

SERGI, S., and A. ASCENZI

1955 "La Mandibola Neandertaliana Circeo III," *Rivista di Anthropologia,* 42:337-404.

SHAW, J. C. MIDDLETON

1931 *The Teeth, the Boney Palate, and the Mandible in the Bantu Races of South Africa.* Bale, Sons, & Danielsson, London.

SICHER, H.

1952 *Oral Anatomy,* Second edition. Mosby, St. Louis.

SIFFRE, A.

1908 "Étude des Dents Humaines du Petit-Puymoyen," *Revue de l'École d'Anthropologie,* 18:66-72.

SILLMAN, J. H.

1964 "Dimensional Changes of the Dental Arches: Longitudinal Study from Birth to 25 Years," *American Journal of Orthodontics,* 50:824-42.

SIMONS, E. L.

1961 "The Phyletic Position of *Ramapithecus,*" *Postilla, Yale Peabody Museum,* 57:1-9.

1963 "Some Fallacies in the Study of Hominid Phylogeny," *Science,* 141:879-89.

1964a "The Early Relatives of Man," *Scientific American,* 211:50-62.

1964b "On the Mandible of *Ramapithecus,*" *Proceedings of the National Academy of Sciences,* 51:528-35.

1965 "The Hunt for Darwin's Third Ape," *Medical Opinion and Review,* 1:71-84.

1967 "The Significance of Primate Paleontology for Anthropological Studies," *American Journal of Physical Anthropology,* 27:307-32.

1968a "Assessment of a Fossil Hominid," *Science,* 160:672-75.

1968b "A Source of Dental Comparison of *Ramapithecus* with *Australopithecus* and *Homo,*" *South African Journal of Science,* 64:92-112.

1968c "Review of the Phyletic Interpretations of Oligocene and Miocene Old World Anthropoidea," *Évolution des Vertèbres.* Colloques Internationaux du Centre Nationale de la Recherche Scientifique, Paris.

1968d "New Fossil Primates: A Review," *Perspectives on Human Evolution* (eds. S. L. Washburn and P. C. Jay), pp.

41-60. Holt, Rinehart, and Winston, New York.

1968e "Recent Advances in Paleoanthropology," *Yearbook of Physical Anthropology:* 1967, 15:14-23.

1969 "Late Miocene Hominid from Fort Ternan, Kenya," *Nature,* 221:448-51.

1970 "*Gigantopithecus,*" *Scientific American,* 222(1):77-85.

SIMONS, E. L., and D. B. PILBEAM

1965 "A Preliminary Revision of the Dryopithecinae," *Folia Primatologica,* 3:81-152.

SIMPSON, G. G.

1953 *The Major Features of Evolution.* Columbia, New York.

1961 *Principles of Animal Taxonomy.* Columbia University, New York.

1963 "The Meaning of Taxonomic Statements." *Classification and Human Evolution* (ed. S. L. Washburn), pp. 1-31. Aldine, Chicago.

SIMPSON, G. G., A. ROE, and R. C. LEWONTIN

1960 *Quantitative Zoology,* Revised edition. Harcourt, Brace, and World, New York.

SMITH, S. A.

1918 "The Human Fossil Skull Found at Talgai, Queensland," *Philosophical Transactions of the Royal Society of London, Series B,* 208:351-87.

SNELL, C.

1948a "Human Skulls from the Urn-Field of Melolo, East Sumba," *Acta Neerlandica Morphologiae Normalis et Pathologicae,* 6:219-37.

1948b "Human Skeletal Remains from Gol bả It, Sungai Siput, Perak, Malay Peninsula," *Acta Neerlandica Morphologiae Normalis et Pathologicae,* 6:363-77.

SOKAL, R. R., and P. H. A. SNEATH

1963 *Principles of Numerical Taxonomy.* Freeman, San Francisco.

SOLECKI, R. S.

1960 "Three Adult Neandertal Skeletons from Shanidar Cave, Northern Iraq," *Smithsonian Institution Annual Report for 1959*:603-35.

1963 "Prehistory in the Shanidar Valley, Northern Iraq," *Science,* 139:179-93.

SOLLAS, W. J.

1924 *Ancient Hunters and their Modern Representatives.* Macmillan, New York.

SPEISER, D.

1923 "Anthropologische Messungen aus dem St. Cruz Inseln," *Archiv für Anthropologie,* 19:89-146.

STEIN, M. R., and J. L. EPSTEIN

1934 "The Molar Teeth of New Britain Melanesians," *Journal of the American Dental Association,* 21:1409-13.

STEWART, T. D.

1958a "First Views of the Restored Shanidar I Skull," *Sumer,* 14:90-96.

1958b "The Restored Shanidar I Skull," *Annual Report of the Smithsonian Institution for 1958*:473-80.

1961a "The Skull of Shanidar II," *Sumer,* 17:97-106.

1961b "The Skull of Shanidar II," *Annual Report of the Smithsonian Institution for 1961*:521-34.

1963 "Shanidar Skeletons IV and VI," *Sumer,* 19:8-25.

STRAUS, W. L., Jr.

1950 "On the Zoological Status of *Telanthropus capensis,*" *American Journal of Physical Anthropology,* 8:495-98.

1963 "The Classification of *Oreopithecus,*" *Classification and Human Evolution* (ed. S. L. Washburn), pp. 146-77. Aldine, Chicago.

SULLIVAN, L. R., and M. HELLMAN

1925 "The Punin Calvarium," *Anthropological Papers of the American Museum of Natural History,* 23:309-40.

SWINDLER, D. R., J. A. GAVAN, and W. M. TURNER

1963 "Molar Tooth Size Variability in African Monkeys," *Human Biology,* 35:104-22.

SZOMBATHY, J.

1902 "Une Crane de la Race de Cro-Magnon trouvée en Moravie," *Congrès Internationale d'Anthropologie et d'Archaeology Préhistoriques, Compte-rendu de la Douzième Session (Paris), 1900:* 133-42.

TANG, YING-CHUN

1964 "Discovery of a New Ape-Man Fossil," *China Reconstructs,* 13:41-43.

TAYLOR, R. M. S.

1934 "Maori Foods and Methods of Preparation," *New Zealand Dental Journal,* 30, Number 147.

1963 "Cause and Effect of Wear of Teeth," *Acta Anatomica,* 53:97-157.

1969a "Variation in the Form of Human Teeth I: An Anthropological and Forensic Study of Maxillary Incisors," *Journal of Dental Research,* 48:5-16.

1969b "Variation in the Form of Human Teeth II: An Anthropological and Forensic Study of Maxillary Canines," *Journal of Dental Research,* 48:173-82.

THOMA, A.

1964 "The Dentition of the Subalyuk Neandertal Child," *Zeitschrift für Morphologie und Anthropologie,* 55:127-50.

1966 "L'Occipital de l'Homme Mindélien de Vertessollos," *L'Anthropologie,* 70:495-534.

1967 "Human Teeth from the Lower Paleolithic of Hungary," *Zeitschrift für Morphologie und Anthropologie,* 58:152-80.

THOMSEN, S.

1955 "Dental Morphology and Occlusion in the People of Tristan da Cunha," *Det Norske Videnskaps-Akademi, Oslo.* Number 25.

THROOP, A. J.

1928 *Mound Builders of Illinois.* Call, East St. Louis.

TOBIAS, P. V.

1962 "Early Members of the Genus *Homo* in Africa," *Evolution und Hominisation* (ed. G. Kurth), pp. 191-204.

1964 "The Early Hominid Remains from Tanganyika: *Australopithecus* and *Homo,*" *Proceedings of the VIIth International Congress of Anthropological and Ethnological Sciences* (Moscow, 1964).

1965a "Early Man in East Africa," *Science,* 149:22-33.

1965b "New Discoveries in Tanganyika: Their Bearing on Hominid Evolution," *Current Anthropology,* 6:391-411.

1965c "*Australopithecus, Homo habilis,* Tool-Using, and Toolmaking," *South African Archaeological Bulletin,* 20:167-92.

1966a "The Distinctiveness of *Homo habilis,*" *Nature,* 209:953-57.

1966b "Fossil Hominid Remains from Ubediya, Israel," *Nature,* 211:130-33.

1966c "Reply to Bielicki (1966)," *Current Anthropology,* 7:579-80.

1966d "The Human Skeletal Remains from the Cave of Hearths, Northern Transvaal," *The Cave of Hearths in Prehistory* (ed. R. J. Mason). University of Witwatersrand, Johannesburg.

1966e "A Reexamination of the Kedung Brubus Mandible," *Zoologische Mededelingen,* 44:307-20.

1967a *Olduvai Gorge, Volume II: The Cranium and Maxillary Dentition of* Australopithecus *(Zinjanthropus)* boisei.

1967b "General Questions Arising from some Lower and Middle Pleistocene Hominids of Olduvai Gorge, Tanganyika," *South African Journal of Science,* 63:41-48.

1967c "Pleistocene Deposits and New Fossil Localities in Kenya," *Nature,* 215:479-80.

1967d "Cultural Hominization among the Earliest African Pleistocene Hominids," *Proceedings of the Prehistoric Society,* 33:367-76.

1969 "The Taxonomy and Phylogeny of the Australopithecines," *Taxonomy and Phylogeny of the Old World Primates with Special Reference to the Origin of Man* (ed. B. Chiarelli), pp. 277-315. Rosenberg and Sellier, Torino.

TOBIAS, P. V., and A. R. HUGHES

1969 "The New Witwatersrand University Excavation at Sterkfontein. Progress Report: some Problems and First Results," *South African Journal of Science,* 24:158-69.

TOBIAS, P. V., and G. H. R. VON KOENIGSWALD

1964 "A Comparison between the Olduvai Hominines and Those of Java, and some Implications for Hominid Phylogeny," *Nature,* 204:515-18.

TURNER, C. G.

1967 "Dental Genetics and Microevolution in Prehistoric and Living Koniag Eskimo," *Journal of Dental Research,* 46:911-17.

TURNER, C. G., and J. D. CADIEN

1969 "Dental Chipping in Aleuts, Eskimos, and Indians," *American Journal of Physical Anthropology,* 31:303-10.

TURNER, W.

1908 "The Craniology, Racial Affinities, and

Descent of the Aborigines of Australia," *Transactions of the Royal Society of Edinburgh,* 46:365-404.
1909 "The Aborigines of Tasmania II," *Transactions of the Royal Society of Edinburgh,* 47:411-54.

TWIESSELMANN, F., and H. BRABRANT
1960 "Recherches sur les Dents et les Maxillaires d'un Population d'Age Franc de Coxyde," *Bulletin du Groupement Internationale pour la Recherche Scientifique en Stomatologie,* 3:99-171, 335-400.

TWIESSELMANN, F., and H. VAN DE POEL
1967 "À Propos des Dents Infériures Chez l'Homme et les Anthropomorphes," *L'Anthropologie,* 71:239-48.

ULRICH, H.
1956a "Paläolische Menschenreste aus der Sowjetunion: Das Mousterian-Kind von Staroselje (Krim)," *Zeitschrift für Morphologie und Anthropologie,* 47:91-8.
1956b "Paläolische Menschenreste aus der Sowjetunion: Das Kinderskelett aus der Grotte Teschik-Tasch," *Zeitschrift für Morphologie und Anthropologie,* 47:99-112.

VALLOIS, H. V.
1941 "Nouvelles Recherches sur le Squelette de Chancelade," *L'Anthropologie,* 50:165-202.
1943 "Les Ossements Humains de Koerhuisbeek," *Verhandlungen der Nederlandsche Akademie van Wetenschappen, Afdeeling Natuurkunde,* 40:1-25.
1945 "L'Homme Fossil de Rabat," *Comptes Rendus de l'Académie des Sciences, Série D,* 221:669-71.
1951 "La Mandibule Humaine Fossile de la Grotte du Porc-Epic près Dire-Daoua (Abyssinie)," *L'Anthropologie,* 55:231-38.
1952 "Les Restes Humains du Gisement Mousterien de Monsempron," *Annales de Paléontologie,* 38:100-120.
1955 "La Mandibule Humaine Premousterienne de Montmaurin," *Comptes Rendus de l'Académie des Sciences,* 240:1577-79.
1956 "The Pre-Mousterien Mandible from Montmaurin," *American Journal of Physical Anthropology,* 14:319-23.
1957 "La Mandibule Prenéandertalienne de Montmaurin," *Mélanges Pittard* (ed. Mme. de Saint-Perier), pp. 395-98. Chastrusse, Brive.
1958a "Les Restes Humains d'Age Aurignacien de la Grotte des Rois, Charente," *Société Anthropologie de Paris, Bulletin et Memoires, Série 10,* 9:138-59.
1958b "Les Restes, le Gisement Aurignacien des Rois à Mouthiers (Charente)," *Gallia,* Supplément 9.
1959 "L'Homme de Rabat," *Bulletin d'Archeologie Marocaine,* 3:87-91.
1962 "La Dent Humaine Levalloiso-Mousterian de Ras-el-Kelb," *Bibliotheca Primatologica,* 1:155-62.

VALLOIS, H. V., and J. ROCHE
1958 "La Mandibule Acheulienne de Temara, Maroc," *Comptes Rendus de l'Académie des Sciences, Série D,* 246:3113-16.

VAN REENEN, J. F.
1966 "Dental Features of a Low-Caries Primitive Population," *Journal of Dental Research,* 45:703-13.

VAN VALEN, L.
1960 "Nonadaptive Aspects of Evolution," *American Naturalist,* 94:305-8.
1963 "Intensities of Selection in Natural Populations," *Proceedings of the 11th International Congress of Genetics,* 1:153-66.

VERNEAU, R.
1899 *L'Homme de la Barma Grande.* Baousse-Rousse.
1906 *Les Grottes de Grimaldi,* Volume II. Anthropologie, Monaco.

VERWORN, M., R. BONNET, and G. STEINMANN
1919 *Der diluvaile Menschenfund von Obercassel bei Bonn.* Bergman, Wiesbaden.

VIRCHOW, H.
1914 "Der Unterkiefer von Ehringsdorf," *Zeitschrift für Ethnologie,* 46:869-79.
1916 "Zahnbogen und Alveolarbogen," *Zeitschrift für Ethnologie,* 48:277-95.
1917 "Der Taubacher Zahn des prähistorischen Museums der Universität Jena," *Praehistorische Zeitschrift,* 9:1-18.
1920 *Die Menschlichen Skeletreste aus dem*

Kämpfe-schen Bruch im Travertin von Ehringsdorf bei Weimar. Fischer, Jena.

VIRCHOW, R.
1882 "Der Kiefer aus der Schipka-Höhle und der Kiefer von La Naulette," *Zeitschrift für Ethnologie,* 14:277-310.

VLECK, E.
1956a "Die Pleistocene Mensch von der Höhle Na Zlatem Kone bei Koneprusy," *Anthropozoikum,* 6:283-312.
1956b "Ein Menschenzahn Pleistozänen Alters von Silika Brezova," *Anthropozoikum,* 6:397-405.
1956c "Novy Nalez Pleistocenniho Cloveka v Jeskyni u Staroselje (SSSR)," *Anthropozoikum,* 6:433-37.
1961 "Nouvelles Trouvailles de l'Homme du Pleistocene Récent de Pavlov (CSSR)," *Anthropos* (Brno), 6.
1964 "Einige in der Ontogenese des modernen Menschen untersuchte Neandertalmerkmale," *Zeitschrift für Morphologie und Anthropologie,* 56:63-83.
1967 "Die Sinus frontales bei europäischen Neandertalern," *Anthropologischer Anzeiger,* 30:166-89.

VOGEL, C.
1966 "Morphologische Studien am Geschichtsschädel Catarrhiner Primaten," *Bibliotheca Primatologica,* 4:1-226.

WALTER, H.
1954 "Einige Bemerkungen zu *Gigantopithecus blacki* und *Sinanthropus officinalis,*" *Zeitschrift für Morphologie und Anthropologie,* 46:297-303.

WASHBURN, S. L.
1959 "Speculations on the Interrelations of the History of Tools and Biological Evolution," *Human Biology,* 31:21-31.
1960 "Tools and Human Evolution," *Scientific American,* 203:63-75.
1963 "Behavior and Human Evolution," *Classification and Human Evolution* (ed. S. L. Washburn), pp. 190-203. Aldine, Chicago.
1968a "On Holloway's 'Tools and Teeth,'" *American Anthropologist,* 70:97-101.
1968b *The Study of Human Evolution.* Condon Lectures, Oregon State System of Higher Education, Eugene.

WASHBURN, S. L., ed.
1961 *The Social Life of Early Man.* Aldine, Chicago.
1963 *Classification and Human Evolution.* Aldine, Chicago.

WASHBURN, S. L., and V. AVIS
1958 "The Evolution of Human Behavior," *Evolution and Behavior* (eds. A. Roe and G. G. Simpson), pp. 421-36. Yale, New Haven.

WASHBURN, S. L., and I. DEVORE
1961a "Social Behavior of Baboons and Early Man," *The Social Life of Early Man* (ed. S. L. Washburn), pp. 91-105. Aldine, Chicago.
1961b "Social Life of Baboons," *Scientific American,* 204:62-71.

WASHBURN, S. L., and D. A. HAMBURG
1965 "The Implications of Primate Research," *Primate Behavior* (ed. I. DeVore), pp. 607-22. Holt, Rinehart, and Winston, New York.

WASHBURN, S. L., and F. C. HOWELL
1960 "Human Evolution and Culture," *Evolution After Darwin,* Volume II: *The Evolution of Man* (ed. S. Tax), pp. 33-56. University of Chicago, Chicago.

WASHBURN, S. L., and P. C. JAY, eds.
1968 *Perspectives on Human Evolution.* Holt, Rinehart, and Winston, New York.

WASHBURN, S. L., and C. S. LANCASTER
1968 "The Evolution of Hunting," *Man the Hunter* (eds. R. B. Lee and I. DeVore), pp. 293-303. Aldine, Chicago.

WATT, D. G., and C. H. M. WILLIAMS
1951 "The Effects of the Physical Consistancy of Food on the Growth and Development of the Mandible and the Maxilla of the Rat," *American Journal of Orthodontics,* 37:895-928.

WAUGH, L. M.
1937a "Influence of Diet on the Jaws and Face of the American Eskimo," *Journal of the American Dental Association,* 24:1640-47.
1937b "Dental Observations among the Eskimos," *Journal of Dental Research,* 16:355-56.

WEIDENREICH, F.
1936 "The Mandibles of *Sinanthropus pekinensis:* A Comparative Study," *Palaeontologia Sinica, Series D,* 7:1-162.

1937a "The Dentition of *Sinanthropus pekinensis:* A Comparative Odontography of the Hominids," *Palaeontologia Sinica, New Series D,* 1(*Whole Series* 101):1-180.

1937b "The Forerunner of *Sinanthropus pekinensis,*" *Bulletin of the Geological Society of China,* 17:137-44.

1941 "The Brain and Its Role in the Phylogenetic Transformation of the Human Skull," *Transactions of the American Philosophical Society,* 31:321-442.

1943 "The Skull of *Sinanthropus pekinensis:* A Comparative Study on a Primitive Hominid Skull," *Palaeontologia Sinica, New Series D,* 10(Whole Series 127):1-484.

1945a "Giant Early Man from Java and South China," *Anthropological Papers of the American Museum of Natural History,* 40:5-138.

1945b "The Keilor Skull: A Wadjak Type from Southeast Australia," *American Journal of Physical Anthropology,* 3:21-32.

WEINERT, H.

1925 *Der Schädel des Eiszeitlichen Menschen von Le Moustier.* Springer, Berlin.

1928 "*Pithecanthropus erectus,*" *Zeitschrift für Anatomie und Entwicklungsgeschichte,* 87:429-547.

1936 "Der Urmenschenschädel von Steinheim," *Zeitschrift für Morphologie und Anthropologie,* 35:463-518.

1939 "*Afrikanthropus njarasensis,*" *Zeitschrift für Morphologie und Anthropologie,* 38:252-308.

1944 *Ursprung der Menschheit.* Enke, Stuttgart.

1950 "Uber die Neuen Vor- und Frühmenschenfunde aus Africa, Java, China, und Frankreich," *Zeitschrift für Morphologie und Anthropologie,* 42:113-48.

1951a "Uber die Vielgestaltigkeit der Summoprimaten vor der Menschwerdung I," *Zeitschrift für Morphologie und Anthropologie,* 42:439-49.

1951b "Uber die Vielgestaltigkeit der Summorprimaten vor der Menschwerdung II," *Zeitschrift für Morphologie und Anthropologie,* 43:73-103.

1951c *Stammesentwicklung der Menschheit.* Vieweg & Sohn, Braunschweig.

1952 "*Australopithecus* und *Paranthropus,*" *Zeitschrift für Morphologie und Anthropologie,* 43:311-30.

WEINMANN, J.

1955 *Bone and Bones,* Second edition. Mosby, St. Louis.

WELLS, L. H.

1947 "A Note on the Broken Maxillary Fragment from the Broken Hill Cave," New Studies on the Rhodesian Man (J. D. Clark *et al.*), pp. 11-12. *Journal of the Royal Anthropological Institute,* 77:7-32.

1957 "The Place of the Broken Hill Skull among Human Types," *Proceedings of the 3rd Pan-African Congress on Prehistory* (ed. J. D. Clark), pp. 172-74. Chatto and Windus, London.

WERTH, E.

1928 *Der Fossile Mensch.* Bortraeger, Berlin.

WHITWORTH, T.

1966 "A Fossil Hominid Skull from Rudoff (Kabua Waterhole)," *South African Archaeological Bulletin,* 21:138-50.

WITKOP, C. J., ed.

1962 *Genetics and Dental Health.* McGraw-Hill, New York.

WOLPOFF, M. H.

1968 "'Telanthropus' and the Single Species Hypothesis," *American Anthropologist,* 70:477-93.

1969a "The Effect of Mutations under Conditions of Reduced Selection," *Social Biology,* 16:11-23.

1969b "Cranial Capacity and Taxonomy of Olduvai Hominid 7," *Nature,* 223:182-83.

1970a "Interstitial Wear," *American Journal of Physical Anthropology* 34 (in press).

1970b "The Evidence for Multiple Hominid Taxa at Swartkrans," *American Anthropologist,* 72:576-607.

WOO, JU-KANG

1954 "New Discoveries about *Sinanthropus pekinensis* in Choukoutien," *Scientia Sinica,* 2:267-88.

1956 "Human Fossils Found in China and their Significance," *Scientia Sinica,* 5:389-98.

1962 "*Gigantopithecus* and Its Phylogenetic

Significance," *Scientia Sinica,* 11:391-96.
1963 "Ape or Man?" *China Reconstructs,* 12:8-10.
1964a "A Newly Discovered Mandible of *Sinanthropus* Type—*Sinanthropus lantianensis,*" *Scientia Sinica,* 13:801-12.
1964b "The Mandible of *Sinanthropus lantianensis,*" *Current Anthropology,* 5:98-101.
1965 "Preliminary Report on a Skull of *Sinanthropus lantianensis* of Lantian, Shensi," *Scientia Sinica,* 14:1032-36.
1966 "The Skull of Lantian Man," *Current Anthropology,* 7:83-86.

WOO, JU-KUNG, and T. K. CHAO
1959 "New Discovery of *Sinanthropus* Mandible from Choukoutien," *Vertebrata Palasiatica,* 3:169-72.

WOO, JU-KANG, and LAN-PO CHIA
1954 "New Discoveries about Sinanthropus pekinensis in Choukoutien," *Scientia Sinica,* 3:335-51.

WOOD-JONES, F., and T. D. CAMPBELL
1924 "Six Hitherto Undescribed Skulls of Tasmanian Natives," *Records of the South Australian Museum,* 2:459-70.

WRAY, D. E.
1952 "Archaeology of the Illinois Valley," *Archaeology of the Eastern United States* (ed. J. B. Griffin), pp. 152-64.

WRIGHT, S.
1952 "The Genetics of Quantitative Variability," *Quantitative Inheritance* (eds. E. C. K. Reeve and C. H. Waddington), pp. 5-41. Allen and Unwin, London.

WUNDERLY, J., W. ADAM, and D. MAHONY
1943 "The Keilor Fossil Skull: Anatomical Description," *Memoirs of the National Museum at Melbourne,* 13:57-69.

WÜST, K.
1950 "Über der Unterkiefer von Mauer im Vergleich zu andern Fossilen und Rezenten Unterkieferen von Anthropoiden und Hominiden," *Zeitschrift für Morphologie und Anthropologie,* 42:1-112.

YAKIMOV, V. P.
1969 "Comment on Neandertal man and *Homo sapiens* in Central and Eastern Europe," (Jelinek), *Current Anthropology,* 10:498.

YAMADA, E.
1932 "The Anthropological Study of the Japanese Teeth," *Journal of the Nippon Dental Association,* 25:15-46, 101-32, 177-208, 255-86, 329-44, 450-81, 528-60, 609-56, 710-44, 774-812.

YULISH, S. M.
1971 "Anterior Tooth Reductions in *Ramapithecus,*" *Primates,* 11:255-63.

ZINGESER, M. R.
1967 "Odontometric Characteristics of the Howler Monkey (*Alouatta caraya*)," *Journal of Dental Research,* 46:975-78.

ZUCKERMAN, S.
1966 "Myths and Methods in Anatomy," *Journal of the Royal College of Surgeons of Edinburgh,* 11:87-114.

ZUHRT, R.
1967 "Gebissegefunde bei Khartoum-Neolithikern vom Jebel Shaqadud (Republik Sudan)," *Zeitschrift für Morphologie und Anthropologie,* 59:36-39.

Appendix

LOWER I1 AUSTRALOPITHECINES

		N	L(M-D)	B(B-L)	L*B	L/B	L+B/2
MLD 18	L	9	4.00	6.80	27.20	58.82	5.40
MLD 18	R	9	5.00	6.00	30.00	83.33	5.50
STS 24	R	43	6.30	6.10	38.43	103.28	6.20
STS 52	R	54	5.90	8.10	47.79	72.84	7.00
NATRON	L	108	5.50	6.10	33.55	90.16	5.80
NATRON	R	108	5.60	6.10	34.16	91.80	5.85
SK 23	L	122	5.60	5.90	33.04	94.92	5.75
SK 23	R	122	5.60	6.30	35.28	88.89	5.95
SK 34	R	132	5.50	6.50	35.75	84.62	6.00
SK 62	R	146	5.40	5.50	29.70	98.18	5.45
SK 63	R	147	5.60	6.90	38.64	81.16	6.25
SK 74	R	156	5.20	6.70	34.84	77.61	5.95
SK 845	R	203	5.50	6.70	36.85	82.09	6.10
OLDUVAI 7	L	305	6.70				
OLDUVAI 7	R	305	6.50				

LOWER I2 AUSTRALOPITHECINES

		N	L(M-D)	B(B-L)	L*B	L/B	L+B/2
MLD 18	L	9	5.20	7.80	40.56	66.67	6.50
MLD 18	R	9	5.50	8.00	44.00	68.75	6.75
STS 24	R	43	7.30	6.80	49.64	107.35	7.05
STS 52	R	54	7.10	8.10	57.51	87.65	7.60
NATRON	L	108	5.90	6.40	37.76	92.19	6.15
NATRON	R	108	6.20	6.50	40.30	95.38	6.35
SK 23	L	122	6.70	6.70	44.89	100.00	6.70
SK 23	R	122	6.60	6.70	44.22	98.51	6.65
SK 34	R	132	6.10	6.80	41.48	89.71	6.45
SK 845	R	203	6.50	7.50	48.75	86.67	7.00
OLDUVAI 7	L	305	7.80				
OLDUVAI 7	R	305	7.50				

LOWER C AUSTRALOPITHECINES

		N	L(M-D)	B(B-L)	L*B	L/B	L+B/2
MLD 18	L	9	9.00	10.70	96.30	84.11	9.85
MLD 18	R	9	9.00	10.30	92.70	87.38	9.65
MLD 40	L	13	8.30	9.50	78.85	87.37	8.90
SE 1937	L	16	8.40	9.00	75.60	93.33	8.70
TM 1516	L	21	9.30	10.00	93.00	93.00	9.65
TM 1528	R	27		9.10			
STS 3	R	32	10.50	12.10	127.05	86.78	11.30
STS 7	L	35	9.20	11.00	101.20	83.64	10.10
STS 36		47	9.50	10.70	101.65	88.79	10.10
STS 51	L	53	8.50	9.20	78.20	92.39	8.85
STS 52	R	54	9.10	10.00	91.00	91.00	9.55
NATRON	L	108	7.30	8.10	59.13	90.12	7.70
NATRON	R	108	7.40	8.30	61.42	89.16	7.85
SK 23	L	122	7.80	7.80	60.84	100.00	7.80
SK 23	R	122	8.10	8.00	64.80	101.25	8.05
SK 29	R	127	7.80	8.10	63.18	96.30	7.95
SK 34	R	132	8.50	8.90	75.65	95.51	8.70
SK 63	R	147	7.50	7.50	56.25	100.00	7.50
SK 87	R	164	7.80	9.20	71.76	84.78	8.50
SK 94	R	167	8.30	8.00	66.40	103.75	8.15
SK 96	L	169	6.90	7.20	49.68	95.83	7.05
SK 82C		176	7.10	7.30	51.83	97.26	7.20
OLDUVAI 7	L	305	9.15	9.05	82.81	101.10	9.10
OLDUVAI 7	R	305	8.95				

LOWER PM3 AUSTRALOPITHECINES

		NUMBER	L(M-D)	B(B-L)	L*B	L/B	L+B/2
MLD 2	L	4	11.50	13.00	149.50	88.46	12.25
MLD 2	R	4	10.00	14.00	140.00	71.43	12.00
MLD 18	L	9	10.00	11.80	118.00	84.75	10.90
MLD 18	R	9	10.00	12.60	126.00	79.37	11.30
MLD 40	L	13	10.00	11.00	110.00	90.91	10.50
STS 7	L	35	8.50	12.00	102.00	70.83	10.25
STS 24	L	43	9.40	10.10	94.94	93.07	9.75
STS 51	R	53	9.20	11.80	108.56	77.97	10.50
STS 52	R	54	9.00	11.70	105.30	76.92	10.35
TM 1517 (TYPE)	L	101	10.00	12.00	120.00	83.33	11.00
TM 1517 (TYPE)	R	101	9.90	11.00	108.90	90.00	10.45
TM 1600	L	103	9.80	12.20	119.56	80.33	11.00
MEGANTHROPUS 1	R	105	10.10	11.70	118.17	86.32	10.90
NATRON	L	108	9.20	13.50	124.20	68.15	11.35
NATRON	R	108	9.90	13.50	133.65	73.33	11.70
SK 6	L	113	10.30	11.10	114.33	92.79	10.70
SK 12	L	117	10.60	13.30	140.98	79.70	11.95
SK 12	R	117	10.20	12.30	125.46	82.93	11.25
SK 23	L	122	9.40	11.40	107.16	82.46	10.40
SK 23	R	122	9.60	11.50	110.40	83.40	10.55
SK 30	L	128	9.50	11.30	107.35	84.07	10.40
SK 34	R	132	9.80	12.80	125.44	76.56	11.3
SK 55	L	143	9.60	11.00	105.60	87.27	10.30
SK 72	L	155	9.50	12.50	118.75	76.00	11.00
SK 74	R	156	9.20	10.60	97.52	86.79	9.90
SK 96	L	169	10.10				
SK 100	R	172	9.90	12.90	127.71	76.74	11.40
SK 827	L	184	10.50	12.20	128.10	86.07	11.35
SK 831	R	188	9.60	11.50	110.40	83.48	10.55
SK 15	L	301	8.60	10.30	88.58	83.50	9.45
OLDUVAI 6	L	304	9.25	9.30	86.02	99.46	9.27
OLDUVAI 7	L	305	9.60	10.30	98.88	93.20	9.95
OLDUVAI 7	R	305	9.90	10.10	99.99	98.02	10.00
HEMANTHROPUS 12		315	11.30				

LOWER PM4 AUSTRALOPITHECINES

		N	L(M-D)	B(B-L)	L*B	L/B	L+B/2
MLD 2	L	4	11.30	12.00	135.60	94.17	11.65
MLD 18	L	9	9.00				
MLD 18	R	9	9.00	12.10	108.90	74.38	10.55
MLD 40	L	13	10.00	14.00	140.00	71.43	12.00
TM 1515	L	20	10.40				
TM 1523	L	25	10.10	11.60	117.16	87.07	10.85
STS 7	L	35	9.50	12.60	119.70	75.40	11.05
STS 52	R	54	9.80	11.70	114.66	83.76	10.75
TM 1517 (TYPE)	L	101	11.00	13.00	143.00	84.62	12.00
TM 1517 (TYPE)	R	101	11.00	13.10	144.10	83.97	12.05
TM 1600	L	103	10.90	11.40	124.26	95.61	11.15
MEGANTHROPUS 1	R	105	9.80	11.90	116.62	82.35	10.85
MEGANTHROPUS 3	R	107	8.50				
NATRON	L	108	14.50	15.20	220.40	95.39	14.85
NATRON	R	108	12.70	14.80	187.96	85.81	13.75
SK 6	L	113	11.00	12.40	136.40	88.71	11.70
SK 6	R	113	10.40				
SK 7	R	114	11.00	12.80	140.80	85.94	11.90
SK 9	L	115	10.80	12.60	136.08	85.71	11.70
SK 12	L	117	12.00	13.50	162.00	88.89	12.75
SK 12	R	117	10.50	12.50	131.25	84.00	11.50
SK 23	L	122	10.50	14.10	148.05	74.47	12.30
SK 23	R	122	10.70	13.50	144.45	79.26	12.10
SK 25	R	124	11.40	13.30	151.62	85.71	12.35
SK 34	R	132	12.00	14.50	174.00	82.76	13.25
SK 74	R	156	10.30	12.00	123.60	85.83	11.15
SK 81	L	159	10.80	13.50	145.80	80.00	12.15
SK 826B	L	183	12.50	13.60	170.00	91.91	13.05
SK 830	L	187	10.60	12.20	129.32	86.89	11.40
SK 1587	L	205	11.10	13.00	144.30	85.38	12.05
SK 1588	R	206	10.80	12.40	133.92	87.10	11.60
OLDUVAI 4	L	303	10.45	11.40	119.13	91.67	10.92
OLDUVAI 7	L	305	10.30	10.70	110.21	96.26	10.50
OLDUVAI 7	R	305	11.10	10.70	118.77	103.74	10.90
HEMANTHROPUS 11		314	11.50	12.50	143.75	92.00	12.00

LOWER M1 AUSTRALOPITHECINES

		N	L(M-D)	B(B-L)	L*B	L/B	L+B/2
TAUNG	L	2	14.00	13.50	189.00	103.70	13.75
TAUNG	R	2	14.00	13.50	189.00	103.70	13.75
MLD 2	L	4	15.00	13.90	208.50	107.91	14.45
MLD 2	R	4	14.60	13.80	201.48	105.80	14.20
MLD 18	R	9	11.60	13.00	150.80	89.23	12.30
MLD 40	L	13	12.80	12.30	157.44	104.07	12.55
STS 4		33	13.10	12.20	159.82	107.38	12.65
STS 7	L	35	12.00	12.70	152.40	94.49	12.35
STS 9		37	14.90	13.00	193.70	114.62	13.95
STS 18	R	40	15.10	13.90	209.89	108.63	14.50
STS 24	R	43	13.30	11.30	150.29	117.70	12.30
STS 37	L	48	16.50	15.00	247.50	110.00	15.75
STS 52	L	54	13.40				
STS 52	R	54	13.00	12.90	167.70	100.78	12.95
TM 1517 (TYPE)	R	101	14.40	13.00	187.20	110.77	13.70
TM 1536	R	102	12.70	11.50	146.05	110.43	12.10
TM 1600	L	103	13.50	13.20	178.20	102.27	13.35
MEGANTHROPUS 1	R	105	14.80	13.60	201.28	108.82	14.20
MEGANTHROPUS 3	R	107	14.00	13.00	182.00	107.69	13.50
NATRON	L	108	16.40	15.30	250.92	107.19	15.85
NATRON	R	108	16.10	15.50	249.55	103.87	15.80
SK 6	L	113	16.00	15.20	243.20	105.26	15.60
SK 6	R	113	16.10	14.60	235.06	110.27	15.35
SK 12	R	117	14.00	13.80	193.20	101.45	13.90
SK 23	L	122	14.80	14.70	217.56	100.68	14.75
SK 23	R	122	14.70	14.60	214.62	100.68	14.65
SK 25	L	124	14.80	13.90	205.72	106.47	14.35
SK 25	R	124	14.50	14.00	203.00	103.57	14.25
SK 34	R	132	14.50	14.40	208.80	100.69	14.45
SK 55	L	143	14.40	13.70	197.28	105.11	14.05
SK 55	R	143	14.30	13.70	195.91	104.38	14.00
SK 61	R	145	15.40	14.60	224.84	105.48	15.00
SK 63	L	147	14.80	13.50	199.80	109.63	14.15
SK 63	R	147	14.90	13.50	201.15	110.37	14.20
SK 104	R	174	15.00	13.70	205.50	109.49	14.35
SK 828	L	185	15.60	14.30	223.08	109.09	14.95
SK 838B	L	196	14.00	13.00	182.00	107.69	13.50
SK 843	L	201	14.60	13.50	197.10	108.15	14.05
SK 845	R	203	15.00	14.50	217.50	103.45	14.75
SK 846	R	204	14.50	13.80	200.10	105.07	14.15
SK 1587	L	205	14.10	13.60	191.76	103.68	13.85
SK 1588	R	206	13.30	13.20	175.56	100.76	13.25
SK 15	L	301	11.90	11.90	141.61	100.00	11.90
SK 45	R	302	11.80	11.50	135.70	102.61	11.65
OLDUVAI 7	L	305	14.30	12.20	174.46	117.21	13.25
OLDUVAI 7	R	305	14.30	12.40	177.32	115.32	13.35
HEMANTHROPUS 9		312	16.30	14.20	231.46	114.79	15.25
HEMANTHROPUS 10		313	15.00	14.00	210.00	107.14	14.50

LOWER M2 AUSTRALOPITHECINES

		N	L(M-D)	B(B-L)	L*B	L/B	L+B/2
MLD 2	L	4	16.70	15.10	252.17	110.60	15.90
MLD 2	R	4	16.50	15.00	247.50	110.00	15.75
MLD 18	L	9	14.70	13.90	204.33	105.76	14.30
MLD 18	R	9	14.40	14.70	211.68	97.96	14.55
MLD 22	L	11	15.30	14.10	215.73	108.51	14.70
MLD 24	L	12	15.60	15.10	235.56	103.31	15.35
MLD 40	L	13	15.00	14.30	214.50	104.90	14.65
TM 1515	L	20	16.80	15.30	257.04	109.80	16.05
STS 4		33	14.30	13.20	188.76	108.33	13.75
STS 6		34	15.30	14.00	214.20	109.29	14.65
STS 7	L	35	15.30	14.60	223.38	104.79	14.95
STS 7	R	35		14.80			
STS 52	L	54	14.80	13.30	196.84	111.28	14.05
STS 52	R	54	14.40	13.40	192.96	107.46	13.90
TM 1517 (TYPE)	R	101	15.20	14.80	224.96	102.70	15.00
MEGANTHROPUS 2	R	106	14.40	13.80	198.72	104.35	14.10
MEGANTHROPUS 3	R	107	14.50	13.00	188.50	111.54	13.75
NATRON	L	108	17.40	16.20	281.88	107.41	16.80
NATRON	R	108	17.20	16.10	276.92	106.83	16.65
SK 1	L	110	17.00	15.30	260.10	111.11	16.15
SK 5	L	112	15.00	14.20	213.00	105.63	14.60
SK 6	L	113	17.10	16.10	275.31	106.21	16.60
SK 6	R	113	17.40	16.20	281.88	107.41	16.80
SK 12	L	117	16.40	14.50	237.80	113.10	15.45
SK 12	R	117	16.10	14.00	225.40	115.00	15.05
SK 23	L	122	15.20	14.80	224.96	102.70	15.00
SK 23	R	122	15.00	14.80	222.00	101.35	14.90
SK 25	R	124	16.70	15.00	250.50	111.33	15.85
SK 34	R	132	16.70	16.20	270.54	103.09	16.45
SK 37	L	134	17.00	14.50	246.50	117.24	15.75
SK 55	R	143	15.70	14.30	224.51	109.79	15.00
SK 845	R	203	16.00	14.60	233.60	109.59	15.30
SK 1587	L	205	15.30	14.20	217.26	107.75	14.75
SK 15	L	301	13.80	13.20	182.16	104.55	13.50
SK 15	R	301	13.60	13.10	178.16	103.82	13.35
SK 45	R	302	13.30	12.30	163.59	108.13	12.80
OLDUVAI 7	L	305	15.60	13.50	210.60	115.56	14.55
HEMANTHROPUS 8		311	17.00	16.20	275.40	104.94	16.60

LOWER M3 — AUSTRALOPITHECINES

		N	L(M-D)	B(B-L)	L*B	L/B	L+B/2
MLD 18	L	9	14.40	14.20	204.48	101.41	14.30
MLD 18	R	9	13.80	14.20	195.96	97.18	14.00
MLD 19	L	10	14.70	13.40	196.98	109.70	14.05
MLD 22	L	11	17.10	15.70	268.47	108.92	16.40
MLD 24	L	12	15.70	14.80	232.36	106.08	15.25
MLD 40	L	13	15.00	14.00	210.00	107.14	14.50
TM 1518	R	22	16.70	14.80	247.16	112.84	15.75
TM 1519	R	23	15.70	13.90	218.23	112.95	14.80
TM 1520	L	24	16.00	13.80	220.80	115.94	14.90
STS 7	L	35	15.40	14.40	221.76	106.94	14.90
STS 41	L	49	15.10	13.10	197.81	115.27	14.10
STS 52	L	54	13.50	12.90	174.15	104.65	13.20
STS 52	R	54	13.70	12.70	173.99	107.87	13.20
STS 55	L	57	15.60	13.50	210.60	115.56	14.55
TM 1517 (TYPE)	R	101	16.40	14.00	229.60	117.14	15.20
TM 1600	L	103	16.10	14.80	238.28	108.78	15.45
MEGANTHROPUS 3	R	107	15.50	13.00	201.50	119.23	14.25
NATRON	L	108	18.80	16.30	306.44	115.34	17.55
NATRON	R	108	18.70	15.70	293.59	119.11	17.20
SK 6	L	113	18.50	15.80	292.30	117.09	17.15
SK 6	R	113	18.10	16.00	289.60	113.12	17.05
SK 12	L	117	16.20	15.20	246.24	106.58	15.70
SK 12	R	117	17.20	15.90	273.48	108.18	16.55
SK 22	R	121	18.20	14.70	267.54	123.81	16.45
SK 23	L	122	16.00	13.00	208.00	123.08	14.50
SK 23	R	122	17.30	14.10	243.93	122.70	15.70
SK 34	R	132	18.00	16.50	297.00	109.09	17.25
SK 55	R	143	15.50	13.70	212.35	113.14	14.60
SK 81	L	159	17.10	14.70	251.37	116.33	15.90
SK 840	L	198	16.00	12.90	206.40	124.03	14.45
SK 841	L	199	15.40	13.70	210.98	112.41	14.55
SK 844	L	202	15.60	13.80	215.28	113.04	14.70
SK 15	L	301	14.30	12.40	177.32	115.32	13.35
SK 15	R	301	13.90	12.30	170.97	113.01	13.10
OLDUVAI 4	L	303	15.10	13.00	196.30	116.15	14.05

UPPER 11 — AUSTRALOPITHECINES

		NUMBER	L(M-D)	B(B-L)	L*B	L/B	L+B/2
STS 52	L	54	9.50	8.20	77.90	115.85	8.85
STS 52	R	54	9.30	8.30	77.19	112.05	8.80
OLDUVAI 5	L	109	10.00	8.00	80.00	125.00	9.00
OLDUVAI 5	R	109	10.10	7.70	77.77	131.16	8.90
SK 6	R	113	9.80	8.10	79.38	120.98	9.00
SK 40	L	136	9.00	7.60	68.40	118.42	8.30
SK 55	L	143	9.70				
SK 55	R	143	9.50				
SK 65	L	149	8.30	7.80	64.74	106.41	8.05
SK 68	L	151	10.90	7.60	82.88	143.42	9.25
SK 69/73	L	152	9.30	7.30	67.89	127.40	8.30
SK 69/73	R	152	9.50	7.50	71.25	126.67	8.50

UPPER 12 — AUSTRALOPITHECINES

		NUMBER	L(M-D)	B(B-L)	L*B	L/B	L+B/2
MLD 11/23	L	8	7.00	7.00	49.00	100.00	7.00
TM 1512	R	18	5.80	5.60	32.48	103.57	5.70
STS 52	L	54	7.30	7.00	51.10	104.29	7.15
STS 52	R	54	6.80	6.10	41.48	111.48	6.45
OLDUVAI 5	L	109	7.00	7.60	53.20	92.10	7.30
OLDUVAI 5	R	109	6.90	7.50	51.75	92.00	7.20
SK 6	R	113	9.20	7.60	69.92	121.05	8.40
SK 27	L	125	7.80	7.60	59.28	102.63	7.70
SK 52	R	142	6.60	6.80	44.88	97.06	6.70
SK 55	L	143	6.80	6.30	42.84	107.94	6.55
SK 65	L	149	5.90	6.50	38.35	90.77	6.20
SK 66	R	150	6.60				
SK 70	L	153	8.10	7.00	56.70	115.71	7.55
SK 71	R	154	6.80	6.90	46.92	98.55	6.9

UPPER C — AUSTRALOPITHECINES

		N	L(M-D)	B(B-L)	L*B	L/B	L+B/2
MLD 11/23	L	8	9.90	9.90	98.01	100.00	9.90
TM 1512	R	18	8.80	9.40	82.72	93.62	9.10
TM 1514	L	19	10.20				
TM 1527	R	26	9.40	8.70	81.78	108.05	9.05
STS 2	L	31	9.50				
STS 48	L	52	9.20	9.50	87.40	96.84	9.35
STS 52	L	54	9.80	9.90	97.02	98.99	9.85
STS 52	R	54	9.90	9.70	96.03	102.06	9.80
OLDUVAI 5	L	109	8.70	9.70	84.39	89.69	9.20
OLDUVAI 5	R	109	8.80	9.90	87.12	88.89	9.35
SK 6	R	113	8.90	10.30	91.67	86.41	9.60
SK 27	R	125	10.60	10.40	110.24	101.92	10.50
SK 38	R	135	9.00	10.00	90.00	90.00	9.50
SK 48	R	140	8.20	8.80	72.16	93.18	8.50
SK 55	L	143	8.30	8.60	71.38	96.51	8.45
SK 55	R	143	8.20	8.90	72.98	92.13	8.55
SK 65	L	149	8.30	10.00	83.00	83.00	9.15
SK 65	R	149	8.50	9.90	84.15	85.86	9.20
SK 83	L	160	8.90	10.30	91.67	86.41	9.60
SK 84		161	9.30	11.10	103.23	83.78	10.20
SK 85/93	L	162	8.50	9.60	81.60	88.54	9.05
SK 85/93	R	162	8.30	9.30	77.19	89.25	8.80
SK 86		163	8.60	8.80	75.68	97.73	8.70
SK 92	R	166	8.10	8.70	70.47	93.10	8.40
SK 95	L	168	8.10	8.40	68.04	96.43	8.25

UPPER PM3 AUSTRALOPITHECINES

		N	L(M-D)	B(B-L)	L*B	L/B	L+B/2
GARUSI	L	1	8.60	12.30	105.78	69.92	10.45
MLD 6	R	6	8.50	11.70	99.45	72.65	10.10
MLD 11/23	L	8	9.10	12.30	111.93	73.98	10.70
TM 1511	L	17	9.30	12.20	113.46	76.23	10.75
TM 1512	R	18	8.90	11.90	105.91	74.79	10.40
STS 1	L	30	9.40	13.50	126.90	69.63	11.45
STS 1	R	30	9.40	13.20	124.08	71.21	11.30
STS 12		38	8.90	12.10	107.69	73.55	10.50
STS 17	L	39	8.70	12.90	112.23	67.44	10.80
STS 42	R	50	8.50	13.00	110.50	65.38	10.75
STS 47		51	8.70	10.70	93.09	81.31	9.70
STS 52	L	54	8.70	12.80	111.36	67.97	10.75
STS 52	R	54	8.60	12.80	110.08	67.19	10.70
STS 54	L	56	8.80	11.70	102.96	75.21	10.25
STS 55	L	57	9.10	13.90	126.49	65.47	11.50
TM 1517 (TYPE)	L	101	10.00	13.70	137.00	72.99	11.85
TM 1517 (TYPE)	R	101	10.20				
OLDUVAI 5	L	109	10.90	17.00	185.30	64.12	13.95
OLDUVAI 5	R	109	10.90	17.00	185.30	64.12	13.95
SK 13/14	L	118	9.70	13.10	127.07	74.05	11.40
SK 13/14	R	118	9.80	13.20	129.36	74.24	11.50
SK 24	L	123	9.60	14.10	135.36	68.09	11.85
SK 27	R	125	9.50	13.40	127.30	70.90	11.45
SK 33		131	10.50	15.00	157.50	70.00	12.75
SK 46	R	138	8.30	13.20	109.56	62.88	10.75
SK 48	R	140	9.20	13.70	126.04	67.15	11.45
SK 52	L	142	10.20	15.00	153.00	68.00	12.60
SK 52	R	142	10.50	15.20	159.60	69.08	12.85
SK 55	L	143	9.50	13.10	124.45	72.52	11.30
SK 55	R	143	9.50	13.50	128.25	70.37	11.50
SK 57	L	144	9.90	15.30	151.47	64.71	12.60
SK 65	L	149	9.00	14.00	126.00	64.29	11.50
SK 74C	R	157	10.10	15.20	153.52	66.45	12.65
SK 83	L	160	8.50	13.90	118.15	61.15	11.20
SK 821	L	177	10.60	14.40	152.64	73.61	12.50
SK 822	L	178	9.70	14.00	135.80	69.29	11.85
SK 823	R	179	10.30	14.20	146.26	72.54	12.25
SK 845	L	203	10.80	14.50	156.60	74.48	12.65

UPPER PM4 AUSTRALOPITHECINES

		N	L(M-D)	B(B-L)	L*B	L/B	L+B/2
GARUSI	L	1	9.10	12.50	113.75	72.80	10.80
MLD 6	R	6	9.40	12.60	118.44	74.60	11.00
MLD 9	R	7	6.00	13.00	78.00	46.15	9.50
MLD 9	R	7	8.00	13.00	104.00	61.54	10.50
MLD 11/23	L	8	9.50	12.50	118.75	76.00	11.00
TM 1511	L	17	8.70	12.60	109.62	69.05	10.65
TM 1511	R	17	8.50	12.50	106.25	68.00	10.50
STS 12		38	9.30	12.20	113.46	76.23	10.75
STS 17	L	39	8.40	13.10	110.04	64.12	10.75
STS 17	R	39	7.20	12.50	90.00	57.60	9.85
STS 30	R	45	10.50	13.90	145.95	75.54	12.20
STS 42	R	50	7.80	13.80	107.64	56.52	10.80
STS 52	L	54	9.10	13.20	120.12	68.94	11.15
STS 52	R	54	9.30	13.30	123.69	69.92	11.30
STS 53	L	55	8.00				
STS 54	L	56	9.90	12.60	124.74	78.57	11.25
TM 1517 (TYPE)	L	101	10.30	15.20	156.56	67.76	12.75
OLDUVAI 5	L	109	11.80	18.00	212.40	65.56	14.90
OLDUVAI 5	R	109	12.00	17.60	211.20	68.18	14.80
SK 11	R	116	10.50	15.00	157.50	70.00	12.75
SK 12	L	117	11.00	16.50	181.50	66.67	13.75
SK 13/14	L	118	10.50	15.10	158.55	69.54	12.80
SK 13/14	R	118	10.50	15.10	158.55	69.54	12.80
SK 28		126	10.50	15.30	160.65	68.63	12.90
SK 32		130	11.00	15.60	171.60	70.51	13.30
SK 46	L	138	9.30	14.60	135.78	63.70	11.95
SK 46	R	138	9.20	14.60	134.32	63.01	11.90
SK 49	L	141	10.80	16.30	176.04	66.26	13.55
SK 49	R	141	12.20	16.10	196.42	75.78	14.15
SK 52	L	142	11.30	16.20	183.06	69.75	13.75
SK 52	R	142	11.50	16.30	187.45	70.55	13.90
SK 57	L	144	10.50	16.20	170.10	64.81	13.35
SK 65	L	149	10.00	15.40	154.00	64.94	12.70
SK 79	R	158	9.30	13.70	127.41	67.88	11.50
SK 83	L	160	11.30	16.70	188.71	67.66	14.00
SK 99	L	171	11.10	15.40	170.94	72.08	13.25
SK 824	L	180	10.40	14.60	151.84	71.23	12.50
SK 825	L	181	10.80	14.50	156.60	74.48	12.65
SK 845	L	203	11.80	15.70	185.26	75.16	13.75

UPPER M1 AUSTRALOPITHECINES

		N	L(M-D)	B(B-L)	L*B	L/B	L+B/2
TAUNG	L	2	12.75	14.00	178.50	91.07	13.37
TAUNG	R	2	12.75	14.00	178.50	91.07	13.37
MLC 1	L	3	14.00	14.50	203.00	96.55	14.25
MLD 6	R	6	12.50	12.80	160.00	97.66	12.65
MLD 9	R	7	13.00	14.00	182.00	92.86	13.50
SE 255	L	14	13.40	13.40	179.56	100.00	13.40
TM 1511	L	17	12.40	13.00	161.20	95.38	12.70
TM 1511	R	17	11.90	13.40	159.46	88.81	12.65
TM 1512	R	18	12.00	13.60	163.20	88.24	12.80
STS 1	L	30	12.50	14.10	176.25	88.65	13.30
STS 8		36	12.40	14.10	174.84	87.94	13.25
STS 17	L	39	12.00	13.10	157.20	91.60	12.55
STS 17	R	39	10.90	13.70	149.33	79.56	12.30
STS 21	R	41	13.20	15.10	199.32	87.42	14.15
STS 22	L	42	12.10	13.70	165.77	88.32	12.90
STS 52	L	54	12.30	14.00	172.20	87.86	13.15
STS 52	R	54	12.20	14.10	172.02	86.52	13.15
STS 53	L	55	11.80	12.60	148.68	93.65	12.20
STS 56		58	12.80	13.40	171.52	95.52	13.10
STS 57	L	59	12.90	13.20	170.28	97.73	13.05
TM 1517 (TYPE)	L	101	13.70	14.60	200.02	93.84	14.15
OLDUVAI 5	L	109	15.20	17.70	269.04	85.88	16.45
OLDUVAI 5	R	109	15.20	17.70	269.04	85.88	16.45
SK 11	R	116		15.90			
SK 13/14	L	118	13.40	14.80	198.32	90.54	14.10
SK 13/14	R	118	13.40	15.00	201.00	89.33	14.20
SK 17	R	120	13.30	14.20	188.86	93.66	13.75
SK 27	L	125	14.00	13.20	184.80	106.06	13.60
SK 46	L	138	12.00				
SK 46	R	138	11.80	15.20	179.36	77.63	13.50
SK 47	R	139	13.10	12.70	166.37	103.15	12.90
SK 48	L	140	13.10	14.00	183.40	93.57	13.55
SK 49	R	141	13.80	15.00	207.00	92.00	14.40
SK 52	R	142	14.40	16.60	239.04	86.75	15.50
SK 55	L	143	14.50	14.40	208.80	100.69	14.45
SK 83	L	160	13.20	14.90	196.68	88.59	14.05
SK 89/90/91	L	165	13.80	14.70	202.86	93.88	14.25
SK 89/90/91	R	165	14.60	15.00	219.00	97.33	14.80
SK 102	L	173	13.70	14.30	195.91	95.80	14.00
SK 829	L	186	13.30	14.00	186.20	95.00	13.65
SK 832	L	190	14.00	14.80	207.20	94.59	14.40
SK 838A	R	195	14.30	14.90	213.07	95.97	14.60
SK 839	R	197	13.20	13.90	183.48	94.96	13.55

UPPER M2 AUSTRALOPITHECINES

		N	L(M-D)	B(B-L)	L*B	L/B	L+B/2
MLC 1	L	3	14.30	15.00	214.50	95.33	14.65
MLD 6	R	6	13.70	14.50	198.65	94.48	14.10
MLD 9	R	7	14.00	16.80	235.20	83.33	15.40
SE 1508	R	15	13.00	15.00	195.00	86.67	14.00
TM 1511	L	17	14.50	15.20	220.40	95.39	14.85
TM 1511	R	17	14.30	15.10	215.93	94.70	14.70
STS 1	L	30	13.30	14.30	190.19	93.01	13.80
STS 8		36	13.80	16.60	229.08	83.13	15.20
STS 12		38	14.30	15.30	218.79	93.46	14.80
STS 17	R	39	12.80	15.20	194.56	84.21	14.00
STS 22	L	42	13.10	15.40	201.74	85.06	14.25
STS 28	R	44	15.10	17.10	258.21	88.30	16.10
STS 32		46	14.10	16.20	228.42	87.04	15.15
STS 37	L	48	14.80	17.00	251.60	87.06	15.90
STS 52	L	54	13.20	15.20	200.64	86.84	14.20
STS 52	R	54	13.30	15.20	202.16	87.50	14.25
STS 53	L	55	13.00	14.60	189.80	89.04	13.80
STS 53	R	55	12.70	14.30	181.61	88.81	13.50
STS 56		58	13.10	13.80	180.78	94.93	13.45
TM 1517 (TYPE)	L	101	13.80	15.90	219.42	86.79	14.85
TM 1517 (TYPE)	R	101	13.80	15.90	219.42	86.79	14.85
OLDUVAI 5	L	109	17.20	21.00	361.20	81.90	19.10
OLDUVAI 5	R	109	17.20	21.00	361.20	81.90	19.10
SK 11	L	116	14.60	16.50	240.90	88.48	15.55
SK 13/14	L	118	15.40	16.50	254.10	93.33	15.95
SK 13/14	R	118	15.60	16.20	252.72	96.30	15.90
SK 27	L	125	14.70	14.20	208.74	103.52	14.45
SK 46	L	138	14.80	16.20	239.76	91.36	15.50
SK 46	R	138	14.40	16.90	243.36	85.21	15.65
SK 47	L	139	14.20	14.50	205.90	97.93	14.35
SK 47	R	139	13.70	14.20	194.54	96.48	13.95
SK 48	L	140	13.60	14.50	197.20	93.79	14.05
SK 49	R	141	14.60	16.40	239.44	89.02	15.50
SK 83	L	160	14.60	16.80	245.28	86.90	15.70
SK 98	L	170	14.90	15.20	226.48	98.03	15.05
SK 826		182	14.80	16.00	236.80	92.50	15.40
SK 831A	L	189	15.70	16.90	265.33	92.90	16.30
SK 834	L	191	14.80	16.50	244.20	89.70	15.65
SK 837	R	194	14.60	16.70	243.82	87.43	15.65
HEMANTHROPUS 6		309	15.70	16.20	254.34	96.91	15.95
HEMANTHROPUS 7		310	14.30	14.70	210.21	97.28	14.50

UPPER M3 — AUSTRALOPITHECINES

		N	L(M-D)	B(B-L)	L*B	L/B	L+B/2
TM 1511	R	17	13.70	15.50	212.35	88.39	14.60
TM 1514	L	19	12.70	14.90	189.23	85.23	13.80
TM 1532	L	28	11.60	14.80	171.68	78.38	13.20
TM 1561	R	29	13.60	15.10	205.36	90.07	14.35
STS 17	R	39	13.40				
STS 28	R	44	15.20	17.90	272.08	84.92	16.55
STS 37	L	48	14.20	16.70	237.14	85.03	15.45
STS 52	R	54	12.50	14.60	182.50	85.62	13.55
STS 53	L	55	12.20	14.80	180.56	82.43	13.50
STS 53	R	55	12.30	14.60	179.58	84.25	13.45
STS 54	R	56	13.00	14.90	193.70	87.25	13.95
TM 1517 (TYPE)	L	101	14.40	16.20	233.28	88.89	15.30
TM 1517 (TYPE)	R	101	14.20	16.10	228.62	88.20	15.15
OLDUVAI 5	L	109	15.70	21.40	335.98	73.36	18.55
OLDUVAI 5	R	109	16.30	20.50	334.15	79.51	18.40
SK 11	L	116	15.10	16.10	243.11	93.79	15.60
SK 13/14	L	118	16.10	17.50	281.75	92.00	16.80
SK 13/14	R	118	15.70	17.40	273.18	90.23	16.55
SK 16	L	119	14.20	16.80	238.56	84.52	15.50
SK 31	R	129	15.40	16.40	252.56	93.90	15.90
SK 36	R	133	15.70	17.00	266.90	92.35	16.35
SK 41	R	137	15.00	16.00	240.00	93.75	15.50
SK 46	L	138	15.60	16.40	255.84	95.12	16.00
SK 46	R	138	15.10	17.20	259.72	87.79	16.15
SK 48	L	140	14.10	15.90	224.19	88.68	15.00
SK 49	L	141	13.90	16.80	233.52	82.74	15.35
SK 49	R	141	12.80	18.20	232.96	70.33	15.50
SK 83	L	160	15.60	16.50	257.40	94.55	16.05
SK 105	L	175	15.60	15.70	244.92	99.36	15.65
SK 831	L	188	16.70	17.80	297.26	93.82	17.25
SK 831A	L	189	17.00	17.80	302.60	95.51	17.40
SK 835	L	192	13.90	16.60	230.74	83.73	15.25
SK 836	L	193	16.10	18.10	291.41	88.95	17.10
SK 837	R	194	15.20	17.00	258.40	89.41	16.10
OLDUVAI 7A		306	13.50	12.75	172.12	105.88	13.12
HEMANTHROPUS 5		308	16.20	15.10	244.62	107.28	15.65

LOWER I1 — H. ERECTUS

		N	L(M-D)	B(B-L)	L*B	L/B	L+B/2
OLDUVAI 16	L	307	7.15				
MAUR (KLAATSCH)	L	404	5.00	7.10	35.50	70.42	6.05
MAUR (KLAATSCH)	R	404	5.50	7.10	39.05	77.46	6.30
RABAT	R	409	6.00	7.00	42.00	85.71	6.50
SINANTHROPUS B1	L	419	6.20	6.10	37.82	101.64	6.15
SINANTHROPUS B1	R	419	6.80	6.50	44.20	104.62	6.65
SINANTHROPUS B5	L	423	6.30	6.70	42.21	94.03	6.50
SINANTHROPUS B5	R	423	6.70	6.20	41.54	108.06	6.45
SINANTHROPUS D1	L	427	6.00	6.40	38.40	93.75	6.20
SINANTHROPUS G1	L	433	6.20	6.80	42.16	91.18	6.50
SINANTHROPUS L4	R	443	6.70	5.80	38.86	115.52	6.25
TERNIFINE 1	R	459	5.60				
TERNIFINE 3	R	461	5.50				

LOWER I2 — H. ERECTUS

		N	L(M-D)	B(B-L)	L*B	L/B	L+B/2
OLDUVAI 16	L	307	8.65				
OLDUVAI 16	R	307	8.80				
MAUR (KLAATSCH)	L	404	6.30	7.70	48.51	81.82	7.00
MAUR (KLAATSCH)	R	404	6.00	7.80	46.80	76.92	6.90
RABAT	R	409	7.00	7.50	52.50	93.33	7.25
SINANTHROPUS A1	L	414	7.20	7.10	51.12	101.41	7.15
SINANTHROPUS B1	L	419	7.00	7.10	49.70	98.59	7.05
SINANTHROPUS B1	R	419	6.80	6.70	45.56	101.49	6.75
SINANTHROPUS B5	L	423	6.80	7.00	47.60	97.14	6.90
SINANTHROPUS B5	R	423	7.00	7.00	49.00	100.00	7.00
SINANTHROPUS C1	R	424	7.20	7.10	51.12	101.41	7.15
SINANTHROPUS D1	L	427	6.40	6.80	43.52	94.12	6.60
SINANTHROPUS G1	L	433	7.00	7.30	51.10	95.89	7.15
SINANTHROPUS H4	R	437		7.30			
SINANTHROPUS K2	R	440	6.30	6.40	40.32	98.44	6.35
UBEIDIYA		463	5.60	5.60	31.36	100.00	5.60

LOWER C — H. ERECTUS

		N	L(M-D)	B(B-L)	L*B	L/B	L+B/2
OLDUVAI 16	L	307		9.40			
LANTIAN	L	402		9.10			
LANTIAN	R	402		9.20			
MAUR (KLAATSCH)	L	404	7.70	9.00	69.30	85.56	8.35
MAUR (KLAATSCH)	R	404	7.60	9.00	68.40	84.44	8.30
OLDUVAI 13	L	406	8.10				
OLDUVAI 13	R	406	7.60	7.85	59.66	96.82	7.72
PITHECAN. C	L	408		7.80			
RABAT	R	409	8.50	9.50	80.75	89.47	9.00
SANGIRAN A		410	10.00	11.00	110.00	90.91	10.50
CASABLANCA	L	413	7.00	9.00	63.00	77.78	8.00
SINANTHROPUS B1	L	419	8.10	8.20	66.42	98.78	8.15
SINANTHROPUS B5	L	423		9.50			
SINANTHROPUS B5	R	423	8.40				
SINANTHROPUS C2	L	425	9.00	10.40	93.60	86.54	9.70
SINANTHROPUS G1	L	433	9.00	10.10	90.90	89.11	9.55
SINANTHROPUS H1	L	434	8.50	8.70	73.95	97.70	8.60
SINANTHROPUS H4	R	437	8.10	8.20	66.42	98.78	8.15
SINANTHROPUS I1	L	438	8.50	8.70	73.95	97.70	8.60
SINANTHROPUS K1	L	439	8.90	9.30	82.77	95.70	9.10
TERNIFINE 1	R	459	7.50	9.00	67.50	83.33	8.25
TERNIFINE 2	L	460	7.00	10.00	70.00	70.00	8.50
TERNIFINE 3	R	461	8.00	11.00	88.00	72.73	9.50

LOWER PM3 H. ERECTUS

		N	L(M-D)	B(B-L)	L*B	L/B	L+B/2
OLDUVAI 16	R	307	9.20	11.00	101.20	83.64	10.10
PITHECAN. A	L	401	5.00	8.40	42.00	59.52	6.70
MAUR (KLAATSCH)	L	404	7.30				
MAUR (KLAATSCH)	R	404	8.10	9.00	72.90	90.00	8.55
OLDUVAI 13	L	406	8.95	9.15	81.89	97.81	9.05
OLDUVAI 13	R	406	9.35	9.70	90.69	96.39	9.52
PITHECAN. C	L	408	8.70	10.70	93.09	81.31	9.70
RABAT	R	409	9.00	10.00	90.00	90.00	9.50
CASABLANCA	L	413	9.00	9.60	86.40	93.75	9.30
SINANTHROPUS A1	L	414	8.30	8.90	73.87	93.26	8.60
SINANTHROPUS 16	L	417	9.20	9.50	87.40	96.84	9.35
SINANTHROPUS 47	L	418	8.20	10.20	83.64	80.39	9.20
SINANTHROPUS B1	R	419	8.80	9.10	80.08	96.70	8.95
SINANTHROPUS B5	R	423	8.80	10.10	88.88	87.13	9.45
SINANTHROPUS C3	R	426	9.30	10.00	93.00	93.00	9.65
SINANTHROPUS D1	R	427	8.20	9.20	75.44	89.13	8.70
SINANTHROPUS F3	L	431	8.40	9.30	78.12	90.32	8.85
SINANTHROPUS G1	L	433	9.10	10.70	97.37	85.05	9.90
SINANTHROPUS G1	R	433	9.00	10.60	95.40	84.91	9.80
SINANTHROPUS H1	L	434	8.20	9.40	77.08	87.23	8.80
SINANTHROPUS H2	R	435	7.90	10.20	80.58	77.45	9.05
SINANTHROPUS H4	R	437	9.00				
SINANTHROPUS K1	L	439	9.80	10.20	99.96	96.08	10.00
SINANTHROPUS M1	L	444	8.20	10.30	84.46	79.61	9.25
SINANTHROPUS M1	R	444	8.10	10.80	87.48	75.00	9.45
S. OFFICINALIS		456	10.00	10.60	106.00	94.34	10.30
TERNIFINE 1	L	459	8.70	8.90	77.43	97.75	8.80
TERNIFINE 1	R	459	8.60	9.80	84.28	87.76	9.20
TERNIFINE 2	L	460	9.00	11.20	100.80	80.36	10.10
TERNIFINE 3	R	461	8.00	10.00	80.00	80.00	9.00

LOWER PM4 H. ERECTUS

		N	L(M-D)	B(B-L)	L*B	L/B	L+B/2
OLDUVAI 16	L	307	8.90	12.00	106.80	74.17	10.45
OLDUVAI 16	R	307	9.90	10.90	107.91	90.83	10.40
LANTIAN	R	402	7.20	9.60	69.12	75.00	8.40
MAUR (KLAATSCH)	R	404	7.50	9.20	69.00	81.52	8.35
OLDUVAI 13	L	406	9.15	8.70	79.60	105.17	8.92
OLDUVAI 13	R	406	8.90	9.80	87.22	90.82	9.35
PITHECAN. B (4)	R	407	9.00	10.90	98.10	82.57	9.95
PITHECAN. C	L	408	8.50	10.50	89.25	80.95	9.50
RABAT	R	409	9.00	9.50	85.50	94.74	9.25
SINANTHROPUS 16	L	417	9.80	10.20	99.96	96.08	10.00
SINANTHROPUS B1	R	419	9.90	8.00	79.20	123.75	8.95
SINANTHROPUS B4	L	422	8.80	9.80	86.24	89.80	9.30
SINANTHROPUS B5	R	423	9.00	9.80	88.20	91.84	9.40
SINANTHROPUS C1	R	424	8.80	11.80	103.84	74.58	10.30
SINANTHROPUS C3	R	426	9.20	11.10	102.12	82.88	10.15
SINANTHROPUS F3	R	431	8.70	9.60	83.52	90.62	9.15
SINANTHROPUS G1	L	433	8.50	11.00	93.50	77.27	9.75
SINANTHROPUS H4	R	437		8.20			
SINANTHROPUS K1	L	439	8.70	10.90	94.83	79.82	9.80
TERNIFINE 1	L	459	8.80	9.80	86.24	89.80	9.30
TERNIFINE 1	R	459	8.50	10.00	85.00	85.00	9.25
TERNIFINE 2	L	460	9.50	10.50	99.75	90.48	10.00
TERNIFINE 3	L	461	7.40	10.00	74.00	74.00	8.70
TERNIFINE 3	R	461	8.60	9.80	84.28	87.76	9.20

LOWER M1 H. ERECTUS

		N	L(M-D)	B(B-L)	L*B	L/B	L+B/2
OLDUVAI 16	R	307	14.70				
LANTIAN	R	402	12.60	11.50	144.90	109.57	12.05
MAUR (KLAATSCH)	L	404	11.10				
MAUR (KLAATSCH)	R	404	11.60	11.20	129.92	103.57	11.40
OLDUVAI 13	R	406	12.70	11.60	147.32	109.48	12.15
PITHECAN. B (4)	R	407	12.80	13.00	166.40	98.46	12.90
RABAT	R	409	13.00	11.00	143.00	118.18	12.00
SANGIRAN 1939	R	411	13.00	13.00	169.00	100.00	13.00
CASABLANCA	R	413	13.00	11.60	150.80	112.07	12.30
SINANTHROPUS A1	L	414	12.20	10.90	132.98	111.93	11.55
SINANTHROPUS A2	R	415	11.80	11.20	132.16	105.36	11.50
SINANTHROPUS A3	R	416	12.50	12.60	157.50	99.21	12.55
SINANTHROPUS 16	L	417	13.90	13.00	180.70	106.92	13.45
SINANTHROPUS 17	L	451	12.70	12.00	152.40	105.83	12.35
SINANTHROPUS B1	R	419	11.90	11.10	132.09	107.21	11.50
SINANTHROPUS B3	R	421	13.60	12.60	171.36	107.94	13.10
SINANTHROPUS C3	L	426	14.10	12.80	180.48	110.16	13.45
SINANTHROPUS C3	R	426		12.00			
SINANTHROPUS F1	R	429	13.40	12.20	163.48	109.84	12.80
SINANTHROPUS G1	L	433	13.20	12.50	165.00	105.60	12.85
SINANTHROPUS H4	R	437	11.30	10.60	119.78	106.60	10.95
SINANTHROPUS I1	L	438	9.90	10.10	99.99	98.02	10.00
SINANTHROPUS K1	L	439	13.00	12.60	163.80	103.17	12.80
SINANTHROPUS L4	L	443	13.00	11.70	152.10	111.11	12.35
SINANTHROPUS O2	L	448	12.30	11.70	143.91	105.13	12.00
S. OFFICINALIS		457	12.80	13.70	175.36	93.43	13.25
TERNIFINE 1	L	459	13.60	12.90	175.44	105.43	13.25
TERNIFINE 1	R	459	13.40	12.70	170.18	105.51	13.05
TERNIFINE 2	L	460	14.00	13.00	182.00	107.69	13.50
TERNIFINE 3	L	461	12.50	11.80	147.50	105.93	12.15
TERNIFINE 3	R	461	12.50	12.00	150.00	104.17	12.25

LOWER M2 H. ERECTUS

		N	L(M-D)	B(B-L)	L*B	L/B	L+B/2
LANTIAN	L	402	12.50	13.00	162.50	96.15	12.75
LANTIAN	R	402	12.60	13.00	163.80	96.92	12.80
MAUR (KLAATSCH)	L	404	12.90				
MAUR (KLAATSCH)	R	404	12.70	12.00	152.40	105.83	12.35
OLDUVAI 13	R	406	13.80	12.20	168.36	113.11	13.00
PITHECAN. B (4)	R	407	13.50	13.40	180.90	100.75	13.45
PITHECAN. C	L	408	14.10	13.10	184.71	107.63	13.60
RABAT	R	409	12.50	11.30	141.25	110.62	11.90
SANGIRAN 1939	R	411	14.10	14.30	201.63	98.60	14.20
CASABLANCA	R	413	14.00	11.20	156.80	125.00	12.60
SINANTHROPUS A2	R	415	11.90	11.40	135.66	104.39	11.65
SINANTHROPUS 16	L	417	12.50	12.50	156.25	100.00	12.50
SINANTHROPUS 17	L	451	12.30	11.80	145.14	104.24	12.05
SINANTHROPUS B1	L	419	12.80	11.10	142.08	115.32	11.95
SINANTHROPUS B4	L	422	13.10	11.50	150.65	113.91	12.30
SINANTHROPUS C1	R	424	12.90	13.00	167.70	99.23	12.95
SINANTHROPUS D1	R	427	12.20	12.00	146.40	101.67	12.10
SINANTHROPUS F1	R	429	13.20	12.70	167.64	103.94	12.95
SINANTHROPUS G1	L	433	12.50	12.70	158.75	98.43	12.60
SINANTHROPUS G1	R	433	12.60	12.90	162.54	97.67	12.75
SINANTHROPUS K1	L	439	12.60	12.60	158.76	100.00	12.60
SINANTHROPUS M3	L	445	11.30	11.50	129.95	98.26	11.40
TERNIFINE 1	L	459	13.50	13.00	175.50	103.85	13.25
TERNIFINE 1	R	459	12.80	13.30	170.24	96.24	13.05
TERNIFINE 2	L	460	14.20	13.70	194.54	103.65	13.95
TERNIFINE 3	L	461	13.00	12.20	158.60	106.56	12.60
TERNIFINE 3	R	461	12.00	12.50	150.00	96.00	12.25

LOWER M3 H. ERECTUS

		N	L(M-D)	B(B-L)	L*B	L/B	L+B/2
OLDUVAI 16	L	307	14.70	14.60	214.62	100.68	14.65
MAUR (KLAATSCH)	L	404	11.30	11.30	127.69	100.00	11.30
MAUR (KLAATSCH)	R	404	10.90	11.90	129.71	91.60	11.40
OLDUVAI 13	L	406	15.20	11.00	167.20	138.18	13.10
OLDUVAI 13	R	406	14.60	12.50	182.50	116.80	13.55
PITHECAN. B (4)	R	407	14.60	12.50	182.50	116.80	13.55
PITHECAN. C	L	408	13.70	13.20	180.84	103.79	13.45
RABAT	R	409	12.50	11.00	137.50	113.64	11.75
CASABLANCA	R	413	12.20	11.30	137.86	107.96	11.75
SINANTHROPUS A2	R	415	10.00	10.00	100.00	100.00	10.00
SINANTHROPUS 16	L	417	14.00	11.20	156.80	125.00	12.60
SINANTHROPUS B2	L	420	13.80	11.80	162.84	116.95	12.80
SINANTHROPUS D1	R	427	12.20	12.10	147.62	100.83	12.15
SINANTHROPUS F1	L	429	12.20	11.40	139.08	107.02	11.80
SINANTHROPUS G1	L	433	12.00	12.30	147.60	97.56	12.15
SINANTHROPUS G1	R	433	12.90	12.40	159.96	104.03	12.65
SINANTHROPUS H1	R	434	10.00	10.20	102.00	98.04	10.10
SINANTHROPUS L4	R	443	12.70	10.80	137.16	117.59	11.75
SINANTHROPUS M1	L	444	10.90	10.80	117.72	100.93	10.85
SINANTHROPUS M3	L	445	10.60	10.70	113.42	99.07	10.65
TERNIFINE 1	L	459	12.80	12.10	154.88	105.79	12.45
TERNIFINE 1	R	459	12.00	12.80	153.60	93.75	12.40
TERNIFINE 2	L	460	13.20	12.50	165.00	105.60	12.85
TERNIFINE 3	L	461	12.30	11.40	140.22	107.89	11.85
TERNIFINE 3	R	461	12.80	12.30	157.44	104.07	12.55

UPPER I1 H. ERECTUS

		NUMBER	L(M-D)	B(B-L)	L*B	L/B	L+B/2
OLDUVAI 16	R	307	11.80				
PITHECAN. B (4)	R	407	10.00				
SINANTHROPUS 17	L	451	10.70	8.10	86.67	132.10	9.40
SINANTHROPUS B1	L	419	9.90	7.60	75.24	130.26	8.75
SINANTHROPUS B1	R	419	9.80	7.90	77.42	124.05	8.85
SINANTHROPUS F4	L	432	10.70	8.10	86.67	132.10	9.40
SINANTHROPUS L1	L	441	10.80	7.50	81.00	144.00	9.15
SINANTHROPUS L2	L	442	7.20	7.50	54.00	96.00	7.35
SINANTHROPUS O1	L	447	8.50	8.20	69.70	103.65	8.40

UPPER I2 H. ERECTUS

		NUMBER	L(M-D)	B(B-L)	L*B	L/B	L+B/2
PITHECAN. B (4)	R	407	10.00	10.40	104.00	96.15	10.20
RABAT	R	409	8.00	8.50	68.00	94.12	8.25
SINANTHROPUS F2	R	430	8.30	8.20	68.06	101.22	8.25
SINANTHROPUS F4	R	432	8.20	8.10	66.42	101.23	8.15
SINANTHROPUS O1	L	447	6.80	8.00	54.40	85.00	7.40
OLDUVAI 16	R	307	7.80				

UPPER C H. ERECTUS

		N	L(M-D)	B(B-L)	L*B	L/B	L+B/2
OLDUVAI 16	R	307	9.40	8.90	83.66	105.62	9.15
PITHECAN. B (4)	L	407	9.50	11.90	113.05	79.83	10.70
PITHECAN. B (4)	R	407	9.50	11.70	111.15	81.20	10.60
RABAT	R	409	9.50	10.00	95.00	95.00	9.75
SINANTHROPUS C1	L	424	9.30	9.90	92.07	93.94	9.60
SINANTHROPUS D1	L	427	9.10	9.80	89.18	92.86	9.45
SINANTHROPUS F4	R	432	10.50	10.40	109.20	100.96	10.45
SINANTHROPUS L1	L	441	9.60	10.40	99.84	92.31	10.00
SINANTHROPUS L1	R	441	9.60	10.60	101.76	90.57	10.10
SINANTHROPUS L2	L	442	8.50	9.80	83.30	86.73	9.15
TERNIFINE 3	R	461	8.70	10.00	87.00	87.00	9.35

UPPER PM3 H. ERECTUS

		N	L(M-D)	B(B-L)	L*B	L/B	L+B/2
OLDUVAI 16	R	307	9.80	13.20	129.36	74.24	11.50
OLDUVAI 13	R	406	8.30	11.40	94.62	72.81	9.85
PITHECAN. B (4)	L	407	8.50	12.40	105.40	68.55	10.45
PITHECAN. B (4)	R	407	8.20	12.40	101.68	66.13	10.30
RABAT	R	409	8.50	12.00	102.00	70.83	10.25
SINANTHROPUS 20	R	452	8.70	11.90	103.53	73.11	10.30
SINANTHROPUS E1	R	428		11.10			
SINANTHROPUS F4	R	432	9.20	12.80	117.76	71.87	11.00
SINANTHROPUS H3	L	436	8.50	12.20	103.70	69.67	10.35
SINANTHROPUS L1	L	441	8.70	12.60	109.62	69.05	10.65
SINANTHROPUS L2	R	442	7.40	10.50	77.70	70.48	8.95
SINANTHROPUS O1	L	447	8.00	11.60	92.80	68.97	9.80
SINANTHROPUS UC	L	449	8.70	11.50	100.05	75.65	10.10

UPPER PM4 H. ERECTUS

		N	L(M-D)	B(B-L)	L*B	L/B	L+B/2
OLDUVAI 16	R	307	8.85	13.80	122.13	64.13	11.32
OLDUVAI 13	R	406	8.70	11.50	100.05	75.65	10.10
PITHECAN. B (4)	L	407	8.50	12.30	104.55	69.11	10.40
PITHECAN. B (4)	R	407	8.20	12.10	99.22	67.77	10.15
RABAT	R	409	8.00	11.00	88.00	72.73	9.50
SINANTHROPUS A1	L	414	7.90	11.30	89.27	69.91	9.60
SINANTHROPUS 20	R	452	8.20	11.70	95.94	70.09	9.95
SINANTHROPUS B1	L	419	8.30	11.20	92.96	74.11	9.75
SINANTHROPUS E1	R	428	7.20	11.20	80.64	64.29	9.20
SINANTHROPUS F2	L	430	8.30	12.10	100.43	68.60	10.20
SINANTHROPUS H3	L	436	7.00	11.00	77.00	63.64	9.00
SINANTHROPUS I1	R	438	7.20	10.30	74.16	69.90	8.75
SINANTHROPUS L1	R	441	7.90	12.50	98.75	63.20	10.20
SINANTHROPUS L2	L	442	7.40	11.20	82.88	66.07	9.30
SINANTHROPUS L2	R	442	7.30	10.80	78.84	67.59	9.05
SINANTHROPUS L4	L	443	8.80	11.70	102.96	75.21	10.25
SINANTHROPUS O1	L	447	7.30	11.10	81.03	65.77	9.20

UPPER M1 H. ERECTUS

		N	L(M-D)	B(B-L)	L*B	L/B	L+B/2
OLDUVAI 16	R	307	13.50	14.70	198.45	91.84	14.10
OLDUVAI 13	R	406	12.50	12.60	157.50	99.21	12.55
PITHECAN. B (4)	L	407	12.30	13.60	167.28	90.44	12.95
PITHECAN. B (4)	R	407	12.10	13.70	165.77	88.32	12.90
RABAT	R	409	12.00	12.00	144.00	100.00	12.00
SINANTHROPUS C2	L	425	13.10				
SINANTHROPUS D1	R	427	11.30	11.70	132.21	96.58	11.50
SINANTHROPUS E1	R	428	10.70	12.20	130.54	87.70	11.45
SINANTHROPUS H3	L	436	10.50	12.00	126.00	87.50	11.25
SINANTHROPUS L1	L	441	12.10	13.40	162.14	90.30	12.75
SINANTHROPUS L2	L	442	10.20	12.30	125.46	82.93	11.25
SINANTHROPUS L2	R	442	10.00	11.70	117.00	85.47	10.85
SINANTHROPUS N1	L	446	11.10	13.70	152.07	81.02	12.40
SINANTHROPUS O1	L	447	10.60	12.40	131.44	85.48	11.50
SINANTHROPUS UC	L	449	11.80	13.00	153.40	90.77	12.40
S. OFFICINALIS		458	12.80	13.70	175.36	93.43	13.25
TERNIFINE 5A		462	12.00	14.40	172.80	83.33	13.20

UPPER M2 H. ERECTUS

		N	L(M-D)	B(B-L)	L*B	L/B	L+B/2
OLDUVAI 16	L	307	12.40	16.30	202.12	76.07	14.35
OLDUVAI 16	R	307	13.30	16.10	214.13	82.61	14.70
OLDUVAI 13	R	406	12.80	13.80	176.64	92.75	13.30
PITHECAN. B (4)	R	407	13.60	15.20	206.72	89.47	14.40
RABAT	R	409	11.50	13.00	149.50	88.46	12.25
SINANTHROPUS A2	R	415	10.50	12.30	129.15	85.37	11.40
SINANTHROPUS B1	L	419	12.20	12.20	148.84	100.00	12.20
SINANTHROPUS B4	L	422	11.10	13.20	146.52	84.09	12.15
SINANTHROPUS D1	R	427	11.40	12.40	141.36	91.94	11.90
SINANTHROPUS E1	R	428	10.00	12.50	125.00	80.00	11.25
SINANTHROPUS H3	L	436	10.00	11.90	119.00	84.03	10.95
SINANTHROPUS L2	L	442	10.20	12.80	130.56	79.69	11.50
SINANTHROPUS L2	R	442	10.30	12.80	131.84	80.47	11.55
SINANTHROPUS O1	L	447	10.60	13.40	142.04	79.10	12.00
SINANTHROPUS UC	L	449	10.00	13.90	139.00	71.94	11.95

UPPER M3 H. ERECTUS

		N	L(M-D)	B(B-L)	L*B	L/B	L+B/2
OLDUVAI 16	L	307	11.70	16.10	188.37	72.67	13.90
OLDUVAI 16	R	307	11.50	16.90	194.35	68.05	14.20
OLDUVAI 13	R	406	12.00	13.10	157.20	91.60	12.55
PITHECAN. B (4)	R	407	10.80	14.00	151.20	77.14	12.40
SANGIRAN 1963	L	412	10.30	12.50	128.75	82.40	11.40
SINANTHROPUS A3	R	416	9.80	12.00	117.60	81.67	10.90
SINANTHROPUS E1	R	428	10.50	11.80	123.90	88.98	11.15
SINANTHROPUS F2	L	430	9.40	11.30	106.22	83.19	10.35
SINANTHROPUS F3	R	431	9.10	10.90	99.19	83.49	10.00
SINANTHROPUS H2	R	435	9.90	12.00	118.80	82.50	10.95
SINANTHROPUS H3	L	436	9.60	11.60	111.36	82.76	10.60
SINANTHROPUS I1	R	438	8.70	10.40	90.48	83.65	9.55
SINANTHROPUS L2	L	442	10.40	12.10	125.84	85.95	11.25
SINANTHROPUS L2	R	442	10.10	12.50	126.25	80.80	11.30
SINANTHROPUS O1	L	447	9.80	12.50	122.50	78.40	11.15
SINANTHROPUS UC	L	449	11.30	15.00	169.50	75.33	13.15
SINANTHROPUS HA		450	9.40	10.50	98.70	89.52	9.95
UBEIDIYA		464	9.60	11.50	110.40	83.48	10.55

LOWER I1 H. NEANDERTAL

		N	L(M-D)	B(B-L)	L*B	L/B	L+B/2
KRAPINA UNTER A	R	507	6.00				
KRAPINA UNTER E	L	511	5.90				
KRAPINA UNTER E	R	511	6.00				
KRAPINA UNTER H	L	514	5.40				
KRAPINA UNTER H	R	514	5.30				
KRAPINA		603	6.20	8.10	50.22	76.54	7.15
KRAPINA		604	7.40	8.20	60.68	90.24	7.80
KRAPINA		605	7.50	8.20	61.50	91.46	7.85
ARCYSLRCURE	R	707	6.00	7.20	43.20	83.33	6.60
EHRINGSCORF CH	L	722	6.40	7.20	46.08	88.89	6.80
EHRINGSCORF CH	R	722	6.30	7.20	45.36	87.50	6.75
EHRINGSFORF AD	L	723	4.50	8.00	36.00	56.25	6.25
LE MOUSTIER	L	746	6.90	7.50	51.75	92.00	7.20
LE MOUSTIER	R	746	6.00	7.20	43.20	83.33	6.60
OCHOZ	L	760	5.00	7.70	38.50	64.94	6.35
OCHOZ	R	760	5.00	7.50	37.50	66.67	6.25
REGOLRCOU	L	764	5.00	7.50	37.50	66.67	6.25
REGOLRCOU	R	764	5.00	7.50	37.50	66.67	6.25
SPIKA	R	776	5.60	7.00	39.20	80.00	6.30
SUBALYUK ADULT	L	782	5.40	7.20	38.88	75.00	6.30
SUBALYUK ADULT	R	782	5.50	7.10	39.05	77.46	6.30
TABUN 1	L	783	5.70				
TABUN 1	R	783	5.70	7.00	39.90	81.43	6.35
TABUN 2	R	784	5.90	8.00	47.20	73.75	6.95
TESHIK TASH	R	809	6.65				
SKHUL 2	L	902	4.50	7.00	31.50	64.29	5.75
SKHUL 4	L	903	4.80	6.50	31.20	73.85	5.65
SKHUL 4	R	903	4.50				
SKHUL 5	L	904	5.00	6.40	32.00	78.12	5.70
SKHUL 5	R	904	5.30				
SKHUL 10	L	907	6.50	7.70	50.05	84.42	7.10

LOWER I2 H. NEANDERTAL

		N	L(M-D)	B(B-L)	L*B	L/B	L+B/2
KRAPINA UNTER B	R	508	6.40				
KRAPINA UNTER C	L	509	7.40				
KRAPINA UNTER D	L	510	6.60				
KRAPINA UNTER E	L	511	7.00	8.30	58.10	84.34	7.65
KRAPINA UNTER H	L	514	6.40				
KRAPINA UNTER H	R	514	6.10				
KRAPINA UNTER I	R	515	7.00	9.10	63.70	76.92	8.05
KRAPINA		606	7.50	8.20	61.50	91.46	7.85
KRAPINA		607	6.60	7.10	46.86	92.96	6.85
KRAPINA		608	7.90	9.00	71.10	87.78	8.45
KRAPINA		609	8.60	10.00	86.00	86.00	9.30
ARCYSURCURE	R	707	7.50	8.20	61.50	91.46	7.85
CIRCEO 3	L	718	6.50				
CIRCEO 3	R	718	7.00				
COMBE GRENAL	R	720	7.80				
EHRINGSDORF CH	L	722	7.20	7.50	54.00	96.00	7.35
EHRINGSDORF CH	R	722	7.30	7.50	54.75	97.33	7.40
EHRINGSFORF AD	L	723	5.80	8.20	47.56	70.73	7.00
JERSEY	R	729	5.80	8.00	46.40	72.50	6.90
LE MOUSTIER	L	746	6.60	7.50	49.50	88.00	7.05
LE MOUSTIER	R	746	6.60	7.80	51.48	84.62	7.20
OCHOZ	L	760	5.50	8.20	45.10	67.07	6.85
OCHOZ	R	760	6.50	8.00	52.00	81.25	7.25
REGOURDOU	L	764	6.00	8.00	48.00	75.00	7.00
REGOURDOU	R	764	6.00	8.00	48.00	75.00	7.00
SHANIDAR 1	L	772		8.20			
SHANIDAR 1	R	772		8.00			
SHANIDAR 3	L	773	6.90	9.00	62.10	76.67	7.95
SHANIDAR 3	R	773	6.90	9.00	62.10	76.67	7.95
SPIKA	L	776	6.50				
SPIKA	R	776	6.00	8.00	48.00	75.00	7.00
SUBALYUK ADULT	L	782	6.80	7.70	52.36	88.31	7.25
SUBALYUK ADULT	R	782	6.90	7.80	53.82	88.46	7.35
TABUN 1	L	783	6.90				
TABUN 1	R	783	6.70	7.60	50.92	88.16	7.15
TABUN 2	L	784	7.00				
TABUN 2	R	784	6.10	8.20	50.02	74.39	7.15
TABUN SERIES 2	R	792	7.20	9.00	64.80	80.00	8.10
TESHIK TASH	R	809	7.15				
SKHUL 4	L	903	6.00				
SKHUL 4	R	903	6.00	7.10	42.60	84.51	6.55
SKHUL 5	L	904	6.60				
SKHUL 5	R	904	6.40	7.00	44.80	91.43	6.70
SKHUL 10	L	907	7.20	8.00	57.60	90.00	7.60

LOWER C H. NEANDERTAL

		N	L(M-D)	B(B-L)	L*B	L/B	L+B/2
KRAPINA UNTER B	R	508	8.00	8.50	68.00	94.12	8.25
KRAPINA UNTER D	L	510	8.00	8.40	67.20	95.24	8.20
KRAPINA UNTER E	L	511	8.30	9.40	78.02	88.30	8.85
KRAPINA UNTER H	L	514	8.20	7.90	64.78	103.80	8.05
KRAPINA UNTER H	R	514	8.00	8.70	69.60	91.95	8.35
KRAPINA UNTER I	L	515	7.80	9.30	72.54	83.87	8.55
KRAPINA UNTER I	R	515	8.50	10.30	87.55	82.52	9.40
KRAPINA		610	8.00	10.00	80.00	80.00	9.00
KRAPINA	R	611	8.40	10.00	84.00	84.00	9.20
KRAPINA		612	8.20	10.00	82.00	82.00	9.10
KRAPINA		613	7.60	8.30	63.08	91.57	7.95
KRAPINA		614	8.20	8.50	69.70	96.47	8.35
KRAPINA		615	8.20	8.20	67.24	100.00	8.20
ARCYSURCURE	L	707	8.10	9.50	76.95	85.26	8.80
ARCYSURCURE	R	707	8.35	10.50	87.67	79.52	9.42
CIRCEO 3	L	718	8.40	8.80	73.92	95.45	8.60
CIRCEO 3	R	718	8.10	9.40	76.14	86.17	8.75
EHRINGSDORF CH	L	722	8.20	8.50	69.70	96.47	8.35
EHRINGSFORF AD	L	723	8.50	8.80	74.80	96.59	8.65
EHRINGSFORF AD	R	723	7.80	9.00	70.20	86.67	8.40
JERSEY	L	729	8.00	10.00	80.00	80.00	9.00
LA FERRASSIE	R	740	5.00	7.50	37.50	66.67	6.25
LA QUINA H5	L	742	8.50	9.00	76.50	94.44	8.75
LE MOUSTIER	L	746	8.00	9.50	76.00	84.21	8.75
LE MOUSTIER	R	746	8.60	9.50	81.70	90.53	9.05
MONSEMPRON B		755	8.00	9.00	72.00	88.89	8.50
OCHOZ	L	760	7.00	9.60	67.20	72.92	8.30
OCHOZ	R	760	7.50	9.50	71.25	78.95	8.50
PETIT PUYMOYEN	L	762	8.50				
REGOURDOU	L	764	7.50	10.00	75.00	75.00	8.75
REGOURDOU	R	764	7.00	10.00	70.00	70.00	8.50
SHANIDAR 3	L	773	7.10	8.20	58.22	86.59	7.65
SHANIDAR 3	R	773	7.10				
SPIKA	R	776	7.00				
SPY 1	L	777	7.30	8.30	60.59	87.95	7.80
SPY 1	R	777	7.50	8.00	60.00	93.75	7.75
SPY 2	R	778	7.50	10.00	75.00	75.00	8.75
SUBALYUK ADULT	L	782	8.00	9.90	79.20	80.81	8.95
SUBALYUK ADULT	R	782	8.00	9.80	78.40	81.63	8.90
TABUN 1	L	783	8.10	8.10	65.61	100.00	8.10
TABUN 1	R	783	8.00	8.30	66.40	96.39	8.15
TABUN 2	L	784	7.80	9.00	70.20	86.67	8.40
TABUN 2	R	784	8.00	9.00	72.00	88.89	8.50
SKHUL 2	L	902	6.90	8.40	57.96	82.14	7.65
SKHUL 2	R	902	6.40	8.20	52.48	78.05	7.30
SKHUL 4	L	903	7.90				
SKHUL 4	R	903	7.30	8.00	58.40	91.25	7.65
SKHUL 5	L	904	8.30	8.90	73.87	93.26	8.60
SKHUL 5	R	904	8.00	9.00	72.00	88.89	8.50
SKHUL 10	L	907	9.10	7.00	63.70	130.00	8.05

LOWER PM3 H. NEANDERTAL

		N	L(M-D)	B(B-L)	L*B	L/B	L+B/2
KRAPINA UNTER B	R	508	8.00				
KRAPINA UNTER D	L	510	8.60	8.80	75.68	97.73	8.70
KRAPINA UNTER E	L	511	8.50	9.20	78.20	92.39	8.85
KRAPINA UNTER H	L	514	7.30	9.00	65.70	81.11	8.15
KRAPINA UNTER H	R	514	7.50	8.70	65.25	86.21	8.10
KRAPINA	L	616	8.10	8.50	68.85	95.29	8.30
KRAPINA		617	8.10	8.50	68.85	95.29	8.30
KRAPINA		618	7.00	9.20	64.40	76.09	8.10
KRAPINA		619	9.00	10.00	90.00	90.00	9.50
KRAPINA		620	9.20	10.00	92.00	92.00	9.60
KRAPINA		621	9.20	8.10	74.52	113.58	8.65
KRAPINA		622	7.80	8.40	65.52	92.86	8.10
KRAPINA		623	8.50	9.30	79.05	91.40	8.90
ARCYSLRCURE		706	8.00	9.00	72.00	88.89	8.50
ARCYSLRCURE	L	707	8.10	9.00	72.90	90.00	8.55
CIRCEO 3	L	718	8.30	9.00	74.70	92.22	8.65
DIREDAWA	R	721	5.00	7.00	35.00	71.43	6.00
EHRINGSDORF CH	L	722	8.30	8.50	70.55	97.65	8.40
EHRINGSFORF AD	L	723	7.80	8.70	67.86	89.66	8.25
EHRINGSFORF AD	R	723	7.30	8.90	64.97	82.02	8.10
JERSEY	L	729	7.80	10.00	78.00	78.00	8.90
L HORTUS		732	10.00	11.30	113.00	88.50	10.65
LA FERRASSIE	R	740	7.00	9.00	63.00	77.78	8.00
LA QUINA H5	L	742	8.30	10.00	83.00	83.00	9.15
LA QUINA H5	R	742	7.20	10.00	72.00	72.00	8.60
LA QUINA 9	L	743	9.00	11.00	99.00	81.82	10.00
LE MOUSTIER	L	746	8.70	8.90	77.43	97.75	8.80
LE MOUSTIER	R	746	8.50	9.20	78.20	92.39	8.85
MAKAPANSGAT	R	749	8.00	8.00	64.00	100.00	8.00
MONSEMPRON B		755	7.50	9.50	71.25	78.95	8.50
OCHOZ	L	760	7.50	9.90	74.25	75.76	8.70
OCHOZ	R	760	7.50	9.60	72.00	78.12	8.55
PETIT PLYMOYEN	L	762	8.30	8.50	70.55	97.65	8.40
RAS EL KELB		763	8.00	9.50	76.00	84.21	8.75
REGOURDOU	L	764	6.50	9.00	58.50	72.22	7.75
REGOURDOU	R	764	7.00	9.00	63.00	77.78	8.00
SHANIDAR 3	L	773	7.20	8.70	62.64	82.76	7.95
SHANIDAR 3	R	773	7.10	7.90	56.09	89.87	7.50
SPIKA	R	776	8.00	8.00	64.00	100.00	8.00
SPY 1	L	777	7.40	8.40	62.16	88.10	7.90
SPY 1	R	777	7.60	8.50	64.60	89.41	8.05
SPY 2	R	778	7.50	9.00	67.50	83.33	8.25
SUBALYUK ADULT	R	782	7.70	9.10	70.07	84.62	8.40
TABUN 1	L	783	7.50	8.00	60.00	93.75	7.75
TABUN 1	R	783	8.00	8.50	68.00	94.12	8.25
TABUN 2	L	784	8.20	9.00	73.80	91.11	8.60
TABUN 2	R	784	7.80	9.00	70.20	86.67	8.40
SKHUL 2	L	902	5.80	7.70	44.66	75.32	6.75
SKHUL 4	L	903	7.60	9.00	68.40	84.44	8.30
SKHUL 4	R	903	7.20	8.00	57.60	90.00	7.60
SKHUL 5	L	904	8.20	9.20	75.44	89.13	8.70
SKHUL 6	L	905	8.90	9.20	81.88	96.74	9.05

LOWER PM4 H. NEANDERTAL

		N	L(M-D)	B(B-L)	L*B	L/B	L+B/2
KRAPINA UNTER D	L	510	8.30	9.70	80.51	85.57	9.00
KRAPINA UNTER E	L	511	8.20	9.00	73.80	91.11	8.60
KRAPINA UNTER F	L	512	8.80	11.00	96.80	80.00	9.90
KRAPINA UNTER H	L	514	7.60	9.00	68.40	84.44	8.30
KRAPINA UNTER H	R	514	7.50	8.90	66.75	84.27	8.20
KRAPINA UNTER I	L	515	7.50	9.30	69.75	80.65	8.40
KRAPINA UNTER I	R	515	7.20	9.30	66.96	77.42	8.25
KRAPINA	L	624	8.40	9.60	80.64	87.50	9.00
KRAPINA		625	8.50	9.90	84.15	85.86	9.20
KRAPINA		626	7.80	8.40	65.52	92.86	8.10
KRAPINA		627	9.20	10.00	92.00	92.00	9.60
KRAPINA		628	7.00	9.30	65.10	75.27	8.15
KRAPINA		629	9.00	10.00	90.00	90.00	9.50
KRAPINA		630	8.10	9.60	77.76	84.37	8.85
ARCYSLRCURE	L	707	7.30	9.70	70.81	75.26	8.50
ARCYSLRCURE	R	707	8.10	11.40	92.34	71.05	9.75
CIRCEO 4	R	719	7.50	8.00	60.00	93.75	7.75
DIREDAWA	R	721	5.50	6.50	35.75	84.62	6.00
EHRINGSDORF CH	L	722	7.50	8.00	60.00	93.75	7.75
EHRINGSFORF AD	L	723	7.00	9.30	65.10	75.27	8.15
EHRINGSFORF AD	R	723	7.30	10.00	73.00	73.00	8.65
JERSEY	L	729	7.00	9.00	63.00	77.78	8.00
L HORTUS		732	10.50	11.30	118.65	92.92	10.90
CROZE DEL DUA	L	739	7.80	8.20	63.96	95.12	8.00
CROZE DEL DUA	R	739	7.60	8.00	60.80	95.00	7.80
LA FERRASSIE	R	740	5.50	8.00	44.00	68.75	6.75
LA QUINA H5	L	742	8.50	10.00	85.00	85.00	9.25
LA QUINA H5	R	742	8.00	10.00	80.00	80.00	9.00
LA QUINA 9	L	743	7.30	9.00	65.70	81.11	8.15
LE MOUSTIER	L	746	8.30	10.20	84.66	81.37	9.25
LE MOUSTIER	R	746	8.20	10.50	86.10	78.10	9.35
LE PLACARD		747	8.40	9.60	80.64	87.50	9.00
MONSEMPRON B		755	8.00	10.00	80.00	80.00	9.00
OCHOZ	L	760	6.50	9.30	60.45	69.89	7.90
OCHOZ	R	760	7.00	9.70	67.90	72.16	8.35
PETIT PUYMOYEN	L	762	7.30	7.50	54.75	97.33	7.40
REGOURDOU	L	764	6.00	8.00	48.00	75.00	7.00
REGOURDOU	R	764	6.00	9.00	54.00	66.67	7.50
SHANIDAR 3	L	773	6.50	9.10	59.15	71.43	7.80
SHANIDAR 3	R	773	6.60	8.50	56.10	77.65	7.55
SPIKA	R	776	7.50	8.00	60.00	93.75	7.75
SPY 1	L	777	7.50	8.10	60.75	92.59	7.80
SPY 1	R	777	7.20	8.00	57.60	90.00	7.60
SPY 2	L	778	7.50	9.00	67.50	83.33	8.25
SPY 2	R	778	7.00	9.00	63.00	77.78	8.00
SUBALYUK ADULT	L	782	7.50	9.00	67.50	83.33	8.25
TABUN 1	L	783	5.70	8.70	49.59	65.52	7.20
TABUN 1	R	783	5.90	8.70	51.33	67.82	7.30
TABUN 2	L	784	7.90	9.50	75.05	83.16	8.70
TABUN 2	R	784	7.90	9.50	75.05	83.16	8.70
VERGISSON 4		813	9.20	8.20	75.44	112.20	8.70
SKHUL 2	L	902	7.20	8.60	61.92	83.72	7.90

LOWER M1 H. NEANDERTAL

		N	L(M-D)	B(B-L)	L*B	L/B	L+B/2
KRAPINA UNTER B	L	508	11.00	10.20	112.20	107.84	10.60
KRAPINA UNTER C	L	509	12.70	11.60	147.32	109.48	12.15
KRAPINA UNTER C	R	509	12.50	11.60	145.00	107.76	12.05
KRAPINA UNTER D	L	510	11.00	10.60	116.60	103.77	10.80
KRAPINA UNTER E	L	511	12.90	12.10	156.09	106.61	12.50
KRAPINA UNTER G	R	513	12.30	11.40	140.22	107.89	11.85
KRAPINA UNTER H	L	514	11.50	11.00	126.50	104.55	11.25
KRAPINA UNTER H	R	514	11.30	10.90	123.17	103.67	11.10
KRAPINA UNTER I	L	515	11.30	11.20	126.56	100.89	11.25
KRAPINA UNTER I	R	515	12.30	12.00	147.60	102.50	12.15
KRAPINA	L	631	13.40	12.40	166.16	108.06	12.90
KRAPINA	L	632	11.50	10.80	124.20	106.48	11.15
KRAPINA	L	633	12.90	11.70	150.93	110.26	12.30
KRAPINA	R	634	12.30	12.00	147.60	102.50	12.15
KRAPINA	R	635	12.40	10.80	133.92	114.81	11.60
KRAPINA		636	13.40	12.20	163.48	109.84	12.80
KRAPINA		637	11.20	10.50	117.60	106.67	10.85
KRAPINA		638	13.60	12.60	171.36	107.94	13.10
KRAPINA		639	11.20	11.00	123.20	101.82	11.10
KRAPINA		640	13.70	12.20	167.14	112.30	12.95
KRAPINA		641	12.00	10.50	126.00	114.29	11.25
KRAPINA		642	13.80	12.40	171.12	111.29	13.10
KRAPINA		643	12.70	11.50	146.05	110.43	12.10
ARCYSLRCURE		706	12.00	11.00	132.00	109.09	11.50
ARCYSLRCURE	L	707	11.00	10.50	115.50	104.76	10.75
ARCYSLRCURE	R	707	10.90	11.80	128.62	92.37	11.35
ARCYSLRCURE B9		713	12.00	10.10	121.20	118.81	11.05
ARCYSLRCURE C15	L	714	12.50	11.50	143.75	108.70	12.00
CIRCEO 3	L	718	11.20	10.00	112.00	112.00	10.60
CIRCEO 3	R	718	10.80	10.50	113.40	102.86	10.65
CIRCEO 4	R	719	10.70	9.60	102.72	111.46	10.15
COMBE GRENAL	R	720	14.00	12.60	176.40	111.11	13.30
DIREDAWA	R	721	9.50	9.00	85.50	105.56	9.25
EHRINGSDORF CH	L	722	12.00	10.50	126.00	114.29	11.25
EHRINGSFORF AD	L	723	11.70	10.90	127.53	107.34	11.30
EHRINGSFORF AD	R	723	11.80	11.00	129.80	107.27	11.40
GIBRALTAR CHILD	L	725	12.50	11.60	145.00	107.76	12.05
LA CHAISE	L	733	12.20	10.60	129.32	115.09	11.40
LA QUINA H5	L	742	12.00	11.50	138.00	104.35	11.75
LA QUINA H5	R	742	12.00	11.50	138.00	104.35	11.75
LA QUINA 9	L	743	11.80	11.90	140.42	99.16	11.85
LE MOUSTIER	L	746	12.40	11.30	140.12	109.73	11.85
LE MOUSTIER	R	746	12.50	11.80	147.50	105.93	12.15
MONTMAURIN	L	759	12.50	10.70	133.75	116.82	11.60
MONTMAURIN	R	759	12.50	10.50	131.25	119.05	11.50
OCHOZ	L	760	12.00	11.20	134.40	107.14	11.60
OCHOZ	R	760	11.50	11.00	126.50	104.55	11.25
PETIT PUYMOYEN	L	762	12.00	10.90	130.80	110.09	11.45
REGOURDOU	L	764	11.00	11.00	121.00	100.00	11.00
REGOURDOU	R	764	11.00	10.50	115.50	104.76	10.75
SHANIDAR 3	L	773	11.30	11.00	124.30	102.73	11.15
SHANIDAR 3	R	773	11.00	11.00	121.00	100.00	11.00

LOWER M1 H. NEANDERTAL

		N	L(M-D)	B(B-L)	L*B	L/B	L+B/2
SHANIDAR 4	R	774	10.10	11.00	111.10	91.82	10.55
SHUKBAH	R	775	11.30	12.70	143.51	88.98	12.00
SPY 1	L	777	11.00	11.00	121.00	100.00	11.00
SPY 1	R	777	11.00	11.00	121.00	100.00	11.00
SPY 2	L	778	11.50	11.80	135.70	97.46	11.65
SPY 2	R	778	11.20	11.70	131.04	95.73	11.45
STAROSELJE	R	779	13.00	11.00	143.00	118.18	12.00
SUBALYUK ADULT	L	782	8.40	10.50	88.20	80.00	9.45
SUBALYUK ADULT	R	782	8.00	10.80	86.40	74.07	9.40
TABUN 1	L	783	10.40	10.20	106.08	101.96	10.30
TABUN 1	R	783	10.00	10.50	105.00	95.24	10.25
TABUN 2	L	784	11.10	11.40	126.54	97.37	11.25
TABUN 2	R	784	11.00	11.00	121.00	100.00	11.00
TABUN SERIES 3	L	798	12.30	11.50	141.45	106.96	11.90
TABUN SERIES 3	R	799	10.80	10.00	108.00	108.00	10.40
TAUBACH	L	807	11.70	9.90	115.83	118.18	10.80
TESHIK TASH	R	809	11.60	11.50	133.40	100.87	11.55
SKHUL 1	R	901	11.60	10.50	121.80	110.48	11.05
SKHUL 4	R	903	11.50	11.20	128.80	102.68	11.35
SKHUL 5	L	904	11.45	11.50	131.67	99.57	11.47
SKHUL 5	R	904	11.30	11.50	129.95	98.26	11.40
SKHUL 7	L	906	10.50				
SKHUL 10	L	907	13.00	11.20	145.60	116.07	12.10

LOWER M2 H. NEANDERTAL

		N	L(M-D)	B(B-L)	L*B	L/B	L+B/2
KRAPINA UNTER C	R	509	13.40	12.00	160.80	111.67	12.70
KRAPINA UNTER E	L	511	12.80	11.50	147.20	111.30	12.15
KRAPINA UNTER G	R	513	12.60	11.40	143.64	110.53	12.00
KRAPINA UNTER H	L	514	11.60	11.50	133.40	100.87	11.55
KRAPINA UNTER H	R	514	12.00	11.50	138.00	104.35	11.75
KRAPINA UNTER I	L	515	11.80	12.50	147.50	94.40	12.15
KRAPINA UNTER I	R	515	12.20	11.40	139.08	107.02	11.80
KRAPINA	R	644	11.00	11.00	121.00	100.00	11.00
KRAPINA	L	645	10.70	10.20	109.14	104.90	10.45
KRAPINA		646	11.30	11.00	124.30	102.73	11.15
KRAPINA		647	12.60	11.60	146.16	108.62	12.10
KRAPINA		648	12.20	11.30	137.86	107.96	11.75
KRAPINA		649	12.10	11.00	133.10	110.00	11.55
KRAPINA		650	11.40	10.60	120.84	107.55	11.00
KRAPINA	L	651	10.30	9.90	101.97	104.04	10.10
KRAPINA		652	13.60	11.40	155.04	119.30	12.50
ARCYSURCURE	L	707	13.70	12.40	169.88	110.48	13.05
ARCYSURCURE	R	707	12.40	11.80	146.32	105.08	12.10
ARCYSURCURE A9		710	12.00	10.10	121.20	118.81	11.05
CIRCEO 2	R	717	11.50	11.00	126.50	104.55	11.25
CIRCEO 3	L	718	12.10	11.00	133.10	110.00	11.55
CIRCEO 3	R	718	11.20	11.00	123.20	101.82	11.10
CIRCEO 4	R	719	11.50	10.00	115.00	115.00	10.75
DIREDAWA	R	721	10.50	10.00	105.00	105.00	10.25
EHRINGSDORF CH	L	722	12.90	10.80	139.32	119.44	11.85
EHRINGSDORF AD	L	723	13.00	11.50	149.50	113.04	12.25
EHRINGSDORF AD	R	723	12.30	10.80	132.84	113.89	11.55
EL WAD	R	724	10.10	10.10	102.01	100.00	10.10
GIBRALTAR CHILD	L	725	11.80	10.10	119.18	116.83	10.95
HAUA FTEAH 1	R	727	11.70	11.40	133.38	102.63	11.55
JERSEY	L	729	12.00	11.80	141.60	101.69	11.90
JERSEY	R	729	12.00	11.50	138.00	104.35	11.75
LA CHAISE	L	733		11.00			
LA QUINA H5	L	742	12.30	12.00	147.60	102.50	12.15
LA QUINA H5	R	742	12.50	12.00	150.00	104.17	12.25
LA QUINA 9	L	743	12.50	12.00	150.00	104.17	12.25
LA VERRERIE		744	12.00	11.00	132.00	109.09	11.50
LE MOUSTIER	L	746	13.00	11.30	146.90	115.04	12.15
LE MOUSTIER	R	746	12.50	11.30	141.25	110.62	11.90
MAKAPANSGAT	R	749	11.50	10.70	123.05	107.48	11.10
MONTMAURIN	L	759	12.50	11.00	137.50	113.64	11.75
MONTMAURIN	R	759	12.00	11.00	132.00	109.09	11.50
OCHOZ	L	760	12.00	11.50	138.00	104.35	11.75
OCHOZ	R	760	12.00	12.20	146.40	98.36	12.10
PETIT PLYMOYEN	L	762	12.00	12.60	151.20	95.24	12.30
REGOURDOU	L	764	10.50	11.00	115.50	95.45	10.75
REGOURDOU	R	764	11.00	11.00	121.00	100.00	11.00
SHANIDAR 3	L	773	12.00	11.20	134.40	107.14	11.60
SHANIDAR 3	R	773	11.00	11.20	123.20	98.21	11.10
SHANIDAR 4	R	774	13.00	12.00	156.00	108.33	12.50
SHUKBAH	R	775	13.50	12.00	162.00	112.50	12.75
SPY 1	L	777	11.00	11.00	121.00	100.00	11.00
SPY 1	R	777	11.00	11.00	121.00	100.00	11.00
SPY 2	L	778	11.50	11.70	134.55	98.29	11.60
SPY 2	R	778	11.20	11.30	126.56	99.12	11.25
SUBALYUK ADULT	L	782	10.80	11.20	120.96	96.43	11.00
SUBALYUK ADULT	R	782		11.40			
TABUN 1	L	783	11.50	10.80	124.20	106.48	11.15
TABUN 1	R	783	11.20	10.60	118.72	105.66	10.90
TABUN 2	L	784	11.20	11.00	123.20	101.82	11.10
TABUN 2	R	784	10.80	11.00	118.80	98.18	10.90
SKHUL 2	L	902	11.30	10.00	113.00	113.00	10.65
SKHUL 4	R	903	10.50	10.70	112.35	98.13	10.60
SKHUL 5	L	904	12.60	11.65	146.79	108.15	12.12
SKHUL 5	R	904	11.60	11.40	132.24	101.75	11.50
SKHUL 7	L	906	10.00	11.00	110.00	90.91	10.50
SKHUL 7	R	906	9.50	10.50	99.75	90.48	10.00

LOWER M2 H. NEANDERTAL

LOWER M3 H. NEANDERTAL

		N	L(M-D)	B(B-L)	L*B	L/B	L+B/2
KRAPINA UNTER G	R	513	11.60	11.00	127.60	105.45	11.30
KRAPINA UNTER H	L	514	12.00	10.50	126.00	114.29	11.25
KRAPINA UNTER H	R	514	12.20	10.80	131.76	112.96	11.50
KRAPINA UNTER I	R	515	11.80	10.90	128.62	108.26	11.35
KRAPINA	R	653	12.00	11.00	132.00	109.09	11.50
KRAPINA	R	654	12.50	11.00	137.50	113.64	11.75
KRAPINA	R	655	11.10	9.90	109.89	112.12	10.50
KRAPINA	R	656	13.00	12.00	156.00	108.33	12.50
KRAPINA		657	11.20	11.00	123.20	101.82	11.10
KRAPINA		658	12.10	11.40	137.94	106.14	11.75
KRAPINA		659	11.70	11.20	131.04	104.46	11.45
KRAPINA		660	13.60				
KRAPINA		661	11.30	10.60	119.78	106.60	10.95
KRAPINA		662	12.70	11.00	139.70	115.45	11.85
KRAPINA		663	11.10	10.00	111.00	111.00	10.55
ARCYSURCURE	R	707	12.00	12.70	152.40	94.49	12.35
ARCYSURCURE A9		709	12.10	10.50	127.05	115.24	11.30
CIRCEO 3	L	718	11.00	10.70	117.70	102.80	10.85
CIRCEO 3	R	718	11.60	11.00	127.60	105.45	11.30
DIRECAWA	R	721	10.00	9.00	90.00	111.11	9.50
EHRINGSDORF CH	L	722	8.30	8.50	70.55	97.65	8.40
EHRINGSFORF AD	L	723	9.50	8.00	76.00	118.75	8.75
EHRINGSFORF AD	R	723	10.20	9.70	98.94	105.15	9.95
HAUA FTEAH 1	R	727	10.60	10.80	114.48	98.15	10.70
JERSEY	R	729	13.00	12.00	156.00	108.33	12.50
LA QUINA H5	L	742	11.50	13.00	149.50	88.46	12.25
LA QUINA H5	R	742	11.50	13.00	149.50	88.46	12.25
LA QUINA 9	L	743	12.60	12.70	160.02	99.21	12.65
LE MOUSTIER	L	746	12.80	11.40	145.92	112.28	12.10
LE MOUSTIER	R	746	13.00	12.00	156.00	108.33	12.50
MONTMAURIN	L	759	13.00	11.00	143.00	118.18	12.00
MONTMAURIN	R	759	13.00	10.70	139.10	121.50	11.85
OCHOZ	L	760	12.00	12.00	144.00	100.00	12.00
REGOURDOU	L	764	11.00	11.00	121.00	100.00	11.00
REGOURDOU	R	764	12.00	11.00	132.00	109.09	11.50
SHANIDAR 3	L	773	12.00	11.00	132.00	109.09	11.50
SHANIDAR 3	R	773	11.00	10.70	117.70	102.80	10.85
SHANIDAR 4	R	774	13.00	12.00	156.00	108.33	12.50
SPY 1	L	777	11.00	10.60	116.60	103.77	10.80
SPY 1	R	777	10.20	11.00	112.20	92.73	10.60
SPY 2	L	778	12.20	11.80	143.96	103.39	12.00
SPY 2	R	778	11.40	11.70	133.38	97.44	11.55
SUBALYUK ADULT	L	782	12.00	11.30	135.60	106.19	11.65
SUBALYUK ADULT	R	782	11.00	11.30	124.30	97.35	11.15
TABUN 1	L	783	10.90	9.80	106.82	111.22	10.35
TABUN 1	R	783	10.30	10.30	106.09	100.00	10.30
TABUN 2	L	784	11.10	9.30	103.23	119.35	10.20
TABUN 2	R	784	11.50	10.80	124.20	106.48	11.15
TABUN SERIES 3	R	797	11.10	9.70	107.67	114.43	10.40
VERGISSON 3	R	812	11.90	11.40	135.66	104.39	11.65
SKHUL 4	R	903	10.60	9.90	104.94	107.07	10.25
SKHUL 5	L	904	11.70	10.95	128.11	106.85	11.32

LOWER M3 H. NEANDERTAL

		N	L(M-D)	B(B-L)	L*B	L/B	L+B/2
SKHUL 5	R	904	11.40	10.50	119.70	108.57	10.95
SKHUL 7	L	906	10.30	10.10	104.03	101.98	10.20
SKHUL 7	R	906	10.70	10.10	108.07	105.94	10.40

UPPER I1 H. NEANDERTAL

		N	L(M-D)	B(B-L)	L*B	L/B	L+B/2
KRAPINA OBER B	L	502	10.00	9.35	93.50	106.95	9.67
KRAPINA OBER B	R	502	10.10	9.20	92.92	109.78	9.65
KRAPINA OBER E	L	505	9.40	8.10	76.14	116.05	8.75
KRAPINA OBER E	R	505	10.00	8.20	82.00	121.95	9.10
KRAPINA OBER F	R	506	9.40	8.80	82.72	106.82	9.10
KRAPINA		543	10.00	9.40	94.00	106.38	9.70
KRAPINA		544	11.00	9.40	103.40	117.02	10.20
KRAPINA		545	10.80	9.40	101.52	114.89	10.10
KRAPINA		546	10.40	8.90	92.56	116.85	9.65
KRAPINA		547	9.90	8.00	79.20	123.75	8.95
KRAPINA		548	10.00	8.10	81.00	123.46	9.05
KRAPINA		549	10.00				
KRAPINA		550	10.40	8.90	92.56	116.85	9.65
KRAPINA		551	10.50				
KRAPINA		552	11.00	9.50	104.50	115.79	10.25
ARCYSURCURE	L	708	9.50	8.00	76.00	118.75	8.75
ARCYSURCURE	R	708	9.40	8.10	76.14	116.05	8.75
ARCYSURCURE B7		712	9.50	8.00	76.00	118.75	8.75
EHRINGSDORF CH	L	722	10.00	8.30	83.00	120.48	9.15
GIBRALTAR ADULT		726	9.20				
LA QUINA CHILD	L	741	10.90				
LA QUINA CHILD	R	741	11.00				
LA QUINA H5	L	742	9.00	8.50	76.50	105.88	8.75
LA VIENNE		745	9.00	8.40	75.60	107.14	8.70
LE MOUSTIER	L	746	11.50	8.00	92.00	143.75	9.75
LE MOUSTIER	R	746	12.00	8.00	96.00	150.00	10.00
MONSEMPRON C		756	9.00	8.50	76.50	105.88	8.75
RHODESIAN 1	L	765	8.00	8.50	68.00	94.12	8.25
RHODESIAN 1	R	765	8.00	8.50	68.00	94.12	8.25
ST BRAIS 2	R	769	10.30	8.60	88.58	119.77	9.45
SHANIDAR 3	L	773	8.20				
TABUN 1	R	783	9.00	8.20	73.80	109.76	8.60
TABUN SERIES 3	L	796	9.20	8.20	75.44	112.20	8.70
TESHIK TASH	L	809	11.10	10.60	117.66	104.72	10.85
TESHIK TASH	R	809	10.80	10.20	110.16	105.88	10.50
SKHUL 1	R	901	10.90	8.70	94.83	125.29	9.80
SKHUL 4	L	903	9.50				
SKHUL 4	R	903	10.00	8.20	82.00	121.95	9.10
SKHUL 5	L	904	8.40	7.50	63.00	112.00	7.95
SKHUL 5	R	904	8.50	7.50	63.75	113.33	8.00
SKHUL 7	L	906	9.20	8.20	75.44	112.20	8.70

UPPER I2 H. NEANDERTAL

		N	L(M-D)	B(B-L)	L*B	L/B	L+B/2
KRAPINA OBER B	R	502	8.30	9.60	79.68	86.46	8.95
KRAPINA OBER C	R	503	8.20	9.55	78.31	85.86	8.87
KRAPINA OBER E	R	505	8.55	8.30	70.96	103.01	8.42
KRAPINA OBER F	R	506	8.50	9.10	77.35	93.41	8.80
KRAPINA		553	8.70				
KRAPINA		554	8.30	9.00	74.70	92.22	8.65
KRAPINA		555	8.20	9.00	73.80	91.11	8.60
KRAPINA		556	9.00	11.20	100.80	80.36	10.10
KRAPINA		557	8.40	8.20	68.88	102.44	8.30
KRAPINA		558	8.20	6.00	49.20	136.67	7.10
KRAPINA		559	8.30	9.00	74.70	92.22	8.65
KRAPINA		560	8.60	8.90	76.54	96.63	8.75
ARCYSURCURE	L	708	6.30	8.10	51.03	77.78	7.20
ARCYSURCURE	R	708	7.10	8.10	57.51	87.65	7.60
ARCYSURCURE D4		711	7.30	7.50	54.75	97.33	7.40
EHRINGSDORF CH	L	722	8.80				
GIBRALTAR ADULT		726	6.00				
LA QUINA CHILD	R	741	8.00				
LA QUINA H5	L	742	8.50	9.00	76.50	94.44	8.75
LE MOUSTIER	L	746	8.50	9.00	76.50	94.44	8.75
LE MOUSTIER	R	746	9.00	9.00	81.00	100.00	9.00
MONSEMPRON H		758	8.00	9.00	72.00	88.89	8.50
RHODESIAN 1	L	765	7.00	8.00	56.00	87.50	7.50
SHANIDAR 3	R	773	7.30				
SPY 1	R	777	7.00	8.00	56.00	87.50	7.50
TABUN 1	L	783	7.30	7.70	56.21	94.81	7.50
TABUN SERIES 1	R	785	7.40	7.80	57.72	94.87	7.60
TABUN SERIES 2	L	791	8.10	8.80	71.28	92.05	8.45
TABUN SERIES 3	L	800	7.40	7.90	58.46	93.67	7.65
TESHIK TASH	L	809	9.00	9.95	89.55	90.45	9.47
TESHIK TASH	R	809	8.65	9.15	79.15	94.54	8.90
SKHUL 1	R	901	8.80	6.20	54.56	141.94	7.50
SKHUL 4	L	903	6.20	7.20	44.64	86.11	6.70
SKHUL 5	L	904	6.40	7.70	49.28	83.12	7.05
SKHUL 5	R	904	7.00	7.20	50.40	97.22	7.10
SKHUL 7	L	906	6.80	8.00	54.40	85.00	7.40

UPPER C H. NEANDERTAL

		N	L(M-D)	B(B-L)	L*B	L/B	L+B/2
KRAPINA OBER B	L	502	9.00	10.55	94.95	85.31	9.77
KRAPINA OBER E	R	505	9.30	9.30	86.49	100.00	9.30
KRAPINA		561	8.00				
KRAPINA		562	9.00	9.60	86.40	93.75	9.30
KRAPINA		563	9.00	10.60	95.40	84.91	9.80
KRAPINA		564	8.40	9.30	78.12	90.32	8.85
KRAPINA		565	8.90	10.50	93.45	84.76	9.70
KRAPINA		566	10.50	11.30	118.65	92.92	10.90
KRAPINA	L	567	9.20	10.00	92.00	92.00	9.60
KRAPINA		568	9.80	10.50	102.90	93.33	10.15
KRAPINA		569	9.20	9.90	91.08	92.93	9.55
AFRICANTHROPUS		704	9.00	9.00	81.00	100.00	9.00
ARCYSURCURE	L	708	8.60	9.90	85.14	86.87	9.25
ARCYSURCURE	R	708	7.70	10.00	77.00	77.00	8.85
GIBRALTAR ADULT		726	7.50				
JEBEL IRHOUND	R	728	9.00	10.00	90.00	90.00	9.50
CROZE DEL DUA	L	736	7.60	8.60	65.36	88.37	8.10
LA FERRASSIE	L	740	6.80	11.20	76.16	60.71	9.00
LA FERRASSIE	R	740	6.50				
LA QUINA H5	L	742	8.50	10.00	85.00	85.00	9.25
LA QUINA H5	R	742	9.00	10.00	90.00	90.00	9.50
LE MOUSTIER	L	746	9.00	10.00	90.00	90.00	9.50
LE MOUSTIER	R	746	9.00	10.00	90.00	90.00	9.50
MONSEMPRON H		758	9.00	9.50	85.50	94.74	9.25
RHODESIAN 1	L	765	10.00	11.00	110.00	90.91	10.50
SACCOPASTORE 2	L	768	8.00	9.20	73.60	86.96	8.60
SACCOPASTORE 2	R	768	8.00	9.20	73.60	86.96	8.60
SHANIDAR 1	R	772	7.70	10.70	82.39	71.96	9.20
SHANIDAR 3	R	773	8.10	8.50	68.85	95.29	8.30
SHANIDAR 4	R	774	7.00	10.00	70.00	70.00	8.50
SPY 1	L	777	7.50	9.00	67.50	83.33	8.25
SPY 1	R	777	7.00	8.00	56.00	87.50	7.50
SPY 2	R	778	8.00	10.00	80.00	80.00	9.00
TABUN 1	R	783	7.90	8.80	69.52	89.77	8.35
TABUN SERIES 1	R	790	8.20	8.90	72.98	92.13	8.55
TANGIER 1	L	805	8.20	10.90	89.38	75.23	9.55
SKHUL 1	L	901	8.70	8.00	69.60	108.75	8.35
SKHUL 2	R	902	7.50	9.00	67.50	83.33	8.25
SKHUL 4	R	903	8.90	8.50	75.65	104.71	8.70
SKHUL 5	L	904	9.20	10.00	92.00	92.00	9.60
SKHUL 5	R	904	8.70	9.50	82.65	91.58	9.10
SKHUL 6	L	905	8.00	9.60	76.80	83.33	8.80

UPPER PM3 H. NEANDERTAL

		N	L(M-D)	B(B-L)	L*B	L/B	L+B/2
KRAPINA OBER D	L	504	8.50	12.00	102.00	70.83	10.25
KRAPINA OBER E	R	505	8.00	10.10	80.80	79.21	9.05
KRAPINA		570	8.00	11.40	91.20	70.18	9.70
KRAPINA		571	8.30	11.40	94.62	72.81	9.85
KRAPINA		572	8.10	10.20	82.62	79.41	9.15
KRAPINA		573	8.20	10.40	85.28	78.85	9.30
AFRICANTHROPUS		703	7.90	10.40	82.16	75.96	9.15
ARCYSLRCURE	L	708	7.10	10.40	73.84	68.27	8.75
ARCYSLRCURE	R	708	7.25	10.00	72.50	72.50	8.62
GIBRALTAR ADULT		726	6.50				
JEBEL IRHOUND	R	728	7.00	11.00	77.00	63.64	9.00
LA FERRASSIE	L	740	6.50	10.00	65.00	65.00	8.25
LA FERRASSIE	R	740	6.30	9.00	56.70	70.00	7.65
LA QUINA H5	L	742	9.00	11.00	99.00	81.82	10.00
LA QUINA H5	R	742	8.30	11.20	92.96	74.11	9.75
LE MOLSTIER	L	746	8.00	10.50	84.00	76.19	9.25
LE MOLSTIER	R	746	8.00	10.50	84.00	76.19	9.25
MONSEMPRON H		758	8.00	11.00	88.00	72.73	9.50
RHODESIAN 1	L	765	7.50	11.00	82.50	68.18	9.25
SACCOPASTORE 2	L	768	7.00	10.00	70.00	70.00	8.50
SHANICAR 1	R	772	8.30	12.00	99.60	69.17	10.15
SHANICAR 3	L	773	7.50	10.40	78.00	72.12	8.95
SHANICAR 3	R	773	7.50	10.30	77.25	72.82	8.90
SHANICAR 4	R	774	6.50	10.00	65.00	65.00	8.25
SPY 1	R	777	7.00	9.80	68.60	71.43	8.40
SPY 2	R	778	7.50	10.50	78.75	71.43	9.00
TABUN 1	R	783	7.50	9.80	73.50	76.53	8.65
TABUN SERIES 1	R	789	7.40	10.10	74.74	73.27	8.75
TABUN SERIES 2	R	795	8.40	10.50	88.20	80.00	9.45
TANGIER 1	L	805	7.70	10.30	79.31	74.76	9.00
TESHIK TASH	R	809		9.20			
SKHUL 4	L	903	6.20	10.30	63.86	60.19	8.25
SKHUL 4	R	903	7.40	10.00	74.00	74.00	8.70
SKHUL 5	L	904	8.20	11.20	91.84	73.21	9.70
SKHUL 5	R	904	8.20	10.80	88.56	75.93	9.50
SKHUL 1C	R	907	8.70	10.50	91.35	82.86	9.60

UPPER PM4 H. NEANDERTAL

		N	L(M-D)	B(B-L)	L*B	L/B	L+B/2
KRAPINA OBER D	L	504	7.60	11.20	85.12	67.86	9.40
KRAPINA OBER E	R	505	8.10	10.50	85.05	77.14	9.30
KRAPINA		574	8.10	10.20	82.62	79.41	9.15
KRAPINA		575	8.30	11.30	93.79	73.45	9.80
KRAPINA		576	8.00	10.40	83.20	76.92	9.20
KRAPINA		577	8.60	11.60	99.76	74.14	10.10
KRAPINA		578	8.20	11.10	91.02	73.87	9.65
ARCYSLRCURE	L	708	6.80	10.30	70.04	66.02	8.55
ARCYSLRCURE	R	708	7.40	10.50	77.70	70.48	8.95
GIBRALTAR ADULT		726	6.00				
JEBEL IRHOUND	R	728	9.00	11.00	99.00	81.82	10.00
JERSEY	L	729	6.50	11.20	72.80	58.04	8.85
LA FERRASSIE	L	740	6.00	9.50	57.00	63.16	7.75
LA FERRASSIE	R	740	6.00	9.70	58.20	61.86	7.85
LA QUINA H5	L	742	7.30	10.50	76.65	69.52	8.90
LA QUINA H5	R	742	8.00	10.60	84.80	75.47	9.30
LE MOLSTIER	L	746	8.00	11.00	88.00	72.73	9.50
LE MOLSTIER	R	746	8.00	11.00	88.00	72.73	9.50
MONSEMPRON H		758	8.00	10.50	84.00	76.19	9.25
SACCOPASTORE 1	L	767	6.10	9.40	57.34	64.89	7.75
SACCOPASTORE 2	L	768	6.30	9.20	57.96	68.48	7.75
SACCOPASTORE 2	R	768	6.50	9.00	58.50	72.22	7.75
SHANICAR 1	R	772	7.50	11.70	87.75	64.10	9.60
SHANICAR 3	L	773	7.20	11.10	79.92	64.86	9.15
SHANICAR 3	R	773	6.50	10.40	67.60	62.50	8.45
SHANICAR 4	L	774	6.60	10.50	69.30	62.86	8.55
SHANICAR 4	R	774	6.20	10.70	66.34	57.94	8.45
SPY 1	R	777	6.30	9.80	61.74	64.29	8.05
SPY 2	R	778	7.30	10.80	78.84	67.59	9.05
STEINHEIM	R	780	7.10	9.30	66.03	76.34	8.20
TABUN 1	R	783	6.50	9.60	62.40	67.71	8.05
TABUN SERIES 1	R	788	7.20	9.70	69.84	74.23	8.45
SKHUL 2	R	902	7.00	11.00	77.00	63.64	9.00
SKHUL 4	L	903	7.50	8.40	63.00	89.29	7.95
SKHUL 5	L	904	7.60	10.75	81.70	70.70	9.17
SKHUL 5	R	904	7.00	10.80	75.60	64.81	8.90

UPPER M1 H. NEANDERTAL

		N	L(M-D)	B(B-L)	L*B	L/B	L+B/2
KRAPINA OBER B	L	502	12.40	12.00	148.80	103.33	12.20
KRAPINA OBER B	R	502	12.50	12.00	150.00	104.17	12.25
KRAPINA OBER C	L	503	13.40	13.20	176.88	101.52	13.30
KRAPINA OBER D	L	504	11.60	12.30	142.68	94.31	11.95
KRAPINA	R	579	10.00	11.60	116.00	86.21	10.80
KRAPINA	L	580	11.80	11.50	135.70	102.61	11.65
KRAPINA	L	581	11.00	12.00	132.00	91.67	11.50
KRAPINA	R	582	11.00	12.50	137.50	88.00	11.75
KRAPINA	L	583	11.20	12.40	138.88	90.32	11.80
KRAPINA	R	584	13.30	13.00	172.90	102.31	13.15
KRAPINA	L	585	13.00	13.40	174.20	97.01	13.20
KRAPINA		586	11.60	12.50	145.00	92.80	12.05
KRAPINA		587	12.60	15.00	189.00	84.00	13.80
KRAPINA		588	12.30	10.70	131.61	114.95	11.50
AFRICANTHROPUS		702	11.50	13.00	149.50	88.46	12.25
ARCYSURCURE	L	708	9.80	11.40	111.72	85.96	10.60
ARCYSURCURE	R	708	9.70	11.20	108.64	86.61	10.45
ARCYSURCURE C20	R	715	10.00	13.00	130.00	76.92	11.50
JERSEY	R	729	11.00	12.40	136.40	88.71	11.70
KSAR AKIL	R	730	12.00	11.00	132.00	109.09	11.50
BAMBINO		731	9.80	11.00	107.80	89.09	10.40
LA CHAPELLE		734	10.00	12.00	120.00	83.33	11.00
CROZE DEL DUA	R	735	10.80	11.20	120.96	96.43	11.00
LA FERRASSIE	L	740	8.20	12.60	103.32	65.08	10.40
LA FERRASSIE	R	740	7.20	12.00	86.40	60.00	9.60
LA QUINA CHILD	L	741	12.30	12.00	147.60	102.50	12.15
LA QUINA CHILD	R	741	12.00	12.00	144.00	100.00	12.00
LA QUINA H5	L	742	10.50	13.00	136.50	80.77	11.75
LA QUINA H5	R	742	10.50	12.50	131.25	84.00	11.50
LE MOUSTIER	L	746	12.00	12.50	150.00	96.00	12.25
LE MOUSTIER	R	746	12.00	12.50	150.00	96.00	12.25
MERIDIONALE D	L	754	12.10	12.10	146.41	100.00	12.10
MONSEMPRON H		758	11.00	12.00	132.00	91.67	11.50
PECH DE L AZE	R	761	12.50	11.60	145.00	107.76	12.05
RHODESIAN 1	R	765	14.00	13.50	189.00	103.70	13.75
SACCOPASTORE 1	L	767	11.30	12.20	137.86	92.62	11.75
SACCOPASTORE 2	L	768	10.00	11.00	110.00	90.91	10.50
SACCOPASTORE 2	R	768	10.00	11.50	115.00	86.96	10.75
SHANIDAR 1	L	772	11.70	11.70	136.89	100.00	11.70
SHANIDAR 1	R	772	12.00	12.50	150.00	96.00	12.25
SHANIDAR 3	L	773	10.50	12.00	126.00	87.50	11.25
SHANIDAR 3	R	773	10.50	12.00	126.00	87.50	11.25
SHANIDAR 4	L	774	11.00	12.00	132.00	91.67	11.50
SHANIDAR 4	R	774	11.00	12.00	132.00	91.67	11.50
SPY 1	R	777	9.50	11.00	104.50	86.36	10.25
SPY 2	R	778	12.30	12.30	151.29	100.00	12.30
STAROSELJE	R	779	12.30	11.40	140.22	107.89	11.85
STEINHEIM	L	780	11.80	12.50	147.50	94.40	12.15
STEINHEIM	R	780	12.30	11.50	141.45	106.96	11.90
TABUN 1	L	783	10.80	11.50	124.20	93.91	11.15
TABUN SERIES 1	R	786	10.10	11.40	115.14	88.60	10.75
TABUN SERIES 1	R	787	11.20	11.30	126.56	99.12	11.25

UPPER M1 H. NEANDERTAL

		N	L(M-D)	B(B-L)	L*B	L/B	L+B/2
TABUN SERIES 2	R	793	11.80	12.30	145.14	95.93	12.05
TABUN SERIES 2	L	794	13.10	9.30	121.83	140.86	11.20
TANGIER 1	L	805	11.70	13.70	160.29	85.40	12.70
TESHIK TASH	L	809	12.45	12.70	158.11	98.03	12.57
TESHIK TASH	R	809	12.80	12.30	157.44	104.07	12.55
SKHUL 1	R	901	12.40	11.30	140.12	109.73	11.85
SKHUL 2	R	902	9.90	11.70	115.83	84.62	10.80
SKHUL 4	L	903	11.30	12.30	138.99	91.87	11.80
SKHUL 4	R	903	11.00	12.50	137.50	88.00	11.75
SKHUL 5	L	904	11.35	12.40	140.74	91.53	11.87
SKHUL 5	R	904	11.00	12.50	137.50	88.00	11.75
SKHUL 6	R	905	11.50	12.20	140.30	94.26	11.85
SKHUL 7	R	906	10.70	11.20	119.84	95.54	10.95
SKHUL 10	R	907	12.00	12.50	150.00	96.00	12.25

UPPER M2 H. NEANDERTAL

		N	L(M-D)	B(B-L)	L*B	L/B	L+B/2
KRAPINA OBER C	L	503	11.40	13.30	151.62	85.71	12.35
KRAPINA OBER D	L	504	10.30	10.60	109.18	97.17	10.45
KRAPINA	L	589	11.30	12.30	138.99	91.87	11.80
KRAPINA	L	590	10.10	11.20	113.12	90.18	10.65
KRAPINA	R	591	12.00	14.00	168.00	85.71	13.00
KRAPINA	R	592	10.20	12.90	131.58	79.07	11.55
KRAPINA		593	11.50	12.30	141.45	93.50	11.90
KRAPINA		594	9.80	12.90	126.42	75.97	11.35
KRAPINA		595	11.80	13.20	155.76	89.39	12.50
KRAPINA		596	8.35	11.30	94.35	73.89	9.82
KRAPINA		597	10.50	13.10	137.55	80.15	11.80
AFRICANTHROPUS		701	10.00	12.10	121.00	82.64	11.05
AFRICANTHROPUS		705	11.50	12.30	141.45	93.50	11.90
ARCYSURCURE	L	708	9.50	13.00	123.50	73.08	11.25
JERSEY	L	729	10.50	13.50	141.75	77.78	12.00
LA FERRASSIE	L	740	9.50	11.90	113.05	79.83	10.70
LA FERRASSIE	R	740	9.50	12.50	118.75	76.00	11.00
LA QUINA CHILD	R	741	9.60	13.60	130.56	70.59	11.60
LA QUINA H5	L	742	10.00	14.00	140.00	71.43	12.00
LA QUINA H5	R	742	10.00	14.00	140.00	71.43	12.00
LE MOUSTIER	L	746	11.50	13.00	149.50	88.46	12.25
LE MOUSTIER	R	746	11.50	13.00	149.50	88.46	12.25
MALTA	R	750	12.00	13.00	156.00	92.31	12.50
MONSEMPRON D		757	11.00	14.50	159.50	75.86	12.75
MONSEMPRON H		758	11.00	13.00	143.00	84.62	12.00
RHODESIAN 1	L	765	13.00	14.00	182.00	92.86	13.50
RHODESIAN 1	R	765	12.20	13.50	164.70	90.37	12.85
RHODESIAN 2	R	766	12.00				
SACCOPASTORE 1	L	767	11.10	11.70	129.87	94.87	11.40
SACCOPASTORE 2	L	768	9.00	11.20	100.80	80.36	10.10
SACCOPASTORE 2	R	768	10.00	11.50	115.00	86.96	10.75
SHANICAR 1	L	772	10.70	12.20	130.54	87.70	11.45
SHANICAR 1	R	772	10.50	12.50	131.25	84.00	11.50
SHANICAR 3	L	773	10.50	12.50	131.25	84.00	11.50
SHANICAR 3	R	773	10.50	12.50	131.25	84.00	11.50
SHANICAR 4	L	774	11.00	12.50	137.50	88.00	11.75
SHANICAR 4	R	774	11.00	13.00	143.00	84.62	12.00
SPY 1	R	777	9.50	11.00	104.50	86.36	10.25
SPY 2	R	778	10.80	12.80	138.24	84.37	11.80
STEINHEIM	L	780	10.80	12.50	135.00	86.40	11.65
STEINHEIM	R	780	11.30	10.00	113.00	113.00	10.65
TABUN 1	R	783	10.50	11.70	122.85	89.74	11.10
TANGIER 2	L	806	11.70	13.70	160.29	85.40	12.70
SKHUL 2	R	902	9.60	11.50	110.40	83.48	10.55
SKHUL 4	L	903	9.30	11.10	103.23	83.78	10.20
SKHUL 4	R	903	9.90	12.20	120.78	81.15	11.05
SKHUL 5	L	904	11.30	11.70	132.21	96.58	11.50
SKHUL 5	R	904	10.80	12.20	131.76	88.52	11.50
SKHUL 7	L	906	9.00	12.30	110.70	73.17	10.65
SKHUL 7	R	906	8.60	12.00	103.20	71.67	10.30
SKHUL 10	R	907	12.20	12.00	146.40	101.67	12.10

UPPER M3 H. NEANDERTAL

		N	L(M-D)	B(B-L)	L*B	L/B	L+B/2
KRAPINA		598	10.00	12.50	125.00	80.00	11.25
KRAPINA		599	10.00	12.50	125.00	80.00	11.25
KRAPINA	L	600	10.20	12.50	127.50	81.60	11.35
KRAPINA	L	601	10.20	12.50	127.50	81.60	11.35
KRAPINA	R	602	12.20	12.00	146.40	101.67	12.10
JERSEY	L	729	9.20	12.30	113.16	74.80	10.75
JERSEY	R	729	9.30	13.20	122.76	70.45	11.25
CROZE DEL DUA	R	737	8.80	11.60	102.08	75.86	10.20
CROZE DEL DUA	R	738	10.10	11.60	117.16	87.07	10.85
LA FERRASSIE	L	740	9.70	11.30	109.61	85.84	10.50
LA FERRASSIE	R	740	8.70	11.00	95.70	79.09	9.85
LA QUINA H5	L	742	9.60	13.50	129.60	71.11	11.55
LA QUINA H5	R	742		14.00			
LE MOUSTIER	L	746	9.00	11.00	99.00	81.82	10.00
LE MOUSTIER	R	746	11.00	12.00	132.00	91.67	11.50
MALTA	R	750	10.70	13.00	139.10	82.31	11.85
RHODESIAN 1	L	765	9.00	12.00	108.00	75.00	10.50
RHODESIAN 2	R	766	10.00	12.00	120.00	83.33	11.00
SACCOPASTORE 1	L	767	8.50	9.60	81.60	88.54	9.05
SACCOPASTORE 2	L	768	8.70	10.90	94.83	79.82	9.80
SACCOPASTORE 2	R	768	9.00	11.20	100.80	80.36	10.10
SHANICAR 1	L	772	10.80	12.30	132.84	87.80	11.55
SHANICAR 1	R	772	11.00	11.70	128.70	94.02	11.35
SHANICAR 3	L	773	10.00	12.00	120.00	83.33	11.00
SHANICAR 3	R	773	10.00	12.00	120.00	83.33	11.00
SHANICAR 4	L	774	9.50	12.50	118.75	76.00	11.00
SHANICAR 4	R	774	10.50	12.50	131.25	84.00	11.50
SPY 1	R	777	9.50	11.00	104.50	86.36	10.25
SPY 2	R	778	10.90	12.00	130.80	90.83	11.45
STEINHEIM	L	780	8.65	10.40	89.96	83.17	9.52
STEINHEIM	R	780	9.00	10.00	90.00	90.00	9.50
TABUN 1	L	783	8.30	10.20	84.66	81.37	9.25
VERGISSON 1	R	810	13.00	9.00	117.00	144.44	11.00
VERGISSON 2	L	811	12.00	10.80	129.60	111.11	11.40
SKHUL 4	L	903	9.30	12.50	116.25	74.40	10.90
SKHUL 4	R	903	9.40	11.10	104.34	84.68	10.25
SKHUL 5	L	904	11.00	12.40	136.40	88.71	11.70
SKHUL 5	R	904	11.90	11.80	140.42	100.85	11.85
SKHUL 7	L	906	8.60	11.00	94.60	78.18	9.80
SKHUL 7	R	906	9.00	11.40	102.60	78.95	10.20

LOWER I1 H. SAPIENS

		N	L(M-D)	B(B-L)	L*B	L/B	L+B/2
PREDMOST 1	L	1009	6.00				
PREDMOST 1	R	1009	6.00				
PREDMOST 4	L	1008	5.40	6.00	32.40	90.00	5.70
PREDMOST 10	L	1014	5.40	5.90	31.86	91.53	5.65
COMBE CHAPELLE	L	1017	5.00	6.00	30.00	83.33	5.50
COMBE CHAPELLE	R	1017	5.00	6.00	30.00	83.33	5.50
BRNO 3	L	1018	4.00	5.80	23.20	68.97	4.90
GRIMALDI ADOL.	L	1019	6.00	7.05	42.30	85.11	6.52
GRIMALDI ADOL.	R	1019	6.20	7.85	48.67	78.98	7.02
ROIS R51-12		1037	6.00	7.00	42.00	85.71	6.50
ROIS R51-13		1038	6.50	7.70	50.05	84.42	7.10
ROIS R51-31		1046	6.50	7.00	45.50	92.86	6.75
ROIS		1054	6.00	7.00	42.00	85.71	6.50
VESTONICE 3	L	1057	3.80	6.10	23.18	62.30	4.95
VESTONICE 3	R	1057	3.80	6.20	23.56	61.29	5.00
A CULOZ 2	L	1101	5.00	6.10	30.50	81.97	5.55
A CULOZ 2	R	1101	5.00	6.10	30.50	81.97	5.55
BUGGISON 2	L	1109	5.00	7.50	37.50	66.67	6.25
BUGGISON 2	R	1109	5.00	7.50	37.50	66.67	6.25
CAP BLAC	L	1110	4.00	5.20	20.80	76.92	4.60
CAP BLAC	R	1110	4.10	5.10	20.91	80.39	4.60
FARINCOURT 3	L	1115	4.40	5.70	25.08	77.19	5.05
FARINCOURT 3	R	1115	4.40	5.60	24.64	78.57	5.00
LACHAUD A	L	1125	5.70	6.20	35.34	91.94	5.95
LACHAUD A	R	1125	5.30	6.30	33.39	84.13	5.80
LAFAYE	L	1128	4.80	6.30	30.24	76.19	5.55
LAFAYE	R	1128	4.40	6.40	28.16	68.75	5.40
MASAT		1130	5.60	5.60	31.36	100.00	5.60
OBERCASSEL 1	L	1132	5.00	6.00	30.00	83.33	5.50
PAS ESTRET 3	L	1134	4.70				
PAS ESTRET 3	R	1134	4.80				
SVAERDBORG	R	1144	5.60	6.00	33.60	93.33	5.80
FRENCHMAN	L	1149	5.50	6.00	33.00	91.67	5.75
FRENCHMAN	R	1149	5.00	6.60	33.00	75.76	5.80
WHITE 55-7740	L	1152	4.60	6.20	28.52	74.19	5.40
ALACA HOYUK 2		1183	5.60	6.40	35.84	87.50	6.00
WADI HALFA	L	1202	6.00	6.10	36.60	98.36	6.05
WADJAK 2	R	1702	6.20	7.20	44.64	86.11	6.70
AUSTRALIAN 39		1708	6.00	6.00	36.00	100.00	6.00
AUSTRALIAN	L	1729	6.50				
AUSTRALIAN	R	1729	6.90				
AUSTRALIAN 8158	L	1730	6.40				
TASMANIAN 2964	L	1763	6.50	6.50	42.25	100.00	6.50
TASMANIAN 2964	R	1763	6.30	7.00	44.10	90.00	6.65
ASSELAR	R	1903	6.50				
NEGRO		1914	5.10	5.60	28.56	91.07	5.35
NEGRO	L	1915	6.40	6.40	40.96	100.00	6.40
NEGRO	R	1915	6.40	6.40	40.96	100.00	6.40
NEGRO	L	1916	6.30	6.50	40.95	96.92	6.40
NEGRO	R	1916	6.50	6.70	43.55	97.01	6.60

LOWER I1 H. SAPIENS

		N	L(M-D)	B(B-L)	L*B	L/B	L+B/2
BANTU 100	L	1917	5.90	7.00	41.30	84.29	6.45
BANTU 100	R	1917	6.00	7.10	42.60	84.51	6.55
NEGRO 2	L	1919	5.40				
NEGRO 2	R	1919	5.10				
NEGRO 29	R	1925	5.50				
BUSHMAN MXD 61	L	1946	6.10	6.45	39.34	94.57	6.27
BUSHMAN MXD 61	R	1946	5.90	6.70	39.53	88.06	6.30
N/HOTTENTOT 6	L	1948	5.25	6.80	35.70	77.21	6.02
N/HOTTENTOT 6	R	1948	5.20	6.70	34.84	77.61	5.95
BUSHMAN MXD 101	L	1949	5.25	5.45	28.61	96.33	5.35
BUSHMAN MXD 101	R	1949	5.50	5.50	30.25	100.00	5.50
MAPUNGUBWE M1A		1951	5.50	6.50	35.75	84.62	6.00
MAPUNGUBWE M2		1952	5.50	6.20	34.10	88.71	5.85
MAPUNGUBWE M3		1953	6.70	7.10	47.57	94.37	6.90
MAPUNGUBWE M9		1955	6.50	7.00	45.50	92.86	6.75
BAMBANDYANALO21		1957	6.10	6.10	37.21	100.00	6.10
BAMBANDYANALO29		1958	6.60	7.00	46.20	94.29	6.80
BAMBANDYANALO31		1959	7.40	7.00	51.80	105.71	7.20
BAMBANDYANALO13		1964	5.70	7.50	42.75	76.00	6.60
BAMBANDYANALO14		1965	6.80	6.60	44.88	103.03	6.70
BUSHMAN		1967	5.00	5.20	26.00	96.15	5.10
FISH HOEK	R	1972	4.50	4.20	18.90	107.14	4.35
N.BRITAIN 43131	L	1308	5.60	6.30	35.28	88.89	5.95
N.BRITAIN 43131	R	1308	5.50	6.00	33.00	91.67	5.75
N.BRITAIN 43137	L	1314	5.90	6.10	35.99	96.72	6.00
N.BRITAIN 43137	R	1314	5.30	6.00	31.80	88.33	5.65
N.BRITAIN 43139	L	1316	5.90	6.50	38.35	90.77	6.20
N.BRITAIN 43141	L	1318	5.10	5.80	29.58	87.93	5.45
N.BRITAIN 43141	R	1318	5.30	5.70	30.21	92.98	5.50
N.BRITAIN 43142	R	1319	4.90	7.10	34.79	69.01	6.00
N.BRITAIN 43146	L	1323	4.60	5.70	26.22	80.70	5.15
N.BRITAIN 43147	L	1324	6.50	5.90	38.35	110.17	6.20
N.BRITAIN 43147	R	1324	6.90	5.80	40.02	118.97	6.35
N.BRITAIN 43151	L	1327	6.10	6.10	37.21	100.00	6.10
N.BRITAIN 43151	R	1327	6.20	6.40	39.68	96.87	6.30
N.BRITAIN 43154	L	1330	5.50	6.70	36.85	82.09	6.10
N.BRITAIN 43154	R	1330	5.70	6.60	37.62	86.36	6.15
N.BRITAIN 43174	L	1331	6.40	7.00	44.80	91.43	6.70
N.BRITAIN 43174	R	1331	5.20	6.20	32.24	83.87	5.70
N.BRITAIN 43193	R	1333	5.50	5.50	30.25	100.00	5.50
N.BRITAIN 43198	L	1335	6.00	6.00	36.00	100.00	6.00
N.BRITAIN 43198	R	1335	6.00	6.50	39.00	92.31	6.25
N.BRITAIN 43199	L	1336	5.10	5.90	30.09	86.44	5.50
N.BRITAIN 43199	R	1336	5.20	6.30	32.76	82.54	5.75
N.BRITAIN 43204	R	1338	5.50	5.60	30.80	98.21	5.55
N.BRITAIN 43226	L	1339	5.40	5.80	31.32	93.10	5.60
N.BRITAIN 43226	R	1339	5.50	5.50	30.25	100.00	5.50
N.BRITAIN 43291	L	1343	5.60	6.50	36.40	86.15	6.05
N.BRITAIN 43291	R	1343		6.40			
N.BRITAIN 43296	L	1345	6.00	6.20	37.20	96.77	6.10

LOWER I1 H. SAPIENS

		N	L(M-D)	B(B-L)	L*B	L/B	L+B/2
N.BRITAIN 43296	R	1345	5.70	6.20	35.34	91.94	5.95
N.BRITAIN	L	1346	5.90				
N.BRITAIN	R	1346	6.10				
HINDU AM 7894	L	2201	5.80	6.20	35.96	93.55	6.00
HINDU (UI)	L	2208	5.55	5.80	32.19	95.69	5.67
HINDU (UI)	R	2208	5.65	5.60	31.64	100.89	5.62
GOL BA IT 98	L	2003		5.50			
GOL BA IT 98	R	2003		5.50			
MELOLC	R	2086	5.00	5.70	28.50	87.72	5.35
MELOLC	L	2087	5.40	5.70	30.78	94.74	5.55
MELOLC	R	2088	6.20	6.60	40.92	93.94	6.40
MINNESOTA MAN	L	1419	5.80	6.40	37.12	90.62	6.10
MINNESOTA MAN	R	1419	5.90	6.40	37.76	92.19	6.15
TARASCC (AM)	L	1422	5.20				
ILLINCIS A-2732	L	1429	5.50	6.00	33.00	91.67	5.75
ILLINCIS A-2732	R	1429	5.70	6.20	35.34	91.94	5.95
ILLINCIS PK9-B4	L	1432	6.10	5.30	32.33	115.09	5.70
ILLINCIS PK9-B4	R	1432	5.70	5.20	29.64	109.62	5.45
ILLINCIS BR19-3	L	1434	5.50	5.80	31.90	94.83	5.65
ILLINCIS BR19-3	R	1434	5.45	5.85	31.88	93.16	5.65
ILLINCIS A-8068	L	1437	4.50	6.70	30.15	67.16	5.60
ILLINCIS A-8068	R	1437	4.80	6.80	32.64	70.59	5.80
DICKSCN MOUND	L	1501	5.00	6.70	33.50	74.63	5.85
DICKSCN MOUND	R	1501	5.25	6.40	33.60	82.03	5.82
DICKSCN MD 242	L	1505	6.05	5.40	32.67	112.04	5.72
DICKSCN MD 242	R	1505	6.00	5.57	33.42	107.72	5.78
DICKSCN MD 256	L	1506	5.26	5.20	27.35	101.15	5.23
DICKSCN MD 256	R	1506	4.80	5.20	24.96	92.31	5.00
DICKSCN MD 262	L	1509	5.80	6.00	34.80	96.67	5.90
DICKSCN MD 262	R	1509	5.80	5.90	34.22	98.31	5.85
DICKSCN MD 266	R	1510	5.90	5.55	32.74	106.31	5.72
DICKSCN MD 276	L	1514	5.50	6.35	34.92	86.61	5.92
DICKSCN MD 276	R	1514	5.80	6.80	39.44	85.29	6.30
DICKSCN MD 319	L	1523	4.60	5.60	25.76	82.14	5.10
DICKSCN MD 319	R	1523	4.60	5.60	25.76	82.14	5.10
DICKSCN MD 327	L	1524	5.00	6.30	31.50	79.37	5.65
DICKSCN MD 327	R	1524	5.10	6.00	30.60	85.00	5.55
DICKSCN MD 348	L	1529	4.80	5.15	24.72	93.20	4.97
DICKSCN MD 348	R	1529	5.05	5.15	26.01	98.06	5.10
DICKSCN MD 349	L	1530	5.85	5.75	33.64	101.74	5.80
DICKSCN MD 349	R	1530	5.65	5.75	32.49	98.26	5.70
DICKSCN MD 352	L	1533	5.85	5.70	33.34	102.63	5.77
DICKSCN MD 352	R	1533	5.75	5.75	33.06	100.00	5.75
DICKSCN MD 355	L	1535	5.55	6.10	33.85	90.98	5.82
DICKSCN MD 355	R	1535	5.35	6.10	32.63	87.70	5.72
DICKSCN MD 362	L	1539	5.90	5.70	33.63	103.51	5.80
DICKSCN MD 362	R	1539	5.85	5.60	32.76	104.46	5.72
DICKSCN MD 365	L	1540	5.30	5.30	28.09	100.00	5.30
DICKSCN MD 365	R	1540	5.30	5.40	28.62	98.15	5.35
DICKSCN MD 371	L	1542	5.40	5.20	28.08	103.85	5.30

LOWER I1 H. SAPIENS

		N	L(M-D)	B(B-L)	L*B	L/B	L+B/2
DICKSCN MD 371	R	1542	5.20	5.20	27.04	100.00	5.20
DICKSCN MD 372	L	1543	5.70	5.90	33.63	96.61	5.80
DICKSCN MD 372	R	1543	5.70	5.90	33.63	96.61	5.80
DICKSCN MD 373	L	1544	4.50	3.75	16.87	120.00	4.12
DICKSCN MD 378	L	1547	5.30	5.35	28.35	99.07	5.32
DICKSCN MD 378	R	1547	5.35	5.10	27.28	104.90	5.22
DICKSCN MD 379	L	1548	5.50	5.75	31.62	95.65	5.62
DICKSCN MD 379	R	1548	5.30	5.80	30.74	91.38	5.55
DICKSCN MD 381	L	1550	5.80	5.60	32.48	103.57	5.70
DICKSCN MD 381	R	1550	5.80	5.60	32.48	103.57	5.70
DICKSCN MD 380	L	1551	5.40	5.60	30.24	96.43	5.50
DICKSCN MD 380	R	1551	5.20	5.70	29.64	91.23	5.45
DICKSCN MD 396	L	1553	5.80	6.80	39.44	85.29	6.30
DICKSCN MD 396	R	1553	5.70	6.60	37.62	86.36	6.15
DICKSCN MD 397	L	1554	5.30	6.20	32.86	85.48	5.75
DICKSCN MD 397	R	1554	5.45	6.20	33.79	87.90	5.82
DICKSCN MD 398	L	1555	5.70	5.50	31.35	103.64	5.60
DICKSCN MD 398	R	1555	5.90	5.80	34.22	101.72	5.85
DICKSCN MD 404	L	1559	5.30	5.85	31.00	90.60	5.57
DICKSCN MD 404	R	1559	5.50	6.50	35.75	84.62	6.00
DICKSCN MD 406	L	1560	5.70	5.10	29.07	111.76	5.40
DICKSCN MD 406	R	1560	5.80	5.35	31.03	108.41	5.57
DICKSCN MD 407	L	1561	6.55	6.30	41.26	103.97	6.42
DICKSCN MD 407	R	1561	6.15	5.90	36.28	104.24	6.02
DICKSCN MD 411	R	1563	6.15	5.65	34.75	108.85	5.90
DICKSCN MD 426	R	1566	5.40	5.30	28.62	101.89	5.35
DICKSCN MD 441	L	1569	5.57	5.45	30.36	102.20	5.51
DICKSCN MD 441	R	1569	5.60	5.40	30.24	103.70	5.50
DICKSCN MD 443	L	1571	6.10	5.80	35.38	105.17	5.95
DICKSCN MD 443	R	1571	5.80	5.70	33.06	101.75	5.75
DICKSCN MD 447	L	1573	5.35	4.95	26.48	108.08	5.15
DICKSCN MD 447	R	1573	5.30	4.90	25.97	108.16	5.10
DICKSCN MD 448	L	1574	5.30	5.14	27.24	103.11	5.22
DICKSCN MD 448	R	1574	5.30	5.12	27.14	103.52	5.21
DICKSCN MD 464	L	1575	5.00	5.70	28.50	87.72	5.35
DICKSCN MD 464	R	1575	5.20	6.10	31.72	85.25	5.65
DICKSCN MD 476	L	1576	5.70	5.55	31.63	102.70	5.62
DICKSCN MD 476	R	1576	5.65	5.35	30.23	105.61	5.50
DICKSCN MD 497	L	1583	5.70	6.35	36.19	89.76	6.02
DICKSCN MD 497	R	1583	5.60	6.50	36.40	86.15	6.05
DICKSCN MD 503	L	1585	5.25	5.90	30.97	88.98	5.57
DICKSCN MD 503	R	1585	5.40	5.95	32.13	90.76	5.67
DICKSCN MD 504	L	1586	7.00				
DICKSCN MD 509	L	1587	5.75	6.24	35.88	92.15	5.99
DICKSCN MD 509	R	1587	5.85	5.90	34.51	99.15	5.87
DICKSCN MD 535	L	1591	5.75	5.20	29.90	110.58	5.47
DICKSCN MD 535	R	1591	5.80	5.30	30.74	109.43	5.55
DICKSCN MD 536	L	1592	5.85	5.25	30.71	111.43	5.55
DICKSCN MD 536	R	1592	5.85	5.25	30.71	111.43	5.55
DICKSCN MD 545	R	1594	5.70	5.90	33.63	96.61	5.80

LOWER I1 H. SAPIENS

			N	L(M-D)	B(B-L)	L*B	L/B	L+B/2
DICKSCN MD	557	L	1596	5.30	5.35	28.35	99.07	5.32
DICKSCN MD	557	R	1596	5.40	5.35	28.89	100.93	5.37
DICKSCN MD	561	R	1597	5.20	5.85	30.42	88.89	5.52
DICKSGN MD	568	L	1599	5.00	6.40	32.00	78.12	5.70
DICKSCN MD	568	R	1599	5.20	6.25	32.50	83.20	5.72
DICKSCN MD	630	L	1603	5.30	5.90	31.27	89.83	5.60
DICKSCN MD	630	R	1603	5.20	5.70	29.64	91.23	5.45
DICKSCN MD	638	L	1606	6.00				
DICKSCN MD	638	R	1606	6.20				
DICKSCN MD	642	L	1607	6.10				
DICKSCN MD	648	L	1609	6.50	6.40	41.60	101.56	6.45
DICKSON MD	648	R	1609	6.40	6.50	41.60	98.46	6.45
DICKSCN MD	652	R	1611	5.30	5.70	30.21	92.98	5.50
DICKSCN MD	667	L	1614	5.80	6.00	34.80	96.67	5.90
DICKSCN MD	667	R	1614	5.75	6.25	35.94	92.00	6.00
DICKSCN MD	681	R	1615	7.20				
DICKSCN MD	694	R	1617	6.60				
DICKSCN MD	722	L	1624	5.45	5.85	31.88	93.16	5.65
DICKSCN MD	722	R	1624	5.40	5.80	31.32	93.10	5.60
DICKSCN MD	724	L	1627	5.90	5.85	34.51	100.85	5.87
DICKSCN MD	724	R	1627	5.56	6.00	33.36	92.67	5.78
DICKSCN MD	746	L	1628	5.00	6.20	31.00	80.65	5.60
DICKSCN MD	746	R	1628	5.10	6.25	31.87	81.60	5.67
DICKSCN MD	749	L	1629	6.00				
DICKSCN MD	749	R	1629	6.04				

LOWER I2 H. SAPIENS

		N	L(M-D)	B(B-L)	L*B	L/B	L+B/2
ARCYSLRCURE C8		1001		8.50			
PREDMCST 1	R	1009	6.50				
PREDMCST 4	R	1008	5.60	6.00	33.60	93.33	5.80
PREDMCST 10	R	1014	6.30	6.00	37.80	105.00	6.15
COMBE CHAPELLE	L	1017	6.00	6.50	39.00	92.31	6.25
COMBE CHAPELLE	R	1017	5.00	6.00	30.00	83.33	5.50
BRNO 3	L	1018	5.00	5.60	28.00	89.29	5.30
BRNO 3	R	1018	5.00	6.00	30.00	83.33	5.50
GRIMALDI ADOL.	L	1019	7.70	7.50	57.75	102.67	7.60
GRIMALDI ADOL.	R	1019	7.85	8.20	64.37	95.73	8.02
ROIS B		1025	7.00	8.00	56.00	87.50	7.50
ROIS R5C-24		1031	7.00	7.00	49.00	100.00	7.00
ROIS R5C-35	R	1033	7.00				
ROIS R51-11		1036	7.00	7.50	52.50	93.33	7.25
ROIS R51-17		1042	7.00	7.00	49.00	100.00	7.00
SALEMAS	L	1056	6.00	6.50	39.00	92.31	6.25
VESTONICE 3	L	1057	4.30	7.00	30.10	61.43	5.65
VESTONICE 3	R	1057	4.70	6.60	31.02	71.21	5.65
A CULOZ 2	L	1101	5.20	6.60	34.32	78.79	5.90
A CULOZ 2	R	1101	6.00	6.50	39.00	92.31	6.25
BUGGISCN 1	L	1108	7.00	7.00	49.00	100.00	7.00
BUGGISCN 1	R	1108	6.00	6.00	36.00	100.00	6.00
BUGGISCN 2	L	1109	7.00	8.00	56.00	87.50	7.50
BUGGISON 2	R	1109	7.00	7.50	52.50	93.33	7.25
CAP BLAC	L	1110	5.00	6.00	30.00	83.33	5.50
CAP BLAC	R	1110	5.00	6.10	30.50	81.97	5.55
FARINCOURT 3	L	1115	5.20	6.40	33.28	81.25	5.80
FARINCOURT 3	R	1115	5.50	6.30	34.65	87.30	5.90
LACHAUD A	L	1125	6.00	7.00	42.00	85.71	6.50
LACHAUD A	R	1125	5.40	6.40	34.56	84.37	5.90
LACHAUD B	R	1126	6.60	7.70	50.82	85.71	7.15
LACHAUD C	L	1127	6.70	6.50	43.55	103.08	6.60
LAFAYE	L	1128	5.50	7.00	38.50	78.57	6.25
LAFAYE	R	1128	5.10	6.80	34.68	75.00	5.95
MASAT		1130	6.30	5.80	36.54	108.62	6.05
OBERCASSEL 1	L	1132	5.00	7.00	35.00	71.43	6.00
OKUZINI		1133	5.90	6.30	37.17	93.65	6.10
PAS ESTRET 3	L	1134	5.70				
PAS ESTRET 3	R	1134	5.30				
PRITZERBER 3	L	1138	6.00	6.50	39.00	92.31	6.25
SVAERDBORG	R	1144	6.00	6.40	38.40	93.75	6.20
FRENCHMAN	L	1149	6.45	6.65	42.89	96.99	6.55
FRENCHMAN	R	1149	5.75	6.60	37.95	87.12	6.17
WHITE 99-7740	L	1152	5.60	6.60	36.96	84.85	6.10
ALACA HOYUK 2		1183	5.70	6.60	37.62	86.36	6.15
WADI HALFA	L	1203	6.10	6.70	40.87	91.04	6.40
WADI HALFA	L	1204	6.40	6.70	42.88	95.52	6.55
WADJAK 2	R	1702	6.80	7.60	51.68	89.47	7.20
AUSTRALIAN 39		1708	6.80	7.00	47.60	97.14	6.90
AUSTRALIAN	L	1729	6.70				

LOWER I2 H. SAPIENS

		N	L(M-D)	B(B-L)	L*B	L/B	L+B/2
AUSTRALIAN	R	1729	7.40				
TASMANIAN 2964	L	1763	6.90	6.30	43.47	109.52	6.60
TASMANIAN 2964	R	1763	7.00	6.70	46.90	104.48	6.85
ASSELAR	R	1903	6.50				
NEGRO		1914	5.90	6.00	35.40	98.33	5.95
NEGRO	L	1915	6.60	6.90	45.54	95.65	6.75
NEGRO	R	1915	6.80	7.00	47.60	97.14	6.90
NEGRO	L	1916	7.50	7.30	54.75	102.74	7.40
NEGRO	R	1916	7.40	7.10	52.54	104.23	7.25
BANTU 100	L	1917	7.30	8.00	58.40	91.25	7.65
BANTU 100	R	1917	6.50	7.70	50.05	84.42	7.10
NEGRO 2	L	1919	6.70				
NEGRO 2	R	1919	6.30				
NEGRO 29	L	1925	6.75				
NEGRO 29	R	1925	6.90				
BUSHMAN MXD 61	L	1946	6.45	7.25	46.76	88.97	6.85
BUSHMAN MXD 61	R	1946	6.10	7.00	42.70	87.14	6.55
BUSHMAN MXD 94	L	1947	5.70				
N/HOTTENTOT 6	L	1948	6.60	7.40	48.84	89.19	7.00
N/HOTTENTOT 6	R	1948	6.90	9.80	67.62	70.41	8.35
BUSHMAN MXD 101	L	1949	6.35	5.40	34.29	117.59	5.87
BUSHMAN MXD 101	R	1949	5.90	5.25	30.97	112.38	5.57
MAPUNGUBWE M1A		1951	6.50	7.00	45.50	92.86	6.75
MAPUNGUBWE M2		1952	6.50	6.90	44.85	94.20	6.70
MAPUNGUBWE M3		1953	6.70	7.10	47.57	94.37	6.90
MAPUNGUBWE M9		1955	6.70	7.30	48.91	91.78	7.00
BAMBANDYANALO21		1957	6.60	6.70	44.22	98.51	6.65
BAMBANDYANALO29		1958	6.50	6.30	40.95	103.17	6.40
BAMBANDYANALO31		1959	6.80	6.50	44.20	104.62	6.65
BAMBANDYANALO 3		1962	6.30	6.20	39.06	101.61	6.25
BAMBANDYANALO13		1964	6.10	6.50	39.65	93.85	6.30
BAMBANDYANALO14		1965	6.30	6.70	42.21	94.03	6.50
BUSHMAN		1967	5.60	5.60	31.36	100.00	5.60
FISH HOEK	R	1972	5.20	4.30	22.36	120.93	4.75
BUSHMAN 30	L	1973	5.70	5.90	33.63	96.61	5.80
N.BRITAIN 43131	L	1308	6.30	6.70	42.21	94.03	6.50
N.BRITAIN 43136	L	1313	6.70	6.20	41.54	108.06	6.45
N.BRITAIN 43137	L	1314	6.30	6.50	40.95	96.92	6.40
N.BRITAIN 43137	R	1314	7.00	6.30	44.10	111.11	6.65
N.BRITAIN 43139	L	1316	6.50	6.40	41.60	101.56	6.45
N.BRITAIN 43141	L	1318	5.50	5.90	32.45	93.22	5.70
N.BRITAIN 43141	R	1318	5.90	5.90	34.81	100.00	5.90
N.BRITAIN 43142	L	1319	6.10	7.30	44.53	83.56	6.70
N.BRITAIN 43142	R	1319	5.70	7.50	42.75	76.00	6.60
N.BRITAIN 43144	L	1321		6.40			
N.BRITAIN 43146	L	1323	6.40	6.70	42.88	95.52	6.55
N.BRITAIN 43146	R	1323	5.50	6.20	34.10	88.71	5.85
N.BRITAIN 43147	L	1324	6.90	6.10	42.09	113.11	6.50
N.BRITAIN 43147	R	1324	6.50	6.10	39.65	106.56	6.30
N.BRITAIN 43151	L	1327	6.60	6.90	45.54	95.65	6.75

LOWER I2 H. SAPIENS

		N	L(M-D)	B(B-L)	L*B	L/B	L+B/2
N.BRITAIN 43151	R	1327	6.80	6.00	40.80	113.33	6.40
N.BRITAIN 43153	L	1329		6.20			
N.BRITAIN 43154	L	1330	6.10	6.10	37.21	100.00	6.10
N.BRITAIN 43154	R	1330	5.90	6.60	38.94	89.39	6.25
N.BRITAIN 43174	L	1331	6.20	6.60	40.92	93.94	6.40
N.BRITAIN 43174	R	1331	5.90	6.40	37.76	92.19	6.15
N.BRITAIN 43179	R	1332	7.60	7.50	57.00	101.33	7.55
N.BRITAIN 43193	L	1333	6.80	6.20	42.16	109.68	6.50
N.BRITAIN 43193	R	1333	5.70	6.10	34.77	93.44	5.90
N.BRITAIN 43198	L	1335	7.10	5.30	37.63	133.96	6.20
N.BRITAIN 43198	R	1335	6.80	6.40	43.52	106.25	6.60
N.BRITAIN 43199	L	1336	6.20	6.40	39.68	96.87	6.30
N.BRITAIN 43199	R	1336	6.10	6.30	38.43	96.83	6.20
N.BRITAIN 43204	R	1338	5.80	6.90	40.02	84.06	6.35
N.BRITAIN 43226	L	1339	6.00	6.30	37.80	95.24	6.15
N.BRITAIN 43226	R	1339	6.20	6.00	37.20	103.33	6.10
N.BRITAIN 43242	R	1341	5.80	7.80	45.24	74.36	6.80
N.BRITAIN 43291	L	1343		6.80			
N.BRITAIN 43296	L	1345	6.80	6.90	46.92	98.55	6.85
N.BRITAIN 43296	R	1345	6.70	7.00	46.90	95.71	6.85
N.BRITAIN	L	1346	6.35				
N.BRITAIN	R	1346	6.40				
HINDU AM 7894	L	2201	6.95	7.30	50.73	95.21	7.12
HINDU (LI)	L	2208	6.25	6.20	38.75	100.81	6.22
HINDU (LI)	R	2208	6.25	6.10	38.12	102.46	6.17
GOL BA IT 98	L	2003		5.90			
GOL BA IT 98	R	2003		5.90			
MELOLO	R	2089	5.60	6.00	33.60	93.33	5.80
MELOLO	L	2090	5.80	6.10	35.38	95.08	5.95
MELOLO	R	2091	6.50	7.20	46.80	90.28	6.85
MINNESOTA MAN	L	1419	6.60	6.60	43.56	100.00	6.60
MINNESOTA MAN	R	1419	6.60	6.60	43.56	100.00	6.60
TARASCO (AM)	L	1422	7.00				
ILLINOIS ME3-10	L	1428	6.15	5.80	35.67	106.03	5.97
ILLINOIS A-2732	L	1429		6.40			
ILLINOIS A-2732	R	1429	6.30	6.40	40.32	98.44	6.35
ILLINOIS PK9-B4	L	1432	6.30	6.00	37.80	105.00	6.15
ILLINOIS PK9-B4	R	1432	6.70	6.00	40.20	111.67	6.35
ILLINOIS BR19-3	L	1434	6.70	6.15	41.20	108.94	6.42
ILLINOIS BR19-3	R	1434	6.65	6.20	41.23	107.26	6.42
ILLINOIS A-8068	L	1437	6.50	6.80	44.20	95.59	6.65
ILLINOIS A-8068	R	1437	6.65	7.05	46.88	94.33	6.85
DICKSON MOUND	L	1501	6.45	6.55	42.25	98.47	6.50
DICKSON MOUND	R	1501	6.50	6.75	43.87	96.30	6.62
DICKSON MD 242	L	1505	6.57	5.80	38.11	113.28	6.18
DICKSON MD 242	R	1505	6.75	5.90	39.82	114.41	6.32
DICKSON MD 256	R	1506	6.25	5.80	36.25	107.76	6.02
DICKSON MD 262	L	1509	6.85	6.25	42.81	109.60	6.55
DICKSON MD 262	R	1509	6.55	6.20	40.61	105.65	6.37
DICKSON MD 266	R	1510	6.50	6.20	40.30	104.84	6.35

LOWER I2 H. SAPIENS

			N	L(M-D)	B(B-L)	L*B	L/B	L+B/2
DICKSCN MD	276	L	1514	6.60	6.70	44.22	98.51	6.65
DICKSCN MD	276	R	1514	6.70	6.80	45.56	98.53	6.75
DICKSON MD	287	L	1516	6.30	6.50	40.95	96.92	6.40
DICKSCN MD	297	L	1520	6.85	6.23	42.68	109.95	6.54
DICKSCN MD	297	R	1520	6.80	6.20	42.16	109.68	6.50
DICKSCN MD	319	L	1523	6.20	6.40	39.68	96.87	6.30
DICKSCN MD	319	R	1523	6.45	6.20	39.99	104.03	6.32
DICKSON MD	327	L	1524	6.40	7.00	44.80	91.43	6.70
DICKSCN MD	327	R	1524	6.30	6.90	43.47	91.30	6.60
DICKSON MD	348	L	1529	5.70	5.90	33.63	96.61	5.80
DICKSON MD	348	R	1529	5.75	5.90	33.92	97.46	5.82
DICKSCN MD	349	L	1530	6.40	6.10	39.04	104.92	6.25
DICKSON MD	349	R	1530	6.40	6.00	38.40	106.67	6.20
DICKSCN MD	352	L	1533	6.65	6.20	41.23	107.26	6.42
DICKSCN MD	352	R	1533	6.85	6.15	42.13	111.38	6.50
DICKSON MD	355	L	1535	6.80	6.80	46.24	100.00	6.80
DICKSON MD	355	R	1535	6.50	6.60	42.90	98.48	6.55
DICKSCN MD	362	L	1539	6.60	6.45	42.57	102.33	6.52
DICKSON MD	362	R	1539	6.55	6.30	41.26	103.97	6.42
DICKSCN MD	365	L	1540	6.00	6.00	36.00	100.00	6.00
DICKSCN MD	365	R	1540	5.90	6.20	36.58	95.16	6.05
DICKSON MD	371	L	1542	6.50	6.50	42.25	100.00	6.50
DICKSON MD	371	R	1542	6.50	6.50	42.25	100.00	6.50
DICKSON MD	372	L	1543	6.70	6.30	42.21	106.35	6.50
DICKSCN MD	372	R	1543	6.70	6.30	42.21	106.35	6.50
DICKSCN MD	378	L	1547	6.00	5.50	33.00	109.09	5.75
DICKSCN MD	378	R	1547	5.95	5.20	30.94	114.42	5.57
DICKSCN MD	379	L	1548	6.45	6.45	41.60	100.00	6.45
DICKSCN MD	379	R	1548	6.50	6.30	40.95	103.17	6.40
DICKSCN MD	381	L	1550	6.20	6.60	40.92	93.94	6.40
DICKSCN MD	381	R	1550	6.20	6.20	38.44	100.00	6.20
DICKSCN MD	380	L	1551	6.00	6.30	37.80	95.24	6.15
DICKSCN MD	380	R	1551	5.85	6.45	37.73	90.70	6.15
DICKSON MD	396	L	1553	6.60	7.10	46.86	92.96	6.85
DICKSON MD	396	R	1553	6.60	7.10	46.86	92.96	6.85
DICKSCN MD	397	L	1554	6.50	6.40	41.60	101.56	6.45
DICKSCN MD	397	R	1554	6.60	6.70	44.22	98.51	6.65
DICKSCN MD	398	L	1555	6.20	6.10	37.82	101.64	6.15
DICKSCN MD	398	R	1555	6.30	6.40	40.32	98.44	6.35
DICKSON MD	404	L	1559	6.30	6.60	41.58	95.45	6.45
DICKSCN MD	406	L	1560	6.50	5.50	35.75	118.18	6.00
DICKSCN MD	406	R	1560	6.80	5.35	36.38	127.10	6.07
DICKSCN MD	407	L	1561	7.15	6.55	46.83	109.16	6.85
DICKSCN MD	407	R	1561	7.00	6.20	43.40	112.90	6.60
DICKSCN MD	411	L	1563	7.23	5.77	41.72	125.30	6.50
DICKSCN MD	411	R	1563	7.15	5.55	39.68	128.83	6.35
DICKSON MD	426	L	1566	6.25	6.20	38.75	100.81	6.22
DICKSCN MD	426	R	1566	6.15	6.30	38.74	97.62	6.22
DICKSCN MD	441	L	1569	6.85	6.10	41.78	112.30	6.47
DICKSCN MD	441	R	1569	7.10	6.15	43.66	115.45	6.62

LOWER I2 H. SAPIENS

			N	L(M-D)	B(B-L)	L*B	L/B	L+B/2
DICKSCN MD	443	L	1571	7.10	5.95	42.24	119.33	6.52
DICKSON MD	443	R	1571	7.05	6.00	42.30	117.50	6.52
DICKSCN MD	446	L	1572	6.10	5.87	35.81	103.92	5.98
DICKSCN MD	447	L	1573	6.00	5.60	33.60	107.14	5.80
DICKSCN MD	447	R	1573	6.14	5.61	34.45	109.45	5.87
DICKSCN MD	448	L	1574	6.27	6.10	38.25	102.79	6.18
DICKSCN MD	448	R	1574	6.22	5.80	36.08	107.24	6.01
DICKSCN MD	464	L	1575	6.60	6.00	39.60	110.00	6.30
DICKSCN MD	464	R	1575	6.60	7.10	46.86	92.96	6.85
DICKSCN MD	476	L	1576	6.50	6.00	39.00	108.33	6.25
DICKSCN MD	476	R	1576	6.75	6.35	42.86	106.30	6.55
DICKSCN MD	497	L	1583	6.85	6.85	46.92	100.00	6.85
DICKSCN MD	497	R	1583	6.90	7.07	48.78	97.60	6.98
DICKSCN MD	503	L	1585	6.50	7.15	46.47	90.91	6.82
DICKSCN MD	503	R	1585	6.60	7.10	46.86	92.96	6.85
DICKSCN MD	504	L	1586	6.20				
DICKSCN MD	509	L	1587	6.50	6.65	43.22	97.74	6.57
DICKSCN MD	509	R	1587	6.64	6.50	43.16	102.15	6.57
DICKSCN MD	535	L	1591	6.70	5.60	37.52	119.64	6.15
DICKSCN MD	535	R	1591	6.85	5.65	38.70	121.24	6.25
DICKSCN MD	536	L	1592	6.60	5.85	38.61	112.82	6.22
DICKSCN MD	536	R	1592	6.80	5.65	38.42	120.35	6.22
DICKSCN MD	545	R	1594	6.50	7.10	46.15	91.55	6.80
DICKSON MD	557	L	1596	6.20	6.10	37.82	101.64	6.15
DICKSCN MD	557	R	1596	6.35	6.15	39.05	103.25	6.25
DICKSCN MD	561	L	1597	6.40	6.35	40.64	100.79	6.37
DICKSON MD	561	R	1597	6.45	6.30	40.63	102.38	6.37
DICKSCN MD	568	L	1599	5.60	6.50	36.40	86.15	6.05
DICKSCN MD	568	R	1599	6.10	6.20	37.82	98.39	6.15
DICKSCN MD	630	L	1603	6.80	6.30	42.84	107.94	6.55
DICKSCN MD	630	R	1603	7.20	6.30	45.36	114.29	6.75
DICKSCN MD	648	L	1609	7.40	6.70	49.58	110.45	7.05
DICKSCN MD	648	R	1609	7.70	6.60	50.82	116.67	7.15
DICKSCN MD	667	L	1614	6.84	7.00	47.88	97.71	6.92
DICKSCN MD	667	R	1614	7.20	6.50	46.80	110.77	6.85
DICKSCN MD	701	L	1620	7.15	6.30	45.04	113.49	6.72
DICKSON MD	722	L	1624	6.30	6.30	39.69	100.00	6.30
DICKSCN MD	722	R	1624	6.40	6.10	39.04	104.92	6.25
DICKSCN MD	724	L	1627	6.60	6.90	45.54	95.65	6.75
DICKSCN MD	724	R	1627	6.45	6.50	41.92	99.23	6.47
DICKSCN MD	746	L	1628	6.10	6.50	39.65	93.85	6.30
DICKSCN MD	746	R	1628	6.20	6.70	41.54	92.54	6.45
DICKSCN MD	749	R	1629	6.75				

LOWER C H. SAPIENS

		N	L(M-D)	B(B-L)	L*B	L/B	L+B/2
ARCYSURCURE C8		1000		9.50			
ARCYSURCURE C10		1004	7.80	9.90	77.22	78.79	8.85
PREDMOST 10	L	1014	7.00	8.40	58.80	83.33	7.70
COMBE CHAPELLE	L	1017	8.00	8.00	64.00	100.00	8.00
COMBE CHAPELLE	R	1017	7.00	9.00	63.00	77.78	8.00
BRNO 3	L	1018	6.70	7.00	46.90	95.71	6.85
BRNO 3	R	1018	6.50	7.00	45.50	92.86	6.75
GRIMALDI ADOL.	L	1019	7.60	8.00	60.80	95.00	7.80
GRIMALDI ADOL.	R	1019	7.20	9.00	64.80	80.00	8.10
ROIS A		1024	7.00	9.00	63.00	77.78	8.00
ROIS B		1025	8.00	9.00	72.00	88.89	8.50
ROIS	R	1048		9.00			
SALEMAS	L	1056	7.00	8.00	56.00	87.50	7.50
VESTONICE 3	L	1057	6.10	8.10	49.41	75.31	7.10
VESTONICE 3	R	1057	6.00	8.00	48.00	75.00	7.00
A CULOZ 2	L	1101	7.00	8.10	56.70	86.42	7.55
A CULOZ 2	R	1101	7.00				
BUGGISON 1	R	1108	8.00	8.00	64.00	100.00	8.00
BUGGISON 2	L	1109	8.00	8.50	68.00	94.12	8.25
BUGGISON 2	R	1109	7.50	8.50	63.75	88.24	8.00
CAP BLAC	L	1110	6.10	7.20	43.92	84.72	6.65
CAP BLAC	R	1110	5.80	7.30	42.34	79.45	6.55
CHANCELADE	L	1111	5.50	7.00	38.50	78.57	6.25
FARINCOURT 3	L	1115	5.10	7.40	37.74	68.92	6.25
FARINCOURT 3	R	1115	5.00	7.30	36.50	68.49	6.15
LACHAUD A	L	1125	7.40	8.30	61.42	89.16	7.85
LACHAUD A	R	1125	7.20	8.20	59.04	87.80	7.70
LAFAYE	L	1128	6.60	8.10	53.46	81.48	7.35
LAFAYE	R	1128	6.20	8.30	51.46	74.70	7.25
MASAT		1130	6.70	8.00	53.60	83.75	7.35
OBERCASSEL 1	L	1132	7.00	8.00	56.00	87.50	7.50
OKUZINI		1133	6.80	7.60	51.68	89.47	7.20
PAS ESTRET 3	L	1134	6.50	7.35	47.77	88.44	6.92
PAS ESTRET 3	R	1134	6.80	7.65	52.02	88.89	7.22
PRITZERBER 3	L	1138	6.00	8.00	48.00	75.00	7.00
SVAERDBORG	R	1144	7.50	8.50	63.75	88.24	8.00
FRENCHMAN	L	1149	7.25	8.45	61.26	85.80	7.85
FRENCHMAN	R	1149	6.75	8.75	59.06	77.14	7.75
WHITE 99-7740	L	1152	6.15	8.35	51.35	73.65	7.25
ALACA HOYUK 2		1183	7.00	7.70	53.90	90.91	7.35
ALACA HOYUK 3		1184	7.10	7.20	51.12	98.61	7.15
WADI HALFA	L	1205	8.50	8.30	70.55	102.41	8.40
WADI HALFA	L	1206	6.90	8.30	57.27	83.13	7.60
WADI HALFA	L	1207	7.10	7.70	54.67	92.21	7.40
WADJAK 2	R	1702	8.40	9.50	79.80	88.42	8.95
AUSTRALIAN 39		1708	8.00	8.00	64.00	100.00	8.00
AUSTRALIAN	L	1729	6.80	9.80	66.64	69.39	8.30
AUSTRALIAN	R	1729	7.55	9.90	74.74	76.26	8.72
TASMANIAN 2964	L	1763	8.00	8.50	68.00	94.12	8.25
TASMANIAN 2964	R	1763	7.90	9.00	71.10	87.78	8.45

LOWER C H. SAPIENS

		N	L(M-D)	B(B-L)	L*B	L/B	L+B/2
ASSELAR	R	1903	6.50	8.00	52.00	81.25	7.25
CAPE FLATS	R	1904	7.00	9.00	63.00	77.78	8.00
NEGRO		1914	7.20	7.40	53.28	97.30	7.30
NEGRO	L	1915	8.00	8.60	68.80	93.02	8.30
NEGRO	R	1915	8.00	8.60	68.80	93.02	8.30
NEGRO	L	1916	8.40	9.00	75.60	93.33	8.70
NEGRO	R	1916	8.50	8.90	75.65	95.51	8.70
NEGRO 2	L	1919	8.20	8.60	70.52	95.35	8.40
NEGRO 29	L	1925	7.90	8.50	67.15	92.94	8.20
NEGRO 29	R	1925	7.60	8.40	63.84	90.48	8.00
N/HOTTENTOT 12	L	1943	6.90	6.70	46.23	102.99	6.80
N/HOTTENTOT 6	L	1944	7.05	9.00	63.45	78.33	8.02
N/HOTTENTOT 6	R	1944	7.20	8.85	63.72	81.36	8.02
BUSHMAN MXD 61	L	1946	7.00	7.90	55.30	88.61	7.45
BUSHMAN MXD 61	R	1946	6.85	7.50	51.37	91.33	7.17
BUSHMAN MXD 94	L	1947	7.10	8.50	60.35	83.53	7.80
N/HOTTENTOT 6	L	1948	7.90	7.70	60.83	102.60	7.80
N/HOTTENTOT 6	R	1948	7.45	7.70	57.36	96.75	7.57
BUSHMAN MXD 101	L	1949	7.00	7.10	49.70	98.59	7.05
BUSHMAN MXD 101	R	1949	6.60	6.50	42.90	101.54	6.55
MAPUNGUBWE M1A		1951	7.00	8.00	56.00	87.50	7.50
MAPUNGUBWE M2		1952	7.50				
MAPUNGUBWE M3		1953	7.90	8.90	70.31	88.76	8.40
MAPUNGUBWE M9		1955	8.00	8.30	66.40	96.39	8.15
BAMBANDYANALO21		1957	6.60	7.50	49.50	88.00	7.05
BAMBANDYANALO29		1958	7.40	7.50	55.50	98.67	7.45
BAMBANDYANALO31		1959	8.00	7.60	60.80	105.26	7.80
BAMBANDYANALO 2		1961	7.30	7.90	57.67	92.41	7.60
BAMBANDYANALO 3		1962	8.10	8.00	64.80	101.25	8.05
BAMBANDYANALO13		1964	8.50	9.00	76.50	94.44	8.75
BAMBANDYANALO14		1965	7.30	8.80	64.24	82.95	8.05
BUSHMAN		1967	6.80	7.00	47.60	97.14	6.90
FISH HOEK	R	1972	6.80	6.00	40.80	113.33	6.40
BUSHMAN 30	L	1973	6.55	6.60	43.23	99.24	6.57
BUSHMAN 30	R	1973	6.45	6.80	43.86	94.85	6.62
N.BRITAIN 43131	L	1308	7.60	8.20	62.32	92.68	7.90
N.BRITAIN 43131	R	1308	7.50	8.00	60.00	93.75	7.75
N.BRITAIN 43136	L	1313	7.40				
N.BRITAIN 43136	R	1313	7.50	7.40	55.50	101.35	7.45
N.BRITAIN 43137	L	1314	7.60	8.40	63.84	90.48	8.00
N.BRITAIN 43137	R	1314	7.40	8.00	59.20	92.50	7.70
N.BRITAIN 43138	L	1315	7.40	8.40	62.16	88.10	7.90
N.BRITAIN 43138	R	1315	6.90	8.70	60.03	79.31	7.80
N.BRITAIN 43139	R	1316	7.60	8.40	63.84	90.48	8.00
N.BRITAIN 43140	L	1317	6.40	8.30	53.12	77.11	7.35
N.BRITAIN 43140	R	1317	7.10	8.10	57.51	87.65	7.60
N.BRITAIN 43141	L	1318	7.20	7.20	51.84	100.00	7.20
N.BRITAIN 43141	R	1318	7.40	7.30	54.02	101.37	7.35
N.BRITAIN 43142	L	1319	7.90	9.30	73.47	84.95	8.60
N.BRITAIN 43142	R	1319	7.90	9.30	73.47	84.95	8.60

LOWER C H. SAPIENS

		N	L(M-D)	B(B-L)	L*B	L/B	L+B/2
N.BRITAIN 43143	L	1320		7.90			
N.BRITAIN 43143	R	1320	7.40	7.30	54.02	101.37	7.35
N.BRITAIN 43144	L	1321	7.00	7.30	51.10	95.89	7.15
N.BRITAIN 43146	R	1323	6.80	7.40	50.32	91.89	7.10
N.BRITAIN 43147	L	1324	7.70	9.40	72.38	81.91	8.55
N.BRITAIN 43147	R	1324	6.80	8.20	55.76	82.93	7.50
N.BRITAIN 43149	L	1325	7.40	8.00	59.20	92.50	7.70
N.BRITAIN 43151	L	1327	7.60	7.20	54.72	105.56	7.40
N.BRITAIN 43151	R	1327	6.90	7.30	50.37	94.52	7.10
N.BRITAIN 43152	L	1328	7.30	7.50	54.75	97.33	7.40
N.BRITAIN 43153	L	1329	7.10	7.60	53.96	93.42	7.35
N.BRITAIN 43153	R	1329		7.30			
N.BRITAIN 43154	L	1330	6.90	7.90	54.51	87.34	7.40
N.BRITAIN 43154	R	1330	7.40	8.00	59.20	92.50	7.70
N.BRITAIN 43174	L	1331	7.50	8.00	60.00	93.75	7.75
N.BRITAIN 43174	R	1331	7.50	7.70	57.75	97.40	7.60
N.BRITAIN 43193	L	1333	7.70	7.80	60.06	98.72	7.75
N.BRITAIN 43193	R	1333	7.50	7.80	58.50	96.15	7.65
N.BRITAIN 43198	L	1335	8.10	7.50	60.75	108.00	7.80
N.BRITAIN 43198	R	1335	8.00	7.70	61.60	103.90	7.85
N.BRITAIN 43199	R	1336	7.40	7.50	55.50	98.67	7.45
N.BRITAIN 43204	L	1338	7.50	9.00	67.50	83.33	8.25
N.BRITAIN 43204	R	1338	7.40	8.90	65.86	83.15	8.15
N.BRITAIN 43226	L	1339	7.10	7.40	52.54	95.95	7.25
N.BRITAIN 43226	R	1339	7.10	7.50	53.25	94.67	7.30
N.BRITAIN 43242	L	1341	7.00	7.40	51.80	94.59	7.20
N.BRITAIN 43242	R	1341	7.00	7.80	54.60	89.74	7.40
N.BRITAIN 43291	L	1343		8.80			
N.BRITAIN 43291	R	1343		8.50			
N.BRITAIN 43296	L	1345	7.2C	8.50	61.20	84.71	7.85
N.BRITAIN 43296	R	1345	7.20	8.60	61.92	83.72	7.90
N.BRITAIN	L	1346	6.70	9.60	64.32	69.79	8.15
N.BRITAIN	R	1346	7.25	9.50	68.87	76.32	8.37
HINDU AM 7894	L	2201	7.65	8.90	68.08	85.96	8.27
HINDU (UI)	L	2208	6.76	6.60	44.62	102.42	6.68
HINDU (UI)	R	2208	6.65	6.35	42.23	104.72	6.50
GOL BA IT 94	L	2001		8.20			
GOL BA IT 94	R	2001		8.10			
GOL BA IT 98	L	2003		7.50			
GOL BA IT 98	R	2003		7.60			
GOL BA IT	R	2010	7.40	7.40	54.76	100.00	7.40
GOL BA IT	L	2011	7.60	7.30	55.48	104.11	7.45
GOL BA IT	R	2012	6.80	6.50	44.20	104.62	6.65
GOL BA IT	L	2013	6.9C	6.60	45.54	104.55	6.75
MELOLO	L	2092	7.40	7.00	51.80	105.71	7.20
MELOLC	R	2093	6.90	7.10	48.99	97.18	7.00
MELOLC	L	2094	7.10	7.20	51.12	98.61	7.15
MELOLO	R	2095	7.50	7.30	54.75	102.74	7.40
MELOLO	L	2096	6.50	7.00	45.50	92.86	6.75
MELOLO	R	2097	6.90	7.40	51.06	93.24	7.15

LOWER C H. SAPIENS

		N	L(M-D)	B(B-L)	L*B	L/B	L+B/2
MELOLC	L	2098	6.70	7.30	48.91	91.78	7.00
MELOLC	R	2099	7.80	9.20	71.76	84.78	8.50
SAINT CRUZ M	L	2204	7.50	8.50	63.75	88.24	8.00
SAINT CRUZ M	R	2204	7.30	8.30	60.59	87.95	7.80
SAINT CRUZ F	L	2205	7.00	7.70	53.90	90.91	7.35
SAINT CRUZ F	R	2205	7.00	7.50	52.50	93.33	7.25
GREENLAND ESK.	R	1403	7.20	8.30	59.76	86.75	7.75
GREENLAND ESK.	R	1404	7.20	7.50	54.00	96.00	7.35
GREENLAND ESK.	R	1405	6.90	7.10	48.99	97.18	7.00
HAIDA	R	1406	7.60	7.40	56.24	102.70	7.50
MINNESOTA MAN	L	1419	7.20	8.30	59.76	86.75	7.75
MINNESOTA MAN	R	1419	7.20	8.30	59.76	86.75	7.75
TARASCO (AM)	L	1422	8.30	9.70	80.51	85.57	9.00
TARASCO (AM)	L	1423	8.25	9.40	77.55	87.77	8.82
ILLINCIS ME3-10	L	1428	6.30	6.75	42.52	93.33	6.52
ILLINCIS A-2732	R	1429	7.35	7.75	56.96	94.84	7.55
ILLINCIS PK9-B4	L	1432	7.00	7.75	54.25	90.32	7.37
ILLINCIS PK9-B4	R	1432	7.00	7.74	54.18	90.44	7.37
ILLINCIS PK9-B1	L	1433	7.00	10.00	70.00	70.00	8.50
ILLINCIS PK9-B1	R	1433	7.20				
ILLINCIS BR19-3	L	1434	7.60	7.23	54.95	105.12	7.41
ILLINCIS BR19-3	R	1434	7.50	7.00	52.50	107.14	7.25
ILLINCIS A-8C68	L	1437	7.60	8.40	63.84	90.48	8.00
ILLINCIS A-8068	R	1437	7.80	8.85	69.03	88.14	8.32
DICKSCN MOUND	L	1501	7.50	8.80	66.00	85.23	8.15
DICKSCN MOUND	R	1501	7.77	8.55	66.43	90.88	8.16
DICKSCN MD 242	L	1505	7.85	7.65	60.05	102.61	7.75
DICKSON MD 242	R	1505	7.85	7.60	59.66	103.29	7.72
DICKSCN MD 256	R	1506	6.80	7.30	49.64	93.15	7.05
DICKSCN MD 261	L	1508	7.40	7.90	58.46	93.67	7.65
DICKSCN MD 261	R	1508	7.15	7.60	54.34	94.08	7.37
DICKSCN MD 276	L	1514	8.40	8.80	73.92	95.45	8.60
DICKSCN MD 276	R	1514	8.10	8.45	68.44	95.86	8.27
DICKSCN MD 278	R	1515	6.80	8.20	55.76	82.93	7.50
DICKSCN MD 287	L	1516	7.30	8.30	60.59	87.95	7.80
DICKSCN MD 287	R	1516	7.10	8.40	59.64	84.52	7.75
DICKSCN MD 297	L	1520	7.36	7.75	57.04	94.97	7.55
DICKSCN MD 297	R	1520	7.40	7.57	56.02	97.75	7.48
DICKSCN MD 302	L	1521	6.75	6.95	46.91	97.12	6.85
DICKSON MD 302	R	1521	6.65	7.10	47.21	93.66	6.87
DICKSCN MD 319	L	1523	7.35	8.65	63.58	84.97	8.00
DICKSCN MD 319	R	1523	7.40	8.30	61.42	89.16	7.85
DICKSCN MD 327	L	1524	7.55	8.40	63.42	89.88	7.97
DICKSCN MD 327	R	1524	7.30	9.55	69.71	76.44	8.42
DICKSON MD 334	L	1525	8.50	9.40	79.90	90.43	8.95
DICKSGN MD 348	L	1529	6.90	7.15	49.33	96.50	7.02
DICKSCN MD 348	R	1529	6.70	7.25	48.57	92.41	6.97
DICKSCN MD 349	L	1530	7.50	7.40	55.50	101.35	7.45
DICKSCN MD 349	R	1530	7.25	7.50	54.37	96.67	7.37
DICKSCN MD 352	L	1533	7.45	7.95	59.23	93.71	7.70

LOWER C H. SAPIENS

			N	L(M-D)	B(B-L)	L*B	L/B	L+B/2
DICKSCN MD	352	R	1533	7.70	8.40	64.68	91.67	8.05
DICKSCN MD	355	L	1535	7.60	7.75	58.90	98.06	7.67
DICKSCN MD	355	R	1535	7.50	7.70	57.75	97.40	7.60
DICKSON MC	362	L	1539	7.50	7.85	58.87	95.54	7.67
DICKSCN MD	362	R	1539	7.20	7.75	55.80	92.90	7.47
DICKSCN MD	365	L	1540	6.70	7.20	48.24	93.06	6.95
DICKSGN MD	365	R	1540	6.50	7.20	46.80	90.28	6.85
DICKSCN MD	467	L	1541	6.90	7.70	53.13	89.61	7.30
DICKSCN MD	371	L	1542	7.60	7.90	60.04	96.20	7.75
DICKSCN MD	371	R	1542	7.60	7.90	60.04	96.20	7.75
DICKSCN MD	372	L	1543	7.40	7.50	55.50	98.67	7.45
DICKSCN MD	372	R	1543	7.55	7.60	57.38	99.34	7.57
DICKSCN MD	378	L	1547	6.15	6.90	42.43	89.13	6.52
DICKSCN MD	378	R	1547	6.20	6.90	42.78	89.86	6.55
DICKSCN MD	379	L	1548	7.45	7.90	58.85	94.30	7.67
DICKSCN MD	379	R	1548	7.20	8.00	57.60	90.00	7.60
DICKSCN MD	381	L	1550	6.80	7.60	51.68	89.47	7.20
DICKSCN MD	381	R	1550	6.80	7.60	51.68	89.47	7.20
DICKSCN MD	380	L	1551	6.70	7.30	48.91	91.78	7.00
DICKSCN MD	380	R	1551	6.80	7.50	51.00	90.67	7.15
DICKSCN MD	396	L	1553	7.90	8.50	67.15	92.94	8.20
DICKSCN MD	396	R	1553	7.90	9.30	73.47	84.95	8.60
DICKSCN MD	397	L	1554	7.50	8.30	62.25	90.36	7.90
DICKSCN MD	397	R	1554	7.70	8.40	64.68	91.67	8.05
DICKSCN MD	398	L	1555	6.80	7.20	48.96	94.44	7.00
DICKSCN MD	398	R	1555	6.80	7.10	48.28	95.77	6.95
DICKSCN MD	399	L	1556	7.25	8.70	63.07	83.33	7.97
DICKSCN MD	399	R	1556	7.20	8.45	60.84	85.21	7.82
DICKSCN MD	402	R	1557	7.60	9.00	68.40	84.44	8.30
DICKSGN MD	404	L	1559	7.35	8.30	61.00	88.55	7.82
DICKSCN MD	404	R	1559	7.20	8.35	60.12	86.23	7.77
DICKSGN MD	406	L	1560	7.25	7.15	51.84	101.40	7.20
DICKSCN MD	406	R	1560	7.20	7.15	51.48	100.70	7.17
DICKSCN MD	407	L	1561	7.53	7.76	58.43	97.04	7.64
DICKSCN MD	407	R	1561	7.40	7.89	58.39	93.79	7.64
DICKSCN MD	409	L	1562	8.15	8.70	70.90	93.68	8.42
DICKSCN MD	409	R	1562	8.20	8.90	72.98	92.13	8.55
DICKSCN MD	411	L	1563	7.50	7.30	54.75	102.74	7.40
DICKSCN MD	411	R	1563	7.70	7.30	56.21	105.48	7.50
DICKSCN MD	414	L	1564	7.28	7.55	54.96	96.42	7.41
DICKSCN MD	414	R	1564	7.22	7.56	54.58	95.50	7.39
DICKSCN MD	415	L	1565	7.62	8.10	61.72	94.07	7.86
DICKSCN MD	426	L	1566	6.90	6.85	47.26	100.73	6.87
DICKSCN MD	426	R	1566	6.67	6.90	46.02	96.67	6.78
DICKSCN MD	432	L	1567	6.50	7.30	47.45	89.04	6.90
DICKSCN MD	432	R	1567	6.30	7.55	47.56	83.44	6.92
DICKSCN MD	443	L	1571	7.98	8.25	65.83	96.73	8.11
DICKSCN MD	443	R	1571	8.10	8.30	67.23	97.59	8.20
DICKSGN MD	446	L	1572	7.25	6.90	50.02	105.07	7.07
DICKSCN MD	446	R	1572	7.15	6.93	49.55	103.17	7.04

LOWER C H. SAPIENS

			N	L(M-D)	B(B-L)	L*B	L/B	L+B/2
DICKSCN MD	447	L	1573	6.83	6.60	45.08	103.48	6.71
DICKSCN MD	448	R	1574	7.00	7.10	49.70	98.59	7.05
DICKSCN MD	464	L	1575	7.26	7.75	56.26	93.68	7.50
DICKSCN MD	464	R	1575	7.40	7.40	54.76	100.00	7.40
DICKSCN MD	476	L	1576	7.48	7.88	58.94	94.92	7.68
DICKSCN MD	476	R	1576	7.20	7.64	55.01	94.24	7.42
DICKSCN MD	480	L	1578	7.05	7.50	52.87	94.00	7.27
DICKSCN MD	480	R	1578	7.05	7.45	52.52	94.63	7.25
DICKSCN MD	497	L	1583	7.30	8.85	64.60	82.49	8.07
DICKSCN MD	497	R	1583	7.25	8.70	63.07	83.33	7.97
DICKSCN MD	503	L	1585	8.20	8.90	72.98	92.13	8.55
DICKSCN MD	503	R	1585	7.95	8.55	67.97	92.98	8.25
DICKSCN MD	509	L	1587	7.50	7.90	59.25	94.94	7.70
DICKSGN MD	509	R	1587	7.65	7.80	59.67	98.08	7.72
DICKSCN MD	535	L	1591	7.50	7.40	55.50	101.35	7.45
DICKSCN MD	535	R	1591	7.40	7.65	56.61	96.73	7.52
DICKSCN MD	536	L	1592	7.35	7.55	55.49	97.35	7.45
DICKSCN MD	536	R	1592	7.50	7.50	56.25	100.00	7.50
DICKSCN MD	545	L	1594	7.85	8.75	68.69	89.71	8.30
DICKSCN MD	545	R	1594	7.80	8.10	63.18	96.30	7.95
DICKSCN MD	557	L	1596	7.00	7.95	55.65	88.05	7.47
DICKSCN MD	557	R	1596	7.20	7.90	56.88	91.14	7.55
DICKSCN MD	561	L	1597	7.50	8.50	63.75	88.24	8.00
DICKSCN MD	561	R	1597	7.55	8.80	66.44	85.80	8.17
DICKSCN MD	567	L	1598	8.17	8.30	67.81	98.43	8.23
DICKSCN MD	567	R	1598	8.10	8.20	66.42	98.78	8.15
DICKSCN MD	568	L	1599	7.30	8.10	59.13	90.12	7.70
DICKSCN MD	568	R	1599	7.65	8.50	65.02	90.00	8.07
DICKSCN MD	589	L	1600	8.10	8.00	64.80	101.25	8.05
DICKSCN MD	589	R	1600		8.50			
DICKSCN MD	599	L	1602	7.70	8.07	62.14	95.42	7.88
DICKSCN MD	599	R	1602	7.90	8.00	63.20	98.75	7.95
DICKSCN MD	630	L	1603	7.50	8.20	61.50	91.46	7.85
DICKSCN MD	630	R	1603	7.40	7.90	58.46	93.67	7.65
DICKSCN MD	643	L	1608		8.50			
DICKSCN MD	643	R	1608		8.80			
DICKSCN MD	648	L	1609	7.80	8.10	63.18	96.30	7.95
DICKSCN MD	648	R	1609	8.10	8.10	65.61	100.00	8.10
DICKSCN MD	658	L	1613	7.10	7.40	52.54	95.95	7.25
DICKSGN MD	658	R	1613	7.10	7.50	53.25	94.67	7.30
DICKSCN MD	667	L	1614	7.90	7.45	58.85	106.04	7.67
DICKSGN MD	667	R	1614	7.80	8.45	65.91	92.31	8.12
CICKSCN MD	722	L	1624	7.40	8.70	64.38	85.06	8.05
DICKSCN MD	722	R	1624	7.40	8.50	62.90	87.06	7.95
DICKSCN MD	724	L	1627	7.52	8.24	61.96	91.26	7.88
DICKSCN MD	724	R	1627	7.52	8.15	61.29	92.27	7.83
DICKSCN MD	746	L	1628	7.40	8.30	61.42	89.16	7.85
CICKSGN MD	746	R	1628	7.40	8.75	64.75	84.57	8.07
DICKSCN MD	749	L	1629	7.30				
DICKSCN MD	749	R	1629	7.40				

LOWER PM3 H. SAPIENS

		N	L(M-D)	B(B-L)	L*B	L/B	L+B/2
PREDMOST 4	L	1008	7.00	7.70	53.90	90.91	7.35
PREDMOST 4	R	1008	7.30	8.00	58.40	91.25	7.65
PREDMOST 10	L	1014	6.70	8.40	56.28	79.76	7.55
PREDMOST 10	R	1014	7.00	8.00	56.00	87.50	7.50
COMBE CHAPELLE	L	1017	6.00	7.00	42.00	85.71	6.50
COMBE CHAPELLE	R	1017	6.00	9.00	54.00	66.67	7.50
BRNO 3	L	1018	6.70	8.40	56.28	79.76	7.55
BRNO 3	R	1018	6.50	8.30	53.95	78.31	7.40
GRIMALDI ADOL.	L	1019	7.50	8.20	61.50	91.46	7.85
GRIMALDI ADOL.	R	1019	7.40	8.40	62.16	88.10	7.90
ROIS A		1024	7.50	8.50	63.75	88.24	8.00
ROIS B		1025	7.50	8.50	63.75	88.24	8.00
ROIS R51-22		1043	8.00	8.50	68.00	94.12	8.25
SALEMAS	L	1056	6.50	7.30	47.45	89.04	6.90
VESTONICE 3	L	1057	5.80	8.30	48.14	69.88	7.05
VESTONICE 3	R	1057	5.80	7.90	45.82	73.42	6.85
A CULOZ 2	L	1101	7.10	9.00	63.90	78.89	8.05
A CULOZ 2	R	1101	7.00	8.60	60.20	81.40	7.80
BUGGISON 1	L	1108	8.00	8.50	68.00	94.12	8.25
BUGGISON 1	R	1108	8.00	9.00	72.00	88.89	8.50
BUGGISON 2	L	1109	8.00	8.00	64.00	100.00	8.00
BUGGISON 2	R	1109	8.00	8.50	68.00	94.12	8.25
CAP BLAC	L	1110	6.00	7.60	45.60	78.95	6.80
CAP BLAC	R	1110	5.80	7.60	44.08	76.32	6.70
CHANCELADE	L	1111	6.00	9.00	54.00	66.67	7.50
FARINCOURT 3	L	1115	6.50	7.00	45.50	92.86	6.75
FARINCOURT 3	R	1115	6.60	7.20	47.52	91.67	6.90
GALLEY HILL	R	1116	7.00	7.20	50.40	97.22	7.10
GARDAR	R	1117	7.10	8.00	56.80	88.75	7.55
HOHLERFELS A	R	1118	7.00	9.00	63.00	77.78	8.00
HOHLERFELS C	R	1119	6.50	8.00	52.00	81.25	7.25
LACHAUD A	L	1125	7.40	7.90	58.46	93.67	7.65
LACHAUD A	R	1125	7.00	7.80	54.60	89.74	7.40
LAFAYE	L	1128	6.90	8.20	56.58	84.15	7.55
LAFAYE	R	1128	6.50	8.30	53.95	78.31	7.40
MASAT		1130	7.10	7.70	54.67	92.21	7.40
OBERCASSEL 1	L	1132	7.00	8.00	56.00	87.50	7.50
OKUZINI		1133	6.70	8.00	53.60	83.75	7.35
PAS ESTRET 3	L	1134	6.70	7.00	46.90	95.71	6.85
PRITZERBER 3	L	1138	6.50	8.00	52.00	81.25	7.25
PRITZERBER 6	R	1141	9.00	6.50	58.50	138.46	7.75
SVAERDBORG	R	1144	8.00	8.20	65.60	97.56	8.10
KAFFIR		1147	7.20	8.20	59.04	87.80	7.70
KAFFIR		1148	7.30	7.50	54.75	97.33	7.40
FRENCHMAN	L	1149	6.75	7.75	52.31	87.10	7.25
FRENCHMAN	R	1149	6.40	8.00	51.20	80.00	7.20
EUROPEAN 344C	R	1150	6.30	7.00	44.10	90.00	6.65
EUROPEAN AJ2	R	1151	6.50	7.10	46.15	91.55	6.80
WHITE 99-7740	L	1152	7.35	8.05	59.17	91.30	7.70
WHITE ZZZ		1153	7.00	7.50	52.50	93.33	7.25

LOWER PM3 H. SAPIENS

		N	L(M-D)	B(B-L)	L*B	L/B	L+B/2
WHITE 14		1154	7.70	7.60	58.52	101.32	7.65
WHITE 4F		1155	7.10	6.80	48.28	104.41	6.95
WHITE 3W		1156	6.20	7.30	45.26	84.93	6.75
WHITE EDNA		1157	6.50	7.80	50.70	83.33	7.15
WHITE H		1158	6.50	7.80	50.70	83.33	7.15
WHITE PG		1159	6.30	7.30	45.99	86.30	6.80
WHITE M		1160	7.50	7.50	56.25	100.00	7.50
WHITE HJB		1161	7.00	8.50	59.50	82.35	7.75
WHITE GT		1162	7.40	7.00	51.80	105.71	7.20
WHITE ANI		1163	7.70	8.40	64.68	91.67	8.05
WHITE BRD		1164	6.80	7.20	48.96	94.44	7.00
WHITE GN		1165	7.50	8.20	61.50	91.46	7.85
WHITE GIVC		1166	7.30	8.20	59.86	89.02	7.75
WHITE BX		1167	7.60	7.50	57.00	101.33	7.55
WHITE CQ		1168	7.40	7.40	54.76	100.00	7.40
WHITE GM		1169	7.50	8.70	65.25	86.21	8.10
WHITE AAD		1170	6.50	8.00	52.00	81.25	7.25
WHITE BIY		1171	7.00	7.50	52.50	93.33	7.25
WHITE AIO		1172	6.50	7.30	47.45	89.04	6.90
WHITE EK	R	1173	7.70	8.40	64.68	91.67	8.05
WHITE 11		1174	6.70	7.30	48.91	91.78	7.00
ALACA HOYUK 2		1183	7.20	7.70	55.44	93.51	7.45
ALACA HOYUK 3		1184	6.90	7.40	51.06	93.24	7.15
WADI HALFA	L	1208	7.50	8.30	62.25	90.36	7.90
WADI HALFA	L	1209	7.40	8.50	62.90	87.06	7.95
WADJAK 2	R	1702	8.50	9.00	76.50	94.44	8.75
AUSTRALIAN 39		1708	7.00	9.00	63.00	77.78	8.00
AUSTRALIAN 8174		1711	7.30	9.20	67.16	79.35	8.25
AUSTRALIAN AM		1712	7.00	7.80	54.60	89.74	7.40
AUSTRALIAN AM		1713	7.00	8.40	58.80	83.33	7.70
AUSTRALIAN AM		1714	7.00	7.80	54.60	89.74	7.40
AUSTRALIAN AM		1715	7.00	8.20	57.40	85.37	7.60
AUSTRALIAN AM		1716	7.20	8.20	59.04	87.80	7.70
AUSTRALIAN AM		1717	6.50	8.00	52.00	81.25	7.25
AUSTRALIAN AM		1718	7.40	9.30	68.82	79.57	8.35
AUSTRALIAN AM		1719	7.20	7.80	56.16	92.31	7.50
AUSTRALIAN AM		1720	7.30	8.50	62.05	85.88	7.90
AUSTRALIAN AM		1721	7.60	8.70	66.12	87.36	8.15
AUSTRALIAN 90	R	1722	7.00	8.50	59.50	82.35	7.75
AUSTRALIAN 54	R	1723		9.00			
AUSTRALIAN 88	L	1724	7.00	8.50	59.50	82.35	7.75
AUSTRALIAN	L	1727	7.50	7.85	58.87	95.54	7.67
AUSTRALIAN	L	1729	7.10	9.00	63.90	78.89	8.05
AUSTRALIAN	R	1729	8.10	9.00	72.90	90.00	8.55
TASMANIAN 310		1754	8.00	9.00	72.00	88.89	8.50
TASMANIAN P3	R	1759	8.00	9.00	72.00	88.89	8.50
TASMANIAN 2964	L	1763	8.00	8.90	71.20	89.89	8.45
ASSELAR	R	1903	7.00	9.00	63.00	77.78	8.00
CAPE FLATS	R	1904	8.00	9.00	72.00	88.89	8.50
NEGRO	L	1906	8.35	8.15	68.05	102.45	8.25

LOWER PM3 H. SAPIENS

		N	L(M-D)	B(B-L)	L*B	L/B	L+B/2
NEGRO AM		1907	7.50	8.20	61.50	91.46	7.85
NEGRO AM		1908	7.50	9.20	69.00	81.52	8.35
NEGRO AM		1909	7.40	8.70	64.38	85.06	8.05
NEGRO AM		1910	8.20	9.50	77.90	86.32	8.85
NEGRO AM		1911	8.00	8.30	66.40	96.39	8.15
NEGRO AM		1912	7.50	9.00	67.50	83.33	8.25
NEGRO		1914	7.30	7.90	57.67	92.41	7.60
NEGRO	L	1915	9.50	9.70	92.15	97.94	9.60
NEGRO	R	1915	9.60	10.00	96.00	96.00	9.80
NEGRO	L	1916	9.20	10.20	93.84	90.20	9.70
NEGRO	R	1916	8.70	9.80	85.26	88.78	9.25
NEGRO 2	L	1919	7.30	8.70	63.51	83.91	8.00
NEGRO 2	R	1919	7.40	8.00	59.20	92.50	7.70
NEGRO 1	L	1920	7.10	8.80	62.48	80.68	7.95
NEGRO 29	L	1925	9.30	9.15	85.09	101.64	9.22
NEGRO 29	R	1925	8.95	8.90	79.65	100.56	8.92
N/HOTTENTOT 12	L	1943	6.15	6.50	39.97	94.62	6.32
N/HOTTENTOT 6	L	1944	8.25	8.75	72.19	94.29	8.50
N/HOTTENTOT 6	R	1944	7.80	9.25	72.15	84.32	8.52
N/BUSHMAN 52	L	1945	7.65				
N/BUSHMAN 52	R	1945	7.75	8.90	68.97	87.08	8.32
BUSHMAN MXD 61	L	1946	6.85	7.60	52.06	90.13	7.22
BUSHMAN MXD 61	R	1946	6.75	7.20	48.60	93.75	6.97
BUSHMAN MXD 94	L	1947	7.10	8.40	59.64	84.52	7.75
BUSHMAN MXD 94	R	1947	6.95	7.50	52.12	92.67	7.22
N/HOTTENTOT 6	L	1948	7.90	8.75	69.12	90.29	8.32
N/HOTTENTOT 6	R	1948	7.70	8.50	65.45	90.59	8.10
BUSHMAN MXD 101	L	1949	7.00	8.20	57.40	85.37	7.60
BUSHMAN MXD 101	R	1949	7.50	7.00	52.50	107.14	7.25
MAPUNGUBWE M1A		1951	7.60	8.90	67.64	85.39	8.25
MAPUNGUBWE M2		1952	8.00	9.50	76.00	84.21	8.75
MAPUNGUBWE M3		1953	7.90	8.90	70.31	88.76	8.40
MAPUNGUBWE M9		1955	8.00	9.20	73.60	86.96	8.60
BAMBANDYANALO21		1957	7.00	8.00	56.00	87.50	7.50
BAMBANDYANALO29		1958	6.90	8.00	55.20	86.25	7.45
BAMBANDYANALO31		1959	8.50	9.00	76.50	94.44	8.75
BAMBANDYANALO33	R	1960	7.60	9.10	69.16	83.52	8.35
BAMBANDYANALO 2		1961	8.30	8.20	68.06	101.22	8.25
BAMBANDYANALO 3		1962	8.20	9.10	74.62	90.11	8.65
BAMBANDYANALO13		1964	7.50	9.20	69.00	81.52	8.35
BAMBANDYANALO14		1965	6.80	8.20	55.76	82.93	7.50
BUSHMAN		1967	6.90	7.60	52.44	90.79	7.25
BUSHMAN AM		1968	7.00	8.00	56.00	87.50	7.50
HOTTENTOT AM		1969	7.00	8.50	59.50	82.35	7.75
HOTTENTOT AM		1970	8.20	9.50	77.90	86.32	8.85
HOTTENTOT AM		1971	8.30	9.20	76.36	90.22	8.75
FISH HOEK	R	1972	6.00	6.00	36.00	100.00	6.00
BUSHMAN 30	L	1973	6.75	7.20	48.60	93.75	6.97
BUSHMAN 30	R	1973	6.90	7.50	51.75	92.00	7.20
GOUNGCU A	L	1975	6.55	8.25	54.04	79.39	7.40

LOWER PM3 H. SAPIENS

		N	L(M-D)	B(B-L)	L*B	L/B	L+B/2
N.BRITAIN 43121	L	1301	7.10	8.60	61.06	82.56	7.85
N.BRITAIN 43127	L	1306	7.20	9.00	64.80	80.00	8.10
N.BRITAIN 43131	L	1308	6.90	8.80	60.72	78.41	7.85
N.BRITAIN 43131	R	1308	6.50	8.70	56.55	74.71	7.60
N.BRITAIN 43135	L	1312	6.40	8.20	52.48	78.05	7.30
N.BRITAIN 43136	L	1313	7.40	7.60	56.24	97.37	7.50
N.BRITAIN 43137	L	1314	8.30	9.20	76.36	90.22	8.75
N.BRITAIN 43137	R	1314	8.20	9.10	74.62	90.11	8.65
N.BRITAIN 43138	L	1315	7.90	9.50	75.05	83.16	8.70
N.BRITAIN 43138	R	1315	7.70	9.60	73.92	80.21	8.65
N.BRITAIN 43141	L	1318	7.20	7.70	55.44	93.51	7.45
N.BRITAIN 43141	R	1318	7.00	7.70	53.90	90.91	7.35
N.BRITAIN 43142	L	1319	7.40	9.40	69.56	78.72	8.40
N.BRITAIN 43143	L	1320	7.30	8.30	60.59	87.95	7.80
N.BRITAIN 43144	L	1321	7.20	8.60	61.92	83.72	7.90
N.BRITAIN 43144	R	1321		7.80			
N.BRITAIN 43147	L	1324	8.00	8.00	64.00	100.00	8.00
N.BRITAIN 43147	R	1324	6.80	8.90	60.52	76.40	7.85
N.BRITAIN 43150	L	1326	7.20	8.00	57.60	90.00	7.60
N.BRITAIN 43150	R	1326	7.40	8.20	60.68	90.24	7.80
N.BRITAIN 43151	L	1327	8.00	7.70	61.60	103.90	7.85
N.BRITAIN 43151	R	1327	7.80	7.80	60.84	100.00	7.80
N.BRITAIN 43153	L	1329		7.40			
N.BRITAIN 43153	R	1329	6.60	7.10	46.86	92.96	6.85
N.BRITAIN 43154	L	1330	7.00	8.70	60.90	80.46	7.85
N.BRITAIN 43154	R	1330	7.10	8.80	62.48	80.68	7.95
N.BRITAIN 43174	L	1331	6.60	9.60	63.36	68.75	8.10
N.BRITAIN 43174	R	1331	7.10	8.30	58.93	85.54	7.70
N.BRITAIN 43179	R	1332	8.20	9.00	73.80	91.11	8.60
N.BRITAIN 43193	R	1333	7.30	9.00	65.70	81.11	8.15
N.BRITAIN 43198	R	1335	7.60	8.50	64.60	89.41	8.05
N.BRITAIN 43199	R	1336	7.20	7.70	55.44	93.51	7.45
N.BRITAIN 43204	L	1338	7.90	9.10	71.89	86.81	8.50
N.BRITAIN 43204	R	1338	7.90	9.30	73.47	84.95	8.60
N.BRITAIN 43226	R	1339	7.10	8.10	57.51	87.65	7.60
N.BRITAIN 43242	R	1341	6.85	8.10	55.48	84.57	7.47
N.BRITAIN 43291	L	1343	7.10	9.00	63.90	78.89	8.05
N.BRITAIN 43291	R	1343	7.40	9.20	68.08	80.43	8.30
N.BRITAIN 43295	L	1344	6.90	9.60	66.24	71.87	8.25
N.BRITAIN 43295	R	1344	7.00	9.30	65.10	75.27	8.15
N.BRITAIN 43296	L	1345	7.10	8.30	58.93	85.54	7.70
N.BRITAIN 43296	R	1345	6.90	8.30	57.27	83.13	7.60
N.BRITAIN	L	1346	7.40	8.70	64.38	85.06	8.05
N.BRITAIN	R	1346	7.80	8.90	69.42	87.64	8.35
HINDU AM 7894	L	2201	7.85	8.30	65.15	94.58	8.07
HINDU (UI)	L	2208	6.10	7.75	47.27	78.71	6.92
HINDU (UI)	R	2208	6.55	7.00	45.85	93.57	6.77
GOL BA IT 98	L	2003		8.20			
GOL BA IT 98	R	2003		8.30			
GOL BA IT	R	2014	7.80	8.80	68.64	88.64	8.30

LOWER PM3 H. SAPIENS

		N	L(M-D)	B(B-L)	L*B	L/B	L+B/2
GOL BA IT	L	2015	7.80	8.60	67.08	90.70	8.20
MELOLO	L	2100	7.40	8.00	59.20	92.50	7.70
MELOLC	R	2101	7.90	8.10	63.99	97.53	8.00
MELOLC	L	2102	7.10	8.00	56.80	88.75	7.55
MELOLC	R	2103	7.70	8.20	63.14	93.90	7.95
MELOLO	L	2104	8.00	9.30	74.40	86.02	8.65
MELOLC	R	2105	8.30	8.90	73.87	93.26	8.60
SAINT CRUZ M	L	2204	6.00	8.00	48.00	75.00	7.00
SAINT CRUZ M	R	2204	7.00	8.00	56.00	87.50	7.50
SAINT CRUZ F	L	2205	7.00	8.00	56.00	87.50	7.50
SAINT CRUZ F	R	2205	6.70	8.00	53.60	83.75	7.35
HAIDA	L	1406	7.40	7.60	56.24	97.37	7.50
HAICA	R	1406	7.70	7.80	60.06	98.72	7.75
INDIAN (AM)		1407	7.90	7.60	60.04	103.95	7.75
INDIAN (AM)		1408	7.40	7.70	56.98	96.10	7.55
INDIAN (AM)		1409	7.20	7.60	54.72	94.74	7.40
INDIAN (AM)		1410	7.40	8.30	61.42	89.16	7.85
INDIAN (AM)		1411	7.40	8.60	63.64	86.05	8.00
INDIAN (AM)		1412	7.30	8.00	58.40	91.25	7.65
INCIAN (AM)		1413	6.40	6.60	42.24	96.97	6.50
INDIAN (AM)		1414	6.10	7.90	48.19	77.22	7.00
INCIAN (AM)		1415	6.50	7.40	48.10	87.84	6.95
INDIAN (AM)		1416	6.30	6.80	42.84	92.65	6.55
MINNESOTA MAN	L	1419	7.30	8.30	60.59	87.95	7.80
MINNESOTA MAN	R	1419	7.30	8.30	60.59	87.95	7.80
TARASCO (AM)	L	1421	7.50	9.10	68.25	82.42	8.30
TARASCO (AM)	L	1422	8.10	8.80	71.28	92.05	8.45
TARASCO (AM)	L	1423	8.40	9.00	75.60	93.33	8.70
ILLINCIS ME3-10	L	1428	6.05	6.40	38.72	94.53	6.22
ILLINCIS A-2732	L	1429	7.50	6.60	49.50	113.64	7.05
ILLINCIS A-2732	R	1429	6.75	7.75	52.31	87.10	7.25
ILLINCIS A-4921	L	1431	7.90				
ILLINOIS A-4921	R	1431	7.70	7.95	61.21	96.86	7.82
ILLINCIS PK9-B4	L	1432	6.00	7.80	46.80	76.92	6.90
ILLINCIS PK9-B4	R	1432	6.35	8.00	50.80	79.37	7.17
ILLINCIS PK9-B1	L	1433	7.00				
ILLINCIS PK9-B1	R	1433	7.40	8.80	65.12	84.09	8.10
ILLINOIS BR19-3	L	1434	8.45	7.55	63.80	111.92	8.00
ILLINOIS BR19-3	R	1434	7.70	7.60	58.52	101.32	7.65
ILLINCIS A-8068	L	1437	7.15				
ILLINOIS A-8068	R	1437	6.70				
DICKSCN MOUND	L	1501	7.23	8.00	57.84	90.37	7.61
DICKSCN MOUND	R	1501	7.10	8.25	58.57	86.06	7.67
DICKSCN MD 242	L	1505	8.00	7.65	61.20	104.58	7.82
DICKSCN MD 242	R	1505	8.25	7.60	62.70	108.55	7.92
DICKSCN MD 256	L	1506	6.60	7.40	48.84	89.19	7.00
DICKSCN MD 256	R	1506	6.65	7.30	48.54	91.10	6.97
DICKSCN MD 261	L	1508	7.40	8.30	61.42	89.16	7.85
DICKSGN MD 261	R	1508	7.35	8.43	61.96	87.19	7.89
DICKSCN MD 262	R	1509	8.35	8.15	68.05	102.45	8.25

LOWER PM3 H. SAPIENS

		N	L(M-D)	B(B-L)	L*B	L/B	L+B/2
DICKSCN MD 266	R	1510	8.00	7.60	60.80	105.26	7.80
CICKSCN MD 276	L	1514	7.60	8.65	65.74	87.86	8.12
DICKSCN MD 276	R	1514	7.66	8.55	65.49	89.59	8.10
DICKSCN MD 278	R	1515	6.40	7.60	48.64	84.21	7.00
DICKSCN MD 287	R	1516	6.75	7.75	52.31	87.10	7.25
DICKSCN MD 297	L	1520	7.32	7.82	57.24	93.61	7.57
DICKSCN MD 297	R	1520	7.56	7.70	58.21	98.18	7.63
DICKSCN MD 302	R	1521	6.60	6.80	44.88	97.06	6.70
DICKSON MD 319	L	1523	6.90	7.30	50.37	94.52	7.10
CICKSCA MD 319	R	1523	6.55	7.55	49.45	86.75	7.05
DICKSCN MD 327	L	1524	7.10	8.90	63.19	79.78	8.00
DICKSCN MD 327	R	1524	7.10	8.95	63.54	79.33	8.02
DICKSCN MD 334	L	1525	7.20	8.40	60.48	85.71	7.80
DICKSCN MD 334	R	1525	7.10	8.50	60.35	83.53	7.80
DICKSCN MD 344	R	1527	7.35	8.40	61.74	87.50	7.87
DICKSCN MD 348	L	1529	6.95	7.70	53.51	90.26	7.32
CICKSCN MD 348	R	1529	6.80	7.70	52.36	88.31	7.25
DICKSCN MD 349	L	1530	7.40	7.75	57.35	95.48	7.57
DICKSCN MD 349	R	1530	7.65	7.50	57.37	102.00	7.57
DICKSCN MD 352	L	1533	7.40	7.95	58.83	93.08	7.67
DICKSCN MD 355	L	1535	7.50	8.30	62.25	90.36	7.90
DICKSCN MD 355	R	1535	8.00	8.45	67.60	94.67	8.22
DICKSCN MD 362	L	1539	7.65	8.10	61.96	94.44	7.87
DICKSCN MD 362	R	1539	7.55	8.40	63.42	89.88	7.97
DICKSCN MD 365	L	1540	7.10	7.70	54.67	92.21	7.40
DICKSCN MD 365	R	1540	7.20	7.90	56.88	91.14	7.55
DICKSCN MD 467	L	1541	6.90	8.00	55.20	86.25	7.45
DICKSCN MD 371	L	1542	7.70	8.40	64.68	91.67	8.05
DICKSCN MD 371	R	1542	7.40	8.50	62.90	87.06	7.95
DICKSCN MD 372	L	1543	7.10	7.65	54.31	92.81	7.37
DICKSCA MD 372	R	1543	6.90	8.00	55.20	86.25	7.45
DICKSCN MD 378	L	1547	6.70	7.20	48.24	93.06	6.95
DICKSCN MD 378	R	1547	6.40	7.40	47.36	86.49	6.90
DICKSCN MD 379	L	1548	7.90	8.55	67.54	92.40	8.22
DICKSCN MD 379	R	1548	7.80	8.40	65.52	92.86	8.10
DICKSCN MD 381	L	1550	7.50	8.40	63.00	89.29	7.95
DICKSCN MD 381	R	1550	7.30	8.50	62.05	85.88	7.90
DICKSON MD 380	L	1551	6.40	7.80	49.92	82.05	7.10
DICKSCN MD 380	R	1551	6.40	7.90	50.56	81.01	7.15
DICKSCN MD 388	R	1552	7.90	8.90	70.31	88.76	8.40
DICKSCN MD 396	L	1553	7.70	8.60	66.22	89.53	8.15
DICKSCN MD 396	R	1553	7.80	8.80	68.64	88.64	8.30
DICKSCN MD 397	L	1554	7.50	7.90	59.25	94.94	7.70
DICKSCN MD 397	R	1554	7.20	8.10	58.32	88.89	7.65
DICKSCN MD 398	L	1555	6.75	7.50	50.62	90.00	7.12
DICKSCN MD 398	R	1555	6.80	7.15	48.62	95.10	6.97
DICKSCN MD 399	L	1556	7.10	7.90	56.09	89.87	7.50
DICKSCN MD 399	R	1556	6.85	7.90	54.11	86.71	7.37
DICKSCN MD 402	R	1557	7.40	8.60	63.64	86.05	8.00
DICKSCN MD 404	L	1559	7.20	8.50	61.20	84.71	7.85

LOWER PM3 H. SAPIENS

			N	L(M-D)	B(B-L)	L*B	L/B	L+B/2
DICKSCN MD	404	R	1559	7.50	8.10	60.75	92.59	7.80
DICKSCN MD	406	R	1560	7.60	7.90	60.04	96.20	7.75
DICKSCN MD	407	L	1561	7.65	8.45	64.64	90.53	8.05
DICKSCN MD	407	R	1561	7.90	8.40	66.36	94.05	8.15
DICKSCN MD	409	R	1562	7.90	8.70	68.73	90.80	8.30
DICKSCN MD	411	L	1563	8.00	8.10	64.80	98.77	8.05
DICKSCN MD	411	R	1563	7.58	8.50	64.43	89.18	8.04
DICKSCN MD	414	L	1564	6.85	7.71	52.81	88.85	7.28
DICKSCN MD	414	R	1564	6.78	7.71	52.27	87.94	7.24
DICKSCN MD	415	L	1565	6.97	7.80	54.37	89.36	7.38
DICKSCN MD	415	R	1565	6.80	7.80	53.04	87.18	7.30
DICKSCN MD	426	L	1566	7.27	7.65	55.62	95.03	7.46
DICKSCN MD	426	R	1566	7.10	7.75	55.02	91.61	7.42
DICKSCN MD	432	L	1567	6.40	6.90	44.16	92.75	6.65
DICKSCN MD	432	R	1567	6.15	6.70	41.20	91.79	6.42
DICKSGN MD	443	L	1571	7.25	7.90	57.27	91.77	7.57
DICKSCN MD	443	R	1571	7.36	8.25	60.72	89.21	7.80
DICKSCN MD	446	L	1572	7.37	7.57	55.79	97.36	7.47
DICKSCN MD	446	R	1572	7.25	7.60	55.10	95.39	7.42
DICKSCN MD	448	L	1574	8.00	6.90	55.20	115.94	7.45
DICKSCN MD	464	L	1575	7.20	7.80	56.16	92.31	7.50
DICKSCN MD	464	R	1575	7.60	7.80	59.28	97.44	7.70
DICKSCN MD	476	L	1576	7.85	8.55	67.12	91.81	8.20
DICKSCN MD	476	R	1576	7.70	8.15	62.75	94.48	7.92
DICKSCN MD	480	L	1578	6.40	7.30	46.72	87.67	6.85
DICKSCN MD	480	R	1578	5.92	7.05	41.74	83.97	6.48
DICKSCN MD	497	L	1583	7.40	8.95	66.23	82.68	8.17
DICKSCN MD	497	R	1583	7.25	8.95	64.89	81.01	8.10
DICKSCN MD	503	L	1585	7.28	7.75	56.42	93.94	7.51
DICKSCN MD	503	R	1585	7.10	7.93	56.30	89.53	7.51
DICKSCN MD	509	L	1587	7.40	8.17	60.46	90.58	7.78
DICKSCN MD	509	R	1587	7.35	8.00	58.80	91.87	7.67
DICKSCN MD	535	L	1591	6.90	7.30	50.37	94.52	7.10
DICKSCN MD	535	R	1591	7.10	7.40	52.54	95.95	7.25
DICKSON MD	536	L	1592	7.15	7.40	52.91	96.62	7.27
DICKSCN MD	536	R	1592	6.88	7.43	51.12	92.60	7.15
DICKSCN MD	545	R	1594	7.92	8.60	68.11	92.09	8.26
DICKSCN MD	557	L	1596	6.85	7.40	50.69	92.57	7.12
DICKSCN MD	557	R	1596	6.80	7.43	50.52	91.52	7.11
DICKSCN MD	561	L	1597	6.90	7.80	53.82	88.46	7.35
DICKSON MD	561	R	1597	7.40	8.30	61.42	89.16	7.85
DICKSCN MD	567	L	1598	7.60	8.73	66.35	87.06	8.16
DICKSCN MD	567	R	1598	7.80	8.70	67.86	89.66	8.25
DICKSCN MD	568	L	1599	6.97	7.67	53.46	90.87	7.32
DICKSCN MD	568	R	1599	6.85	7.85	53.77	87.26	7.35
DICKSCN MD	589	L	1600	6.90	8.00	55.20	86.25	7.45
DICKSCN MD	589	R	1600	7.40	8.00	59.20	92.50	7.70
DICKSCN MD	599	L	1602	7.50	8.30	62.25	90.36	7.90
DICKSCN MD	599	R	1602	7.35	8.17	60.05	89.96	7.76
DICKSCN MD	630	L	1603	7.70	8.10	62.37	95.06	7.90

LOWER PM3 H. SAPIENS

			N	L(M-D)	B(B-L)	L*B	L/B	L+B/2
DICKSCN MD	630	R	1603	7.60	8.10	61.56	93.83	7.85
DICKSCN MD	643	L	1608	7.30	8.90	64.97	82.02	8.10
DICKSGN MD	643	R	1608	7.00	8.80	61.60	79.55	7.90
DICKSCN MD	648	R	1609	7.60	8.00	60.80	95.00	7.80
DICKSCN MD	652	L	1611	7.60	7.70	58.52	98.70	7.65
DICKSCN MD	658	L	1613	7.50	8.50	63.75	88.24	8.00
DICKSCN MD	667	L	1614	7.25	8.25	59.81	87.88	7.75
DICKSCN MD	667	R	1614	7.48	8.45	63.21	88.52	7.96
DICKSCN MD	709	L	1623	6.95	7.75	53.86	89.68	7.35
DICKSCN MD	722	L	1624	6.60	8.05	53.13	81.99	7.32
DICKSCN MD	722	R	1624	7.05	8.10	57.10	87.04	7.57
DICKSCN MD	724	L	1627	7.90	8.70	68.73	90.80	8.30
DICKSCN MD	724	R	1627	7.67	8.40	64.43	91.31	8.03
DICKSCN MD	746	L	1628	7.20	8.22	59.18	87.59	7.71
DICKSCN MD	746	R	1628	7.10	8.15	57.86	87.12	7.62
DICKSCN MD	749	L	1629	8.70	7.85	68.29	110.83	8.27
DICKSCN MD	749	R	1629	8.65	7.90	68.33	109.49	8.27

LOWER PM4 H. SAPIENS

		N	L(M-D)	B(B-L)	L*B	L/B	L+B/2
ARCYSLRCURE C9		1003	8.50	10.10	85.85	84.16	9.30
PREDMCST 4	L	1008	7.20	8.30	59.76	86.75	7.75
PREDMCST 4	R	1008	7.30	8.00	58.40	91.25	7.65
PREDMOST 10	L	1014	7.00	9.00	63.00	77.78	8.00
PREDMOST 10	R	1014	7.50	8.80	66.00	85.23	8.15
COMBE CHAPELLE	L	1017	7.00	8.00	56.00	87.50	7.50
COMBE CHAPELLE	R	1017	7.00	9.50	66.50	73.68	8.25
BRNO 3	L	1018	6.70	8.80	58.96	76.14	7.75
BRNO 3	R	1018	6.40	8.50	54.40	75.29	7.45
GRIMALDI ADOL.	L	1019	6.80	9.50	64.60	71.58	8.15
GRIMALDI ADOL.	R	1019	7.30	9.30	67.89	78.49	8.30
ROIS A		1024	8.50				
ROIS B		1025	8.00	9.00	72.00	88.89	8.50
ROIS R51-23		1044	8.00	8.50	68.00	94.12	8.25
ROIS		1053	7.50	8.50	63.75	88.24	8.00
SALEMAS	L	1056	7.00	8.30	58.10	84.34	7.65
VESTONICE 3	L	1057	6.30	8.40	52.92	75.00	7.35
VESTONICE 3	R	1057	6.60	8.60	56.76	76.74	7.60
A CULCZ 2	L	1101	7.00	9.00	63.00	77.78	8.00
A CULCZ 2	R	1101	7.10	9.00	63.90	78.89	8.05
BUGGISON 1	L	1108	8.00	9.00	72.00	88.89	8.50
BUGGISON 1	R	1108	8.00	8.50	68.00	94.12	8.25
BUGGISON 2	L	1109	7.50	8.00	60.00	93.75	7.75
CAP BLAC	L	1110	6.20	8.10	50.22	76.54	7.15
CAP BLAC	R	1110	6.00	8.50	51.00	70.59	7.25
CHANCELADE	L	1111	6.00	9.00	54.00	66.67	7.50
CHANCELADE	R	1111	6.00	9.00	54.00	66.67	7.50
EGOLZWIL 1	L	1112	6.40	7.20	46.08	88.89	6.80
FARINCOURT 3	L	1115	6.50	7.00	45.50	92.86	6.75
FARINCOURT 3	R	1115	6.50	7.30	47.45	89.04	6.90
GALLEY HILL	R	1116	7.00	8.00	56.00	87.50	7.50
GARDAR	R	1117	7.20	8.00	57.60	90.00	7.60
HOHLERFELS A	L	1118		8.00			
HOHLERFELS A	R	1118	7.00	8.90	62.30	78.65	7.95
HOHLERFELS C	R	1119	7.10	8.10	57.51	87.65	7.60
LACHALC A	L	1125	7.50	8.10	60.75	92.59	7.80
LACHALC A	R	1125	7.00	8.00	56.00	87.50	7.50
LAFAYE	L	1128	6.90	8.90	61.41	77.53	7.90
LAFAYE	R	1128	6.30	8.70	54.81	72.41	7.50
MASAT		1130	7.60	8.20	62.32	92.68	7.90
OBERCASSEL 1	L	1132	6.50	8.50	55.25	76.47	7.50
OKUZINI		1133	7.40	8.70	64.38	85.06	8.05
PRITZERBER 3	L	1138	7.00	8.00	56.00	87.50	7.50
PRITZERBER 5	R	1140	10.00	8.50	85.00	117.65	9.25
PRITZERBER 6	L	1141	10.00	9.00	90.00	111.11	9.50
PRITZERBER 6	R	1141	10.50	9.50	99.75	110.53	10.00
SVAERCBORG	R	1144	7.50	8.80	66.00	85.23	8.15
KAFFIR		1147	6.90	8.20	56.58	84.15	7.55
KAFFIR		1148	7.50	8.80	66.00	85.23	8.15
FRENCHMAN	L	1149	7.10	8.25	58.57	86.06	7.67

LOWER PM4 H. SAPIENS

		N	L(M-D)	B(B-L)	L*B	L/B	L+B/2
FRENCHMAN	R	1149	6.00	8.80	52.80	68.18	7.40
EUROPEAN 344C	R	1150	6.30	7.60	47.88	82.89	6.95
EUROPEAN AJ2	R	1151	6.50	7.50	48.75	86.67	7.00
WHITE 99-7740	L	1152	6.90	7.15	49.33	96.50	7.02
WHITE ZZZ		1153	8.00	8.60	68.80	93.02	8.30
WHITE 14		1154	7.20	8.60	61.92	83.72	7.90
WHITE 4F		1155	7.30	8.40	61.32	86.90	7.85
WHITE 3W		1156	6.40	7.80	49.92	82.05	7.10
WHITE EDNA		1157	7.00	8.30	58.10	84.34	7.65
WHITE H		1158	6.80	8.30	56.44	81.93	7.55
WHITE PG		1159	6.60	7.80	51.48	84.62	7.20
WHITE M		1160	6.60	8.30	54.78	79.52	7.45
WHITE HJB		1161	6.80	8.70	59.16	78.16	7.75
WHITE GT		1162	6.60	8.80	58.08	75.00	7.70
WHITE ANI		1163	6.70	9.00	60.30	74.44	7.85
WHITE BRD		1164	6.50	7.60	49.40	85.53	7.05
WHITE GN		1165	7.00	9.00	63.00	77.78	8.00
WHITE GIVC		1166	7.30	8.70	63.51	83.91	8.00
WHITE BX		1167	7.00	8.50	59.50	82.35	7.75
WHITE CQ		1168	7.50	8.50	63.75	88.24	8.00
WHITE GM		1169	8.00	9.60	76.80	83.33	8.80
WHITE AAD		1170	7.20	8.70	62.64	82.76	7.95
WHITE BIY		1171	7.20	7.80	56.16	92.31	7.50
WHITE AIO		1172	6.80	8.20	55.76	82.93	7.50
WHITE EK	R	1173	6.70	9.00	60.30	74.44	7.85
WHITE 11		1174	6.70	7.30	48.91	91.78	7.00
ALACA HOYUK 2		1183	7.20	8.00	57.60	90.00	7.60
ALACA HOYUK 3		1184	7.00	7.80	54.60	89.74	7.40
WADI HALFA	L	1210	6.70	8.00	53.60	83.75	7.35
WADI HALFA	L	1211	8.10	8.80	71.28	92.05	8.45
WADJAK 2	R	1702	8.00	8.40	67.20	95.24	8.20
AUSTRALIAN 39		1708	8.00	9.00	72.00	88.89	8.50
AUSTRALIAN 8158		1710	7.40	9.50	70.30	77.89	8.45
AUSTRALIAN 8174		1711	9.30	9.00	83.70	103.33	9.15
AUSTRALIAN AM		1712	7.40	9.00	66.60	82.22	8.20
AUSTRALIAN AM		1713	7.00	8.40	58.80	83.33	7.70
AUSTRALIAN AM		1714	7.50	8.60	64.50	87.21	8.05
AUSTRALIAN AM		1715	7.00	9.00	63.00	77.78	8.00
AUSTRALIAN AM		1716	8.20	9.20	75.44	89.13	8.70
AUSTRALIAN AM		1717	7.20	9.50	68.40	75.79	8.35
AUSTRALIAN AM		1718	7.00	8.50	59.50	82.35	7.75
AUSTRALIAN AM		1719	7.80	8.50	66.30	91.76	8.15
AUSTRALIAN AM		1720	7.00	7.70	53.90	90.91	7.35
AUSTRALIAN AM		1721	7.60	9.00	68.40	84.44	8.30
AUSTRALIAN 90	R	1722	8.00	9.50	76.00	84.21	8.75
AUSTRALIAN 54	R	1723	8.00	9.80	78.40	81.63	8.90
AUSTRALIAN 88	L	1724	8.00	7.50	60.00	106.67	7.75
AUSTRALIAN	L	1727	8.00	8.40	67.20	95.24	8.20
AUSTRALIAN	L	1729	8.20	9.30	76.26	88.17	8.75
AUSTRALIAN	R	1729	8.00	9.00	72.00	88.89	8.50

LOWER PM4 H. SAPIENS

		N	L(M-D)	B(B-L)	L*B	L/B	L+B/2
AUSTRALIAN 8158	L	1730	8.30	9.20	76.36	90.22	8.75
AUSTRALIAN AM	L	1731	8.00	9.30	74.40	86.02	8.65
TASMANIAN 310		1754	7.00	9.00	63.00	77.78	8.00
TASMANIAN 2964	L	1763	8.80	9.80	86.24	89.80	9.30
TASMANIAN 2964	R	1763	8.20	10.10	82.82	81.19	9.15
ASSELAR	R	1903	7.50	8.00	60.00	93.75	7.75
CAPE FLATS	R	1904	7.50	9.00	67.50	83.33	8.25
NEGRO	L	1906	7.50	9.20	69.00	81.52	8.35
NEGRO AM		1907	8.00	9.80	78.40	81.63	8.90
NEGRO AM		1908	6.70	8.20	54.94	81.71	7.45
NEGRO AM		1909	7.70	8.80	67.76	87.50	8.25
NEGRO AM		1910	7.60	9.70	73.72	78.35	8.65
NEGRO AM		1911	7.80	9.00	70.20	86.67	8.40
NEGRO AM		1912	7.30	9.50	69.35	76.84	8.40
NEGRO AM		1913	7.30	9.50	69.35	76.84	8.40
NEGRO		1914	7.10	8.20	58.22	86.59	7.65
NEGRO	L	1915	10.50	10.00	105.00	105.00	10.25
NEGRO	R	1915	10.00	9.20	92.00	108.70	9.60
NEGRO 2	L	1919	8.40	10.00	84.00	84.00	9.20
NEGRO 2	R	1919	8.00	9.80	78.40	81.63	8.90
NEGRO 1	L	1920	7.80	8.70	67.86	89.66	8.25
NEGRO 1	R	1920	7.50	9.60	72.00	78.12	8.55
NEGRO 5	R	1922	8.20	9.00	73.80	91.11	8.60
NEGRO 29	L	1925	8.80	8.25	72.60	106.67	8.52
NEGRO 29	R	1925	8.00	8.80	70.40	90.91	8.40
N/HOTTENTOT 12	L	1943	6.75	7.00	47.25	96.43	6.87
N/HOTTENTOT 12	R	1943	6.15	6.90	42.43	89.13	6.52
N/HOTTENTOT 6	L	1944	8.00	8.50	68.00	94.12	8.25
N/HOTTENTOT 6	R	1944	7.20	8.50	61.20	84.71	7.85
N/BUSHMAN 52	L	1945	8.15				
BUSHMAN MXD 61	L	1946	7.65	8.20	62.73	93.29	7.92
BUSHMAN MXD 61	R	1946	7.10	8.10	57.51	87.65	7.60
BUSHMAN MXD 94	L	1947	7.10	8.90	63.19	79.78	8.00
BUSHMAN MXD 94	R	1947	7.30	8.25	60.22	88.48	7.77
N/HOTTENTOT 6	L	1948	8.00	8.75	70.00	91.43	8.37
N/HOTTENTOT 6	R	1948	7.95	8.50	67.57	93.53	8.22
MAPUNGUBWE	L	1950	7.20	8.05	57.96	89.44	7.62
MAPUNGUBWE	R	1950	7.40	8.45	62.53	87.57	7.92
MAPUNGUBWE M1A		1951	7.70	9.00	69.30	85.56	8.35
MAPUNGUBWE M9		1955	8.00	10.00	80.00	80.00	9.00
BAMBANDYANALO21		1957	7.40	8.40	62.16	88.10	7.90
BAMBANDYANALO29		1958	6.70	8.70	58.29	77.01	7.70
BAMBANDYANALO31		1959	8.20	9.60	78.72	85.42	8.90
BAMBANDYANALO33	R	1960	7.60	8.90	67.64	85.39	8.25
BAMBANDYANALO 2		1961	9.10	9.30	84.63	97.85	9.20
BAMBANDYANALO 3		1962	7.50	9.00	67.50	83.33	8.25
BAMBANDYANALO13		1964	8.50	8.90	75.65	95.51	8.70
BAMBANDYANALO14		1965	9.00	11.90	107.10	75.63	10.45
BUSHMAN		1967	7.00	7.80	54.60	89.74	7.40
BUSHMAN AM		1968	7.20	7.70	55.44	93.51	7.45

LOWER PM4 H. SAPIENS

		N	L(M-D)	B(B-L)	L*B	L/B	L+B/2
HOTTENTOT AM		1969	7.00	8.70	60.90	80.46	7.85
HOTTENTOT AM		1970	8.30	9.70	80.51	85.57	9.00
HOTTENTOT AM		1971	8.40	9.50	79.80	88.42	8.95
FISH HOEK	R	1972	6.10	6.50	39.65	93.85	6.30
BUSHMAN 30	L	1973	7.50	8.00	60.00	93.75	7.75
BUSHMAN 30	R	1973	7.65	8.25	63.11	92.73	7.95
N.BRITAIN 43121	L	1301	7.00	8.80	61.60	79.55	7.90
N.BRITAIN 43127	L	1306	7.80	7.80	60.84	100.00	7.80
N.BRITAIN 43130	R	1307	8.00	9.80	78.40	81.63	8.90
N.BRITAIN 43131	L	1308	7.90	9.80	77.42	80.61	8.85
N.BRITAIN 43131	R	1308	7.90	9.90	78.21	79.80	8.90
N.BRITAIN 43135	R	1312	6.30	8.30	52.29	75.90	7.30
N.BRITAIN 43136	L	1313	10.90	9.10	99.19	119.78	10.00
N.BRITAIN 43136	R	1313	10.40	9.50	98.80	109.47	9.95
N.BRITAIN 43137	L	1314	7.70	9.40	72.38	81.91	8.55
N.BRITAIN 43137	R	1314	7.70	8.90	68.53	86.52	8.30
N.BRITAIN 43138	L	1315	8.30	9.70	80.51	85.57	9.00
N.BRITAIN 43138	R	1315	8.20	10.20	83.64	80.39	9.20
N.BRITAIN 43139	R	1316	7.40	9.00	66.60	82.22	8.20
N.BRITAIN 43141	L	1318	7.20	8.40	60.48	85.71	7.80
N.BRITAIN 43141	R	1318	7.50	8.80	66.00	85.23	8.15
N.BRITAIN 43142	R	1319	7.30	9.40	68.62	77.66	8.35
N.BRITAIN 43143	L	1320	6.70	8.10	54.27	82.72	7.40
N.BRITAIN 43144	L	1321	7.20	8.50	61.20	84.71	7.85
N.BRITAIN 43145	L	1322	8.00	9.70	77.60	82.47	8.85
N.BRITAIN 43145	R	1322	7.70	9.50	73.15	81.05	8.60
N.BRITAIN 43146	L	1323	11.30	11.20	126.56	100.89	11.25
N.BRITAIN 43146	R	1323	11.10	10.00	111.00	111.00	10.55
N.BRITAIN 43147	L	1324	9.20	8.50	78.20	108.24	8.85
N.BRITAIN 43147	R	1324	9.20	8.70	80.04	105.75	8.95
N.BRITAIN 43150	L	1326	7.30	8.30	60.59	87.95	7.80
N.BRITAIN 43150	R	1326	7.60	8.40	63.84	90.48	8.00
N.BRITAIN 43151	L	1327	8.00	8.50	68.00	94.12	8.25
N.BRITAIN 43151	R	1327	7.60	8.30	63.08	91.57	7.95
N.BRITAIN 43152	R	1328	8.00	8.30	66.40	96.39	8.15
N.BRITAIN 43153	R	1329	7.20	8.10	58.32	88.89	7.65
N.BRITAIN 43154	L	1330	7.50	9.10	68.25	82.42	8.30
N.BRITAIN 43154	R	1330	7.20	9.20	66.24	78.26	8.20
N.BRITAIN 43174	L	1331	7.40	8.90	65.86	83.15	8.15
N.BRITAIN 43174	R	1331	7.80	8.90	69.42	87.64	8.35
N.BRITAIN 43179	R	1332	8.30	9.60	79.68	86.46	8.95
N.BRITAIN 43193	R	1333	8.20	9.60	78.72	85.42	8.90
N.BRITAIN 43198	R	1335	7.70	8.90	68.53	86.52	8.30
N.BRITAIN 43199	L	1336	7.40	8.70	64.38	85.06	8.05
N.BRITAIN 43199	R	1336	7.20	8.20	59.04	87.80	7.70
N.BRITAIN 43202	R	1337	7.20	8.70	62.64	82.76	7.95
N.BRITAIN 43204	L	1338	7.80	9.60	74.88	81.25	8.70
N.BRITAIN 43204	R	1338	7.60	9.40	71.44	80.85	8.50
N.BRITAIN 43226	R	1339	7.10	9.10	64.61	78.02	8.10
N.BRITAIN 43242	L	1341	7.00	9.20	64.40	76.09	8.10

LOWER PM4 H. SAPIENS

	N	L(M-D)	B(B-L)	L*B	L/B	L+B/2
N.BRITAIN 43242 R	1341	7.20	9.10	65.52	79.12	8.15
N.BRITAIN 43291 R	1343	7.30	8.80	64.24	82.95	8.05
N.BRITAIN 43295 L	1344	8.20	10.30	84.46	79.61	9.25
N.BRITAIN 43295 R	1344	8.20	10.30	84.46	79.61	9.25
N.BRITAIN 43296 L	1345	7.00	7.90	55.30	88.61	7.45
N.BRITAIN 43296 R	1345	6.90	7.90	54.51	87.34	7.40
N.BRITAIN L	1346	8.25	8.80	72.60	93.75	8.52
N.BRITAIN R	1346	7.70	9.20	70.84	83.70	8.45
HINDU AM 7894 L	2201	6.90	8.30	57.27	83.13	7.60
HINDU AM R	2202	6.6C	7.70	50.82	85.71	7.15
HINDU (UI) L	2208	7.40	7.30	54.02	101.37	7.35
HINDU (UI) R	2208	7.20	7.50	54.00	96.00	7.35
GOL BA IT 98 L	2003		8.50			
GOL BA IT 98 R	2003		8.50			
GOL BA IT L	2016	8.50	8.90	75.65	95.51	8.70
GOL BA IT R	2017	8.90	8.70	77.43	102.30	8.80
MELOLC L	2106	7.10	7.90	56.09	89.87	7.50
MELOLC R	2107	7.60	8.10	61.56	93.83	7.85
MELOLC L	2108	7.60	8.70	66.12	87.36	8.15
MELOLC R	2109	7.70	8.70	66.99	88.51	8.20
MELOLC L	2110	7.00	8.90	62.30	78.65	7.95
MELOLC R	2111	7.40	7.30	54.02	101.37	7.35
MELOLC L	2112	7.60	8.50	64.60	89.41	8.05
MELOLC R	2113	7.40	8.60	63.64	86.05	8.00
MELOLC L	2114	7.80	9.50	74.10	82.11	8.65
MELOLC R	2115	8.00	9.30	74.40	86.02	8.65
SAINT CRUZ M L	2204	10.50	9.50	99.75	110.53	10.00
SAINT CRUZ M R	2204	8.00	9.00	72.00	88.89	8.50
SAINT CRUZ F L	2205	7.30	8.50	62.05	85.88	7.90
SAINT CRUZ F R	2205	7.50	8.50	63.75	88.24	8.00
HAICA L	1406	7.00	7.90	55.30	88.61	7.45
HAICA R	1406	6.60	8.00	52.80	82.50	7.30
INDIAN (AM)	1407	7.00	8.00	56.00	87.50	7.50
INDIAN (AM)	1408	6.50	7.50	48.75	86.67	7.00
INDIAN (AM)	1409	6.50	8.20	53.30	79.27	7.35
INDIAN (AM)	1410	6.00	7.70	46.20	77.92	6.85
INDIAN (AM)	1411	7.00	8.00	56.00	87.50	7.50
INDIAN (AM)	1412	6.70	7.70	51.59	87.01	7.20
INDIAN (AM)	1413	7.00	8.20	57.40	85.37	7.60
INDIAN (AM)	1414	7.00	9.30	65.10	75.27	8.15
INDIAN (AM)	1415	7.50	9.20	69.00	81.52	8.35
INDIAN (AM)	1416	8.20	9.30	76.26	88.17	8.75
INDIAN (AM)	1417	6.10	7.70	46.97	79.22	6.90
INDIAN (AM)	1418	7.30	7.60	55.48	96.05	7.45
MINNESOTA MAN L	1419	8.00	8.80	70.40	90.91	8.40
MINNESOTA MAN R	1419	7.80	8.70	67.86	89.66	8.25
TARASCO (AM) L	1421	7.75	9.25	71.69	83.78	8.50
TARASCO (AM) L	1422	8.80	9.45	83.16	93.12	9.12
TARASCO (AM) L	1423	7.90	8.70	68.73	90.80	8.30
ILLINCIS ME3-10 L	1428	6.60	7.70	50.82	85.71	7.15

LOWER PM4 H. SAPIENS

	N	L(M-D)	B(B-L)	L*B	L/B	L+B/2
ILLINCIS A-2732 L	1429	6.90	8.30	57.27	83.13	7.60
ILLINCIS A-2732 R	1429	7.10	7.90	56.09	89.87	7.50
ILLINCIS A-6890 L	1430	6.10	7.85	47.88	77.71	6.97
ILLINCIS A-6890 R	1430	6.50	8.15	52.97	79.75	7.32
ILLINCIS A-4921 L	1431	8.10	8.50	68.85	95.29	8.30
ILLINCIS A-4921 R	1431	8.30	9.00	74.70	92.22	8.65
ILLINCIS PK9-B4 L	1432	7.55	8.60	64.93	87.79	8.07
ILLINCIS PK9-B4 R	1432	7.40	8.50	62.90	87.06	7.95
ILLINCIS PK9-B1 L	1433	7.00	8.70	60.90	80.46	7.85
ILLINCIS PK9-B1 R	1433	7.00	9.10	63.70	76.92	8.05
ILLINCIS BR19-3 L	1434	7.30	8.70	63.51	83.91	8.00
ILLINCIS BR19-3 R	1434	6.85	8.50	58.22	80.59	7.67
ILLINCIS A-8068 L	1437	7.15	7.95	56.84	89.94	7.55
ILLINCIS A-8068 R	1437	6.70	8.40	56.28	79.76	7.55
DICKSCN MOUND L	1501	7.15	8.25	58.99	86.67	7.70
DICKSCN MOUND R	1501	7.25	9.00	65.25	80.56	8.12
DICKSCN MD 242 L	1505	8.27	8.75	72.36	94.51	8.51
DICKSCN MD 242 R	1505	8.15	8.70	70.90	93.68	8.42
DICKSCN MD 256 L	1506	7.50	7.90	59.25	94.94	7.70
DICKSCN MD 256 R	1506	7.40	8.00	59.20	92.50	7.70
DICKSCN MD 261 L	1508	7.80	8.90	69.42	87.64	8.35
DICKSCN MD 261 R	1508	8.13	8.70	70.73	93.45	8.41
DICKSCN MD 276 L	1514	8.55	9.67	82.68	88.42	9.11
DICKSCN MD 276 R	1514	8.04	9.42	75.74	85.35	8.73
DICKSON MD 278 R	1515	7.20	8.50	61.20	84.71	7.85
DICKSCN MD 287 L	1516	7.40	8.30	61.42	89.16	7.85
DICKSCN MD 287 R	1516	7.25	8.05	58.36	90.06	7.65
DICKSCN MD 297 L	1520	7.77	8.20	63.71	94.76	7.98
DICKSCN MD 297 R	1520	7.50	7.95	59.62	94.34	7.72
DICKSON MD 302 L	1521	6.70	7.35	49.24	91.16	7.02
DICKSON MD 302 R	1521	6.55	7.00	45.85	93.57	6.77
DICKSCN MD 310 L	1522	10.75	9.25	99.44	116.22	10.00
DICKSCN MD 319 L	1523	6.90	8.10	55.89	85.19	7.50
DICKSCN MD 319 R	1523	6.90	8.05	55.54	85.71	7.47
DICKSCN MD 327 L	1524	7.50	8.80	66.00	85.23	8.15
DICKSCN MD 327 R	1524	7.60	9.00	68.40	84.44	8.30
DICKSCN MD 334 L	1525	8.05	8.80	70.84	91.48	8.42
DICKSCN MD 334 R	1525	8.00	8.80	70.40	90.91	8.40
DICKSCN MD 344 R	1527	6.90	9.00	62.10	76.67	7.95
DICKSON MD 348 L	1529	7.20	8.10	58.32	88.89	7.65
DICKSCN MD 348 R	1529	7.20	8.10	58.32	88.89	7.65
DICKSCN MD 349 L	1530	8.20	8.70	71.34	94.25	8.45
DICKSCN MD 349 R	1530	8.20	8.85	72.57	92.66	8.52
DICKSCN MD 355 L	1535	8.30	9.20	76.36	90.22	8.75
DICKSCN MD 355 R	1535	7.90	8.70	68.73	90.80	8.30
DICKSCN MD 362 L	1539	8.45	8.80	74.36	96.02	8.62
DICKSCN MD 362 R	1539	8.50	8.25	70.12	103.03	8.37
DICKSCN MD 365 L	1540	7.20	8.10	58.32	88.89	7.65
DICKSCN MD 365 R	1540	7.60	8.10	61.56	93.83	7.85
DICKSCN MD 467 L	1541	7.00	8.00	56.00	87.50	7.50

LOWER PM4 H. SAPIENS

		N	L(M-D)	B(B-L)	L*B	L/B	L+B/2
DICKSON MD	371 L	1542	8.00	9.00	72.00	88.89	8.50
DICKSON MD	371 R	1542	7.70	9.00	69.30	85.56	8.35
DICKSON MD	372 L	1543	7.00	8.30	58.10	84.34	7.65
DICKSON MD	372 R	1543	7.05	8.30	58.51	84.94	7.67
DICKSON MD	378 L	1547	7.30	8.20	59.86	89.02	7.75
DICKSON MD	378 R	1547	7.15	7.75	55.41	92.26	7.45
DICKSON MD	379 L	1548	7.60	8.75	66.50	86.86	8.17
DICKSON MD	379 R	1548	7.70	9.20	70.84	83.70	8.45
DICKSON MD	381 L	1550	7.80	8.70	67.86	89.66	8.25
DICKSON MD	381 R	1550	7.30	7.50	54.75	97.33	7.40
DICKSON MD	380 L	1551	6.80	8.10	55.08	83.95	7.45
DICKSON MD	380 R	1551	6.70	8.00	53.60	83.75	7.35
DICKSON MD	396 L	1553	7.70	8.70	66.99	88.51	8.20
DICKSON MD	396 R	1553	8.00	9.30	74.40	86.02	8.65
DICKSON MD	397 L	1554	7.50	8.30	62.25	90.36	7.90
DICKSON MD	397 R	1554	7.50	7.80	58.50	96.15	7.65
DICKSON MD	398 L	1555	7.50	8.20	61.50	91.46	7.85
DICKSON MD	398 R	1555	6.90	7.80	53.82	88.46	7.35
DICKSON MD	399 L	1556	7.70	8.85	68.14	87.01	8.27
DICKSON MD	399 R	1556	7.20	8.70	62.64	82.76	7.95
DICKSON MD	402 R	1557	7.60	9.30	70.68	81.72	8.45
DICKSON MD	404 L	1559	7.65	8.50	65.02	90.00	8.07
DICKSON MD	404 R	1559	7.50	8.40	63.00	89.29	7.95
DICKSON MD	406 L	1560	7.00	8.20	57.40	85.37	7.60
DICKSON MD	406 R	1560	7.30	8.20	59.86	89.02	7.75
DICKSON MD	407 L	1561	8.55	9.15	78.23	93.44	8.85
DICKSON MD	407 R	1561	8.15	8.85	72.13	92.09	8.50
DICKSON MD	409 R	1562	8.20	9.27	76.01	88.46	8.73
DICKSON MD	411 L	1563	7.86	8.55	67.20	91.93	8.20
DICKSON MD	411 R	1563	7.95	8.25	65.59	96.36	8.10
DICKSON MD	414 L	1564	7.00	7.85	54.95	89.17	7.42
DICKSON MD	414 R	1564	6.74	7.89	53.18	85.42	7.31
DICKSON MD	415 L	1565	6.75	7.48	50.49	90.24	7.11
DICKSON MD	415 R	1565	6.90	7.60	52.44	90.79	7.25
DICKSON MD	426 L	1566	7.48	8.42	62.98	88.84	7.95
DICKSON MD	426 R	1566	7.32	8.12	59.44	90.15	7.72
DICKSON MD	432 L	1567	7.25	7.40	53.65	97.97	7.32
DICKSON MD	432 R	1567	6.40	7.70	49.28	83.12	7.05
DICKSON MD	443 L	1571	8.31	8.75	72.71	94.97	8.53
DICKSON MD	443 R	1571	8.23	8.90	73.25	92.47	8.56
DICKSON MD	446 L	1572	7.93	7.57	60.03	104.76	7.75
DICKSON MD	446 R	1572	7.90	8.10	63.99	97.53	8.00
DICKSON MD	464 L	1575	7.50	8.43	63.22	88.97	7.96
DICKSON MD	464 R	1575	7.45	8.80	65.56	84.66	8.12
DICKSON MD	476 L	1576	8.02	9.00	72.18	89.11	8.51
DICKSON MD	480 L	1578	6.55	7.75	50.76	84.52	7.15
DICKSON MD	485 L	1579	8.45	10.30	87.03	82.04	9.37
DICKSON MD	497 L	1583	8.10	9.85	79.78	82.23	8.97
DICKSON MD	497 R	1583	8.10	10.00	81.00	81.00	9.05
DICKSON MD	503 L	1585	8.50	8.75	74.37	97.14	8.62

LOWER PM4 H. SAPIENS

		N	L(M-D)	B(B-L)	L*B	L/B	L+B/2
DICKSON MD	503 R	1585	8.42	8.70	73.25	96.78	8.56
DICKSON MD	509 L	1587	7.30	7.75	56.57	94.19	7.52
DICKSON MD	509 R	1587	7.25	7.93	57.49	91.42	7.59
DICKSON MD	535 L	1591	7.25	8.25	59.81	87.88	7.75
DICKSON MD	535 R	1591	7.30	8.35	60.95	87.43	7.82
DICKSON MD	536 L	1592	7.20	8.35	60.12	86.23	7.77
DICKSON MD	536 R	1592	7.40	8.35	61.79	88.62	7.87
DICKSON MD	557 L	1596	7.22	7.85	56.68	91.97	7.53
DICKSON MD	557 R	1596	6.97	7.80	54.37	89.36	7.38
DICKSON MD	561 L	1597	7.82	8.80	68.82	88.86	8.31
DICKSON MD	561 R	1597	7.80	8.88	69.26	87.84	8.34
DICKSON MD	567 L	1598	8.15	9.60	78.24	84.90	8.87
DICKSON MD	567 R	1598	7.92	9.50	75.24	83.37	8.71
DICKSON MD	568 L	1599	7.48	8.37	62.61	89.37	7.92
DICKSON MD	568 R	1599	7.50	8.40	63.00	89.29	7.95
DICKSON MD	589 L	1600	7.80	8.80	68.64	88.64	8.30
DICKSON MD	589 R	1600	7.40	8.60	63.64	86.05	8.00
DICKSON MD	599 L	1602	7.80	8.80	68.64	88.64	8.30
DICKSON MD	599 R	1602	7.95	8.45	67.18	94.08	8.20
DICKSON MD	630 L	1603	7.50	8.20	61.50	91.46	7.85
DICKSON MD	630 R	1603	7.40	7.80	57.72	94.87	7.60
DICKSON MD	643 L	1608	7.30	9.00	65.70	81.11	8.15
DICKSON MD	643 R	1608	7.00	9.10	63.70	76.92	8.05
DICKSON MD	658 L	1613	6.70	8.60	57.62	77.91	7.65
DICKSON MD	658 R	1613	7.70	8.80	67.76	87.50	8.25
DICKSON MD	667 L	1614	8.15	8.10	66.01	100.62	8.12
DICKSON MD	667 R	1614	7.90	8.65	68.33	91.33	8.27
DICKSON MD	709 L	1623	6.80	7.95	54.06	85.53	7.37
DICKSON MD	722 L	1624	7.90	9.05	71.49	87.29	8.47
DICKSON MD	722 R	1624	7.85	8.85	69.47	88.70	8.35
DICKSON MD	724 L	1627	8.25	8.80	72.60	93.75	8.52
DICKSON MD	724 R	1627	8.15	8.80	71.72	92.61	8.47
DICKSON MD	746 L	1628	7.50	8.90	66.75	84.27	8.20
DICKSON MD	746 R	1628	7.40	8.55	63.27	86.55	7.97

LOWER M1 H. SAPIENS

		N	L(M-D)	B(B-L)	L*B	L/B	L+B/2
ARCYSURCURE C10		1005	12.50	11.70	146.25	106.84	12.10
PREDMOST 1	L	1009	12.00	10.00	120.00	120.00	11.00
PREDMOST 1	R	1009	12.60	10.65	134.19	118.31	11.62
PREDMOST 2	L	1010	12.80	11.00	140.80	116.36	11.90
PREDMOST 2	R	1010	12.70	11.00	139.70	115.45	11.85
PREDMOST 3	L	1007	12.50	11.40	142.50	109.65	11.95
PREDMOST 3	R	1007	11.80	11.50	135.70	102.61	11.65
PREDMOST 4	L	1008	10.50	10.80	113.40	97.22	10.65
PREDMOST 4	R	1008	10.50	11.00	115.50	95.45	10.75
PREDMOST 5	L	1011	11.50	11.00	126.50	104.55	11.25
PREDMOST 5	R	1011	12.00	11.20	134.40	107.14	11.60
PREDMOST 7	L	1012	12.00	10.80	129.60	111.11	11.40
PREDMOST 9	L	1013	13.00	11.50	149.50	113.04	12.25
PREDMOST 9	R	1013	12.80	11.80	151.04	108.47	12.30
PREDMOST 10	L	1014	11.20	10.20	114.24	109.80	10.70
PREDMOST 10	R	1014	11.00	10.20	112.20	107.84	10.60
PREDMOST 14	L	1015	12.50	11.00	137.50	113.64	11.75
PREDMOST 14	R	1015	12.30	11.20	137.76	109.82	11.75
PREDMOST 18	L	1016	12.50	11.80	147.50	105.93	12.15
PREDMOST 18	R	1016	12.50	12.00	150.00	104.17	12.25
PREDMOST 259	R	1058	11.80	11.00	129.80	107.27	11.40
PREDMOST 476	L	1059	11.00	10.40	114.40	105.77	10.70
PREDMOST 476	R	1059	11.50	10.50	120.75	109.52	11.00
PREDMOST 3070	R	1060	10.30	10.00	103.00	103.00	10.15
COMBE CHAPELLE	L	1017	12.00	11.00	132.00	109.09	11.50
COMBE CHAPELLE	R	1017	12.00	12.00	144.00	100.00	12.00
BRNO 3	L	1018	10.70	11.00	117.70	97.27	10.85
BRNO 3	R	1018	10.50	10.80	113.40	97.22	10.65
GRIMALDI ADOL.	L	1019	12.45	11.00	136.95	113.18	11.72
GRIMALDI ADOL.	R	1019	12.40	11.20	138.88	110.71	11.80
KLATY KLN	L	1020	10.00	10.50	105.00	95.24	10.25
KLATY KLN	R	1020	10.50	11.00	115.50	95.45	10.75
LA ROCHETTE B	L	1022	10.00	10.10	101.00	99.01	10.05
ROIS A		1024	10.00	9.50	95.00	105.26	9.75
ROIS R51-14	R	1039	12.00	10.00	120.00	120.00	11.00
ROIS R51-30		1045	11.50	11.00	126.50	104.55	11.25
SALEMAS	L	1056	11.00	11.00	121.00	100.00	11.00
VESTONICE 3	L	1057	10.00	11.70	117.00	85.47	10.85
VESTONICE 3	R	1057	10.10	11.20	113.12	90.18	10.65
A CULOZ 2	L	1101	11.00	11.50	126.50	95.65	11.25
A CULOZ 2	R	1101	11.00	11.60	127.60	94.83	11.30
ARLAY	L	1104	10.20	10.50	107.10	97.14	10.35
ARLAY	R	1104	10.50	10.00	105.00	105.00	10.25
BUGGISON 1	L	1108	12.00	11.00	132.00	109.09	11.50
BUGGISON 1	R	1108	12.50	11.00	137.50	113.64	11.75
BUGGISON 2	L	1109	12.50	11.00	137.50	113.64	11.75
BUGGISON 2	R	1109	12.00	11.00	132.00	109.09	11.50
CAP BLAC	L	1110	10.20	10.20	104.04	100.00	10.20
CAP BLAC	R	1110	9.80	10.30	100.94	95.15	10.05
EGOLZWIL 1	L	1112	10.00	10.90	109.00	91.74	10.45

LOWER M1 H. SAPIENS

		N	L(M-D)	B(B-L)	L*B	L/B	L+B/2
EGOLZWIL 1	R	1112	10.60	10.80	114.48	98.15	10.70
FARINCOURT 3	L	1115	10.30	9.30	95.79	110.75	9.80
FARINCOURT 3	R	1115	10.00	9.50	95.00	105.26	9.75
GALLEY HILL	R	1116	11.00	11.10	122.10	99.10	11.05
GARDAR	R	1117	12.40	11.50	142.60	107.83	11.95
HOHLERFELS A	L	1118	12.00	12.10	145.20	99.17	12.05
HOHLERFELS A	R	1118	12.00	12.00	144.00	100.00	12.00
HOHLERFELS C	R	1119	12.00	11.00	132.00	109.09	11.50
ISTURITZ 3		1122	11.50	11.50	132.25	100.00	11.50
LACHAUD A	L	1125	11.10	10.40	115.44	106.73	10.75
LACHAUD A	R	1125	11.00	10.30	113.30	106.80	10.65
LACHAUD B	L	1126	11.20	11.00	123.20	101.82	11.10
LACHAUD B	R	1126	11.60	10.90	126.44	106.42	11.25
LAFAYE	L	1128	10.40	10.90	113.36	95.41	10.65
LAFAYE	R	1128	10.40	10.80	112.32	96.30	10.60
MASAT		1130	10.90	10.40	113.36	104.81	10.65
MECHTA	R	1131	12.50	11.25	140.62	111.11	11.87
OBERCASSEL 1	L	1132	10.00	11.00	110.00	90.91	10.50
OBERCASSEL 1	R	1132	10.00	11.00	110.00	90.91	10.50
OKUZINI		1133	10.60	9.90	104.94	107.07	10.25
PAS ESTRET 3	L	1134	10.00	10.35	103.50	96.62	10.17
PAS ESTRET 3	R	1134	10.40	10.35	107.64	100.48	10.37
PAS ESTRET 4	L	1135	11.40	11.70	133.38	97.44	11.55
PAS ESTRET 4	R	1135	11.40	11.60	132.24	98.28	11.50
PRITZERBER 3	L	1138	11.00	11.00	121.00	100.00	11.00
PRITZERBER 3	R	1138	11.00	11.00	121.00	100.00	11.00
PRITZERBER 4	L	1139	11.50	10.50	120.75	109.52	11.00
PRITZERBER 4	R	1139	11.00	11.00	121.00	100.00	11.00
SILICKA BREZOVA	R	1143	11.00	10.00	110.00	110.00	10.50
SVAERCBORG	R	1144	12.20	11.50	140.30	106.09	11.85
KAFFIR		1147	10.80	11.00	118.80	98.18	10.90
KAFFIR		1148	10.60	10.60	112.36	100.00	10.60
FRENCHMAN	L	1149	10.20	9.75	99.45	104.62	9.97
FRENCHMAN	R	1149	10.80	9.40	101.52	114.89	10.10
EUROPEAN 344C	L	1150	11.00	10.00	110.00	110.00	10.50
EUROPEAN 344C	R	1150	11.00	10.10	111.10	108.91	10.55
EUROPEAN AJ2	L	1151	11.00	10.00	110.00	110.00	10.50
EUROPEAN AJ2	R	1151	11.00	10.10	111.10	108.91	10.55
WHITE 99-7740	L	1152	10.50	10.10	106.05	103.96	10.30
WHITE ZZZ		1153	10.60	10.60	112.36	100.00	10.60
WHITE 14		1154	11.00	11.00	121.00	100.00	11.00
WHITE 4F		1155	11.20	11.00	123.20	101.82	11.10
WHITE 3W		1156	9.80	9.20	90.16	106.52	9.50
WHITE EDNA		1157	11.50	11.00	126.50	104.55	11.25
WHITE H		1158	11.00	10.30	113.30	106.80	10.65
WHITE PG		1159	10.60	10.00	106.00	106.00	10.30
WHITE M		1160	11.20	10.50	117.60	106.67	10.85
WHITE HJB		1161	11.00	10.40	114.40	105.77	10.70
WHITE BRD		1164	11.00	10.20	112.20	107.84	10.60
WHITE GN		1165	11.80	10.70	126.26	110.28	11.25

LOWER M1 H. SAPIENS

		N	L(M-D)	B(B-L)	L*B	L/B	L+B/2
WHITE GIVC		1166	11.70	10.50	122.85	111.43	11.10
WHITE BX		1167	11.40	10.60	120.84	107.55	11.00
WHITE CQ		1168	11.00	10.50	115.50	104.76	10.75
WHITE GM		1169	11.50	10.50	120.75	109.52	11.00
WHITE AAD		1170	11.00	11.00	121.00	100.00	11.00
WHITE BIY		1171	10.30	9.70	99.91	106.19	10.00
WHITE AIO		1172	10.50	9.50	99.75	110.53	10.00
WHITE 99-7740		1175	10.60	10.00	106.00	106.00	10.30
WHITE 99-7743		1176	10.40	11.00	114.40	94.55	10.70
ALACA HOYUK 2		1183	11.60	10.60	122.96	109.43	11.10
ALACA HOYUK 3		1184	11.10	9.80	108.78	113.27	10.45
ALACA HOYUK 8		1185	11.40	10.20	116.28	111.76	10.80
BEDOUIN		1188	10.20	10.20	104.04	100.00	10.20
BELT CAVE	R	1189	11.70	11.60	135.72	100.86	11.65
WADI HALFA	L	1212	12.50	12.70	158.75	98.43	12.60
WADJAK 2	L	1702	13.70	12.00	164.40	114.17	12.85
WADJAK 2	R	1702	13.70	12.50	171.25	109.60	13.10
AUSTRALIAN 9801	R	1706	11.50	12.00	138.00	95.83	11.75
AUSTRALIAN 9800	L	1707	10.20	11.50	117.30	88.70	10.85
AUSTRALIAN 9800	R	1707	10.00	11.50	115.00	86.96	10.75
AUSTRALIAN 39		1708	11.50	11.00	126.50	104.55	11.25
AUSTRALIAN 8157		1709	12.00	11.70	140.40	102.56	11.85
AUSTRALIAN 8174		1711	12.00	12.80	153.60	93.75	12.40
AUSTRALIAN AM		1712	11.00	11.80	129.80	93.22	11.40
AUSTRALIAN AM		1713	11.00	10.90	119.90	100.92	10.95
AUSTRALIAN AM		1714	11.00	11.50	126.50	95.65	11.25
AUSTRALIAN AM		1715	10.50	11.50	120.75	91.30	11.00
AUSTRALIAN AM		1716	10.50	10.70	112.35	98.13	10.60
AUSTRALIAN AM		1717	11.50	12.00	138.00	95.83	11.75
AUSTRALIAN AM		1718	11.50	11.50	132.25	100.00	11.50
AUSTRALIAN AM		1719	11.50	11.30	129.95	101.77	11.40
AUSTRALIAN AM		1720	11.50	11.50	132.25	100.00	11.50
AUSTRALIAN AM		1721	12.00	11.90	142.80	100.84	11.95
AUSTRALIAN 90	R	1722	13.00	13.00	169.00	100.00	13.00
AUSTRALIAN 54	R	1723	13.00	12.50	162.50	104.00	12.75
AUSTRALIAN 88	L	1724	11.30	11.00	124.30	102.73	11.15
AUSTRALIAN	L	1727	11.90	12.10	143.99	98.35	12.00
AUSTRALIAN	L	1729	13.50	12.90	174.15	104.65	13.20
AUSTRALIAN	R	1729	13.60	12.60	171.36	107.94	13.10
AUSTRALIAN 8158	L	1730	12.35	10.70	132.14	115.42	11.52
AUSTRALIAN AM	L	1731	12.30	12.10	148.83	101.65	12.20
TASMANIAN 1406	L	1751	12.50	11.80	147.50	105.93	12.15
TASMANIAN 1406	R	1751	12.50	11.50	143.75	108.70	12.00
TASMANIAN 310		1754	11.00	11.00	121.00	100.00	11.00
TASMANIAN 707	L	1760	11.50	12.00	138.00	95.83	11.75
TASMANIAN 2964	L	1763	12.90	11.70	150.93	110.26	12.30
BOSKOP		1902	12.50	12.00	150.00	104.17	12.25
ASSELAR	R	1903	10.00	11.00	110.00	90.91	10.50
CAPE FLATS	R	1904	11.80	11.80	139.24	100.00	11.80
NEGRO	L	1906	12.50	11.65	145.62	107.30	12.07

LOWER M1 H. SAPIENS

		N	L(M-D)	B(B-L)	L*B	L/B	L+B/2
NEGRO AM		1907	12.00	11.70	140.40	102.56	11.85
NEGRO AM		1908	11.00	10.80	118.80	101.85	10.90
NEGRO AM		1909	11.50	11.20	128.80	102.68	11.35
NEGRO AM		1910	12.40	11.70	145.08	105.98	12.05
NEGRO AM		1911	11.60	11.00	127.60	105.45	11.30
NEGRO AM		1912	12.00	12.00	144.00	100.00	12.00
NEGRO AM		1913	12.50	11.40	142.50	109.65	11.95
NEGRO		1914	11.00	10.30	113.30	106.80	10.65
NEGRO	L	1915	13.60				
NEGRO	R	1915	14.00	12.80	179.20	109.37	13.40
BANTU 100	L	1917	13.60	11.80	160.48	115.25	12.70
BANTU 100	R	1917	13.50	12.40	167.40	108.87	12.95
NEGRO 2	L	1919	12.60	11.50	144.90	109.57	12.05
NEGRO 2	R	1919	12.50	11.00	137.50	113.64	11.75
NEGRO 1	L	1920	11.30	10.80	122.04	104.63	11.05
NEGRO 1	R	1920	11.50	11.50	132.25	100.00	11.50
NEGRO 3091	L	1921	12.30	10.80	132.84	113.89	11.55
NEGRO 3091	R	1921	11.40	11.40	129.96	100.00	11.40
NEGRO 5	R	1922	12.60	11.30	142.38	111.50	11.95
NEGRO 9	R	1924	10.50	10.20	107.10	102.94	10.35
NEGRO 29	L	1925	12.25	11.25	137.81	108.89	11.75
NEGRO 29	R	1925	12.10	11.10	134.31	109.01	11.60
N/HOTTENTOT 12	L	1943	9.50	8.80	83.60	107.95	9.15
N/HOTTENTOT 12	R	1943	9.90	9.30	92.07	106.45	9.60
N/HOTTENTOT 6	L	1944	11.50	11.00	126.50	104.55	11.25
N/HOTTENTOT 6	R	1944	11.90	10.70	127.33	111.21	11.30
N/BUSHMAN 52	L	1945	10.80	11.90	128.52	90.76	11.35
N/BUSHMAN 52	R	1945	10.75	11.50	123.62	93.48	11.12
BUSHMAN MXD 61	L	1946	11.40	10.40	118.56	109.62	10.90
BUSHMAN MXD 61	R	1946	11.50	10.90	125.35	105.50	11.20
BUSHMAN MXD 94	L	1947	11.40	11.30	128.82	100.88	11.35
BUSHMAN MXD 94	R	1947	11.50	11.40	131.10	100.88	11.45
N/HOTTENTOT 6	L	1948	12.90	12.00	154.80	107.50	12.45
N/HOTTENTOT 6	R	1948	13.00	11.25	146.25	115.56	12.12
MAPUNGUBWE	L	1950	11.00	10.40	114.40	105.77	10.70
MAPUNGUBWE	R	1950	10.75	10.70	115.02	100.47	10.72
MAPUNGUBWE M1A		1951	12.10	11.30	136.73	107.08	11.70
MAPUNGUBWE M2		1952	13.00	11.30	146.90	115.04	12.15
MAPUNGUBWE M3		1953	12.00	13.00	156.00	92.31	12.50
MAPUNGUBWE M5		1954	12.00	11.00	132.00	109.09	11.50
MAPUNGUBWE M9		1955	12.50	12.00	150.00	104.17	12.25
BAMBANDYANALO21		1957	11.20	10.50	117.60	106.67	10.85
BAMBANDYANALO29		1958	11.90	11.30	134.47	105.31	11.60
BAMBANDYANALO31		1959	12.00	11.90	142.80	100.84	11.95
BAMBANDYANALO33	R	1960	12.40	11.90	147.56	104.20	12.15
BAMBANDYANALO 2		1961	12.80	12.10	154.88	105.79	12.45
BAMBANDYANALO 3		1962	11.60	11.40	132.24	101.75	11.50
BAMBANDYANALO 5		1963	14.10	12.50	176.25	112.80	13.30
BAMBANDYANALO13		1964	11.20	11.60	129.92	96.55	11.40
BAMBANDYANALO14		1965	11.40	10.70	121.98	106.54	11.05

LOWER M1 H. SAPIENS

Specimen	Side	N	L(M-D)	B(B-L)	L*B	L/B	L+B/2
BUSHMAN		1967	10.90	10.20	111.18	106.86	10.55
BUSHMAN AM		1968	11.30	11.20	126.56	100.89	11.25
HOTTENTOT AM		1969	10.50	10.70	112.35	98.13	10.60
HOTTENTOT AM		1970	11.60	11.50	133.40	100.87	11.55
HOTTENTOT AM		1971	12.20	11.40	139.08	107.02	11.80
FISH HOEK	R	1972	11.30	9.50	107.35	118.95	10.40
BUSHMAN 30	L	1973	10.40	10.00	104.00	104.00	10.20
BUSHMAN 30	R	1973	10.60	10.00	106.00	106.00	10.30
N.BRITAIN 43121	L	1301	11.60	11.40	132.24	101.75	11.50
N.BRITAIN 43122	L	1302	11.40	11.20	127.68	101.79	11.30
N.BRITAIN 43122	R	1302	11.40	11.10	126.54	102.70	11.25
N.BRITAIN 43130	L	1307	11.80	11.90	140.42	99.16	11.85
N.BRITAIN 43130	R	1307	12.00	12.10	145.20	99.17	12.05
N.BRITAIN 43131	L	1308	11.20	12.10	135.52	92.56	11.65
N.BRITAIN 43131	R	1308	11.30	12.00	135.60	94.17	11.65
N.BRITAIN 43132	L	1309	12.70	12.20	154.94	104.10	12.45
N.BRITAIN 43132	R	1309	12.70	12.30	156.21	103.25	12.50
N.BRITAIN 43133	L	1310	11.20	11.00	123.20	101.82	11.10
N.BRITAIN 43133	R	1310	11.00	10.80	118.80	101.85	10.90
N.BRITAIN 43134	L	1311	10.80	11.20	120.96	96.43	11.00
N.BRITAIN 43134	R	1311	11.10	11.70	129.87	94.87	11.40
N.BRITAIN 43135	L	1312	10.40	10.40	108.16	100.00	10.40
N.BRITAIN 43135	R	1312	10.00	10.30	103.00	97.09	10.15
N.BRITAIN 43136	L	1313	11.80	11.10	130.98	106.31	11.45
N.BRITAIN 43136	R	1313	11.70	11.00	128.70	106.36	11.35
N.BRITAIN 43137	L	1314	11.70	11.30	132.21	103.54	11.50
N.BRITAIN 43137	R	1314	11.90	11.20	133.28	106.25	11.55
N.BRITAIN 43138	L	1315	11.00	11.40	125.40	96.49	11.20
N.BRITAIN 43138	R	1315	10.80	11.00	118.80	98.18	10.90
N.BRITAIN 43139	L	1316	11.30				
N.BRITAIN 43139	R	1316	11.90	11.80	140.42	100.85	11.85
N.BRITAIN 43141	L	1318	11.30	10.80	122.04	104.63	11.05
N.BRITAIN 43141	R	1318	11.50	11.30	129.95	101.77	11.40
N.BRITAIN 43142	L	1319	11.90	11.80	140.42	100.85	11.85
N.BRITAIN 43142	R	1319	11.70	11.90	139.23	98.32	11.80
N.BRITAIN 43143	L	1320	11.20	11.40	127.68	98.25	11.30
N.BRITAIN 43143	R	1320	11.00	11.30	124.30	97.35	11.15
N.BRITAIN 43144	L	1321	11.30	11.70	132.21	96.58	11.50
N.BRITAIN 43144	R	1321	11.30	11.70	132.21	96.58	11.50
N.BRITAIN 43145	L	1322	12.00	11.90	142.80	100.84	11.95
N.BRITAIN 43145	R	1322	11.70	12.20	142.74	95.90	11.95
N.BRITAIN 43146	L	1323	10.80				
N.BRITAIN 43146	R	1323	11.20	11.00	123.20	101.82	11.10
N.BRITAIN 43147	L	1324	12.80	12.20	156.16	104.92	12.50
N.BRITAIN 43147	R	1324	12.70	12.20	154.94	104.10	12.45
N.BRITAIN 43149	L	1325	12.50	11.90	148.75	105.04	12.20
N.BRITAIN 43149	R	1325	12.00	12.30	147.60	97.56	12.15
N.BRITAIN 43150	L	1326	11.20	10.50	117.60	106.67	10.85
N.BRITAIN 43150	R	1326	11.10	10.60	117.66	104.72	10.85
N.BRITAIN 43151	L	1327	12.20	10.90	132.98	111.93	11.55

LOWER M1 H. SAPIENS

Specimen	Side	N	L(M-D)	B(B-L)	L*B	L/B	L+B/2
N.BRITAIN 43151	R	1327	12.00	11.00	132.00	109.09	11.50
N.BRITAIN 43152	L	1328	10.60	11.30	119.78	93.81	10.95
N.BRITAIN 43152	R	1328	11.80	11.30	133.34	104.42	11.55
N.BRITAIN 43153	L	1329		10.40			
N.BRITAIN 43153	R	1329	10.80	10.40	112.32	103.85	10.60
N.BRITAIN 43154	L	1330	12.20	11.80	143.96	103.39	12.00
N.BRITAIN 43154	R	1330	11.50	12.00	138.00	95.83	11.75
N.BRITAIN 43174	L	1331	11.90	11.60	138.04	102.59	11.75
N.BRITAIN 43174	R	1331	12.20	11.20	136.64	108.93	11.70
N.BRITAIN 43179	L	1332	13.50	12.60	170.10	107.14	13.05
N.BRITAIN 43179	R	1332	13.60	12.50	170.00	108.80	13.05
N.BRITAIN 43193	R	1333	11.30	11.80	133.34	95.76	11.55
N.BRITAIN 43194	L	1334	12.60	10.90	137.34	115.60	11.75
N.BRITAIN 43194	R	1334	12.40	10.60	131.44	116.98	11.50
N.BRITAIN 43198	L	1335	12.30	12.00	147.60	102.50	12.15
N.BRITAIN 43198	R	1335	12.50	11.40	142.50	109.65	11.95
N.BRITAIN 43199	L	1336	11.30	11.00	124.30	102.73	11.15
N.BRITAIN 43199	R	1336	11.50	10.90	125.35	105.50	11.20
N.BRITAIN 43202	L	1337	12.60	11.50	144.90	109.57	12.05
N.BRITAIN 43202	R	1337	12.80	11.20	143.36	114.29	12.00
N.BRITAIN 43204	L	1338	12.00	11.30	135.60	106.19	11.65
N.BRITAIN 43204	R	1338	12.00	11.40	136.80	105.26	11.70
N.BRITAIN 43226	L	1339	11.30	10.50	118.65	107.62	10.90
N.BRITAIN 43226	R	1339	11.00	10.30	113.30	106.80	10.65
N.BRITAIN 43242	L	1341	11.00	10.10	111.10	108.91	10.55
N.BRITAIN 43242	R	1341	11.30	10.20	115.26	110.78	10.75
N.BRITAIN 43290	L	1342	12.00	11.00	132.00	109.09	11.50
N.BRITAIN 43290	R	1342	11.70	11.10	129.87	105.41	11.40
N.BRITAIN 43291	L	1343	11.60	10.60	122.96	109.43	11.10
N.BRITAIN 43291	R	1343	12.00	10.40	124.80	115.38	11.20
N.BRITAIN 43295	L	1344	12.90	11.60	149.64	111.21	12.25
N.BRITAIN 43295	R	1344	12.70	12.20	154.94	104.10	12.45
N.BRITAIN 43296	L	1345	12.00	11.30	135.60	106.19	11.65
N.BRITAIN 43296	R	1345	11.70	11.40	133.38	102.63	11.55
N.BRITAIN	L	1346	12.90	12.10	156.09	106.61	12.50
N.BRITAIN	R	1346	12.80	12.00	153.60	106.67	12.40
NIAH CAVE	R	2207	10.20	12.30	125.46	82.93	11.25
HINDU AM 7894	L	2201	11.90	10.70	127.33	111.21	11.30
HINDU AM	R	2202	11.60	11.80	136.88	98.31	11.70
HINDU (UI)	L	2208	11.40	10.15	115.71	112.32	10.77
HINDU (UI)	R	2208	11.25	10.15	114.19	110.84	10.70
HARAPPA 2	L	1802	10.50	11.00	115.50	95.45	10.75
HARAPPA 2	R	1802	10.50	11.00	115.50	95.45	10.75
HARAPPA 4	L	1804	10.00	9.00	90.00	111.11	9.50
HARAPPA 4	R	1804	11.00	9.00	99.00	122.22	10.00
HARAPPA 5	R	1805	10.50	10.50	110.25	100.00	10.50
HARAPPA 10	R	1807	10.00	10.50	105.00	95.24	10.25
HARAPPA 12	L	1809	10.00	10.00	100.00	100.00	10.00
HARAPPA 12	R	1809	10.00	10.50	105.00	95.24	10.25
HARAPPA 14	L	1811	9.00	11.50	103.50	78.26	10.25

LOWER M1 H. SAPIENS

		N	L(M-D)	B(B-L)	L*B	L/B	L+B/2
HARAPPA 15	L	1812	10.50	11.00	115.50	95.45	10.75
HARAPPA 15	R	1812	11.00	11.00	121.00	100.00	11.00
HARAPPA 16	L	1813	11.50	10.00	115.00	115.00	10.75
HARAPPA 16	R	1813	11.00	10.00	110.00	110.00	10.50
HARAPPA 27	L	1820	10.00	10.50	105.00	95.24	10.25
HARAPPA 27	R	1820	10.00	10.50	105.00	95.24	10.25
HARAPPA 15	L	1812	10.00	11.00	110.00	90.91	10.50
HARAPPA 15	R	1812	10.00	11.00	110.00	90.91	10.50
HARAPPA 35	L	1823	10.50	10.00	105.00	105.00	10.25
HARAPPA 35	R	1823	10.00	11.00	110.00	90.91	10.50
HARAPPA 37	L	1825	11.50	12.00	138.00	95.83	11.75
HARAPPA 37	R	1825	10.00	12.00	120.00	83.33	11.00
HARAPPA 42	L	1830	10.00	10.00	100.00	100.00	10.00
HARAPPA 42	R	1830	10.00	10.00	100.00	100.00	10.00
HARAPPA 54	L	1841	11.00	10.00	110.00	110.00	10.50
HARAPPA 54	R	1841	11.50	10.00	115.00	115.00	10.75
HARAPPA 58	L	1844	11.00	10.50	115.50	104.76	10.75
HARAPPA 58	R	1844	10.50	9.50	99.75	110.53	10.00
HARAPPA 60	L	1846	10.50	10.00	105.00	105.00	10.25
HARAPPA 60	R	1846	10.50	9.50	99.75	110.53	10.00
HARAPPA 62	L	1848	11.00	10.50	115.50	104.76	10.75
HARAPPA 62	R	1848	11.00	10.50	115.50	104.76	10.75
HARAPPA 63	L	1849	10.00	10.00	100.00	100.00	10.00
HARAPPA 63	R	1849	10.50	10.50	110.25	100.00	10.50
HARAPPA 66	L	1852	10.50	10.50	110.25	100.00	10.50
HARAPPA 66	R	1852	10.00	10.00	100.00	100.00	10.00
HARAPPA 69	L	1853	12.50	11.50	143.75	108.70	12.00
HARAPPA 69	R	1853	11.50	11.00	126.50	104.55	11.25
HARAPPA 71	R	1855	10.50	11.50	120.75	91.30	11.00
HARAPPA 74	L	1857	11.00	9.50	104.50	115.79	10.25
HARAPPA 74	R	1857	10.50	10.00	105.00	105.00	10.25
HARAPPA 75	L	1858	10.00	11.00	110.00	90.91	10.50
HARAPPA 88	L	1861	11.00	10.50	115.50	104.76	10.75
HARAPPA 88	R	1861	11.00	10.00	110.00	110.00	10.50
HARAPPA 91	L	1863	11.00	10.00	110.00	110.00	10.50
HARAPPA 91	R	1863	11.00	10.00	110.00	110.00	10.50
HARAPPA 93	L	1864	10.50				
HARAPPA 93	R	1864	10.00	9.00	90.00	111.11	9.50
HARAPPA 95	L	1865	11.00	8.50	93.50	129.41	9.75
HARAPPA 95	R	1865	11.00	9.00	99.00	122.22	10.00
GOL BA IT 95	L	2002		10.60			
GOL BA IT 95	R	2002		10.70			
GOL BA IT 98	L	2003		10.30			
GOL BA IT 98	R	2003		10.10			
GOL BA IT	R	2018	11.60	11.20	129.92	103.57	11.40
MELOLC	L	2116	11.30	10.70	120.91	105.61	11.00
MELOLC	R	2117	12.00	10.60	127.20	113.21	11.30
MELOLC	L	2118	12.20	10.80	131.76	112.96	11.50
MELOLC	R	2119	11.90	11.30	134.47	105.31	11.60
MELOLC	L	2120	10.70	10.50	112.35	101.90	10.60

LOWER M1 H. SAPIENS

		N	L(M-D)	B(B-L)	L*B	L/B	L+B/2
MELOLC	R	2121	12.10	10.80	130.68	112.04	11.45
MELOLC	L	2122	11.40	10.20	116.28	111.76	10.80
MELOLC	R	2123	11.30	10.20	115.26	110.78	10.75
MELOLC	L	2124	11.50	10.40	119.60	110.58	10.95
MELOLC	R	2125	11.70	10.70	125.19	109.35	11.20
MELOLC	L	2126	11.70	10.80	126.36	108.33	11.25
MELOLC	R	2127	12.10	10.80	130.68	112.04	11.45
MELOLC	L	2128	12.50	11.60	145.00	107.76	12.05
SAINT CRUZ M	L	2204	12.50	11.00	137.50	113.64	11.75
SAINT CRUZ M	R	2204	11.70	11.20	131.04	104.46	11.45
SAINT CRUZ F	L	2205	11.40	10.60	120.84	107.55	11.00
SAINT CRUZ F	R	2205	11.30	10.30	116.39	109.71	10.80
GREENLAND ESK.	L	1402	11.50	10.30	118.45	111.65	10.90
GREENLAND ESK.	R	1402	11.50	10.00	115.00	115.00	10.75
HAIDA	L	1406	12.40	12.30	152.52	100.81	12.35
HAIDA	R	1406	12.30	12.30	151.29	100.00	12.30
INDIAN (AM)		1407	11.70	11.40	133.38	102.63	11.55
INDIAN (AM)		1408	11.80	11.00	129.80	107.27	11.40
INDIAN (AM)		1409	11.30	11.00	124.30	102.73	11.15
INDIAN (AM)		1410	10.80	10.00	108.00	108.00	10.40
INDIAN (AM)		1411	11.00	10.60	116.60	103.77	10.80
INDIAN (AM)		1412	10.60	10.50	111.30	100.95	10.55
INDIAN (AM)		1413	10.70	10.20	109.14	104.90	10.45
INDIAN (AM)		1414	11.50	11.00	126.50	104.55	11.25
INDIAN (AM)		1415	12.00	11.60	139.20	103.45	11.80
INDIAN (AM)		1416	12.00	11.80	141.60	101.69	11.90
INDIAN (AM)		1417	12.30	11.70	143.91	105.13	12.00
INDIAN (AM)		1418	12.30	11.70	143.91	105.13	12.00
MINNESOTA MAN	L	1419	12.90	12.30	158.67	104.88	12.60
MINNESOTA MAN	R	1419	12.90	12.30	158.67	104.88	12.60
TARASCO (AM)	L	1421	12.80	11.90	152.32	107.56	12.35
TARASCO (AM)	L	1422	13.30	12.20	162.26	109.02	12.75
TARASCO (AM)	L	1423	12.70	10.70	135.89	118.69	11.70
TARASCO (AM)	L	1424	12.30	10.70	131.61	114.95	11.50
TARASCO (AM)	L	1425	11.20	11.10	124.32	100.90	11.15
ILLINOIS ME3-10	L	1428	10.55	10.25	108.14	102.93	10.40
ILLINOIS A-2732	R	1429	12.00	11.65	139.80	103.00	11.82
ILLINOIS A-6890	L	1430	10.80	10.70	115.56	100.93	10.75
ILLINOIS A-6890	R	1430	10.95	10.70	117.16	102.34	10.82
ILLINOIS A-4921	L	1431	10.00	11.55	115.50	86.58	10.77
ILLINOIS A-4921	R	1431	11.60	11.80	136.88	98.31	11.70
ILLINOIS PK9-B4	L	1432	10.80	10.40	112.32	103.85	10.60
ILLINOIS PK9-B4	R	1432	10.80	11.00	118.80	98.18	10.90
ILLINOIS PK9-B1	L	1433	12.50	12.30	153.75	101.63	12.40
ILLINOIS PK9-B1	R	1433	12.00	12.45	149.40	96.39	12.22
ILLINOIS BR19-3	L	1434	11.35	11.40	129.39	99.56	11.37
ILLINOIS BR19-3	R	1434	11.40	11.10	126.54	102.70	11.25
ILLINOIS PIKE C	L	1436	11.80	11.60	136.88	101.72	11.70
ILLINOIS PIKE C	R	1436	11.95	11.60	138.62	103.02	11.77
ILLINOIS A-8068	L	1437	11.30				

LOWER M1 H. SAPIENS

		N	L(M-D)	B(B-L)	L*B	L/B	L+B/2
ILLINCIS A-8068	R	1437	11.90	11.45	136.25	103.93	11.67
DICKSCN MOUND	L	1501	11.85	10.60	125.61	111.79	11.22
DICKSCN MOUND	R	1501	11.90	10.60	126.14	112.26	11.25
DICKSCN MD 242	L	1505	12.15	11.50	139.72	105.65	11.82
DICKSON MD 242	R	1505	12.00	11.40	136.80	105.26	11.70
DICKSCN MD 256	L	1506	11.40	10.90	124.26	104.59	11.15
DICKSCN MD 256	R	1506	11.60	11.35	131.66	102.20	11.47
DICKSON MD 258	L	1507	10.80	10.20	110.16	105.88	10.50
DICKSON MD 258	R	1507	10.80	9.90	106.92	109.09	10.35
DICKSON MD 261	L	1508	11.20	11.00	123.20	101.82	11.10
DICKSCN MD 261	R	1508	11.20	11.00	123.20	101.82	11.10
DICKSON MD 262	L	1509	12.45	11.25	140.06	110.67	11.85
DICKSCN MD 262	R	1509	12.33	11.00	135.63	112.09	11.66
DICKSON MD 266	R	1510	11.90	11.20	133.28	106.25	11.55
DICKSCN MD 276	L	1514	13.05	12.45	162.47	104.82	12.75
DICKSCN MD 276	R	1514	12.55	12.35	154.99	101.62	12.45
DICKSON MD 278	R	1515	11.00	10.90	119.90	100.92	10.95
DICKSCN MD 287	L	1516	11.80	11.50	135.70	102.61	11.65
DICKSCN MD 287	R	1516	11.50	10.05	115.57	114.43	10.77
DICKSCN MD 297	L	1520	12.35	11.65	143.88	106.01	12.00
DICKSCN MD 297	R	1520	12.10	11.02	133.34	109.80	11.56
DICKSON MD 302	L	1521	11.05	10.20	112.71	108.33	10.62
DICKSCN MD 302	R	1521	10.45	10.05	105.02	103.98	10.25
DICKSCN MD 319	L	1523	11.40	11.32	129.05	100.71	11.36
DICKSCN MD 319	R	1523	11.60	11.35	131.66	102.20	11.47
DICKSON MD 327	L	1524	11.1C	10.90	120.99	101.83	11.00
DICKSON MD 327	R	1524	11.05	10.95	121.00	100.91	11.00
DICKSCN MD 334	L	1525	12.20	10.70	130.54	114.02	11.45
DICKSON MD 334	R	1525	11.70	11.90	139.23	98.32	11.80
DICKSCN MD 344	R	1527	10.30	10.90	112.27	94.50	10.60
DICKSON MD 348	L	1529	10.60	10.10	107.06	104.95	10.35
DICKSCN MD 348	R	1529	10.90	10.20	111.18	106.86	10.55
DICKSCN MD 349	L	1530	11.70	10.80	126.36	108.33	11.25
DICKSON MD 349	R	1530	10.80	10.60	114.48	101.89	10.70
DICKSCN MD 350	R	1531	12.30	11.50	141.45	106.96	11.90
DICKSCN MD 352	L	1533	12.20	11.20	136.64	108.93	11.70
DICKSON MD 352	R	1533	12.05	10.90	131.34	110.55	11.47
DICKSON MD 353	L	1534	11.30	11.10	125.43	101.80	11.20
DICKSCN MD 355	L	1535	12.10	11.75	142.17	102.98	11.92
DICKSON MD 355	R	1535	12.40	11.90	147.56	104.20	12.15
DICKSCN MD 357	L	1536	10.75	11.20	120.40	95.98	10.97
DICKSON MD 357	R	1536	11.20	11.00	123.20	101.82	11.10
DICKSON MD 362	L	1539	11.80	11.20	132.16	105.36	11.50
DICKSCN MD 362	R	1539	11.65	11.50	133.97	101.30	11.57
DICKSON MD 365	L	1540	11.20	10.50	117.60	106.67	10.85
DICKSCN MD 365	R	1540	10.30	10.40	107.12	99.04	10.35
DICKSCN MD 371	L	1542	11.70	11.50	134.55	101.74	11.60
DICKSON MD 371	R	1542	11.30	11.80	133.34	95.76	11.55
DICKSCN MD 372	L	1543	10.60	11.00	116.60	96.36	10.80
DICKSCN MD 372	R	1543	10.70	11.20	119.84	95.54	10.95

LOWER M1 H. SAPIENS

		N	L(M-D)	B(B-L)	L*B	L/B	L+B/2
DICKSCN MD 378	L	1547	11.00	9.80	107.80	112.24	10.40
DICKSCN MD 378	R	1547	11.00	10.20	112.20	107.84	10.60
DICKSCN MD 379	L	1548	11.20	11.15	124.88	100.45	11.17
DICKSCN MD 379	R	1548	11.50	11.00	126.50	104.55	11.25
DICKSON MD 381	R	1550	11.40	11.30	128.82	100.88	11.35
DICKSON MD 380	R	1551	9.90	10.00	99.00	99.00	9.95
DICKSON MD 388	L	1552	11.80	11.50	135.70	102.61	11.65
DICKSON MD 388	R	1552	12.00	11.50	138.00	104.35	11.75
DICKSCN MD 397	L	1554	12.30	11.70	143.91	105.13	12.00
DICKSCN MD 397	R	1554	12.30	11.80	145.14	104.24	12.05
DICKSON MD 399	L	1556	10.80	11.15	120.42	96.86	10.97
DICKSON MD 399	R	1556	10.90	11.10	120.99	98.20	11.00
DICKSON MD 402	L	1557	12.70	11.80	149.86	107.63	12.25
DICKSON MD 402	R	1557	12.50	12.40	155.00	100.81	12.45
DICKSCN MD 403	L	1558	12.60	11.00	138.60	114.55	11.80
DICKSON MD 406	L	1560	10.90	10.80	117.72	100.93	10.85
DICKSON MD 407	L	1561	12.44	12.20	151.77	101.97	12.32
DICKSCN MD 407	R	1561	12.00	11.43	137.16	104.99	11.71
DICKSON MD 409	L	1562	11.55	12.20	140.91	94.67	11.87
DICKSCN MD 409	R	1562	11.50	11.90	136.85	96.64	11.70
DICKSON MD 414	L	1564	11.10	10.96	121.66	101.28	11.03
DICKSCN MD 414	R	1564	10.80	11.20	120.96	96.43	11.00
DICKSCN MD 415	L	1565	11.88	11.10	131.87	107.03	11.49
DICKSCN MD 415	R	1565	11.90	11.10	132.09	107.21	11.50
DICKSCN MD 426	L	1566	11.45	11.20	128.24	102.23	11.32
DICKSCN MD 432	L	1567	10.05	10.40	104.52	96.63	10.22
DICKSON MD 432	R	1567	10.20	10.50	107.10	97.14	10.35
DICKSCN MD 441	L	1569	11.50	11.00	126.50	104.55	11.25
DICKSON MD 441	R	1569	11.60	10.85	125.86	106.91	11.22
DICKSCN MD 443	L	1571	12.62	12.31	155.35	102.52	12.46
DICKSON MD 443	R	1571	12.18	11.44	139.34	106.47	11.81
DICKSON MD 446	L	1572	11.05	11.35	125.42	97.36	11.20
DICKSCN MD 446	R	1572	11.38	11.20	127.46	101.61	11.29
DICKSCN MD 447	L	1573	10.85	10.20	110.67	106.37	10.52
DICKSON MD 447	R	1573	10.52	10.01	105.31	105.09	10.26
DICKSCN MD 448	L	1574	11.97	10.70	128.08	111.87	11.33
DICKSON MD 448	R	1574	12.83	10.30	132.15	124.56	11.56
DICKSON MD 464	L	1575	11.50	11.00	126.50	104.55	11.25
DICKSON MD 464	R	1575	11.55	11.10	128.20	104.05	11.32
DICKSCN MD 476	L	1576	12.40	11.55	143.22	107.36	11.97
DICKSCN MD 476	R	1576	12.00	11.55	138.60	103.90	11.77
DICKSCN MD 478	L	1577	13.10	11.70	153.27	111.97	12.40
DICKSCN MD 485	L	1579	12.90	12.85	165.76	100.39	12.87
DICKSCN MD 497	L	1583	11.90	11.80	140.42	100.85	11.85
DICKSCN MD 497	R	1583	11.45	12.18	139.46	94.01	11.81
DICKSCN MD 503	L	1585	11.85	11.55	136.87	102.60	11.70
DICKSCN MD 503	R	1585	11.95	11.40	136.23	104.82	11.67
DICKSON MD 509	L	1587	12.15	11.20	136.08	108.48	11.67
DICKSCN MD 509	R	1587	12.00	11.12	133.44	107.91	11.56
DICKSCN MD 535	L	1591	11.95	11.60	138.62	103.02	11.77

LOWER M1 H. SAPIENS

		N	L(M-D)	B(B-L)	L*B	L/B	L+B/2
DICKSON MD	535 R	1591	12.50	10.85	135.62	115.21	11.67
DICKSON MD	536 L	1592	12.00	12.00	144.00	100.00	12.00
DICKSON MD	536 R	1592	12.10	11.20	135.52	108.04	11.65
DICKSON MD	542 R	1593	12.50	11.60	145.00	107.76	12.05
DICKSON MD	545 R	1594	12.55	12.03	150.98	104.32	12.29
DICKSON MD	557 L	1596	11.42	10.90	124.48	104.77	11.16
DICKSON MD	557 R	1596	11.20	10.85	121.52	103.23	11.02
DICKSON MD	561 L	1597	11.85	11.60	137.46	102.16	11.72
DICKSON MD	561 R	1597	12.70	11.85	150.49	107.17	12.27
DICKSON MD	568 L	1599	11.95	11.00	131.45	108.64	11.47
DICKSON MD	568 R	1599	11.80	11.45	135.11	103.06	11.62
DICKSON MD	589 R	1600	11.60	10.90	126.44	106.42	11.25
DICKSON MD	594 L	1601	11.10	11.20	124.32	99.11	11.15
DICKSON MD	594 R	1601	11.10	11.20	124.32	99.11	11.15
DICKSON MD	599 L	1602	12.20	11.70	142.74	104.27	11.95
DICKSON MD	599 R	1602	12.25	11.50	140.87	106.52	11.87
DICKSON MD	630 L	1603	12.10	11.80	142.78	102.54	11.95
DICKSON MD	630 R	1603	12.20	11.60	141.52	105.17	11.90
DICKSON MD	642 R	1607	11.80	11.00	129.80	107.27	11.40
DICKSON MD	643 L	1608	11.00	10.80	118.80	101.85	10.90
DICKSON MD	643 R	1608	11.40	11.20	127.68	101.79	11.30
DICKSON MD	652 L	1611	11.00	10.60	116.60	103.77	10.80
DICKSON MD	658 R	1613	12.00	11.10	133.20	108.11	11.55
DICKSON MD	667 L	1614	11.85	10.90	129.16	108.72	11.37
DICKSON MD	667 R	1614	12.00	11.15	133.80	107.62	11.57
DICKSON MD	709 L	1623	11.15	10.70	119.30	104.21	10.92
DICKSON MD	709 R	1623	11.80	10.90	128.62	108.26	11.35
DICKSON MD	722 L	1624	11.75	11.10	130.42	105.86	11.42
DICKSON MD	722 R	1624	11.50	11.10	127.65	103.60	11.30
DICKSON MD	724 L	1627	11.25	11.70	131.62	96.15	11.47
DICKSON MD	724 R	1627	11.32	11.95	135.27	94.73	11.63
DICKSON MD	746 R	1628	12.00	11.25	135.00	106.67	11.62
DICKSON MD	749 L	1629	12.70	11.32	143.76	112.19	12.01
DICKSON MD	749 R	1629	12.70	11.15	141.60	113.90	11.92
DICKSON MD	767 R	1631	11.90	10.35	123.16	114.98	11.12

LOWER M2 H. SAPIENS

		N	L(M-D)	B(B-L)	L*B	L/B	L+B/2
PREDMOST 1	L	1009	11.00	11.00	121.00	100.00	11.00
PREDMOST 1	R	1009	10.80	10.20	110.16	105.88	10.50
PREDMOST 3	L	1007	12.50	11.90	148.75	105.04	12.20
PREDMOST 3	R	1007	11.80	11.50	135.70	102.61	11.65
PREDMOST 4	L	1008	9.20	10.00	92.00	92.00	9.60
PREDMOST 4	R	1008	9.80	10.30	100.94	95.15	10.05
PREDMOST 5	L	1011	10.40	10.60	110.24	98.11	10.50
PREDMOST 5	R	1011	11.00	10.70	117.70	102.80	10.85
PREDMOST 7	L	1012	11.00	10.80	118.80	101.85	10.90
PREDMOST 7	R	1012	11.40	10.00	114.00	114.00	10.70
PREDMOST 9	L	1013	12.80	11.60	148.48	110.34	12.20
PREDMOST 9	R	1013	12.80	12.40	158.72	103.23	12.60
PREDMOST 10	L	1014	10.40	9.90	102.96	105.05	10.15
PREDMOST 10	R	1014	10.50	10.20	107.10	102.94	10.35
PREDMOST 14	L	1015	12.00	12.00	144.00	100.00	12.00
PREDMOST 18	L	1016	12.50	12.00	150.00	104.17	12.25
PREDMOST 476	L	1059	11.00	10.00	110.00	110.00	10.50
PREDMOST 3070	R	1060	9.50	10.00	95.00	95.00	9.75
COMBE CHAPELLE	L	1017	11.50	11.00	126.50	104.55	11.25
COMBE CHAPELLE	R	1017	12.00	11.50	138.00	104.35	11.75
BRNO 3	L	1018	10.20	10.80	110.16	94.44	10.50
BRNO 3	R	1018	10.00	11.00	110.00	90.91	10.50
GRIMALDI ADOL.	L	1019	13.00	10.90	141.70	119.27	11.95
GRIMALDI ADOL.	R	1019	13.30	10.80	143.64	123.15	12.05
KLATY KLN	L	1020	11.00	11.00	121.00	100.00	11.00
KLATY KLN	R	1020	11.00	11.00	121.00	100.00	11.00
ROIS A		1024	11.50	11.00	126.50	104.55	11.25
ROIS R5C-3		1026	11.50	10.00	115.00	115.00	10.75
ROIS R5C-31		1032	10.00	10.00	100.00	100.00	10.00
ROIS R5C-40		1034	12.50	11.00	137.50	113.64	11.75
ROIS		1049	11.00	10.50	115.50	104.76	10.75
ROIS		1050	11.50	11.00	126.50	104.55	11.25
VESTONICE 3	L	1057	10.90	11.10	120.99	98.20	11.00
VESTONICE 3	R	1057	10.80	11.10	119.88	97.30	10.95
A CULOZ 2	L	1101	10.90	11.00	119.90	99.09	10.95
A CULOZ 2	R	1101	11.00	11.10	122.10	99.10	11.05
BUGGISON 1	L	1108	11.00	11.00	121.00	100.00	11.00
BUGGISON 1	R	1108	11.50	11.00	126.50	104.55	11.25
BUGGISON 2	L	1109	11.00	10.50	115.50	104.76	10.75
BUGGISON 2	R	1109	12.00	11.00	132.00	109.09	11.50
CAP BLAC	L	1110	9.10	10.10	91.91	90.10	9.60
CAP BLAC	R	1110	9.20	10.10	92.92	91.09	9.65
CHANCELADE	L	1111	9.50	12.00	114.00	79.17	10.75
EGOLZWIL 1	L	1112	9.70				
EGOLZWIL 1	R	1112	9.80	10.70	104.86	91.59	10.25
FARINCOURT 3	L	1115	9.80	8.70	85.26	112.64	9.25
FARINCOURT 3	R	1115	9.40	8.70	81.78	108.05	9.05
GALLEY HILL	R	1116	10.30	11.30	116.39	91.15	10.80
GARDAR	R	1117	11.60	10.20	118.32	113.73	10.90
HOHLERFELS A	L	1118	11.50	11.50	132.25	100.00	11.50

LOWER M2 H. SAPIENS

		N	L(M-D)	B(B-L)	L*B	L/B	L+B/2
HOHLERFELS A	R	1118	11.50	12.00	138.00	95.83	11.75
HOHLERFELS C	R	1119	12.10	11.00	133.10	110.00	11.55
KABUA 1		1123	12.00	12.20	146.40	98.36	12.10
LACHAUD A	L	1125	11.20	9.70	108.64	115.46	10.45
LACHAUD A	R	1125	11.10	9.60	106.56	115.62	10.35
LACHAUD B	L	1126	12.10	11.50	139.15	105.22	11.80
LACHAUD B	R	1126	11.60	10.60	122.96	109.43	11.10
LAFAYE	L	1128	10.70	10.80	115.56	99.07	10.75
LAFAYE	R	1128	10.70	11.80	126.26	90.68	11.25
MASAT		1130	10.80	10.00	108.00	108.00	10.40
MECHTA	R	1131	12.00	12.50	150.00	96.00	12.25
OBERCASSEL 1	L	1132	10.50	11.00	115.50	95.45	10.75
OBERCASSEL 1	R	1132	10.00	10.50	105.00	95.24	10.25
OKUZINI		1133	10.00	10.00	100.00	100.00	10.00
PAS ESTRET 3	L	1134	10.70	10.10	108.07	105.94	10.40
PAS ESTRET 3	R	1134	11.10	9.90	109.89	112.12	10.50
PAS ESTRET 4	L	1135	12.20	11.40	139.08	107.02	11.80
PRITZERBER 3	L	1138	11.00	11.00	121.00	100.00	11.00
PRITZERBER 3	R	1138	10.50	11.00	115.50	95.45	10.75
PRITZERBER 4	L	1139	11.50	11.00	126.50	104.55	11.25
PRITZERBER 4	R	1139	11.00	10.50	115.50	104.76	10.75
SILICKA BREZOVA	R	1143	11.00	10.00	110.00	110.00	10.50
SVAERCBORG	R	1144	12.20	11.20	136.64	108.93	11.70
KAFFIR		1147	9.80	10.60	103.88	92.45	10.20
KAFFIR		1148	11.30	10.40	117.52	108.65	10.85
FRENCHMAN	L	1149	10.35	10.30	106.60	100.49	10.32
FRENCHMAN	R	1149	10.00	9.90	99.00	101.01	9.95
EUROPEAN 344C	L	1150	10.00	9.50	95.00	105.26	9.75
EUROPEAN 344C	R	1150	10.00	9.50	95.00	105.26	9.75
EUROPEAN AJ2	L	1151	10.00	10.00	100.00	100.00	10.00
EUROPEAN AJ2	R	1151	10.00	10.00	100.00	100.00	10.00
WHITE 99-7740	L	1152	10.50	10.60	111.30	99.06	10.55
WHITE ZZZ		1153	11.00	9.80	107.80	112.24	10.40
WHITE 14		1154	10.50	9.80	102.90	107.14	10.15
WHITE 4F		1155	10.50	10.50	110.25	100.00	10.50
WHITE 3W		1156	8.70	8.70	75.69	100.00	8.70
WHITE EDNA		1157	11.00	10.80	118.80	101.85	10.90
WHITE F		1158	9.70	10.00	97.00	97.00	9.85
WHITE PG		1159	10.30	10.00	103.00	103.00	10.15
WHITE M		1160	10.40	10.00	104.00	104.00	10.20
WHITE HJB		1161	9.40	10.40	97.76	90.38	9.90
WHITE GT		1162	10.20	10.00	102.00	102.00	10.10
WHITE ANI		1163	11.40	11.20	127.68	101.79	11.30
WHITE BRD		1164	10.00	9.50	95.00	105.26	9.75
WHITE GN		1165	11.00	10.50	115.50	104.76	10.75
WHITE GIVC		1166	11.00	11.00	121.00	100.00	11.00
WHITE BX		1167	10.70	10.40	111.28	102.88	10.55
WHITE CQ		1168	11.00	10.30	113.30	106.80	10.65
WHITE GM		1169	10.50	10.50	110.25	100.00	10.50
WHITE AAD		1170	11.00	11.00	121.00	100.00	11.00

LOWER M2 H. SAPIENS

		N	L(M-D)	B(B-L)	L*B	L/B	L+B/2
WHITE BIY		1171	9.80	9.60	94.08	102.08	9.70
WHITE AIO		1172	9.60	9.00	86.40	106.67	9.30
WHITE EK	R	1173	11.40	11.20	127.68	101.79	11.30
WHITE 99-7740		1175	10.50	10.20	107.10	102.94	10.35
WHITE 99-7743		1176	12.30	11.20	137.76	109.82	11.75
ALACA HOYUK 2		1183	11.10	10.00	111.00	111.00	10.55
ALACA HOYUK 3		1184	11.00	9.70	106.70	113.40	10.35
BEDOUIN		1188	10.70	10.50	112.35	101.90	10.60
BELT CAVE	R	1189	11.80	10.00	118.00	118.00	10.90
WADJAK 1		1701	12.00	11.00	132.00	109.09	11.50
WADJAK 2	L	1702	11.60	10.70	124.12	108.41	11.15
WADJAK 2	R	1702	11.70	11.00	128.70	106.36	11.35
AUSTRALIAN 9801	L	1706	11.60	11.80	136.88	98.31	11.70
AUSTRALIAN 9801	R	1706	11.80	12.00	141.60	98.33	11.90
AUSTRALIAN 9800	L	1707	11.00	11.00	121.00	100.00	11.00
AUSTRALIAN 9800	R	1707	11.20	11.00	123.20	101.82	11.10
AUSTRALIAN 39		1708	13.20	11.20	147.84	117.86	12.20
AUSTRALIAN 8158		1710	12.10	11.40	137.94	106.14	11.75
AUSTRALIAN 8174		1711	11.60	12.00	139.20	96.67	11.80
AUSTRALIAN AM		1712	11.70	11.40	133.38	102.63	11.55
AUSTRALIAN AM		1713	11.30	10.40	117.52	108.65	10.85
AUSTRALIAN AM		1714	11.00	11.30	124.30	97.35	11.15
AUSTRALIAN AM		1715	10.50	10.50	110.25	100.00	10.50
AUSTRALIAN AM		1716	11.40	11.00	125.40	103.64	11.20
AUSTRALIAN AM		1717	10.60	11.00	116.60	96.36	10.80
AUSTRALIAN AM		1718	10.40	10.50	109.20	99.05	10.45
AUSTRALIAN AM		1719	10.60	10.60	112.36	100.00	10.60
AUSTRALIAN AM		1720	11.60	11.00	127.60	105.45	11.30
AUSTRALIAN AM		1721	10.70	10.40	111.28	102.88	10.55
AUSTRALIAN 90	R	1722	14.00	12.50	175.00	112.00	13.25
AUSTRALIAN 54	R	1723	12.50	12.00	150.00	104.17	12.25
AUSTRALIAN 88	L	1724	10.00	10.60	106.00	94.34	10.30
AUSTRALIAN	L	1727	12.05	11.90	143.39	101.26	11.97
AUSTRALIAN	L	1729	13.25	12.10	160.32	109.50	12.67
AUSTRALIAN	R	1729	12.60	12.30	154.98	102.44	12.45
AUSTRALIAN 8158	L	1730	12.20	11.70	142.74	104.27	11.95
AUSTRALIAN AM	L	1731	11.30	11.00	124.30	102.73	11.15
TASMANIAN 1406	L	1751	13.00	12.00	156.00	108.33	12.50
TASMANIAN 1406	R	1751	12.50	11.50	143.75	108.70	12.00
TASMANIAN	R	1752	12.00	11.00	132.00	109.09	11.50
TASMANIAN	R	1753	10.70	12.60	134.82	84.92	11.65
TASMANIAN 310		1754	12.00	11.00	132.00	109.09	11.50
TASMANIAN P3	R	1759	12.00	11.50	138.00	104.35	11.75
TASMANIAN 707	R	1760	12.00	12.00	144.00	100.00	12.00
TASMANIAN 2964	L	1763	13.40	11.40	152.76	117.54	12.40
TASMANIAN 2964	R	1763	12.90	11.40	147.06	113.16	12.15
BOSKOP		1902	11.00	11.50	126.50	95.65	11.25
ASSELAR	R	1903	11.00	11.00	121.00	100.00	11.00
CAPE FLATS	R	1904	11.50	12.00	138.00	95.83	11.75
NEGRO	L	1906	13.50	11.65	157.27	115.88	12.57

LOWER M2 H. SAPIENS

		N	L(M-D)	B(B-L)	L*B	L/B	L+B/2
NEGRO AM		1907	12.00	11.80	141.60	101.69	11.90
NEGRO AM		1908	10.80	10.40	112.32	103.85	10.60
NEGRO AM		1909	11.00	10.80	118.80	101.85	10.90
NEGRO AM		1911	12.00	11.00	132.00	109.09	11.50
NEGRO AM		1912	12.30	12.00	147.60	102.50	12.15
NEGRO		1914	11.10	10.30	114.33	107.77	10.70
NEGRO	L	1915	14.40	12.80	184.32	112.50	13.60
NEGRO	R	1915	15.40	13.20	203.28	116.67	14.30
NEGRO	L	1916	13.70	12.60	172.62	108.73	13.15
NEGRO	R	1916	13.50	12.30	166.05	109.76	12.90
NEGRO 2	L	1919	11.80	10.60	125.08	111.32	11.20
NEGRO 2	R	1919	11.40	11.00	125.40	103.64	11.20
NEGRO 1	L	1920	10.40	10.70	111.28	97.20	10.55
NEGRO 1	R	1920	10.80	10.20	110.16	105.88	10.50
NEGRO 3C91	L	1921	10.50	10.60	111.30	99.06	10.55
NEGRO 3C91	R	1921	10.50	9.50	99.75	110.53	10.00
NEGRO 5	R	1922	12.00	11.00	132.00	109.09	11.50
NEGRO 6	L	1923	11.20	10.60	118.72	105.66	10.90
NEGRO 9	L	1924	10.10	10.00	101.00	101.00	10.05
NEGRO 9	R	1924	10.40	9.80	101.92	106.12	10.10
NEGRO 29	L	1925	12.40	10.70	132.68	115.89	11.55
NEGRO 29	R	1925	12.00	11.60	139.20	103.45	11.80
N/HOTTENTOT 12	L	1943	10.00	9.65	96.50	103.63	9.82
N/HOTTENTOT 12	R	1943	9.50	9.60	91.20	98.96	9.55
N/HOTTENTOT 6	L	1944	12.40	12.25	151.90	101.22	12.32
N/HOTTENTOT 6	R	1944	12.60	11.30	142.38	111.50	11.95
N/BUSHMAN 52	L	1945	12.10	11.20	135.52	108.04	11.65
N/BUSHMAN 52	R	1945	12.10	11.20	135.52	108.04	11.65
BUSHMAN MXD 61	L	1946	11.10	10.10	112.11	109.90	10.60
BUSHMAN MXD 61	R	1946	11.25	10.25	115.31	109.76	10.75
BUSHMAN MXD 94	L	1947	11.25	11.30	127.12	99.56	11.27
BUSHMAN MXD 94	R	1947	12.40	10.90	135.16	113.76	11.65
N/HOTTENTOT 6	L	1948	12.20	11.30	137.86	107.96	11.75
N/HOTTENTOT 6	R	1948	12.25	11.70	143.32	104.70	11.97
MAPUNGUBWE	L	1950	10.60	10.25	108.65	103.41	10.42
MAPUNGUBWE	R	1950	10.90	10.25	111.72	106.34	10.57
MAPUNGUBWE M3		1953	12.50	11.00	137.50	113.64	11.75
MAPUNGUBWE M5		1954	12.00	11.50	138.00	104.35	11.75
MAPUNGUBWE M9		1955	13.00	12.00	156.00	108.33	12.50
BAMBANDYANALO21		1957	10.50	10.00	105.00	105.00	10.25
BAMBANDYANALO29		1958	11.60	10.10	117.16	114.85	10.85
BAMBANDYANALO31		1959	12.00	11.20	134.40	107.14	11.60
BAMBANDYANALO33	R	1960	11.60	11.00	127.60	105.45	11.30
BAMBANDYANALO 3		1962	11.30	11.20	126.56	100.89	11.25
BAMBANDYANALO 5		1963	14.10	12.60	177.66	111.90	13.35
BAMBANDYANALO13		1964	11.40	11.70	133.38	97.44	11.55
BAMBANDYANALO14		1965	10.70	10.40	111.28	102.88	10.55
BUSHMAN		1967	10.60	10.10	107.06	104.95	10.35
BUSHMAN AM		1968	11.10	10.70	118.77	103.74	10.90
HOTTENTOT AM		1969	10.40	10.50	109.20	99.05	10.45

LOWER M2 H. SAPIENS

		N	L(M-D)	B(B-L)	L*B	L/B	L+B/2
HOTTENTOT AM		1970	12.00	11.00	132.00	109.09	11.50
HOTTENTOT AM		1971	12.00	10.80	129.60	111.11	11.40
FISH HOEK	R	1972	10.00	9.00	90.00	111.11	9.50
BUSHMAN 30	L	1973	10.65	11.00	117.15	96.82	10.82
BUSHMAN 30	R	1973	10.40	10.65	110.76	97.65	10.52
GOUNGOU A	L	1975		9.80			
GOUNGOU C	R	1976	13.15	11.94	157.01	110.13	12.54
N.BRITAIN 43122	L	1302	11.00	10.90	119.90	100.92	10.95
N.BRITAIN 43130	R	1307	12.10	11.90	143.99	101.68	12.00
N.BRITAIN 43131	L	1308	11.40	11.50	131.10	99.13	11.45
N.BRITAIN 43131	R	1308	11.70	11.30	132.21	103.54	11.50
N.BRITAIN 43133	L	1310	10.80	10.40	112.32	103.85	10.60
N.BRITAIN 43134	L	1311	12.10	11.40	137.94	106.14	11.75
N.BRITAIN 43134	R	1311	11.20	11.50	128.80	97.39	11.35
N.BRITAIN 43135	L	1312	9.20	10.20	93.84	90.20	9.70
N.BRITAIN 43135	R	1312	9.30	10.40	96.72	89.42	9.85
N.BRITAIN 43136	L	1313	11.80	10.50	123.90	112.38	11.15
N.BRITAIN 43136	R	1313	11.60	10.70	124.12	108.41	11.15
N.BRITAIN 43137	L	1314	11.00	11.10	122.10	99.10	11.05
N.BRITAIN 43137	R	1314	11.70	11.10	129.87	105.41	11.40
N.BRITAIN 43138	L	1315	11.10	11.00	122.10	100.91	11.05
N.BRITAIN 43138	R	1315	10.40	11.00	114.40	94.55	10.70
N.BRITAIN 43139	L	1316	10.90	11.20	122.08	97.32	11.05
N.BRITAIN 43139	R	1316	11.50	11.00	126.50	104.55	11.25
N.BRITAIN 43140	R	1317	11.10	10.80	119.88	102.78	10.95
N.BRITAIN 43141	L	1318	10.40	10.60	110.24	98.11	10.50
N.BRITAIN 43141	R	1318	11.10	10.60	117.66	104.72	10.85
N.BRITAIN 43142	L	1319	11.60	11.60	134.56	100.00	11.60
N.BRITAIN 43142	R	1319	12.00	11.50	138.00	104.35	11.75
N.BRITAIN 43143	L	1320	11.30	11.00	124.30	102.73	11.15
N.BRITAIN 43143	R	1320	11.50	10.70	123.05	107.48	11.10
N.BRITAIN 43144	L	1321	10.50	10.60	111.30	99.06	10.55
N.BRITAIN 43144	R	1321	10.40	10.70	111.28	97.20	10.55
N.BRITAIN 43145	L	1322	12.00	11.90	142.80	100.84	11.95
N.BRITAIN 43145	R	1322	12.30	11.90	146.37	103.36	12.10
N.BRITAIN 43146	L	1323	12.10				
N.BRITAIN 43146	R	1323	11.10	11.20	124.32	99.11	11.15
N.BRITAIN 43147	L	1324	12.30	11.90	146.37	103.36	12.10
N.BRITAIN 43147	R	1324	12.10	11.90	143.99	101.68	12.00
N.BRITAIN 43149	L	1325	11.10	11.00	122.10	100.91	11.05
N.BRITAIN 43149	R	1325	10.50	11.80	123.90	88.98	11.15
N.BRITAIN 43150	R	1326	10.50	10.40	109.20	100.96	10.45
N.BRITAIN 43151	L	1327	11.10	10.30	114.33	107.77	10.70
N.BRITAIN 43151	R	1327	11.20	10.60	118.72	105.66	10.90
N.BRITAIN 43152	L	1328	10.40	10.30	107.12	100.97	10.35
N.BRITAIN 43152	R	1328	10.40	10.40	108.16	100.00	10.40
N.BRITAIN 43153	L	1329	10.80	10.00	108.00	108.00	10.40
N.BRITAIN 43153	R	1329	10.80				
N.BRITAIN 43154	L	1330	11.20	10.90	122.08	102.75	11.05
N.BRITAIN 43154	R	1330	11.40	11.30	128.82	100.88	11.35

LOWER M2 H. SAPIENS

		N	L(M-D)	B(B-L)	L*B	L/B	L+B/2
N.BRITAIN 43174	L	1331	11.50	11.10	127.65	103.60	11.30
N.BRITAIN 43174	R	1331	11.90	11.40	135.66	104.39	11.65
N.BRITAIN 43179	L	1332	13.10	12.50	163.75	104.80	12.80
N.BRITAIN 43179	R	1332	13.00	12.10	157.30	107.44	12.55
N.BRITAIN 43193	R	1333	10.70	11.40	121.98	93.86	11.05
N.BRITAIN 43194	L	1334	12.20	11.00	134.20	110.91	11.60
N.BRITAIN 43194	R	1334	12.40	10.70	132.68	115.89	11.55
N.BRITAIN 43198	R	1335	12.10	11.30	136.73	107.08	11.70
N.BRITAIN 43202	L	1337	11.20	11.00	123.20	101.82	11.10
N.BRITAIN 43202	R	1337	10.90	11.30	123.17	96.46	11.10
N.BRITAIN 43204	L	1338	11.50	10.90	125.35	105.50	11.20
N.BRITAIN 43204	R	1338	12.10	11.20	135.52	108.04	11.65
N.BRITAIN 43226	L	1339	10.30	10.10	104.03	101.98	10.20
N.BRITAIN 43226	R	1339	11.10	10.10	112.11	109.90	10.60
N.BRITAIN 43242	L	1341	10.20	9.50	96.90	107.37	9.85
N.BRITAIN 43242	R	1341	9.60	9.50	91.20	101.05	9.55
N.BRITAIN 43290	R	1342	11.20	10.30	115.36	108.74	10.75
N.BRITAIN 43291	L	1343	11.40	10.60	120.84	107.55	11.00
N.BRITAIN 43291	R	1343	11.80	10.40	122.72	113.46	11.10
N.BRITAIN 43295	L	1344	12.00	11.30	135.60	106.19	11.65
N.BRITAIN 43296	L	1345	10.50	10.00	105.00	105.00	10.25
N.BRITAIN 43296	R	1345	9.90	9.90	98.01	100.00	9.90
N.BRITAIN	L	1346	12.50	11.90	148.75	105.04	12.20
N.BRITAIN	R	1346	12.00	12.00	144.00	100.00	12.00
NIAH CAVE	R	2207	10.70	13.00	139.10	82.31	11.85
HINDU AM 7894	L	2201	11.30	10.30	116.39	109.71	10.80
HINDU AM	R	2202	10.10	11.40	115.14	88.60	10.75
HINDU AM	L	2202	11.00	10.70	117.70	102.80	10.85
HINDU (UI)	L	2208	10.30	9.55	98.36	107.85	9.92
HINDU (UI)	R	2208	10.40	9.40	97.76	110.64	9.90
HARAPPA 2	L	1802	11.00	11.00	121.00	100.00	11.00
HARAPPA 2	R	1802	10.00	10.50	105.00	95.24	10.25
HARAPPA 4	L	1804	10.00	7.50	75.00	133.33	8.75
HARAPPA 4	R	1804	9.00	7.50	67.50	120.00	8.25
HARAPPA 5	L	1805	11.00	10.50	115.50	104.76	10.75
HARAPPA 5	R	1805	11.00	10.50	115.50	104.76	10.75
HARAPPA 10	R	1807	10.50	9.50	99.75	110.53	10.00
HARAPPA 12	L	1809	10.00	9.00	90.00	111.11	9.50
HARAPPA 12	R	1809	10.00	9.00	90.00	111.11	9.50
HARAPPA 15	L	1812	9.00	10.50	94.50	85.71	9.75
HARAPPA 15	R	1812	9.00	10.50	94.50	85.71	9.75
HARAPPA 16	L	1813	10.50	9.00	94.50	116.67	9.75
HARAPPA 16	R	1813	10.00	9.00	90.00	111.11	9.50
HARAPPA 17	L	1814	9.00	7.50	67.50	120.00	8.25
HARAPPA 17	R	1814	9.00	7.50	67.50	120.00	8.25
HARAPPA 27	R	1820	10.00				
HARAPPA 15	L	1812	9.00	10.50	94.50	85.71	9.75
HARAPPA 15	R	1812	9.00	11.00	99.00	81.82	10.00
HARAPPA 35	L	1823	9.00	10.50	94.50	85.71	9.75
HARAPPA 35	R	1823	10.00	10.50	105.00	95.24	10.25

LOWER M2 H. SAPIENS

		N	L(M-D)	B(B-L)	L*B	L/B	L+B/2
HARAPPA 37	L	1825	11.00	12.00	132.00	91.67	11.50
HARAPPA 37	R	1825	11.00	12.00	132.00	91.67	11.50
HARAPPA 42	L	1830	9.00	9.50	85.50	94.74	9.25
HARAPPA 42	R	1830	9.50	9.00	85.50	105.56	9.25
HARAPPA 54	L	1841	10.00	9.00	90.00	111.11	9.50
HARAPPA 54	R	1841	9.00	9.50	85.50	94.74	9.25
HARAPPA 58	L	1844	11.00	9.50	104.50	115.79	10.25
HARAPPA 58	R	1844	10.50	10.00	105.00	105.00	10.25
HARAPPA 60	L	1846	10.00	9.00	90.00	111.11	9.50
HARAPPA 60	R	1846	9.50	9.00	85.50	105.56	9.25
HARAPPA 62	L	1848	9.00	9.00	81.00	100.00	9.00
HARAPPA 62	R	1848	9.50	9.00	85.50	105.56	9.25
HARAPPA 63	L	1849	10.00	9.50	95.00	105.26	9.75
HARAPPA 63	R	1849	9.50	10.50	99.75	90.48	10.00
HARAPPA 65	R	1851	10.00	10.00	100.00	100.00	10.00
HARAPPA 66	L	1852	9.00	10.00	90.00	90.00	9.50
HARAPPA 66	R	1852	10.00	9.00	90.00	111.11	9.50
HARAPPA 69	L	1853	11.00	11.50	126.50	95.65	11.25
HARAPPA 69	R	1853	10.50	11.00	115.50	95.45	10.75
HARAPPA 71	R	1855	11.50	10.50	120.75	109.52	11.00
HARAPPA 73	R	1856	11.00	12.00	132.00	91.67	11.50
HARAPPA 74	L	1857	10.00	8.50	85.00	117.65	9.25
HARAPPA 74	R	1857	9.00	8.50	76.50	105.88	8.75
HARAPPA 75	L	1858	9.00	9.50	85.50	94.74	9.25
HARAPPA 88	L	1861	10.00	10.00	100.00	100.00	10.00
HARAPPA 88	R	1861	10.00	10.00	100.00	100.00	10.00
HARAPPA 89	R	1862	10.50	9.00	94.50	116.67	9.75
HARAPPA 91	L	1863	10.00	8.00	80.00	125.00	9.00
HARAPPA 91	R	1863	10.00	9.00	90.00	111.11	9.50
HARAPPA 93	L	1864	10.00	9.50	95.00	105.26	9.75
HARAPPA 93	R	1864	10.00				
HARAPPA 95	L	1865	10.00	8.00	80.00	125.00	9.00
HARAPPA 95	R	1865	10.00	7.00	70.00	142.86	8.50
GOL BA IT 98	L	2003		10.30			
GOL BA IT 98	R	2003		10.30			
GOL BA IT	R	2019	11.60	10.40	120.64	111.54	11.00
MELOLO	R	2129	10.30	9.60	98.88	107.29	9.95
MELOLO	L	2130	10.90	9.80	106.82	111.22	10.35
MELOLO	R	2131	10.90	10.20	111.18	106.86	10.55
MELOLO	L	2132	11.20	10.80	120.96	103.70	11.00
MELOLO	R	2133	9.50	10.20	96.90	93.14	9.85
MELOLO	L	2134	11.60	10.50	121.80	110.48	11.05
MELOLO	R	2135	11.20	9.60	107.52	116.67	10.40
MELOLO	L	2136	11.10	10.00	111.00	111.00	10.55
MELOLO	R	2137	11.20	9.80	109.76	114.29	10.50
MELOLO	L	2138	10.80	10.00	108.00	108.00	10.40
MELOLO	R	2139	11.20	10.40	116.48	107.69	10.80
MELOLO	L	2140	11.80	10.90	128.62	108.26	11.35
MELOLO	R	2141	11.50	10.60	121.90	108.49	11.05
MELOLO	L	2142	11.80	11.00	129.80	107.27	11.40

LOWER M2 H. SAPIENS

		N	L(M-D)	B(B-L)	L*B	L/B	L+B/2
MELOLC	R	2143	12.20	10.20	124.44	119.61	11.20
MELOLO	L	2144	10.90	11.60	126.44	93.97	11.25
SAINT CRUZ M	L	2204	10.70	10.50	112.35	101.90	10.60
SAINT CRUZ M	R	2204	11.3C	10.90	123.17	103.67	11.10
SAINT CRUZ F	L	2205	10.80	10.40	112.32	103.85	10.60
SAINT CRUZ F	R	2205	11.00	10.5C	115.50	104.76	10.75
TING TS,UN		2206	11.20	10.10	113.12	110.89	10.65
GREENLAND ESK.	L	1402	11.5C	11.00	126.50	104.55	11.25
GREENLAND ESK.	R	1402	10.50	11.00	115.50	95.45	10.75
HAIDA	L	1406	12.00	11.40	136.80	105.26	11.70
HAIDA	R	1406		11.10			
INDIAN (AM)		1407	11.00	11.00	121.00	100.00	11.00
INDIAN (AM)		1408	11.70	10.3C	120.51	113.59	11.00
INDIAN (AM)		1409	10.8C	10.6C	114.48	101.89	10.70
INDIAN (AM)		141C	10.00	9.50	95.00	105.26	9.75
INDIAN (AM)		1411	10.2C	10.00	102.00	102.00	10.10
INDIAN (AM)		1412	10.2C	10.20	104.04	100.00	10.20
INDIAN (AM)		1413	10.7C	10.2C	109.14	104.90	10.45
INDIAN (AM)		1414	11.30	1C.70	120.91	105.61	11.00
INDIAN (AM)		1415	11.8C	10.70	126.26	110.28	11.25
INDIAN (AM)		1416	11.80	11.00	129.80	107.27	11.40
INDIAN (AM)		1417	11.00	10.60	116.60	103.77	10.80
MINNESOTA MAN	L	1419	12.00	12.10	145.20	99.17	12.05
MINNESOTA MAN	R	1419	12.0C	12.10	145.20	99.17	12.05
TARASCO (AM)	L	1421	11.90	11.55	137.44	103.03	11.72
TARASCO (AM)	L	1422	12.7C	12.10	153.67	104.96	12.40
TARASCO (AM)	L	1423	12.00	12.3C	147.60	97.56	12.15
TARASCO (AM)	L	1425	11.90	10.50	124.95	113.33	11.20
ILLINCIS A-6890	L	143C	9.00	10.45	94.05	86.12	9.72
ILLINCIS A-6890	R	143C	9.65	10.10	97.46	95.54	9.87
ILLINCIS A-4921	L	1431	11.10	11.40	126.54	97.37	11.25
ILLINOIS A-4921	R	1431	11.50	11.35	130.52	101.32	11.42
ILLINCIS PK9-B4	L	1432	11.00	10.15	111.65	108.37	10.57
ILLINCIS PK9-B4	R	1432	11.00	10.45	114.95	105.26	10.72
ILLINCIS PK9-B1	R	1433	11.75	11.70	137.47	100.43	11.72
ILLINCIS BR19-3	L	1434	10.65	10.80	115.02	98.61	10.72
ILLINCIS BR19-3	R	1434	10.55	10.50	110.77	100.48	10.52
ILLINCIS A-8068	L	1437	10.40	10.55	109.72	98.58	10.47
ILLINCIS A-8C68	R	1437	10.65	1C.40	110.76	102.40	10.52
DICKSCN MOUND	L	1501	11.75	10.2C	119.85	115.20	10.97
DICKSCN MOUND	R	1501	11.65	10.2C	118.83	114.22	10.92
DICKSON MD 242	L	1505	12.50	11.05	138.12	113.12	11.77
DICKSCN MD 242	R	1505	12.40	11.18	138.63	110.91	11.79
DICKSCN MD 256	L	1506	11.95	11.05	132.05	108.14	11.50
DICKSON MD 256	R	1506	11.50	10.85	124.77	105.99	11.17
DICKSON MD 261	L	1508	10.00	1C.90	109.00	91.74	10.45
DICKSCN MC 261	R	1508	11.68	10.95	127.90	106.67	11.31
DICKSCN MD 276	L	1514	13.20	12.20	161.04	108.20	12.70
DICKSCN MD 276	R	1514	13.50	12.60	170.10	107.14	13.05
DICKSCN MD 278	R	1515	10.90	10.55	114.99	103.32	10.72

LOWER M2 H. SAPIENS

		N	L(M-D)	B(B-L)	L*B	L/B	L+B/2
DICKSCN MD 287	L	1516	11.60	11.06	128.30	104.88	11.33
DICKSCN MD 287	R	1516	11.95	10.50	125.47	113.81	11.22
DICKSCN MD 297	L	1520	11.90	11.40	135.66	104.39	11.65
DICKSCN MD 297	R	152C	12.30	12.10	148.83	101.65	12.20
DICKSCN MD 302	L	1521	10.85	10.10	109.58	107.43	10.47
CICKSCN MD 302	R	1521	10.45	10.20	106.59	102.45	1C.32
DICKSON MD 319	L	1523	11.20	10.60	118.72	105.66	10.90
DICKSON MD 319	R	1523	11.65	10.65	124.07	109.39	11.15
CICKSCN MD 327	L	1524	11.45	11.05	126.52	103.62	11.25
DICKSCN MD 327	R	1524	11.30	10.95	123.73	103.20	11.12
DICKSCN MD 334	L	1525	12.20	12.00	146.40	101.67	12.10
DICKSCN MD 334	R	1525	12.40	12.10	150.04	102.48	12.25
DICKSCN MD 344	L	1527	11.30	1C.75	121.47	105.12	11.02
DICKSCN MD 344	R	1527	11.00	11.00	121.00	100.00	11.00
DICKSCN MD 348	L	1529	11.75	10.60	124.55	110.85	11.17
DICKSCN MD 348	R	1529	11.15	10.00	111.50	111.50	10.57
DICKSCN MD 349	L	1530	11.80	10.60	125.08	111.32	11.20
DICKSON MD 349	R	1530	11.10	10.40	115.44	106.73	10.75
DICKSON MD 353	L	1534	9.60	10.30	98.88	93.20	9.95
DICKSCN MD 355	R	1535	11.30	11.10	125.43	101.80	11.20
DICKSON MD 357	R	1536	10.70	10.30	110.21	103.88	10.50
DICKSCN MD 365	L	1540	10.60	9.70	102.82	109.28	10.15
DICKSCN MD 365	R	1540	9.80	9.70	95.06	101.03	9.75
DICKSCN MD 371	L	1542	12.30	11.50	141.45	106.96	11.90
DICKSCN MD 371	R	1542	11.50	11.90	136.85	96.64	11.70
DICKSCN MD 372	L	1543	11.00	10.90	119.90	100.92	10.95
DICKSCN MD 372	R	1543	10.70	11.20	119.84	95.54	10.95
DICKSCN MD 378	L	1547	10.90	9.70	105.73	112.37	10.30
DICKSCN MD 378	R	1547	10.70	9.80	104.86	109.18	10.25
DICKSON MD 379	L	1548	10.50	10.10	106.05	103.96	10.30
DICKSCN MD 379	R	1548	11.00	10.45	114.95	105.26	10.72
DICKSON MD 380	L	1551	9.80	10.00	98.00	98.00	9.90
DICKSCN MD 380	R	1551	9.90	9.90	98.01	100.00	9.90
DICKSON MD 388	L	1552	12.80	11.60	148.48	110.34	12.20
DICKSCN MD 388	R	1552	12.60	11.40	143.64	110.53	12.00
DICKSCN MD 396	L	1553	12.10	11.10	134.31	109.01	11.60
DICKSCN MD 396	R	1553	12.20	11.20	136.64	108.93	11.70
DICKSCN MD 397	L	1554	12.30	11.20	137.76	109.82	11.75
DICKSCN MD 397	R	1554	12.70	11.55	146.68	109.96	12.12
DICKSON MD 398	L	1555	11.20	10.30	115.36	108.74	10.75
DICKSON MD 398	R	1555	12.50	10.10	126.25	123.76	11.30
DICKSCN MD 399	L	1556	11.20	10.60	118.72	105.66	10.90
DICKSCN MD 399	R	1556	11.00	10.70	117.70	102.80	10.85
DICKSCN MD 402	L	1557	12.90	12.10	156.09	106.61	12.50
DICKSON MD 402	R	1557	12.30	12.20	150.06	100.82	12.25
DICKSCN MD 404	L	1559	12.40	10.75	133.30	115.35	11.57
DICKSCN MD 406	R	1560	11.20	10.30	115.36	108.74	10.75
DICKSCN MD 407	L	1561	12.20	11.25	137.25	108.44	11.72
DICKSCN MD 407	R	1561	12.50	11.30	141.25	110.62	11.90
DICKSON MD 409	L	1562	12.20	11.45	139.69	106.55	11.82

LOWER M2 H. SAPIENS

			N	L(M-D)	B(B-L)	L*B	L/B	L+B/2
DICKSCN MD	409	R	1562	12.55	11.80	148.09	106.36	12.17
DICKSCN MD	411	L	1563	11.75	10.45	122.79	112.44	11.10
DICKSCN MD	411	R	1563	11.78	10.40	122.51	113.27	11.09
DICKSCN MD	414	L	1564	11.32	10.43	118.07	108.53	10.87
DICKSCN MD	414	R	1564	11.50	10.18	117.07	112.97	10.84
DICKSCN MD	415	L	1565	10.55	10.25	108.14	102.93	10.40
DICKSCN MD	415	R	1565	10.45	10.20	106.59	102.45	10.32
DICKSCN MD	426	L	1566	11.20	10.50	117.60	106.67	10.85
DICKSCN MD	426	R	1566	10.90	10.24	111.62	106.45	10.57
DICKSCN MD	432	L	1567	9.70	10.20	98.94	95.10	9.95
DICKSCN MD	432	R	1567	10.50	10.40	109.20	100.96	10.45
DICKSCN MD	443	L	1571	11.92	11.50	137.08	103.65	11.71
DICKSCN MD	443	R	1571	12.12	10.90	132.11	111.19	11.51
DICKSCN MD	446	L	1572	11.25	10.55	118.69	106.64	10.90
DICKSCN MD	464	L	1575	11.70	10.50	122.85	111.43	11.10
DICKSCN MD	464	R	1575	11.90	10.70	127.33	111.21	11.30
DICKSCN MD	476	L	1576	11.90	11.50	136.85	103.48	11.70
DICKSCN MD	476	R	1576	12.00	11.03	132.36	108.79	11.51
DICKSCN MD	478	L	1577	12.50	12.10	151.25	103.31	12.30
DICKSCN MD	480	L	1578	10.20	9.90	100.98	103.03	10.05
DICKSCN MD	480	R	1578	10.00	9.65	96.50	103.63	9.82
DICKSCN MD	497	L	1583	13.00	11.15	144.95	116.59	12.07
DICKSCN MD	497	R	1583	12.05	11.75	141.59	102.55	11.90
DICKSCN MD	509	L	1587	10.62	10.33	109.70	102.81	10.47
DICKSCN MD	509	R	1587	10.70	9.77	104.54	109.52	10.23
DICKSCN MD	535	L	1591	11.40	10.45	119.13	109.09	10.92
DICKSCN MD	535	R	1591	11.60	10.50	121.80	110.48	11.05
DICKSCN MD	536	L	1592	11.50	10.35	119.02	111.11	10.92
DICKSCN MD	536	R	1592	11.75	10.42	122.43	112.76	11.08
DICKSCN MD	545	R	1594	12.49	11.94	149.13	104.61	12.21
DICKSCN MD	557	L	1596	10.75	10.80	116.10	99.54	10.77
DICKSCN MD	557	R	1596	11.20	10.60	118.72	105.66	10.90
DICKSCN MD	561	L	1597	11.50	11.50	132.25	100.00	11.50
DICKSCN MD	561	R	1597	12.20	11.85	144.57	102.95	12.02
DICKSCN MD	567	L	1598	12.00	11.30	135.60	106.19	11.65
DICKSCN MD	567	R	1598	11.90	11.55	137.44	103.03	11.72
DICKSCN MD	568	L	1599	11.20	10.00	112.00	112.00	10.60
DICKSCN MD	568	R	1599	11.30	10.30	116.39	109.71	10.80
DICKSCN MD	589	R	1600	11.70				
DICKSCN MD	594	R	1601	9.90	10.20	100.98	97.06	10.05
DICKSCN MD	599	L	1602	12.10	11.25	136.12	107.56	11.67
DICKSCN MD	599	R	1602	11.65	11.15	129.90	104.48	11.40
DICKSCN MD	630	L	1603	11.80	10.40	122.72	113.46	11.10
DICKSCN MD	630	R	1603	12.00	10.70	128.40	112.15	11.35
DICKSCN MD	643	L	1608	11.20	10.90	122.08	102.75	11.05
DICKSCN MD	643	R	1608	10.70	11.40	121.98	93.86	11.05
DICKSCN MD	658	L	1613	11.90	11.10	132.09	107.21	11.50
DICKSCN MD	658	R	1613	11.00	10.70	117.70	102.80	10.85
DICKSCN MD	667	L	1614	12.30	11.20	137.76	109.82	11.75
DICKSCN MD	667	R	1614	12.30	10.52	129.40	116.92	11.41

LOWER M2 H. SAPIENS

			N	L(M-D)	B(B-L)	L*B	L/B	L+B/2
DICKSCN MD	709	L	1623	11.05	10.70	118.23	103.27	10.87
DICKSCN MD	709	R	1623	11.00	10.90	119.90	100.92	10.95
DICKSCN MD	722	L	1624	11.80	11.25	132.75	104.89	11.52
DICKSCN MD	724	L	1627	11.45	11.15	127.67	102.69	11.30
DICKSCN MD	724	R	1627	11.95	11.00	131.45	108.64	11.47
DICKSCN MD	746	L	1628	11.25	10.80	121.50	104.17	11.02
DICKSCA MD	746	R	1628	11.45	10.80	123.66	106.02	11.12

LOWER M3 H. SAPIENS

		N	L(M-D)	B(B-L)	L*B	L/B	L+B/2
ARCYSURCURE C10	R	1006	13.00	11.00	143.00	118.18	12.00
PREDMOST 3	R	1007	12.70	11.40	144.78	111.40	12.05
PREDMOST 4	L	1008	10.20	9.90	100.98	103.03	10.05
PREDMOST 4	R	1008	9.80	10.00	98.00	98.00	9.90
PREDMOST 9	L	1013	12.80	11.80	151.04	108.47	12.30
PREDMOST 9	R	1013	12.50	11.80	147.50	105.93	12.15
PREDMOST 10	L	1014	11.20	10.20	114.24	109.80	10.70
PREDMOST 10	R	1014	10.70	10.20	109.14	104.90	10.45
PREDMOST 3070	R	1060	10.10	10.00	101.00	101.00	10.05
COMBE CHAPELLE	L	1017	11.00	11.00	121.00	100.00	11.00
COMBE CHAPELLE	R	1017	10.00	10.00	100.00	100.00	10.00
BRNO 3	L	1018	10.80	10.60	114.48	101.89	10.70
BRNO 3	R	1018	10.50	10.30	108.15	101.94	10.40
GRIMALDI ADOL.	L	1019	12.70	10.50	133.35	120.95	11.60
GRIMALDI ADOL.	R	1019	12.60	9.30	117.18	135.48	10.95
ROIS A		1024	11.00	11.00	121.00	100.00	11.00
ROIS R5C-9		1029	11.00	10.00	110.00	110.00	10.50
ROIS R51-15		1040	12.00	11.00	132.00	109.09	11.50
VESTONICE 3	L	1057	10.90	10.50	114.45	103.81	10.70
VESTONICE 3	R	1057	10.90	10.50	114.45	103.81	10.70
A CULOZ 2	L	1101	10.90	10.40	113.36	104.81	10.65
A CULOZ 2	R	1101	10.20	10.20	104.04	100.00	10.20
ARLAY	L	1104	10.00	10.00	100.00	100.00	10.00
ARLAY	R	1104	10.00	9.80	98.00	102.04	9.90
ARLAY	L	1105	10.00	10.00	100.00	100.00	10.00
ARLAY	R	1105	10.00	9.80	98.00	102.04	9.90
ABRI BLACHARD	R	1106	9.50	9.30	88.35	102.15	9.40
BUGGISON 1	L	1108	12.00	11.00	132.00	109.09	11.50
BUGGISON 1	R	1108	12.50	11.00	137.50	113.64	11.75
BUGGISON 2	L	1109	12.50	11.00	137.50	113.64	11.75
BUGGISON 2	R	1109	11.50	11.00	126.50	104.55	11.25
CHANCELADE	L	1111	11.50	12.50	143.75	92.00	12.00
CHANCELADE	R	1111	10.50	11.00	115.50	95.45	10.75
EGOLZWIL 1	L	1112	9.70	9.20	89.24	105.43	9.45
EGOLZWIL 1	R	1112	9.00	9.10	81.90	98.90	9.05
FARINCOURT 3	L	1115	9.30	9.10	84.63	102.20	9.20
FARINCOURT 3	R	1115	8.90	9.10	80.99	97.80	9.00
GALLEY HILL	R	1116	10.20	11.50	117.30	88.70	10.85
GARDAR	R	1117	11.00	10.40	114.40	105.77	10.70
HOHLERFELS A	L	1118	11.50	11.10	127.65	103.60	11.30
HOHLERFELS A	R	1118	11.50	11.10	127.65	103.60	11.30
HOHLERFELS C	R	1119	12.00	11.10	133.20	108.11	11.55
ISTURITZ 1	L	1120	11.00	11.00	121.00	100.00	11.00
ISTURITZ 3		1122	11.00	11.00	121.00	100.00	11.00
KABUA 1		1123	11.70	11.50	134.55	101.74	11.60
LACHAUD A	L	1125	11.80	9.40	110.92	125.53	10.60
LACHAUD A	R	1125	11.20	9.60	107.52	116.67	10.40
LAFAYE	L	1128	9.60	10.20	97.92	94.12	9.90
LAFAYE	R	1128	7.70	7.80	60.06	98.72	7.75
LES VACHONS	R	1129	11.80	11.10	130.98	106.31	11.45

LOWER M3 H. SAPIENS

		N	L(M-D)	B(B-L)	L*B	L/B	L+B/2
MASAT		1130	10.20	9.20	93.84	110.87	9.70
MECHTA	L	1131	11.25	12.50	140.62	90.00	11.87
MECHTA	R	1131	11.25	12.50	140.62	90.00	11.87
OBERCASSEL 1	L	1132	10.00	11.00	110.00	90.91	10.50
OBERCASSEL 1	R	1132	11.00	10.00	110.00	110.00	10.50
PRITZERBER 3	L	1138	11.00	10.00	110.00	110.00	10.50
PRITZERBER 3	R	1138	11.00	10.50	115.50	104.76	10.75
PRITZERBER 4	L	1139	10.50	10.00	105.00	105.00	10.25
PRITZERBER 4	R	1139	10.00	10.00	100.00	100.00	10.00
TERRASSON A	L	1145	11.80	9.40	110.92	125.53	10.60
TERRASSON A	R	1145	11.20	9.60	107.52	116.67	10.40
TERRASSON B	R	1146	11.50	10.40	119.60	110.58	10.95
KAFFIR		1148	10.50	13.50	141.75	77.78	12.00
FRENCHMAN	L	1149	10.85	9.95	107.96	109.05	10.40
FRENCHMAN	R	1149	10.50	10.10	106.05	103.96	10.30
EUROPEAN 344C	L	1150	9.80	9.10	89.18	107.69	9.45
EUROPEAN 344C	R	1150	9.80	9.40	92.12	104.26	9.60
EUROPEAN AJ2	L	1151	10.00	9.50	95.00	105.26	9.75
EUROPEAN AJ2	R	1151	10.00	9.50	95.00	105.26	9.75
WHITE 59-7740	L	1152	10.35	10.40	107.64	99.52	10.37
WHITE 14		1154	9.20	8.90	81.88	103.37	9.05
WHITE HJB		1161	10.80	10.20	110.16	105.88	10.50
WHITE GT		1162	9.80	9.50	93.10	103.16	9.65
WHITE ANI		1163	10.30	10.30	106.09	100.00	10.30
WHITE EK	L	1173	10.80	9.50	102.60	113.68	10.15
WHITE EK	R	1173	10.80	10.50	113.40	102.86	10.65
WHITE 59-7740		1175	9.60	9.40	90.24	102.13	9.50
BEDOUIN		1188	9.70	9.30	90.21	104.30	9.50
WADI HALFA	L	1213	11.30	10.90	123.17	103.67	11.10
WADI HALFA	L	1214	11.20	11.60	129.92	96.55	11.40
WADJAK 1		1701	13.00	11.00	143.00	118.18	12.00
WADJAK 2	L	1702	12.00	13.30	159.60	90.23	12.65
AUSTRALIAN 9801	L	1706	12.30	12.20	150.06	100.82	12.25
AUSTRALIAN 9801	R	1706	13.00	12.60	163.80	103.17	12.80
AUSTRALIAN 9800	L	1707	11.20	11.00	123.20	101.82	11.10
AUSTRALIAN 9800	R	1707	11.40	12.80	145.92	89.06	12.10
AUSTRALIAN 39		1708	12.00	11.00	132.00	109.09	11.50
AUSTRALIAN 8157		1709	11.00	10.90	119.90	100.92	10.95
AUSTRALIAN 8174		1711	11.20	11.40	127.68	98.25	11.30
AUSTRALIAN AM		1712	11.50	11.00	126.50	104.55	11.25
AUSTRALIAN AM		1713	11.00	10.40	114.40	105.77	10.70
AUSTRALIAN AM		1714	10.00	9.80	98.00	102.04	9.90
AUSTRALIAN AM		1715	11.40	10.80	123.12	105.56	11.10
AUSTRALIAN AM		1716	11.00	10.50	115.50	104.76	10.75
AUSTRALIAN AM		1717	11.00	11.20	123.20	98.21	11.10
AUSTRALIAN AM		1718	10.80	11.00	118.80	98.18	10.90
AUSTRALIAN AM		1719	11.40	10.70	121.98	106.54	11.05
AUSTRALIAN AM		1720	10.60	10.00	106.00	106.00	10.30
AUSTRALIAN AM		1721	12.00	11.80	141.60	101.69	11.90
AUSTRALIAN 90	R	1722	13.00	13.00	169.00	100.00	13.00

LOWER M3 H. SAPIENS

		N	L(M-D)	B(B-L)	L*B	L/B	L+B/2
AUSTRALIAN 54	R	1723	12.50	11.50	143.75	108.70	12.00
AUSTRALIAN 88	L	1724	10.00	10.00	100.00	100.00	10.00
AUSTRALIAN	L	1727	11.40	11.10	126.54	102.70	11.25
AUSTRALIAN	L	1729	12.00	12.10	145.20	99.17	12.05
AUSTRALIAN	R	1729	12.40	10.70	132.68	115.89	11.55
AUSTRALIAN 8158	L	1730	10.90	11.50	125.35	94.78	11.20
AUSTRALIAN AM	L	1731	13.00	12.00	156.00	108.33	12.50
TASMANIAN 1406	L	1751	11.10	12.50	138.75	88.80	11.80
TASMANIAN 1406	R	1751	11.80	11.50	135.70	102.61	11.65
TASMANIAN 310		1754	10.00	10.00	100.00	100.00	10.00
TASMANIAN P3	R	1759	13.00	11.50	149.50	113.04	12.25
TASMANIAN 2964	L	1763	12.20	11.00	134.20	110.91	11.60
TASMANIAN 2964	R	1763	12.40	11.00	136.40	112.73	11.70
ASSELAR	R	1903	11.00	10.50	115.50	104.76	10.75
CAPE FLATS	R	1904	11.30	11.50	129.95	98.26	11.40
NEGRO	L	1906	12.30	10.70	131.61	114.95	11.50
NEGRO AM		1907	10.50	10.50	110.25	100.00	10.50
NEGRO AM		1908	10.30	10.30	106.09	100.00	10.30
NEGRO AM		1909	12.50	11.00	137.50	113.64	11.75
NEGRO AM		1910	12.40	11.80	146.32	105.08	12.10
NEGRO AM		1911	12.00	11.00	132.00	109.09	11.50
NEGRO AM		1912	12.50	12.00	150.00	104.17	12.25
NEGRO		1914	11.20	10.40	116.48	107.69	10.80
NEGRO	L	1915	13.40				
NEGRO	R	1915	12.00				
NEGRO	L	1916	14.60	12.90	188.34	113.18	13.75
NEGRO	R	1916	14.50	12.50	181.25	116.00	13.50
NEGRO 2	L	1919	10.40	10.90	113.36	95.41	10.65
NEGRO 2	R	1919	11.40	11.00	125.40	103.64	11.20
NEGRO 1	L	1920	10.40	10.60	110.24	98.11	10.50
NEGRO 1	R	1920	10.50	10.20	107.10	102.94	10.35
NEGRO 3C91	L	1921	9.60	8.20	78.72	117.07	8.90
NEGRO 3C91	R	1921	10.00	9.70	97.00	103.09	9.85
NEGRO 6	L	1923	11.00	11.00	121.00	100.00	11.00
NEGRO 6	R	1923	10.80	11.20	120.96	96.43	11.00
NEGRO 9	L	1924	8.50	9.80	83.30	86.73	9.15
NEGRO 9	R	1924	10.40	10.20	106.08	101.96	10.30
NEGRO 29	L	1925	12.40	12.90	159.96	96.12	12.65
NEGRO 29	R	1925	12.70	11.90	151.13	106.72	12.30
N/HOTTENTOT 12	R	1943	9.70	9.25	89.72	104.86	9.47
N/HOTTENTOT 6	L	1944	11.25	10.60	119.25	106.13	10.92
N/HOTTENTOT 6	R	1944	11.25	11.30	127.12	99.56	11.27
N/BUSHMAN 52	L	1945	11.25	10.75	120.94	104.65	11.00
N/BUSHMAN 52	R	1945	12.30	11.25	138.37	109.33	11.77
BUSHMAN MXD 61	L	1946	9.60	11.10	106.56	86.49	10.35
BUSHMAN MXD 61	R	1946	10.90	9.50	103.55	114.74	10.20
N/HOTTENTOT 6	L	1948	12.00	11.90	142.80	100.84	11.95
N/HOTTENTOT 6	R	1948	11.00	10.75	118.25	102.33	10.87
MAPUNGUBWE	L	1950	9.40	9.90	93.06	94.95	9.65
MAPUNGUBWE	R	1950	9.60	10.00	96.00	96.00	9.80

LOWER M3 H. SAPIENS

		N	L(M-D)	B(B-L)	L*B	L/B	L+B/2
MAPUNGUBWE M5		1954	11.70	11.00	128.70	106.36	11.35
MAPUNGUBWE M10		1956	12.50	11.50	143.75	108.70	12.00
BAMBANDYANALO21		1957	10.00	9.60	96.00	104.17	9.80
BAMBANDYANALO29		1958	11.90	10.50	124.95	113.33	11.20
BAMBANDYANALO31		1959	11.00	10.50	115.50	104.76	10.75
BAMBANDYANALO 3		1962	11.60	11.00	127.60	105.45	11.30
BAMBANDYANALO13		1964	11.10	11.20	124.32	99.11	11.15
BAMBANDYANALO14		1965	11.50	11.00	126.50	104.55	11.25
ZITZIKAMA		1966	9.50	8.00	76.00	118.75	8.75
BUSHMAN		1967	9.90	9.60	95.04	103.12	9.75
BUSHMAN AM		1968	10.80	10.80	116.64	100.00	10.80
HOTTENTOT AM		1969	11.00	10.50	115.50	104.76	10.75
HOTTENTOT AM		1970	11.00	11.00	121.00	100.00	11.00
HOTTENTOT AM		1971	12.50	11.70	146.25	106.84	12.10
FISH HOEK	R	1972	10.00	8.00	80.00	125.00	9.00
BUSHMAN 30	L	1973	9.75	10.10	98.47	96.53	9.92
BUSHMAN 30	R	1973	9.25	9.65	89.26	95.85	9.45
N.BRITAIN 43122	L	1302	11.30	10.70	120.91	105.61	11.00
N.BRITAIN 43130	L	1307	11.50	12.50	143.75	92.00	12.00
N.BRITAIN 43130	R	1307	12.70	12.10	153.67	104.96	12.40
N.BRITAIN 43132	L	1309	11.90	12.00	142.80	99.17	11.95
N.BRITAIN 43132	R	1309	13.10	11.60	151.96	112.93	12.35
N.BRITAIN 43133	L	1310	12.00				
N.BRITAIN 43134	L	1311	10.00	10.10	101.00	99.01	10.05
N.BRITAIN 43134	R	1311	11.60	10.50	121.80	110.48	11.05
N.BRITAIN 43135	L	1312	11.10	10.20	113.22	108.82	10.65
N.BRITAIN 43135	R	1312	10.50	10.00	105.00	105.00	10.25
N.BRITAIN 43137	L	1314	10.80	11.20	120.96	96.43	11.00
N.BRITAIN 43137	R	1314	11.10	11.00	122.10	100.91	11.05
N.BRITAIN 43138	L	1315	11.60	11.10	128.76	104.50	11.35
N.BRITAIN 43138	R	1315	11.90	11.10	132.09	107.21	11.50
N.BRITAIN 43139	L	1316	11.80	11.60	136.88	101.72	11.70
N.BRITAIN 43139	R	1316	12.40	11.40	141.36	108.77	11.90
N.BRITAIN 43140	R	1317	11.80	11.00	129.80	107.27	11.40
N.BRITAIN 43141	L	1318	11.40	10.80	123.12	105.56	11.10
N.BRITAIN 43141	R	1318	11.30	10.60	119.78	106.60	10.95
N.BRITAIN 43142	L	1319	13.00	12.00	156.00	108.33	12.50
N.BRITAIN 43142	R	1319	12.00				
N.BRITAIN 43143	L	1320	10.70	11.80	126.26	90.68	11.25
N.BRITAIN 43143	R	1320	10.50	11.20	117.60	93.75	10.85
N.BRITAIN 43144	L	1321	10.40	10.50	109.20	99.05	10.45
N.BRITAIN 43144	R	1321	10.20	11.00	112.20	92.73	10.60
N.BRITAIN 43147	L	1324	11.70	11.60	135.72	100.86	11.65
N.BRITAIN 43147	R	1324	11.60	11.50	133.40	100.87	11.55
N.BRITAIN 43149	L	1325	10.20	10.30	105.06	99.03	10.25
N.BRITAIN 43149	R	1325	10.70	10.70	114.49	100.00	10.70
N.BRITAIN 43150	R	1326	10.70	11.70	125.19	91.45	11.20
N.BRITAIN 43151	L	1327	11.50	11.20	128.80	102.68	11.35
N.BRITAIN 43151	R	1327	11.90	11.00	130.90	108.18	11.45
N.BRITAIN 43152	R	1328	13.40	9.90	132.66	135.35	11.65

LOWER M3 H. SAPIENS

		N	L(M-D)	B(B-L)	L*B	L/B	L+B/2
N.BRITAIN 43153	L	1329	9.90	9.60	95.04	103.12	9.75
N.BRITAIN 43153	R	1329	9.80				
N.BRITAIN 43154	L	1330	11.60	11.50	133.40	100.87	11.55
N.BRITAIN 43154	R	1330	11.60	11.20	129.92	103.57	11.40
N.BRITAIN 43174	L	1331	11.90	10.70	127.33	111.21	11.30
N.BRITAIN 43174	R	1331	11.90	10.20	121.38	116.67	11.05
N.BRITAIN 43179	L	1332	14.00	12.00	168.00	116.67	13.00
N.BRITAIN 43179	R	1332	13.30	12.00	159.60	110.83	12.65
N.BRITAIN 43193	R	1333	10.60	11.00	116.60	96.36	10.80
N.BRITAIN 43194	L	1334	11.30	10.10	114.13	111.88	10.70
N.BRITAIN 43194	R	1334	11.40	10.30	117.42	110.68	10.85
N.BRITAIN 43198	L	1335	12.10	11.00	133.10	110.00	11.55
N.BRITAIN 43198	R	1335	12.00	11.20	134.40	107.14	11.60
N.BRITAIN 43199	R	1336	12.50	10.80	135.00	115.74	11.65
N.BRITAIN 43202	L	1337	11.30	10.50	118.65	107.62	10.90
N.BRITAIN 43202	R	1337	11.30	10.40	117.52	108.65	10.85
N.BRITAIN 43204	L	1338	11.90	10.90	129.71	109.17	11.40
N.BRITAIN 43204	R	1338	12.20	10.50	128.10	116.19	11.35
N.BRITAIN 43226	L	1339	11.80	9.90	116.82	119.19	10.85
N.BRITAIN 43226	R	1339	10.80	9.90	106.92	109.09	10.35
N.BRITAIN 43242	L	1341	11.20	10.80	120.96	103.70	11.00
N.BRITAIN 43242	R	1341	9.30	11.30	105.09	82.30	10.30
N.BRITAIN 43290	R	1342	11.30	9.80	110.74	115.31	10.55
N.BRITAIN 43291	L	1343	12.40	10.80	133.92	114.81	11.60
N.BRITAIN 43291	R	1343	11.60	10.50	121.80	110.48	11.05
N.BRITAIN 43295	L	1344	11.70	11.20	131.04	104.46	11.45
N.BRITAIN 43296	L	1345	11.50	10.60	121.90	108.49	11.05
N.BRITAIN 43296	R	1345	11.60	10.50	121.80	110.48	11.05
N.BRITAIN	L	1346	11.40	11.30	128.82	100.88	11.35
N.BRITAIN	R	1346	12.20	11.30	137.86	107.96	11.75
NIAH CAVE	R	2207	11.50	12.40	142.60	92.74	11.95
HINDU AM 7894	L	2201	11.70	10.05	117.58	116.42	10.87
HINDU AM	R	2202	11.50	11.10	127.65	103.60	11.30
HINDU (UI)	R	2208	10.50	10.00	105.00	105.00	10.25
HARAPPA 2	L	1802	10.00	11.00	110.00	90.91	10.50
HARAPPA 2	R	1802	10.00	10.00	100.00	100.00	10.00
HARAPPA 4	L	1804	8.50	7.50	63.75	113.33	8.00
HARAPPA 4	R	1804	9.00	7.50	67.50	120.00	8.25
HARAPPA 5	L	1805	12.00	10.50	126.00	114.29	11.25
HARAPPA 5	R	1805	11.50	10.50	120.75	109.52	11.00
HARAPPA 10	R	1807	8.00	9.50	76.00	84.21	8.75
HARAPPA 12	L	1809	10.50	9.00	94.50	116.67	9.75
HARAPPA 12	R	1809	10.50	9.00	94.50	116.67	9.75
HARAPPA 14	L	1811	10.50	9.00	94.50	116.67	9.75
HARAPPA 15	L	1812	9.00	9.50	85.50	94.74	9.25
HARAPPA 15	R	1812	8.50	9.00	76.50	94.44	8.75
HARAPPA 17	L	1814	9.00	7.00	63.00	128.57	8.00
HARAPPA 17	R	1814	8.50	7.00	59.50	121.43	7.75
HARAPPA 27	L	1820	10.00	9.00	90.00	111.11	9.50
HARAPPA 15	L	1812	7.50	8.00	60.00	93.75	7.75

LOWER M3 H. SAPIENS

		N	L(M-D)	B(B-L)	L*B	L/B	L+B/2
HARAPPA 15	R	1812	8.50	9.00	76.50	94.44	8.75
HARAPPA 35	L	1823	9.00	10.00	90.00	90.00	9.50
HARAPPA 35	R	1823	10.00	10.00	100.00	100.00	10.00
HARAPPA 37	L	1825	10.00	11.00	110.00	90.91	10.50
HARAPPA 37	R	1825	10.50	11.50	120.75	91.30	11.00
HARAPPA 42	L	1830	9.50	8.50	80.75	111.76	9.00
HARAPPA 42	R	1830	9.50	8.50	80.75	111.76	9.00
HARAPPA 54	L	1841	10.00	9.00	90.00	111.11	9.50
HARAPPA 54	R	1841	9.00	9.00	81.00	100.00	9.00
HARAPPA 56	R	1843	10.00	8.50	85.00	117.65	9.25
HARAPPA 58	L	1844	10.50	9.50	99.75	110.53	10.00
HARAPPA 60	L	1846	10.00	9.00	90.00	111.11	9.50
HARAPPA 60	R	1846	10.00	8.50	85.00	117.65	9.25
HARAPPA 62	L	1848	11.00	8.50	93.50	129.41	9.75
HARAPPA 62	R	1848	10.00	9.50	95.00	105.26	9.75
HARAPPA 63	L	1849	10.00	9.50	95.00	105.26	9.75
HARAPPA 63	R	1849	10.00	10.00	100.00	100.00	10.00
HARAPPA 66	L	1852	9.00	8.50	76.50	105.88	8.75
HARAPPA 69	L	1853	9.50	10.50	99.75	90.48	10.00
HARAPPA 69	R	1853	10.50	11.00	115.50	95.45	10.75
HARAPPA 73	R	1856	9.00	11.00	99.00	81.82	10.00
HARAPPA 74	R	1857	9.50	9.00	85.50	105.56	9.25
HARAPPA 75	L	1858	9.50	9.50	90.25	100.00	9.50
HARAPPA 88	L	1861	9.50	9.00	85.50	105.56	9.25
HARAPPA 88	R	1861	10.50	9.50	99.75	110.53	10.00
HARAPPA 89	L	1862	9.50				
HARAPPA 89	R	1862	10.00	9.00	90.00	111.11	9.50
HARAPPA 93	L	1864	9.50	9.00	85.50	105.56	9.25
HARAPPA 93	R	1864	9.50	9.00	85.50	105.56	9.25
GOL BA IT 95	L	2002		11.20			
GOL BA IT 95	R	2002		10.60			
GOL BA IT 98	L	2003		10.60			
GOL BA IT 98	R	2003		10.30			
MELOLO	L	2145	9.90	9.80	97.02	101.02	9.85
MELOLO	R	2146	9.70	9.70	94.09	100.00	9.70
MELOLO	L	2147	10.20	10.40	106.08	98.08	10.30
MELOLO	R	2148	12.20	10.70	130.54	114.02	11.45
MELOLO	L	2149	10.30	10.20	105.06	100.98	10.25
MELOLO	L	2150	10.20	9.90	100.98	103.03	10.05
MELOLO	L	2151	9.60	10.10	96.96	95.05	9.85
SAINT CRUZ M	L	2204	12.00	11.00	132.00	109.09	11.50
SAINT CRUZ M	R	2204	11.70	10.70	125.19	109.35	11.20
SAINT CRUZ F	L	2205	10.00	10.00	100.00	100.00	10.00
SAINT CRUZ F	R	2205	10.40	10.40	108.16	100.00	10.40
SAINT CRUZ F	L	2205	9.60	10.80	103.68	88.89	10.20
DELEWARE INDIAN	R	1401	13.50	12.00	162.00	112.50	12.75
HAIDA	L	1406	12.00	11.40	136.80	105.26	11.70
INDIAN (AM)		1407	11.30	11.00	124.30	102.73	11.15
INDIAN (AM)		1408	11.50	11.00	126.50	104.55	11.25
INDIAN (AM)		1409	11.00	10.20	112.20	107.84	10.60

LOWER M3 H. SAPIENS

	N	L(M-D)	B(B-L)	L*B	L/B	L+B/2
INDIAN (AM)	1410	9.50	9.50	90.25	100.00	9.50
INDIAN (AM)	1411	11.00	10.30	113.30	106.80	10.65
INDIAN (AM)	1412	11.40	10.00	114.00	114.00	10.70
INDIAN (AM)	1413	10.70	10.30	110.21	103.88	10.50
INDIAN (AM)	1414	10.50	10.20	107.10	102.94	10.35
INDIAN (AM)	1415	12.00	10.70	128.40	112.15	11.35
INDIAN (AM)	1416	11.40	10.80	123.12	105.56	11.10
INDIAN (AM)	1417	11.50	10.50	120.75	109.52	11.00
MINNESOTA MAN L	1419	12.80	11.80	151.04	108.47	12.30
MINNESOTA MAN R	1419	13.10	11.60	151.96	112.93	12.35
TARASCO (AM) L	1421	12.10	11.10	134.31	109.01	11.60
TARASCO (AM) L	1422	12.50	10.70	133.75	116.82	11.60
TARASCO (AM) L	1423	11.20	10.50	117.60	106.67	10.85
ILLINOIS A-2732 R	1429	11.30	11.40	128.82	99.12	11.35
ILLINOIS A-6890 L	1430	10.40	10.65	110.76	97.65	10.52
ILLINOIS A-6890 R	1430	10.60	11.25	119.25	94.22	10.92
ILLINOIS A-4921 L	1431	12.60	12.00	151.20	105.00	12.30
ILLINOIS A-4921 R	1431	12.00	11.60	139.20	103.45	11.80
ILLINOIS PK9-B4 L	1432	10.00	9.35	93.50	106.95	9.67
ILLINOIS PK9-B4 R	1432	9.30	10.25	95.32	90.73	9.77
ILLINOIS PK9-B1 L	1433	11.00	12.30	135.30	89.43	11.65
ILLINOIS PK9-B1 R	1433	11.85	11.10	131.53	106.76	11.47
ILLINOIS BR19-3 L	1434	10.74	10.50	112.77	102.29	10.62
ILLINOIS BR19-3 R	1434	10.20	10.55	107.61	96.68	10.37
ILLINOIS PIKE C L	1436	11.50	11.80	135.70	97.46	11.65
ILLINOIS A-8068 L	1437	11.05	11.00	121.55	100.45	11.02
ILLINOIS A-8068 R	1437	10.80	10.90	117.72	99.08	10.85
DICKSON MOUND L	1501	12.10	10.60	128.26	114.15	11.35
DICKSON MOUND R	1501	11.30	10.25	115.82	110.24	10.77
DICKSON MD 256 L	1506	13.80	10.05	138.69	137.31	11.92
DICKSON MD 256 R	1506	13.90	10.10	140.39	137.62	12.00
DICKSON MD 261 L	1508	11.40	10.50	119.70	108.57	10.95
DICKSON MD 261 R	1508	10.85	10.40	112.84	104.33	10.62
DICKSON MD 276 L	1514	12.65	12.20	154.33	103.69	12.42
DICKSON MD 276 R	1514	13.25	12.05	159.66	109.96	12.65
DICKSON MD 278 R	1515	11.10	9.85	109.33	112.69	10.47
DICKSON MD 287 L	1516	12.10	10.90	131.89	111.01	11.50
DICKSON MD 287 R	1516	11.85	10.60	125.61	111.79	11.22
DICKSON MD 297 L	1520	11.30	10.40	117.52	108.65	10.85
DICKSON MD 297 R	1520	11.28	10.33	116.52	109.20	10.80
DICKSON MD 302 L	1521	10.05	8.10	81.40	124.07	9.07
DICKSON MD 302 R	1521	10.70	8.80	94.16	121.59	9.75
DICKSON MD 319 L	1523	10.80	10.35	111.78	104.35	10.57
DICKSON MD 319 R	1523	10.50	10.00	105.00	105.00	10.25
DICKSON MD 327 L	1524	12.00	11.00	132.00	109.09	11.50
DICKSON MD 327 R	1524	12.10	11.10	134.31	109.01	11.60
DICKSON MD 334 L	1525	9.20	10.05	92.46	91.54	9.62
DICKSON MD 334 R	1525	10.10	10.60	107.06	95.28	10.35
DICKSON MD 348 L	1529	10.20	9.70	98.94	105.15	9.95
DICKSON MD 348 R	1529	10.45	10.00	104.50	104.50	10.22

LOWER M3 H. SAPIENS

	N	L(M-D)	B(B-L)	L*B	L/B	L+B/2
DICKSON MD 349 L	1530	11.95	10.15	121.29	117.73	11.05
DICKSON MD 349 R	1530	11.50	9.90	113.85	116.16	10.70
DICKSON MD 355 L	1535	12.20	11.05	134.81	110.41	11.62
DICKSON MD 355 R	1535	12.15	11.20	136.08	108.48	11.67
DICKSON MD 357 R	1536	9.90	10.50	103.95	94.29	10.20
DICKSON MD 362 L	1539	11.25	9.70	109.12	115.98	10.47
DICKSON MD 365 L	1540	10.00	9.60	96.00	104.17	9.80
DICKSON MD 365 R	1540	10.40	10.40	108.16	100.00	10.40
DICKSON MD 371 L	1542	11.80	11.00	129.80	107.27	11.40
DICKSON MD 371 R	1542	10.30	11.50	118.45	89.57	10.90
DICKSON MD 372 L	1543	11.00	10.60	116.60	103.77	10.80
DICKSON MD 372 R	1543	10.60	10.70	113.42	99.07	10.65
DICKSON MD 379 L	1548	10.60	10.20	108.12	103.92	10.40
DICKSON MD 379 R	1548	11.45	11.20	128.24	102.23	11.32
DICKSON MD 381 L	1550	11.30	11.30	127.69	100.00	11.30
DICKSON MD 381 R	1550	13.80	11.00	151.80	125.45	12.40
DICKSON MD 380 L	1551	9.60	9.70	93.12	98.97	9.65
DICKSON MD 380 R	1551	9.90	9.80	97.02	101.02	9.85
DICKSON MD 396 L	1553	11.80	10.30	121.54	114.56	11.05
DICKSON MD 396 R	1553	12.50	10.90	136.25	114.68	11.70
DICKSON MD 397 R	1554	10.90	10.90	118.81	100.00	10.90
DICKSON MD 398 R	1555	10.30	10.90	112.27	94.50	10.60
DICKSON MD 399 L	1556	10.65	11.00	117.15	96.82	10.82
DICKSON MD 399 R	1556	10.65	10.70	113.95	99.53	10.67
DICKSON MD 402 R	1557	13.50	12.30	166.05	109.76	12.90
DICKSON MD 404 L	1559	11.40	10.65	121.41	107.04	11.02
DICKSON MD 407 L	1561	11.60	10.85	125.86	106.91	11.22
DICKSON MD 407 R	1561	12.35	10.50	129.67	117.62	11.42
DICKSON MD 409 L	1562	11.00	11.10	122.10	99.10	11.05
DICKSON MD 409 R	1562	11.70	11.10	129.87	105.41	11.40
DICKSON MD 411 L	1563	10.10	9.85	99.48	102.54	9.97
DICKSON MD 411 R	1563	10.55	9.80	103.39	107.65	10.17
DICKSON MD 414 L	1564	10.30	9.80	100.94	105.10	10.05
DICKSON MD 415 L	1565	10.03	9.90	99.30	101.31	9.96
DICKSON MD 426 L	1566	10.48	10.10	105.85	103.76	10.29
DICKSON MD 426 R	1566	10.50	10.25	107.62	102.44	10.37
DICKSON MD 432 L	1567	9.05	9.25	83.71	97.84	9.15
DICKSON MD 432 R	1567	8.65	8.45	73.09	102.37	8.55
DICKSON MD 443 R	1571	12.04	11.00	132.44	109.45	11.52
DICKSON MD 446 L	1572	10.50	10.20	107.10	102.94	10.35
DICKSON MD 446 R	1572	10.70	9.85	105.39	108.63	10.27
DICKSON MD 464 R	1575	10.40	9.50	98.80	109.47	9.95
DICKSON MD 476 L	1576	12.80	11.15	142.72	114.80	11.97
DICKSON MD 476 R	1576	12.60	11.15	140.49	113.00	11.87
DICKSON MD 480 L	1578	10.20	9.70	98.94	105.15	9.95
DICKSON MD 480 R	1578	10.40	9.85	102.44	105.58	10.12
DICKSON MD 485 L	1579	13.30	12.65	168.24	105.14	12.97
DICKSON MD 497 R	1583	11.70	11.40	133.38	102.63	11.55
DICKSON MD 503 L	1585	12.05	11.50	138.57	104.78	11.77
DICKSON MD 503 R	1585	12.10	11.02	133.34	109.80	11.56

LOWER M3 H. SAPIENS

		N	L(M-D)	B(B-L)	L*B	L/B	L+B/2
DICKSCN MD 535	L	1591	11.05	10.25	113.26	107.80	10.65
DICKSON MD 535	R	1591	11.35	9.90	112.36	114.65	10.62
DICKSON MD 536	L	1592	11.15	10.15	113.17	109.85	10.65
DICKSCN MD 536	R	1592	11.45	8.90	101.90	128.65	10.17
DICKSON MD 545	L	1594	12.97	11.55	149.80	112.29	12.26
DICKSCN MD 545	R	1594	11.35	10.65	120.88	106.57	11.00
DICKSCN MD 557	L	1596	10.65	10.70	113.95	99.53	10.67
DICKSCN MD 557	R	1596	10.40	10.44	108.58	99.62	10.42
DICKSON MD 561	L	1597	10.90	11.40	124.26	95.61	11.15
DICKSCN MD 561	R	1597	11.60	11.50	133.40	100.87	11.55
DICKSCN MD 567	L	1598	12.45	11.50	143.17	108.26	11.97
DICKSCN MD 567	R	1598	12.25	11.90	145.77	102.94	12.07
DICKSCN MD 589	R	1600	12.20	10.80	131.76	112.96	11.50
DICKSCN MD 599	R	1602	11.70	10.00	117.00	117.00	10.85
DICKSON MD 630	L	1603	12.40	10.80	133.92	114.81	11.60
DICKSON MD 630	R	1603	12.30	11.30	138.99	108.85	11.80
DICKSON MD 643	L	1608	11.80	10.90	128.62	108.26	11.35
DICKSGN MD 643	R	1608	12.00	10.90	130.80	110.09	11.45
DICKSON MD 658	L	1613	12.10	11.00	133.10	110.00	11.55
DICKSON MD 658	R	1613	10.90	12.90	140.61	84.50	11.90
DICKSON MD 667	R	1614	10.75	10.65	114.49	100.94	10.70
DICKSON MD 709	L	1623	11.15	10.70	119.30	104.21	10.92
DICKSCN MD 709	R	1623	12.05	10.30	124.11	116.99	11.17
DICKSON MD 722	R	1624	11.80	11.00	129.80	107.27	11.40
DICKSCN MD 724	L	1627	11.65	10.50	122.32	110.95	11.07
DICKSON MD 724	R	1627	10.80	11.95	129.06	90.38	11.37
DICKSGN MD 746	L	1628	11.40	10.40	118.56	109.62	10.90
DICKSCN MD 746	R	1628	11.00	10.30	113.30	106.80	10.65

UPPER I1 H. SAPIENS

		N	L(M-D)	B(B-L)	L*B	L/B	L+B/2
PREDMOST 3	L	1007	9.00	8.35	75.15	107.78	8.67
PREDMOST 3	R	1007	9.30	8.45	78.58	110.06	8.87
PREDMOST 4	L	1008	8.35	7.85	65.55	106.37	8.10
COMBE CHAPELLE	L	1017	9.00	7.50	67.50	120.00	8.25
COMBE CHAPELLE	R	1017	9.00	6.80	61.20	132.35	7.90
BRNO 3	L	1018	6.50	7.00	45.50	92.86	6.75
BRNO 3	R	1018	6.00	7.00	42.00	85.71	6.50
GRIMALDI ADOL.	L	1019	9.20	9.10	83.72	101.10	9.15
GRIMALDI ADOL.	R	1019	8.80	8.70	76.56	101.15	8.75
ROIS R5C-5		1027	9.50	7.50	71.25	126.67	8.50
ROIS	R	1028	10.00				
ROIS R5C-45		1035	10.00	7.00	70.00	142.86	8.50
ROIS		1055	10.50	8.00	84.00	131.25	9.25
VESTONICE 3	L	1057	6.20	7.40	45.88	83.78	6.80
VESTONICE 3	R	1057	6.60	6.80	44.88	97.06	6.70
ALAMANN 5	L	1102	8.50	8.00	68.00	106.25	8.25
ALAMANN 5	R	1102	8.50	8.00	68.00	106.25	8.25
ALAMANN 1288	R	1103	8.00	7.00	56.00	114.29	7.50
BUGGISON 1	L	1108	8.50	8.00	68.00	106.25	8.25
BUGGISON 1	R	1108	8.50	8.00	68.00	106.25	8.25
CAP BLAC	L	1110	7.00	7.00	49.00	100.00	7.00
CAP BLAC	R	1110	7.20	7.00	50.40	102.86	7.10
KABUA 1		1123	6.50	7.50	48.75	86.67	7.00
LAFAYE	L	1128	7.10	7.60	53.96	93.42	7.35
LAFAYE	R	1128	7.60	7.90	60.04	96.20	7.75
MASAT		1130	8.60	6.80	58.48	126.47	7.70
OKUZINI		1133	8.70	7.60	66.12	114.47	8.15
PAS ESTRET 4	L	1135	9.70	7.90	76.63	122.78	8.80
SVAERDBORG	R	1144	8.70	7.80	67.86	111.54	8.25
FRENCHMAN	L	1149	7.50				
FRENCHMAN	R	1149	8.10				
ALACA HOYUK 2		1183	8.70	7.20	62.64	120.83	7.95
ALACA HOYUK 3		1184	9.00	7.10	63.90	126.76	8.05
IRAN(SIALK)	L	1191	8.80	8.50	74.80	103.53	8.65
JARMO 28	R	1193	8.05	6.40	51.52	125.78	7.22
WADI HALFA	L	1196	10.30	8.10	83.43	127.16	9.20
WADI HALFA	L	1197	9.70	6.90	66.93	140.58	8.30
WADI HALFA	L	1198	9.60	7.10	68.16	135.21	8.35
KEILOR	R	1703	7.50	7.50	56.25	100.00	7.50
TALGAI	L	1704	10.90	8.60	93.74	126.74	9.75
AUSTRALIAN 39		1708	11.00	8.00	88.00	137.50	9.50
AUSTRALIAN	L	1728	8.80	10.10	88.88	87.13	9.45
AUSTRALIAN	R	1728	9.00	10.60	95.40	84.91	9.80
AUSTRALIAN 179	L	1732	8.60	6.20	53.32	138.71	7.40
AUSTRALIAN 179	R	1732	8.00	6.40	51.20	125.00	7.20
TASMANIAN 3637	L	1755	10.15	8.95	90.84	113.41	9.55
TASMANIAN 3637	R	1755	9.80	8.70	85.26	112.64	9.25
NEGRO		1914	9.10	7.00	63.70	130.00	8.05
NEGRO	L	1915	9.80	8.60	84.28	113.95	9.20
NEGRO	R	1915	9.70	8.70	84.39	111.49	9.20

UPPER I1 H. SAPIENS

		N	L(M-D)	B(B-L)	L*B	L/B	L+B/2
NEGRO	L	1916	10.20	8.10	82.62	125.93	9.15
NEGRO	R	1916	10.20	8.20	83.64	124.39	9.20
BANTU 100	L	1917	10.40	9.50	98.80	109.47	9.95
BANTU 100	R	1917	9.90	9.30	92.07	106.45	9.60
BANTU 118	L	1918	9.55	8.00	76.40	119.37	8.77
BANTU 118	R	1918	9.35	8.30	77.60	112.65	8.82
BUSHMAN MXD 101	R	1949	7.90				
MAPUNGUBWE M2		1952	9.00	8.00	72.00	112.50	8.50
MAPUNGUBWE M3		1953	9.70	8.00	77.60	121.25	8.85
MAPUNGUBWE M5		1954	7.50	7.00	52.50	107.14	7.25
MAPUNGUBWE M9		1955	9.50	8.30	78.85	114.46	8.90
BAMBANDYANALO21		1957	9.90	6.90	68.31	143.48	8.40
BAMBANDYANALO29		1958	9.30	8.40	78.12	110.71	8.85
BAMBANDYANALO31		1959	10.60	7.40	78.44	143.24	9.00
BAMBANDYANALO13		1964	8.30	7.60	63.08	109.21	7.95
BAMBANDYANALO14		1965	9.00	8.40	75.60	107.14	8.70
BUSHMAN		1967	8.30	6.50	53.95	127.69	7.40
FISH HOEK	R	1972	8.00	6.00	48.00	133.33	7.00
N.BRITAIN 43142	R	1319	9.50	8.80	83.60	107.95	9.15
N.BRITAIN 43144	L	1321		7.50			
N.BRITAIN 43144	R	1321	9.50	7.50	71.25	126.67	8.50
N.BRITAIN 43146	R	1323	7.80	7.00	54.60	111.43	7.40
N.BRITAIN 43147	R	1324	10.00	7.60	76.00	131.58	8.80
N.BRITAIN 43150	L	1326	8.60	8.00	68.80	107.50	8.30
N.BRITAIN 43150	R	1326	8.70	7.70	66.99	112.99	8.20
N.BRITAIN 43151	L	1327	9.20	7.00	64.40	131.43	8.10
N.BRITAIN 43151	R	1327	9.10	7.20	65.52	126.39	8.15
N.BRITAIN 43153	L	1329		7.00			
N.BRITAIN 43154	L	1330	8.80	7.70	67.76	114.29	8.25
N.BRITAIN 43154	R	1330	8.30	7.60	63.08	109.21	7.95
N.BRITAIN 43174	L	1331	8.70	7.90	68.73	110.13	8.30
N.BRITAIN 43174	R	1331	8.80	7.90	69.52	111.39	8.35
N.BRITAIN 43179	L	1332	9.20	7.40	68.08	124.32	8.30
N.BRITAIN 43179	R	1332	9.30	7.40	68.82	125.68	8.35
N.BRITAIN 43193	L	1333	9.30	7.50	69.75	124.00	8.40
N.BRITAIN 43193	R	1333	9.30	7.60	70.68	122.37	8.45
N.BRITAIN 43194	L	1334	9.00	7.00	63.00	128.57	8.00
N.BRITAIN 43194	R	1334		6.70			
N.BRITAIN 43199	L	1336	9.00	7.90	71.10	113.92	8.45
N.BRITAIN 43202	R	1337	9.50	8.40	79.80	113.10	8.95
N.BRITAIN 43204	L	1338	9.20	7.80	71.76	117.95	8.50
N.BRITAIN 43204	R	1338	9.10	7.70	70.07	118.18	8.40
N.BRITAIN 43226	L	1339	8.90	7.00	62.30	127.14	7.95
N.BRITAIN 43290	L	1342	9.10	7.70	70.07	118.18	8.40
N.BRITAIN 43290	R	1342	8.90	7.90	70.31	112.66	8.40
N.BRITAIN 43291	R	1343		7.30			
N.BRITAIN 43295	L	1344	8.50	7.80	66.30	108.97	8.15
N.BRITAIN 43295	R	1344	8.90	7.80	69.42	114.10	8.35
N.BRITAIN	L	1346	9.40				
N.BRITAIN	R	1346	8.50				

UPPER I1 H. SAPIENS

		N	L(M-D)	B(B-L)	L*B	L/B	L+B/2
HINDU (UI)	L	2208	9.05	6.95	62.90	130.22	8.00
HINDU (UI)	R	2208	8.90	7.00	62.30	127.14	7.95
GOL BA IT 99	L	2004	9.50	8.20	77.90	115.85	8.85
MELOLO	L	2022	8.20	7.20	59.04	113.89	7.70
MELOLO	R	2023	8.30	6.90	57.27	120.29	7.60
MELOLO	L	2024	9.10	8.00	72.80	113.75	8.55
MELOLO	R	2025	9.10	7.90	71.89	115.19	8.50
TING TS,UN	R	2206	8.30	6.40	53.12	129.69	7.35
HAIDA	L	1406	9.10	7.50	68.25	121.33	8.30
HAIDA	R	1406	8.90	7.40	65.86	120.27	8.15
MINNESOTA MAN	L	1419	8.50	7.60	64.60	111.84	8.05
MINNESOTA MAN	R	1419	8.50	7.60	64.60	111.84	8.05
ILLINOIS T25-2	L	1427	8.00	7.50	60.00	106.67	7.75
ILLINOIS A-4921	L	1431	8.90	7.10	63.19	125.35	8.00
ILLINOIS A-4921	R	1431	8.80	7.30	64.24	120.55	8.05
ILLINOIS PK9-B4	L	1432	8.75	7.60	66.50	115.13	8.17
ILLINOIS PK9-B4	R	1432	8.45	8.05	68.02	104.97	8.25
ILLINOIS BR19-3	L	1434	8.35	7.25	60.54	115.17	7.80
ILLINOIS BR19-3	R	1434	8.10	7.25	58.72	111.72	7.67
DICKSON MOUND	L	1501	8.30	7.15	59.34	116.08	7.72
DICKSON MOUND	R	1501	8.80	7.40	65.12	118.92	8.10
DICKSON MD 242	L	1505	9.95	7.00	69.65	142.14	8.47
DICKSON MD 242	R	1505	9.63	7.20	69.34	133.75	8.41
DICKSON MD 256	L	1506	8.85	7.10	62.83	124.65	7.97
DICKSON MD 256	R	1506	8.90	7.10	63.19	125.35	8.00
DICKSON MD 258	R	1507	8.30	6.60	54.78	125.76	7.45
DICKSON MD 261	L	1508	9.15	7.05	64.51	129.79	8.10
DICKSON MD 261	R	1508	9.25	7.00	64.75	132.14	8.12
DICKSON MD 262	L	1509	9.00	7.15	64.35	125.87	8.07
DICKSON MD 262	R	1509	9.20	7.55	69.46	121.85	8.37
DICKSON MD 266	L	1510	9.25	7.55	69.84	122.52	8.40
DICKSON MD 276	L	1514	9.30	8.10	75.33	114.81	8.70
DICKSON MD 276	R	1514	9.45	7.85	74.18	120.38	8.65
DICKSON MD 287	L	1516	8.35	7.40	61.79	112.84	7.87
DICKSON MD 287	R	1516	8.50	7.50	63.75	113.33	8.00
DICKSON MD 291	R	1518	9.02	7.15	64.49	126.15	8.08
DICKSON MD 292	R	1519	8.45				
DICKSON MD 302	L	1521	8.20	6.40	52.48	128.12	7.30
DICKSON MD 319	L	1523	8.35	7.40	61.79	112.84	7.87
DICKSON MD 319	R	1523	8.35	7.50	62.62	111.33	7.92
DICKSON MD 327	L	1524	8.75	7.40	64.75	118.24	8.07
DICKSON MD 327	R	1524	8.75	7.20	63.00	121.53	7.97
DICKSON MD 334	L	1525	9.30	8.30	77.19	112.05	8.80
DICKSON MD 347	R	1528	9.45	7.60	71.82	124.34	8.52
DICKSON MD 348	R	1529	8.20	6.70	54.94	122.39	7.45
DICKSON MD 349	L	1530	9.20	7.50	69.00	122.67	8.35
DICKSON MD 349	R	1530	8.30	7.20	59.76	115.28	7.75
DICKSON MD 351	L	1532	8.90	7.50	66.75	118.67	8.20
DICKSON MD 355	L	1535	9.70	7.90	76.63	122.78	8.80
DICKSON MD 355	R	1535	9.55	7.90	75.44	120.89	8.72

UPPER I1 H. SAPIENS

		N	L(M-D)	B(B-L)	L*B	L/B	L+B/2
DICKSCN MD	361 L	1538	7.90	7.00	55.30	112.86	7.45
DICKSON MD	361 R	1538	7.85	7.00	54.95	112.14	7.42
DICKSCN MD	362 L	1539	8.70	7.20	62.64	120.83	7.95
DICKSCN MD	362 R	1539	8.90	7.60	67.64	117.11	8.25
DICKSCN MD	365 L	1540	8.10	6.70	54.27	120.90	7.40
DICKSON MD	365 R	1540	8.20	6.50	53.30	126.15	7.35
DICKSCN MD	371 R	1542	9.00	7.10	63.90	126.76	8.05
DICKSCN MD	378 L	1547	8.20	6.10	50.02	134.43	7.15
DICKSCN MD	378 R	1547	8.10	6.10	49.41	132.79	7.10
DICKSCN MD	379 L	1548	9.00	7.20	64.80	125.00	8.10
DICKSCN MD	379 R	1548	8.90	7.60	67.64	117.11	8.25
DICKSCN MD	380 L	1549	8.70	7.60	66.12	114.47	8.15
DICKSCN MD	380 R	1549	8.50	7.50	63.75	113.33	8.00
DICKSCN MD	380 L	1551	8.40	7.00	58.80	120.00	7.70
DICKSCN MD	380 R	1551	8.40	7.20	60.48	116.67	7.80
DICKSCN MD	396 L	1553	9.80	7.80	76.44	125.64	8.80
DICKSCN MD	396 R	1553	9.70	7.80	75.66	124.36	8.75
DICKSCN MD	397 L	1554	8.90	8.00	71.20	111.25	8.45
DICKSCN MD	397 R	1554	8.70	7.80	67.86	111.54	8.25
DICKSCN MD	398 L	1555	9.40	7.20	67.68	130.56	8.30
DICKSCN MD	398 R	1555	9.60	7.40	71.04	129.73	8.50
DICKSCN MD	399 L	1556	8.30	7.30	60.59	113.70	7.80
DICKSCN MD	399 R	1556	8.00	7.60	60.80	105.26	7.80
DICKSCN MD	404 L	1559	8.65	7.00	60.55	123.57	7.82
DICKSCN MD	404 R	1559	8.80	7.13	62.74	123.42	7.96
DICKSCN MD	406 L	1560	8.75	6.50	56.87	134.62	7.62
DICKSCN MD	406 R	1560	8.80	6.65	58.52	132.33	7.72
DICKSON MD	407 L	1561	9.20	7.60	69.92	121.05	8.40
DICKSCN MD	407 R	1561	9.05	7.80	70.59	116.03	8.42
DICKSCN MD	411 L	1563	9.05	6.87	62.17	131.73	7.96
DICKSCN MD	411 R	1563	9.00	6.70	60.30	134.33	7.85
DICKSCN MD	415 R	1565	8.30	7.10	58.93	116.90	7.70
DICKSON MD	426 R	1566	8.80	6.90	60.72	127.54	7.85
DICKSCN MD	443 L	1571	9.45	7.37	69.65	128.22	8.41
DICKSCN MD	443 R	1571	9.40	7.67	72.10	122.56	8.53
DICKSCN MD	447 L	1573	8.40	6.35	53.34	132.28	7.37
DICKSCN MD	447 R	1573	8.00	6.45	51.60	124.03	7.22
DICKSCN MD	448 L	1574	9.07	7.20	65.30	125.97	8.13
DICKSCN MD	448 R	1574	8.60	6.80	58.48	126.47	7.70
DICKSCN MD	464 L	1575	8.45	7.00	59.15	120.71	7.72
DICKSCN MD	464 R	1575	8.55	7.80	66.69	109.62	8.17
DICKSCN MD	476 L	1576	9.25	6.90	63.82	134.06	8.07
DICKSON MD	476 R	1576	9.35	7.06	66.01	132.44	8.20
DICKSCN MD	480 L	1578	8.17	6.80	55.56	120.15	7.48
DICKSCN MD	480 R	1578	8.20	6.55	53.71	125.19	7.37
DICKSCN MD	497 L	1583	9.30	8.15	75.79	114.11	8.72
DICKSCN MD	497 R	1583	9.25	8.20	75.85	112.80	8.72
DICKSCN MD	489 L	1584	8.65				
DICKSCN MD	489 R	1584	8.82				
DICKSON MD	503 L	1585	9.20	8.07	74.24	114.00	8.63

UPPER I1 H. SAPIENS

		N	L(M-D)	B(B-L)	L*B	L/B	L+B/2
DICKSCN MD	503 R	1585	9.40	8.75	82.25	107.43	9.07
DICKSCN MD	509 L	1587	9.14	7.52	68.73	121.54	8.33
DICKSCN MD	509 R	1587	8.80	7.56	66.53	116.40	8.18
DICKSCN MD	527 R	1589	9.45				
DICKSCN MD	535 L	1591	8.80	6.80	59.84	129.41	7.80
DICKSCN MD	535 R	1591	8.88	6.80	60.38	130.59	7.84
DICKSCN MD	536 L	1592	9.00	7.00	63.00	128.57	8.00
DICKSCN MD	536 R	1592	8.95	6.85	61.31	130.66	7.90
DICKSCN MD	542 R	1593	9.30				
DICKSCN MD	557 R	1596	8.50	7.30	62.05	116.44	7.90
DICKSCN MD	561 R	1597	8.40	7.40	62.16	113.51	7.90
DICKSCN MD	599 L	1602	9.10	8.25	75.07	110.30	8.67
DICKSCN MD	599 R	1602	9.15	8.10	74.11	112.96	8.62
DICKSCN MD	630 L	1603	9.10	7.70	70.07	118.18	8.40
DICKSCN MD	630 R	1603	9.40	7.60	71.44	123.68	8.50
DICKSCN MD	638 R	1606	8.90				
DICKSCN MD	642 L	1607	9.10	7.60	69.16	119.74	8.35
DICKSCN MD	648 L	1609	9.60	8.10	77.76	118.52	8.85
DICKSCN MD	648 R	1609	9.50	8.00	76.00	118.75	8.75
DICKSCN MD	651 L	1610	8.65	6.80	58.82	127.21	7.72
DICKSCN MD	651 R	1610	8.45	6.45	54.50	131.01	7.45
DICKSCN MD	652 R	1611	8.90	7.20	64.08	123.61	8.05
DICKSCN MD	667 L	1614	9.61	7.40	71.11	129.86	8.50
DICKSCN MD	667 R	1614	9.55	7.20	68.76	132.64	8.37
DICKSCN MD	694 L	1617	9.85				
DICKSCN MD	694 R	1617	9.65				
DICKSCN MD	722 L	1624	9.05	7.90	71.49	114.56	8.47
DICKSCN MD	722 R	1624	9.05	7.75	70.14	116.77	8.40
DICKSCN MD	724 L	1627	9.50	7.42	70.49	128.03	8.46
DICKSCN MD	724 R	1627	9.60	7.43	71.33	129.21	8.51
DICKSON MD	746 L	1628	9.10	7.70	70.07	118.18	8.40
DICKSON MD	746 R	1628	9.10	7.70	70.07	118.18	8.40
DICKSCN MD	749 L	1629	9.45	8.22	77.68	114.96	8.83
DICKSCN MD	749 R	1629	9.15	8.00	73.20	114.37	8.57

UPPER I2 H. SAPIENS

		N	L(M-D)	B(B-L)	L*B	L/B	L+B/2
PREDMOST 3	L	1007	7.85	8.25	64.76	95.15	8.05
PREDMOST 3	R	1007	7.65	8.25	63.11	92.73	7.95
PREDMOST 4	L	1008	7.30	7.60	55.48	96.05	7.45
COMBE CHAPELLE	L	1017	6.00	6.00	36.00	100.00	6.00
COMBE CHAPELLE	R	1017	5.00	6.00	30.00	83.33	5.50
BRNO 3	L	1018	5.40	6.30	34.02	85.71	5.85
BRNO 3	R	1018	5.20	6.30	32.76	82.54	5.75
GRIMALDI ADOL.	L	1019	8.85	8.70	76.99	101.72	8.77
GRIMALDI ADOL.	R	1019	8.70	8.50	73.95	102.35	8.60
VESTONICE 3	L	1057	6.30	6.70	42.21	94.03	6.50
VESTONICE 3	R	1057	6.30	7.20	45.36	87.50	6.75
ALAMANN 5	L	1102	7.00	8.00	56.00	87.50	7.50
BUGGISON 1	L	1108	7.50	7.00	52.50	107.14	7.25
BUGGISON 1	R	1108	7.50	8.00	60.00	93.75	7.75
CAP BLAC	L	1110	6.00	6.20	37.20	96.77	6.10
CAP BLAC	R	1110	6.10	6.10	37.21	100.00	6.10
KABUA 1		1123	5.30	6.20	32.86	85.48	5.75
KOERHUISBEEK C1	L	1124	7.00	7.00	49.00	100.00	7.00
LAFAYE	L	1128	5.50	7.20	39.60	76.39	6.35
LAFAYE	R	1128	6.10	7.00	42.70	87.14	6.55
MASAT		1130	6.60	6.20	40.92	106.45	6.40
OKUZINI		1133	6.50	6.50	42.25	100.00	6.50
SVAERDBORG	L	1144	7.20	6.20	44.64	116.13	6.70
FRENCHMAN	L	1149	6.60				
FRENCHMAN	R	1149	6.10				
ALACA HOYUK 2		1183	6.30	6.70	42.21	94.03	6.50
ALACA HOYUK 3		1184	7.00	6.70	46.90	104.48	6.85
IRAN(SIALK)	L	1191	6.00	8.20	49.20	73.17	7.10
JARMO 28	R	1193	6.90	6.50	44.85	106.15	6.70
WADI HALFA	L	1196	8.10	6.80	55.08	119.12	7.45
KEILOR	R	1703	6.00	6.00	36.00	100.00	6.00
AUSTRALIAN 39		1708	6.00	7.00	42.00	85.71	6.50
AUSTRALIAN	L	1728	7.50	8.80	66.00	85.23	8.15
AUSTRALIAN	R	1728	7.90	8.80	69.52	89.77	8.35
AUSTRALIAN 179	L	1732	6.00	6.70	40.20	89.55	6.35
AUSTRALIAN 179	R	1732	6.00	6.00	36.00	100.00	6.00
TASMANIAN 3637	L	1755	8.80	8.10	71.28	108.64	8.45
TASMANIAN 3637	R	1755	8.50	7.80	66.30	108.97	8.15
TASMANIAN 2964	L	1763	8.90	7.60	67.64	117.11	8.25
TASMANIAN 2964	R	1763		7.90			
NEGRO		1914	6.80	6.00	40.80	113.33	6.40
NEGRO	L	1915	8.40	7.90	66.36	106.33	8.15
NEGRO	R	1915	8.20	8.20	67.24	100.00	8.20
NEGRO	L	1916	9.30	8.00	74.40	116.25	8.65
NEGRO	R	1916	9.50	8.00	76.00	118.75	8.75
BANTU 100	L	1917	9.10	9.40	85.54	96.81	9.25
BANTU 118	L	1918	8.00	6.90	55.20	115.94	7.45
BANTU 118	R	1918	8.20	7.00	57.40	117.14	7.60
MAPUNGUBWE M2		1952	8.00	7.00	56.00	114.29	7.50
MAPUNGUBWE M3		1953	7.50	7.00	52.50	107.14	7.25

UPPER I2 H. SAPIENS

		N	L(M-D)	B(B-L)	L*B	L/B	L+B/2
MAPUNGUBWE M9		1955	8.20	7.90	64.78	103.80	8.05
MAPUNGUBWE M10		1956	8.00	7.30	58.40	109.59	7.65
BAMBANDYANALO21		1957	7.50	6.50	48.75	115.38	7.00
BAMBANDYANALO29		1958	7.70	7.50	57.75	102.67	7.60
BAMBANDYANALO31		1959	10.30	6.90	71.07	149.28	8.60
BAMBANDYANALO13		1964	7.00	6.60	46.20	106.06	6.80
BAMBANDYANALO14		1965	7.90	8.00	63.20	98.75	7.95
BUSHMAN		1967	6.70	6.00	40.20	111.67	6.35
FISH HOEK	R	1972	7.00	6.00	42.00	116.67	6.50
GOUNGOU A	L	1975	7.60	7.10	53.96	107.04	7.35
N.BRITAIN 43121	L	1301	6.90	7.10	48.99	97.18	7.00
N.BRITAIN 43136	R	1313	7.20	5.90	42.48	122.03	6.55
N.BRITAIN 43137	L	1314	6.90	6.70	46.23	102.99	6.80
N.BRITAIN 43138	L	1315	7.20	7.00	50.40	102.86	7.10
N.BRITAIN 43138	R	1315	7.30	7.10	51.83	102.82	7.20
N.BRITAIN 43146	R	1323	7.10	6.50	46.15	109.23	6.80
N.BRITAIN 43147	L	1324	8.20	6.60	54.12	124.24	7.40
N.BRITAIN 43147	R	1324	8.20	6.60	54.12	124.24	7.40
N.BRITAIN 43150	L	1326	6.50	7.10	46.15	91.55	6.80
N.BRITAIN 43150	R	1326	7.00	7.00	49.00	100.00	7.00
N.BRITAIN 43151	L	1327	7.80	6.70	52.26	116.42	7.25
N.BRITAIN 43151	R	1327	7.80	6.40	49.92	121.87	7.10
N.BRITAIN 43154	L	1330		6.90			
N.BRITAIN 43154	R	1330	7.00	7.00	49.00	100.00	7.00
N.BRITAIN 43174	L	1331	7.40	6.30	46.62	117.46	6.85
N.BRITAIN 43174	R	1331	7.70	6.90	53.13	111.59	7.30
N.BRITAIN 43179	L	1332	8.00	7.00	56.00	114.29	7.50
N.BRITAIN 43179	R	1332	7.90	7.00	55.30	112.86	7.45
N.BRITAIN 43193	L	1333	7.10	7.00	49.70	101.43	7.05
N.BRITAIN 43193	R	1333	8.00	6.70	53.60	119.40	7.35
N.BRITAIN 43194	L	1334	8.20	6.60	54.12	124.24	7.40
N.BRITAIN 43194	R	1334	6.90	6.60	45.54	104.55	6.75
N.BRITAIN 43199	L	1336	7.40	6.10	45.14	121.31	6.75
N.BRITAIN 43199	R	1336	6.90	6.50	44.85	106.15	6.70
N.BRITAIN 43202	L	1337	7.40	7.50	55.50	98.67	7.45
N.BRITAIN 43202	R	1337	7.50	7.50	56.25	100.00	7.50
N.BRITAIN 43204	R	1338	7.80	7.30	56.94	106.85	7.55
N.BRITAIN 43226	L	1339	6.90	6.20	42.78	111.29	6.55
N.BRITAIN 43242	L	1341	7.20	6.30	45.36	114.29	6.75
N.BRITAIN 43242	R	1341	7.00	6.70	46.90	104.48	6.85
N.BRITAIN 43290	L	1342	6.20	6.60	40.92	93.94	6.40
N.BRITAIN 43290	R	1342	6.10	6.80	41.48	89.71	6.45
N.BRITAIN 43295	R	1344	7.50	7.00	52.50	107.14	7.25
N.BRITAIN	L	1346	7.00				
N.BRITAIN	R	1346	7.50				
HINDU (UI)	L	2208	6.95	6.20	43.09	112.10	6.57
HINDU (UI)	R	2208	7.00	6.40	44.80	109.37	6.70
TING TS,UN	R	2206	7.00	8.00	56.00	87.50	7.50
HAIDA	L	1406	7.60	7.10	53.96	107.04	7.35
MINNESOTA MAN	R	1419	7.50	6.80	51.00	110.29	7.15

UPPER I2 H. SAPIENS

	N	L(M-D)	B(B-L)	L*B	L/B	L+B/2
ILLINCIS PK2-B1 L	1426	7.85	7.20	56.52	109.03	7.52
ILLINCIS T25-2 L	1427	4.90	4.40	21.56	111.36	4.65
ILLINCIS A-2732 L	1429		6.30			
ILLINCIS A-4921 L	1431	8.00	6.85	54.80	116.79	7.42
ILLINCIS A-4921 R	1431	7.60	7.10	53.96	107.04	7.35
ILLINCIS PK9-B4 L	1432	7.50	6.50	48.75	115.38	7.00
ILLINCIS PK9-B4 R	1432	7.30	6.20	45.26	117.74	6.75
ILLINCIS BR19-3 L	1434	8.40	6.65	55.86	126.32	7.52
ILLINCIS BR19-3 R	1434	7.95	6.35	50.48	125.20	7.15
DICKSCN MOUND L	1501	8.02	7.30	58.55	109.86	7.66
DICKSCN MOUND R	1501	8.15	7.20	58.68	113.19	7.67
DICKSCN MD 242 L	1505	7.95	7.25	57.64	109.66	7.60
DICKSON MD 242 R	1505	7.60	6.80	51.68	111.76	7.20
DICKSCN MD 256 L	1506	6.50	6.25	40.62	104.00	6.37
DICKSCN MD 256 R	1506	6.00	5.75	34.50	104.35	5.87
DICKSCN MD 261 L	1508	7.80	6.60	51.48	118.18	7.20
DICKSCN MD 261 R	1508	7.50	6.80	51.00	110.29	7.15
DICKSCN MD 262 L	1509	7.65	7.25	55.46	105.52	7.45
DICKSCN MD 262 R	1509	7.16	6.55	46.90	109.31	6.85
DICKSCN MD 266 L	1510	7.70	6.40	49.28	120.31	7.05
DICKSCN MD 276 L	1514	6.65	6.15	40.90	108.13	6.40
DICKSCN MD 276 R	1514	6.65	6.15	40.90	108.13	6.40
DICKSCN MD 287 L	1516	7.45	6.85	51.03	108.76	7.15
DICKSCN MD 287 R	1516	7.25	6.40	46.40	113.28	6.82
DICKSCN MD 291 R	1518	7.40	7.00	51.80	105.71	7.20
DICKSCN MD 297 L	1520	7.50	6.65	49.87	112.78	7.07
DICKSCN MD 319 L	1523	7.10	5.80	41.18	122.41	6.45
DICKSCN MD 319 R	1523	7.50	6.50	48.75	115.38	7.00
DICKSCN MD 327 L	1524	6.65	6.60	43.89	100.76	6.62
DICKSCN MD 327 R	1524	6.70	5.80	38.86	115.52	6.25
DICKSCN MD 348 L	1529	7.10	6.25	44.37	113.60	6.67
DICKSCN MD 348 R	1529	6.90	6.20	42.78	111.29	6.55
DICKSCN MD 349 R	1530	7.40	6.10	45.14	121.31	6.75
DICKSCN MD 351 L	1532	8.20	7.50	61.50	109.33	7.85
DICKSCN MD 351 R	1532	8.30	6.90	57.27	120.29	7.60
DICKSCN MD 352 L	1533	7.40	6.60	48.84	112.12	7.00
DICKSCN MD 355 L	1535	8.10	7.60	61.56	106.58	7.85
DICKSCN MD 355 R	1535	8.50	7.50	63.75	113.33	8.00
DICKSCN MD 361 L	1538	6.95	6.70	46.56	103.73	6.82
DICKSCN MD 361 R	1538	6.85	6.60	45.21	103.79	6.72
DICKSCN MD 362 L	1539	7.50	7.20	54.00	104.17	7.35
DICKSCN MD 362 R	1539	7.60	7.25	55.10	104.83	7.42
DICKSCN MD 365 L	1540	7.50	6.70	50.25	111.94	7.10
DICKSCN MD 365 R	1540	7.50	6.80	51.00	110.29	7.15
DICKSCN MD 371 R	1542	7.50	6.50	48.75	115.38	7.00
DICKSCN MD 378 L	1547	6.60	5.60	36.96	117.86	6.10
DICKSCN MD 379 L	1548	7.75	7.15	55.41	108.39	7.45
DICKSCN MD 379 R	1548	7.65	7.20	55.08	106.25	7.42
DICKSCN MD 380 L	1549	6.80	6.60	44.88	103.03	6.70
DICKSCN MD 380 R	1549	6.90	6.60	45.54	104.55	6.75

UPPER I2 H. SAPIENS

	N	L(M-D)	B(B-L)	L*B	L/B	L+B/2
DICKSCN MD 381 L	1550	8.00	6.60	52.80	121.21	7.30
DICKSCN MD 381 R	1550	7.80	6.70	52.26	116.42	7.25
DICKSCN MD 380 L	1551	7.20	6.40	46.08	112.50	6.80
DICKSCN MD 396 L	1553	7.70	7.20	55.44	106.94	7.45
DICKSCN MD 396 R	1553	7.60	7.00	53.20	108.57	7.30
DICKSON MD 397 L	1554	7.40	6.90	51.06	107.25	7.15
DICKSCN MD 397 R	1554	7.20	7.00	50.40	102.86	7.10
DICKSCN MD 398 L	1555	7.85	6.40	50.24	122.66	7.12
DICKSCN MD 398 R	1555	7.90	6.20	48.98	127.42	7.05
DICKSCN MD 399 L	1556	6.90	7.00	48.30	98.57	6.95
DICKSON MD 399 R	1556	7.10	6.70	47.57	105.97	6.90
DICKSCN MD 404 L	1559	7.30	6.80	49.64	107.35	7.05
DICKSCN MD 404 R	1559	7.38	6.90	50.92	106.96	7.14
DICKSCN MD 406 L	1560	7.75	6.63	51.38	116.89	7.19
DICKSCN MD 406 R	1560	7.80	6.70	52.26	116.42	7.25
DICKSON MD 407 L	1561	7.33	7.15	52.41	102.52	7.24
DICKSCN MD 407 R	1561	7.60	6.60	50.16	115.15	7.10
DICKSCN MD 411 L	1563	8.05	6.32	50.88	127.37	7.18
DICKSCN MD 411 R	1563	7.95	6.60	52.47	120.45	7.27
DICKSCN MD 414 L	1564	7.35	6.15	45.20	119.51	6.75
DICKSON MD 426 L	1566	7.20	6.85	49.32	105.11	7.02
DICKSCN MD 426 R	1566	7.24	6.85	49.59	105.69	7.04
DICKSCN MD 443 L	1571	7.18	7.10	50.98	101.13	7.14
DICKSCN MD 443 R	1571	7.54	6.85	51.65	110.07	7.19
DICKSCN MD 447 L	1573	7.60	6.00	45.60	126.67	6.80
DICKSCN MD 447 R	1573	7.10	6.25	44.37	113.60	6.67
DICKSON MD 448 L	1574	7.70	6.35	48.89	121.26	7.02
DICKSCN MD 448 R	1574	7.80	5.88	45.86	132.65	6.84
DICKSCN MD 464 L	1575	7.30	6.90	50.37	105.80	7.10
DICKSCN MD 464 R	1575	6.75	6.40	43.20	105.47	6.57
DICKSCN MD 476 L	1576	8.13	6.67	54.23	121.89	7.40
DICKSCN MD 476 R	1576	8.75	6.35	55.56	137.80	7.55
DICKSCN MD 478 L	1577	7.64	7.00	53.48	109.14	7.32
DICKSON MD 480 L	1578	6.60	6.25	41.25	105.60	6.42
DICKSCN MD 480 R	1578	6.80	6.40	43.52	106.25	6.60
DICKSCN MD 497 L	1583	8.05	7.92	63.76	101.64	7.98
DICKSCN MD 497 R	1583	8.10	7.30	59.13	110.96	7.70
DICKSCN MD 503 L	1585	7.50	7.50	56.25	100.00	7.50
DICKSCN MD 503 R	1585	8.00	7.50	60.00	106.67	7.75
DICKSCN MD 509 L	1587	8.15	6.72	54.77	121.28	7.43
DICKSCN MD 509 R	1587	7.82	7.03	54.97	111.24	7.42
DICKSCN MD 535 L	1591	7.43	6.10	45.32	121.80	6.76
DICKSCN MD 535 R	1591	6.95	5.80	40.31	119.83	6.37
DICKSCN MD 536 L	1592	7.40	6.25	46.25	118.40	6.82
DICKSCN MD 536 R	1592	6.90	5.80	40.02	118.97	6.35
DICKSCN MD 557 L	1596	7.14	6.18	44.13	115.53	6.66
DICKSCN MD 557 R	1596	7.55	6.15	46.43	122.76	6.85
DICKSCN MD 567 R	1598	7.25	6.75	48.94	107.41	7.00
DICKSCN MD 594 L	1601	7.40	6.70	49.58	110.45	7.05
DICKSCN MD 599 L	1602	7.65	6.70	51.25	114.18	7.17

UPPER I2 H. SAPIENS

		N	L(M-D)	B(B-L)	L*B	L/B	L+B/2
DICKSON MD 599	R	1602	7.70	6.75	51.97	114.07	7.22
DICKSCN MD 630	L	1603	8.20	6.90	56.58	118.84	7.55
DICKSCN MD 630	R	1603	8.10	6.90	55.89	117.39	7.50
DICKSCN MD 642	L	1607	8.10				
DICKSCN MD 648	L	1609	8.10	6.70	54.27	120.90	7.40
DICKSCN MD 648	R	1609	8.60	7.40	63.64	116.22	8.00
DICKSCN MD 667	L	1614	9.00	7.00	63.00	128.57	8.00
DICKSCN MD 667	R	1614	8.93	6.50	58.04	137.38	7.71
DICKSON MD 687	R	1616	6.70	5.90	39.53	113.56	6.30
DICKSCN MD 722	L	1624	7.70	7.30	56.21	105.48	7.50
DICKSCN MD 722	R	1624	7.65	7.15	54.70	106.99	7.40
DICKSCN MD 724	L	1627	7.30	6.55	47.81	111.45	6.92
DICKSCN MD 724	R	1627	7.40	6.60	48.84	112.12	7.00
DICKSON MD 746	L	1628	8.00	6.80	54.40	117.65	7.40
DICKSCN MD 746	R	1628	7.65	7.00	53.55	109.29	7.32
DICKSCN MD 749	L	1629	7.70	7.00	53.90	110.00	7.35
DICKSCN MD 749	R	1629	7.85	7.55	59.27	103.97	7.70

UPPER C H. SAPIENS

		N	L(M-D)	B(B-L)	L*B	L/B	L+B/2
PREDMOST 3	L	1007	8.62	9.40	81.03	91.70	9.01
PREDMOST 3	R	1007	8.50	9.30	79.05	91.40	8.90
PREDMCST 4	L	1008	8.65	7.70	66.60	112.34	8.17
PREDMOST 7	L	1012	8.20	9.00	73.80	91.11	8.60
COMBE CHAPELLE	L	1017	8.00	9.00	72.00	88.89	8.50
COMBE CHAPELLE	R	1017	7.00	9.00	63.00	77.78	8.00
BRNO 3	L	1018	8.00	8.30	66.40	96.39	8.15
BRNO 3	R	1018	7.50	7.50	56.25	100.00	7.50
GRIMALDI ADOL.	L	1019	9.35	10.45	97.71	89.47	9.90
GRIMALDI ADOL.	R	1019	8.90	10.50	93.45	84.76	9.70
LA ROCHETTE A	L	1021	7.80	9.00	70.20	86.67	8.40
VESTONICE 3	L	1057	7.90	9.00	71.10	87.78	8.45
VESTONICE 3	R	1057	7.90	8.60	67.94	91.86	8.25
A CULOZ 2	L	1101	8.00	9.00	72.00	88.89	8.50
ALAMANN 5	R	1102	7.00	8.00	56.00	87.50	7.50
ALAMANN 1288	L	1103	7.00	7.50	52.50	93.33	7.25
ALAMANN 1288	R	1103	7.00	8.00	56.00	87.50	7.50
BUGGISON 1	L	1108	9.00	9.00	81.00	100.00	9.00
BUGGISON 1	R	1108	9.00	9.00	81.00	100.00	9.00
BUGGISON 2	L	1109	8.00	8.50	68.00	94.12	8.25
CAP BLAC	L	1110	7.00	8.10	56.70	86.42	7.55
CAP BLAC	R	1110	7.00	8.00	56.00	87.50	7.50
FARINCOURT 2		1114	8.00	9.50	76.00	84.21	8.75
KABUA 1		1123	7.00	8.30	58.10	84.34	7.65
KOERHUISBEEK C1	L	1124	8.00	9.00	72.00	88.89	8.50
KOERHUISBEEK C1	R	1124	8.00	8.00	64.00	100.00	8.00
LAFAYE	L	1128	7.60	8.40	63.84	90.48	8.00
LAFAYE	R	1128	7.20	8.20	59.04	87.80	7.70
MASAT		1130	7.00	8.60	60.20	81.40	7.80
OKUZINI		1133	7.60	8.40	63.84	90.48	8.00
SVAERDBORG	R	1144	8.40	8.70	73.08	96.55	8.55
FRENCHMAN	L	1149	8.80	10.50	92.40	83.81	9.65
FRENCHMAN	R	1149	8.40	9.30	78.12	90.32	8.85
ALACA HOYUK 2		1183	7.80	8.50	66.30	91.76	8.15
ALACA HOYUK 3		1184	7.80	8.20	63.96	95.12	8.00
IRAN(SIALK)	L	1190		7.40			
IRAN(SIALK)	L	1191	6.90	8.50	58.65	81.18	7.70
IRAN(SIALK)	L	1192	7.50	8.00	60.00	93.75	7.75
JARMO 28	R	1193	8.70	8.30	72.21	104.82	8.50
WADI HALFA	L	1196	7.80	8.90	69.42	87.64	8.35
WADI HALFA	L	1199	7.20	8.40	60.48	85.71	7.80
WADI HALFA	L	1200	8.00	8.70	69.60	91.95	8.35
WADI HALFA	L	1201	7.30	7.90	57.67	92.41	7.60
WADJAK 2	L	1702	9.20	10.20	93.84	90.20	9.70
WADJAK 2	R	1702	9.70	10.20	98.94	95.10	9.95
KEILOR	R	1703	9.00	10.50	94.50	85.71	9.75
TALGAI	L	1704	9.60	10.90	104.64	88.07	10.25
TALGAI	R	1704	10.00				
COHUNA	L	1705	10.40	11.50	119.60	90.43	10.95
COHUNA	R	1705	10.20	11.40	116.28	89.47	10.80

UPPER C H. SAPIENS

	N	L(M-D)	B(B-L)	L*B	L/B	L+B/2
AUSTRALIAN 39	1708	8.00	10.50	84.00	76.19	9.25
AUSTRALIAN L	1728	8.00	10.90	87.20	73.39	9.45
AUSTRALIAN R	1728	8.50	10.90	92.65	77.98	9.70
AUSTRALIAN 179 L	1732	8.00	7.50	60.00	106.67	7.75
AUSTRALIAN 179 R	1732	7.80	7.40	57.72	105.41	7.60
TASMANIAN 3637 L	1755	8.00	9.30	74.40	86.02	8.65
TASMANIAN 3637 R	1755	8.35	8.90	74.31	93.82	8.62
TASMANIAN 2964 L	1763	9.20	10.50	96.60	87.62	9.85
TASMANIAN 2964 R	1763	9.30	10.40	96.72	89.42	9.85
ASSELAR R	1903	7.50	8.50	63.75	88.24	8.00
CAPE FLATS R	1904	7.50	9.50	71.25	78.95	8.50
NEGRO	1914	7.60	8.10	61.56	93.83	7.85
NEGRO L	1915	9.10	9.80	89.18	92.86	9.45
NEGRO R	1915	9.00	9.80	88.20	91.84	9.40
NEGRO L	1916	9.30	9.60	89.28	96.87	9.45
NEGRO R	1916	9.30	9.70	90.21	95.88	9.50
MAPUNGUBWE M3	1953	9.00	9.60	86.40	93.75	9.30
MAPUNGUBWE M5	1954	8.00	9.50	76.00	84.21	8.75
MAPUNGUBWE M9	1955	9.00	9.50	85.50	94.74	9.25
BAMBANDYANALO21	1957	8.50	8.80	74.80	96.59	8.65
BAMBANDYANALO29	1958	8.40	8.20	68.88	102.44	8.30
BAMBANDYANALO31	1959	8.50	8.60	73.10	98.84	8.55
BAMBANDYANALO13	1964	8.50	9.50	80.75	89.47	9.00
BAMBANDYANALO14	1965	8.00	9.30	74.40	86.02	8.65
BUSHMAN	1967	7.50	7.80	58.50	96.15	7.65
FISH HOEK R	1972	6.00	6.80	40.80	88.24	6.40
GOUNGOU A L	1975	8.35	8.70	72.64	95.98	8.52
N.BRITAIN 43131 R	1308	9.00	9.20	82.80	97.83	9.10
N.BRITAIN 43134 L	1311	8.50	8.50	72.25	100.00	8.50
N.BRITAIN 43135 R	1312	7.70	8.30	63.91	92.77	8.00
N.BRITAIN 43136 L	1313	7.80	7.60	59.28	102.63	7.70
N.BRITAIN 43136 R	1313	8.40	7.80	65.52	107.69	8.10
N.BRITAIN 43138 L	1315	7.80	8.50	66.30	91.76	8.15
N.BRITAIN 43138 R	1315	8.20	8.80	72.16	93.18	8.50
N.BRITAIN 43139 L	1316	7.80	7.60	59.28	102.63	7.70
N.BRITAIN 43141 L	1318	8.10	8.50	68.85	95.29	8.30
N.BRITAIN 43142 L	1319	9.00	9.30	83.70	96.77	9.15
N.BRITAIN 43143 R	1320	8.20	8.10	66.42	101.23	8.15
N.BRITAIN 43146 L	1323	8.50	8.10	68.85	104.94	8.30
N.BRITAIN 43146 R	1323	8.30	8.50	70.55	97.65	8.40
N.BRITAIN 43147 R	1324	8.30	9.10	75.53	91.21	8.70
N.BRITAIN 43150 L	1326	8.40	8.70	73.08	96.55	8.55
N.BRITAIN 43150 R	1326	7.90	8.80	69.52	89.77	8.35
N.BRITAIN 43151 L	1327	8.70	8.50	73.95	102.35	8.60
N.BRITAIN 43151 R	1327	8.80	8.60	75.68	102.33	8.70
N.BRITAIN 43152 R	1328		8.20			
N.BRITAIN 43154 R	1330	8.90	9.10	80.99	97.80	9.00
N.BRITAIN 43174 L	1331	9.10	8.30	75.53	109.64	8.70
N.BRITAIN 43179 L	1332	8.70	8.50	73.95	102.35	8.60
N.BRITAIN 43179 R	1332	8.50	8.60	73.10	98.84	8.55

UPPER C H. SAPIENS

	N	L(M-D)	B(B-L)	L*B	L/B	L+B/2
N.BRITAIN 43193 L	1333	8.80	8.20	72.16	107.32	8.50
N.BRITAIN 43193 R	1333	8.60	8.20	70.52	104.88	8.40
N.BRITAIN 43194 L	1334	8.20	8.00	65.60	102.50	8.10
N.BRITAIN 43198 R	1335	9.10	9.20	83.72	98.91	9.15
N.BRITAIN 43199 L	1336	8.30	8.00	66.40	103.75	8.15
N.BRITAIN 43199 R	1336	8.40	8.00	67.20	105.00	8.20
N.BRITAIN 43202 L	1337	9.10	9.50	86.45	95.79	9.30
N.BRITAIN 43202 R	1337	9.20	10.00	92.00	92.00	9.60
N.BRITAIN 43204 L	1338	8.30	9.60	79.68	86.46	8.95
N.BRITAIN 43204 R	1338	9.10	9.70	88.27	93.81	9.40
N.BRITAIN 43226 L	1339	7.40	8.50	62.90	87.06	7.95
N.BRITAIN 43226 R	1339	7.60	8.20	62.32	92.68	7.90
N.BRITAIN 43242 L	1341	7.70	8.20	63.14	93.90	7.95
N.BRITAIN 43242 R	1341	7.70	8.10	62.37	95.06	7.90
N.BRITAIN 43290 L	1342	8.10	8.40	68.04	96.43	8.25
N.BRITAIN 43290 R	1342	8.90	8.80	78.32	101.14	8.85
N.BRITAIN 43291 L	1343	8.60	9.20	79.12	93.48	8.90
N.BRITAIN 43291 R	1343	8.40	9.40	78.96	89.36	8.90
N.BRITAIN 43295 R	1344	8.40	8.10	68.04	103.70	8.25
N.BRITAIN L	1346	8.10	10.45	84.64	77.51	9.27
N.BRITAIN R	1346	8.20	10.50	86.10	78.10	9.35
HINDU (UI) L	2208	7.30	8.25	60.22	88.48	7.77
HINDU (UI) R	2208	7.45	8.30	61.83	89.76	7.87
GOL BA IT 99 L	2004	8.90	9.60	85.44	92.71	9.25
GOL BA IT R	2005	7.70	8.30	63.91	92.77	8.00
GOL BA IT L	2006	7.80	8.30	64.74	93.98	8.05
SAINT CRUZ M L	2204	8.30	9.70	80.51	85.57	9.00
SAINT CRUZ M R	2204	8.30	9.30	77.19	89.25	8.80
SAINT CRUZ F L	2205	7.70	8.50	65.45	90.59	8.10
SAINT CRUZ F R	2205	7.50	8.00	60.00	93.75	7.75
HAIDA L	1406	8.40	8.30	69.72	101.20	8.35
HAIDA R	1406	8.00	8.40	67.20	95.24	8.20
MINNESOTA MAN L	1419	8.70	9.40	81.78	92.55	9.05
MINNESOTA MAN R	1419	8.40	9.40	78.96	89.36	8.90
PUNIN (EQUADOR) R	1420	8.95	9.30	83.23	96.24	9.12
ILLINOIS PK2-B1 L	1426	8.70	9.85	85.69	88.32	9.27
ILLINOIS PK2-B1 R	1426	9.00	9.80	88.20	91.84	9.40
ILLINOIS T25-2 L	1427	8.00	8.10	64.80	98.77	8.05
ILLINOIS T25-2 R	1427	7.80	8.40	65.52	92.86	8.10
ILLINOIS A-2732 L	1429	8.60	8.20	70.52	104.88	8.40
ILLINOIS A-2732 R	1429	8.65	8.00	69.20	108.12	8.32
ILLINOIS A-6890 R	1430	7.90	8.40	66.36	94.05	8.15
ILLINOIS A-4921 L	1431	8.30	9.10	75.53	91.21	8.70
ILLINOIS A-4921 R	1431	8.20	9.20	75.44	89.13	8.70
ILLINOIS PK9-B4 R	1432	7.90	7.80	61.62	101.28	7.85
ILLINOIS PK9-B1 R	1433		9.60			
ILLINOIS BR19-3 L	1434	8.30	8.10	67.23	102.47	8.20
ILLINOIS BR19-3 R	1434	8.55	8.00	68.40	106.87	8.27
ILLINOIS BLUFFS L	1435	8.10	8.00	64.80	101.25	8.05
DICKSON MOUND L	1501	8.65	8.60	74.39	100.58	8.62

UPPER C H. SAPIENS

	N	L(M-D)	B(B-L)	L*B	L/B	L+B/2
DICKSCN MOUND R	1501	8.63	8.95	77.24	96.42	8.79
DICKSCN MD 242 L	1505	8.85	7.65	67.70	115.69	8.25
DICKSCN MD 242 R	1505	8.85	7.90	69.91	112.03	8.37
DICKSON MD 256 L	1506	7.70	8.30	63.91	92.77	8.00
DICKSCN MD 256 R	1506	7.90	8.20	64.78	96.34	8.05
DICKSCN MD 261 L	1508	8.25	8.20	67.65	100.61	8.22
DICKSCN MD 261 R	1508	8.20	8.50	69.70	96.47	8.35
DICKSCN MD 262 R	1509	8.80	8.90	78.32	98.88	8.85
DICKSCN MD 266 L	1510	8.64	8.78	75.86	98.41	8.71
DICKSCN MD 266 R	1510	8.55	9.00	76.95	95.00	8.77
DICKSCN MD 276 L	1514	9.00	9.85	88.65	91.37	9.42
DICKSGN MD 276 R	1514	9.18	10.15	93.18	90.44	9.66
DICKSCN MD 287 L	1516	8.05	8.80	70.84	91.48	8.42
DICKSCN MD 287 R	1516	8.10	8.80	71.28	92.05	8.45
DICKSCN MD 297 L	1520	8.50	8.20	69.70	103.66	8.35
DICKSCN MD 302 L	1521	7.70	7.62	58.67	101.05	7.66
DICKSCN MD 302 R	1521	7.55	7.75	58.51	97.42	7.65
DICKSCN MD 319 L	1523	8.80	9.35	82.28	94.12	9.07
DICKSCN MD 319 R	1523	8.80	8.95	78.76	98.32	8.87
DICKSCN MD 327 L	1524	8.55	8.80	75.24	97.16	8.67
DICKSCN MD 327 R	1524	8.50	8.80	74.80	96.59	8.65
DICKSCN MD 334 L	1525	8.60	9.60	82.56	89.58	9.10
DICKSCN MD 334 R	1525	8.70	9.20	80.04	94.57	8.95
DICKSGN MD 348 L	1529	7.85	7.95	62.41	98.74	7.90
DICKSCN MD 348 R	1529	7.90	7.90	62.41	100.00	7.90
DICKSON MD 349 R	1530	8.10	8.10	65.61	100.00	8.10
DICKSCN MD 355 L	1535	8.90	8.65	76.98	102.89	8.77
DICKSCN MD 355 R	1535	9.25	9.00	83.25	102.78	9.12
DICKSON MD 361 L	1538	8.20	8.80	72.16	93.18	8.50
DICKSCN MD 361 R	1538	8.10	8.65	70.06	93.64	8.37
DICKSCN MD 362 L	1539	8.75	8.45	73.94	103.55	8.60
DICKSCN MD 362 R	1539	8.50	8.40	71.40	101.19	8.45
DICKSCN MD 365 L	1540	7.90	7.90	62.41	100.00	7.90
DICKSCN MD 365 R	1540	7.50	7.80	58.50	96.15	7.65
DICKSCN MD 467 L	1541	7.40	8.90	65.86	83.15	8.15
DICKSCN MD 371 L	1542	8.80	9.00	79.20	97.78	8.90
DICKSCN MD 371 R	1542	8.90	8.80	78.32	101.14	8.85
DICKSCN MD 372 R	1543	8.40	8.40	70.56	100.00	8.40
DICKSCN MD 378 L	1547	7.10	7.45	52.89	95.30	7.27
DICKSCN MD 378 R	1547	7.20	7.55	54.36	95.36	7.37
DICKSCN MD 379 L	1548	8.25	8.20	67.65	100.61	8.22
DICKSCN MD 379 R	1548	8.30	8.40	69.72	98.81	8.35
DICKSON MD 380 L	1549	8.10	8.90	72.09	91.01	8.50
DICKSCN MD 380 R	1549	8.00	8.70	69.60	91.95	8.35
DICKSCN MD 381 L	1550	7.80	8.00	62.40	97.50	7.90
DICKSCN MD 381 R	1550	7.90	8.40	66.36	94.05	8.15
DICKSCN MD 380 L	1551	7.90	8.20	64.78	96.34	8.05
DICKSCN MD 380 R	1551	7.60	8.30	63.08	91.57	7.95
DICKSCN MD 396 L	1553	9.00	9.10	81.90	98.90	9.05
DICKSCN MD 396 R	1553	8.80	9.20	80.96	95.65	9.00

UPPER C H. SAPIENS

	N	L(M-D)	B(B-L)	L*B	L/B	L+B/2
DICKSON MD 397 L	1554	8.40	9.40	78.96	89.36	8.90
DICKSCN MD 397 R	1554	8.40	8.80	73.92	95.45	8.60
DICKSCN MD 398 R	1555	8.00	8.00	64.00	100.00	8.00
DICKSCN MD 399 L	1556	8.00	8.65	69.20	92.49	8.32
DICKSCN MD 399 R	1556	8.10	8.70	70.47	93.10	8.40
DICKSCN MD 404 L	1559	8.70	9.05	78.73	96.13	8.87
DICKSCN MD 404 R	1559	8.35	8.90	74.31	93.82	8.62
DICKSCN MD 406 L	1560	8.20	8.05	66.01	101.86	8.12
DICKSCN MD 406 R	1560	8.04	8.09	65.04	99.38	8.06
DICKSCN MD 407 L	1561	8.35	8.60	71.81	97.09	8.47
DICKSGN MD 407 R	1561	8.85	8.85	78.32	100.00	8.85
DICKSCN MD 411 L	1563	8.85	8.30	73.45	106.63	8.57
DICKSCN MD 411 R	1563	8.73	8.50	74.20	102.71	8.61
DICKSCN MD 414 L	1564	8.20	8.16	66.91	100.49	8.18
DICKSCN MD 415 L	1565	8.70	8.70	75.69	100.00	8.70
DICKSCN MD 415 R	1565	8.55	8.20	70.11	104.27	8.37
DICKSCN MD 426 L	1566	7.70	7.55	58.13	101.99	7.62
DICKSGN MD 426 R	1566	7.95	7.60	60.42	104.61	7.77
DICKSCN MD 443 L	1571	8.98	9.05	81.27	99.23	9.01
DICKSCN MD 443 R	1571	8.92	8.85	78.94	100.79	8.88
DICKSCN MD 446 L	1572	8.17	7.67	62.66	106.52	7.92
DICKSCN MD 446 R	1572	8.25	7.92	65.34	104.17	8.08
DICKSCN MD 464 L	1575	9.10	8.10	73.71	112.35	8.60
DICKSCN MD 464 R	1575	9.40	8.20	77.08	114.63	8.80
DICKSCN MD 476 L	1576	8.80	8.90	78.32	98.88	8.85
DICKSCN MD 476 R	1576	8.55	8.90	76.09	96.07	8.72
DICKSCN MD 480 L	1578	7.95	7.75	61.61	102.58	7.85
DICKSON MD 480 R	1578	8.50	8.00	68.00	106.25	8.25
DICKSCN MD 497 L	1583	8.53	9.46	80.69	90.17	8.99
DICKSCN MD 497 R	1583	8.41	9.50	79.89	88.53	8.95
DICKSCN MD 503 L	1585	9.15	9.68	88.57	94.52	9.41
DICKSCN MD 503 R	1585	8.95	9.50	85.02	94.21	9.22
DICKSCN MD 509 L	1587	8.38	7.98	66.87	105.01	8.18
DICKSCN MD 509 R	1587	8.41	8.06	67.78	104.34	8.23
DICKSCN MD 535 L	1591	8.20	8.20	67.24	100.00	8.20
DICKSCN MD 535 R	1591	8.35	8.10	67.63	103.09	8.22
DICKSCN MD 536 L	1592	8.30	8.30	68.89	100.00	8.30
DICKSCN MD 536 R	1592	8.30	8.10	67.23	102.47	8.20
DICKSCN MD 557 L	1596	8.10	8.16	66.10	99.26	8.13
DICKSON MD 557 R	1596	8.13	8.30	67.48	97.95	8.21
DICKSCN MD 561 L	1597	7.95	9.55	75.92	83.25	8.75
DICKSCN MD 567 R	1598	8.65	9.15	79.15	94.54	8.90
DICKSCN MD 594 L	1601	7.75	8.10	62.77	95.68	7.92
DICKSCN MD 594 R	1601	7.50	8.35	62.62	89.82	7.92
DICKSCN MD 599 L	1602	8.85	9.25	81.86	95.68	9.05
DICKSCN MD 599 R	1602	8.90	9.30	82.77	95.70	9.10
DICKSCN MD 630 L	1603	8.30	8.50	70.55	97.65	8.40
DICKSCN MD 630 R	1603	8.50	8.30	70.55	102.41	8.40
DICKSCN MD 648 L	1609	9.00	8.90	80.10	101.12	8.95
DICKSCN MD 648 R	1609	8.80	8.80	77.44	100.00	8.80

UPPER C H. SAPIENS

	N	L(M-D)	B(B-L)	L*B	L/B	L+B/2
DICKSON MD 658 R	1613	8.00	8.60	68.80	93.02	8.30
DICKSON MD 667 L	1614	8.70	9.20	80.04	94.57	8.95
DICKSON MD 667 R	1614	9.15	9.30	85.09	98.39	9.22
DICKSON MD 687 R	1616	7.60	7.70	58.52	98.70	7.65
DICKSON MD 709 L	1623	8.85	8.10	71.68	109.26	8.47
DICKSON MD 722 L	1624	8.40	9.10	76.44	92.31	8.75
DICKSON MD 722 R	1624	8.35	9.20	76.82	90.76	8.77
DICKSON MD 724 L	1627	7.50	9.30	69.75	80.65	8.40
DICKSON MD 724 R	1627	8.18	9.05	74.03	90.39	8.61
DICKSON MD 746 L	1628	8.50	8.90	75.65	95.51	8.70
DICKSON MD 746 R	1628	8.45	9.10	76.89	92.86	8.77
DICKSON MD 749 L	1629	8.30	8.05	66.81	103.11	8.17

UPPER PM3 H. SAPIENS

		N	L(M-D)	B(B-L)	L*B	L/B	L+B/2
PREDMOST 3	L	1007	7.65	8.90	68.08	85.96	8.27
PREDMOST 3	R	1007	7.85	10.70	83.99	73.36	9.27
PREDMOST 4	L	1008	6.70	8.25	55.27	81.21	7.47
PREDMOST 4	R	1008	6.50	9.90	64.35	65.66	8.20
COMBE CHAPELLE	L	1017	6.00	9.00	54.00	66.67	7.50
COMBE CHAPELLE	R	1017	6.00	9.00	54.00	66.67	7.50
BRNO 3	L	1018	6.00	9.30	55.80	64.52	7.65
BRNO 3	R	1018	6.00	8.80	52.80	68.18	7.40
GRIMALDI ADOL.	L	1019	7.85	10.55	82.82	74.41	9.20
GRIMALDI ADOL.	R	1019	8.35	10.60	88.51	78.77	9.47
LA ROCHETTE A	L	1021	7.10	9.90	70.29	71.72	8.50
LA ROCHETTE A	R	1021	7.10	9.90	70.29	71.72	8.50
ROIS		1051	6.00	9.00	54.00	66.67	7.50
ROIS		1052	6.50	9.50	61.75	68.42	8.00
VESTONICE 3	L	1057	6.50	9.40	61.10	69.15	7.95
VESTONICE 3	R	1057	5.90	9.20	54.28	64.13	7.55
A CULOZ 2	L	1101	7.10	10.20	72.42	69.61	8.65
ALAMANN 5	L	1102	6.50	9.00	58.50	72.22	7.75
ALAMANN 5	R	1102	7.00	9.00	63.00	77.78	8.00
ALAMANN 1288	L	1103	6.00	8.00	48.00	75.00	7.00
ALAMANN 1288	R	1103	6.00	8.00	48.00	75.00	7.00
BUGGISON 1	L	1108	8.00	10.50	84.00	76.19	9.25
BUGGISON 1	R	1108	8.50	10.50	89.25	80.95	9.50
BUGGISON 2	L	1109	8.00	11.00	88.00	72.73	9.50
BUGGISON 2	R	1109	8.00	11.00	88.00	72.73	9.50
CAP BLAC	L	1110	5.50	9.20	50.60	59.78	7.35
CAP BLAC	R	1110	6.30	9.20	57.96	68.48	7.75
EGOLZWIL 1	R	1112	5.90	8.00	47.20	73.75	6.95
KABUA 1		1123	6.00	10.00	60.00	60.00	8.00
KOERHLISBEEK C1	L	1124	7.00	9.50	66.50	73.68	8.25
KOERHLISBEEK C1	R	1124	7.00	9.00	63.00	77.78	8.00
LAFAYE	L	1128	5.80	9.30	53.94	62.37	7.55
LAFAYE	R	1128	6.20	9.60	59.52	64.58	7.90
MASAT		1130	7.80	9.30	72.54	83.87	8.55
OKUZINI		1133	6.70	9.50	63.65	70.53	8.10
RHUNDA	R	1142	4.50	8.10	36.45	55.56	6.30
SVAERDBORG	R	1144	7.50	10.00	75.00	75.00	8.75
FRENCHMAN	L	1149	6.85	9.30	63.70	73.66	8.07
FRENCHMAN	R	1149	7.05	8.90	62.74	79.21	7.97
ALACA HOYUK 2		1183	7.20	9.30	66.96	77.42	8.25
ALACA HOYUK 3		1184	7.00	8.70	60.90	80.46	7.85
IRAN(SIALK)	L	1190	6.70	8.25	55.27	81.21	7.47
IRAN(SIALK)	L	1191	6.60	9.50	62.70	69.47	8.05
IRAN(SIALK)	L	1192	6.30	8.60	54.18	73.26	7.45
JARMO 2B	L	1193	7.00	9.40	65.80	74.47	8.20
JARMO 2B	R	1193	7.50	9.25	69.37	81.08	8.37
WADJAK 1		1701	9.00	9.40	84.60	95.74	9.20
WADJAK 2	L	1702	8.00	10.70	85.60	74.77	9.35
WADJAK 2	R	1702	8.30	11.00	91.30	75.45	9.65
KEILOR	R	1703	6.00	10.50	63.00	57.14	8.25

UPPER PM3 H. SAPIENS

		N	L(M-D)	B(B-L)	L*B	L/B	L+B/2
TALGAI	L	1704	8.60	12.30	105.78	69.92	10.45
COHUNA	L	1705	8.50	11.00	93.50	77.27	9.75
COHUNA	R	1705	9.60	11.25	108.00	85.33	10.42
AUSTRALIAN 39		1708	7.50	10.80	81.00	69.44	9.15
AUSTRALIAN	L	1726	6.90	8.90	61.41	77.53	7.90
AUSTRALIAN	L	1728	7.25	10.50	76.12	69.05	8.87
AUSTRALIAN	R	1728	7.30	10.20	74.46	71.57	8.75
AUSTRALIAN 179	L	1732	6.90	8.00	55.20	86.25	7.45
AUSTRALIAN 179	R	1732	7.00	9.40	65.80	74.47	8.20
TASMANIAN 310		1754	8.00	10.00	80.00	80.00	9.00
TASMANIAN 3637	L	1755	7.75	8.95	69.36	86.59	8.35
TASMANIAN 3637	R	1755	7.95	9.40	74.73	84.57	8.67
TASMANIAN P1	R	1757	7.50	10.50	78.75	71.43	9.00
TASMANIAN P2	L	1758	9.00	12.00	108.00	75.00	10.50
TASMANIAN P2	R	1758	9.00	12.00	108.00	75.00	10.50
TASMANIAN 2966	R	1762		9.70			
TASMANIAN 2964	L	1763	8.50	11.10	94.35	76.58	9.80
TASMANIAN 2964	R	1763	8.50	11.10	94.35	76.58	9.80
ASSELAR	R	1903	7.00	9.00	63.00	77.78	8.00
CAPE FLATS	R	1904	7.50	10.50	78.75	71.43	9.00
NEGRO	L	1905	8.45	10.75	90.84	78.60	9.60
NEGRO		1914	6.90	9.10	62.79	75.82	8.00
NEGRO	L	1915	8.70	11.00	95.70	79.09	9.85
NEGRO	R	1915	8.50	10.90	92.65	77.98	9.70
NEGRO	L	1916	8.90	11.70	104.13	76.07	10.30
NEGRO	R	1916	9.00	11.60	104.40	77.59	10.30
BANTU 100	L	1917	8.80	10.60	93.28	83.02	9.70
BANTU 100	R	1917	8.80	10.70	94.16	82.24	9.75
MAPUNGUBWE	L	1950	7.00	9.20	64.40	76.09	8.10
MAPUNGUBWE	R	1950	6.90				
MAPUNGUBWE M2		1952	8.00	10.70	85.60	74.77	9.35
MAPUNGUBWE M3		1953	8.00	10.50	84.00	76.19	9.25
MAPUNGUBWE M9		1955	8.00	11.00	88.00	72.73	9.50
BAMBANDYANALO21		1957	7.20	9.30	66.96	77.42	8.25
BAMBANDYANALO29		1958	7.20	8.90	64.08	80.90	8.05
BAMBANDYANALO31		1959	8.20	9.60	78.72	85.42	8.90
BAMBANDYANALO13		1964	8.20	10.60	86.92	77.36	9.40
BAMBANDYANALO14		1965	7.00	9.70	67.90	72.16	8.35
BUSHMAN		1967	6.80	8.60	58.48	79.07	7.70
FISH HOEK	R	1972	6.20	6.80	42.16	91.18	6.50
GOUNGOU A	L	1975	6.70	8.90	59.63	75.28	7.80
N.BRITAIN 43126	L	1305	7.30	10.20	74.46	71.57	8.75
N.BRITAIN 43127	L	1306		10.80			
N.BRITAIN 43127	R	1306	8.40	10.50	88.20	80.00	9.45
N.BRITAIN 43132	L	1309	6.30	9.40	59.22	67.02	7.85
N.BRITAIN 43132	R	1309	6.70	9.70	64.99	69.07	8.20
N.BRITAIN 43133	L	1310	7.00	9.80	68.60	71.43	8.40
N.BRITAIN 43134	L	1311	7.30	9.90	72.27	73.74	8.60
N.BRITAIN 43134	R	1311	7.70	10.50	80.85	73.33	9.10
N.BRITAIN 43135	L	1312	7.20	9.90	71.28	72.73	8.55

UPPER PM3 H. SAPIENS

		N	L(M-D)	B(B-L)	L*B	L/B	L+B/2
N.BRITAIN 43136	L	1313	7.10	9.10	64.61	78.02	8.10
N.BRITAIN 43136	R	1313	7.40	9.20	68.08	80.43	8.30
N.BRITAIN 43137	R	1314	6.90	9.70	66.93	71.13	8.30
N.BRITAIN 43138	R	1315	7.80	9.80	76.44	79.59	8.80
N.BRITAIN 43139	L	1316	7.60	9.80	74.48	77.55	8.70
N.BRITAIN 43142	L	1319	8.10	11.00	89.10	73.64	9.55
N.BRITAIN 43142	R	1319	7.90	10.60	83.74	74.53	9.25
N.BRITAIN 43144	L	1321	7.20	10.30	74.16	69.90	8.75
N.BRITAIN 43146	L	1323	7.70	10.30	79.31	74.76	9.00
N.BRITAIN 43146	R	1323	7.50	10.20	76.50	73.53	8.85
N.BRITAIN 43147	R	1324	8.30	10.40	86.32	79.81	9.35
N.BRITAIN 43150	L	1326	8.00	10.50	84.00	76.19	9.25
N.BRITAIN 43150	R	1326	8.40	10.70	89.88	78.50	9.55
N.BRITAIN 43151	L	1327	8.50	10.40	88.40	81.73	9.45
N.BRITAIN 43151	R	1327	9.00	10.50	94.50	85.71	9.75
N.BRITAIN 43152	L	1328	7.80	10.80	84.24	72.22	9.30
N.BRITAIN 43152	R	1328	7.50	10.60	79.50	70.75	9.05
N.BRITAIN 43154	L	1330	7.20	10.60	76.32	67.92	8.90
N.BRITAIN 43154	R	1330	7.20	10.40	74.88	69.23	8.80
N.BRITAIN 43174	L	1331	7.60	10.40	79.04	73.08	9.00
N.BRITAIN 43179	L	1332	7.40	10.00	74.00	74.00	8.70
N.BRITAIN 43179	R	1332	7.10	9.70	68.87	73.20	8.40
N.BRITAIN 43193	L	1333	8.10	10.20	82.62	79.41	9.15
N.BRITAIN 43193	R	1333	7.90	10.10	79.79	78.22	9.00
N.BRITAIN 43194	L	1334	7.80	10.40	81.12	75.00	9.10
N.BRITAIN 43194	R	1334	7.80	10.50	81.90	74.29	9.15
N.BRITAIN 43198	L	1335	7.80	10.50	81.90	74.29	9.15
N.BRITAIN 43198	R	1335	7.50	10.50	78.75	71.43	9.00
N.BRITAIN 43199	L	1336	6.80	9.40	63.92	72.34	8.10
N.BRITAIN 43199	R	1336	6.90	9.40	64.86	73.40	8.15
N.BRITAIN 43202	L	1337	8.10	10.40	84.24	77.88	9.25
N.BRITAIN 43202	R	1337	8.00	10.50	84.00	76.19	9.25
N.BRITAIN 43204	L	1338	7.60	10.80	82.08	70.37	9.20
N.BRITAIN 43204	R	1338	7.80	11.00	85.80	70.91	9.40
N.BRITAIN 43226	L	1339	7.40	9.30	68.82	79.57	8.35
N.BRITAIN 43226	R	1339	7.10	9.30	66.03	76.34	8.20
N.BRITAIN 43329	L	1340	8.10	11.20	90.72	72.32	9.65
N.BRITAIN 43329	R	1340	8.40	11.10	93.24	75.68	9.75
N.BRITAIN 43242	R	1341	7.20	9.80	70.56	73.47	8.50
N.BRITAIN 43290	L	1342	7.50	10.50	78.75	71.43	9.00
N.BRITAIN 43290	R	1342	7.00	10.50	73.50	66.67	8.75
N.BRITAIN 43291	L	1343	7.30	10.10	73.73	72.28	8.70
N.BRITAIN 43291	R	1343	7.50	10.10	75.75	74.26	8.80
N.BRITAIN 43295	L	1344	7.70	10.10	77.77	76.24	8.90
N.BRITAIN 43295	R	1344	7.60	9.56	72.66	79.50	8.58
N.BRITAIN	L	1346	6.85	9.90	67.81	69.19	8.37
N.BRITAIN	R	1346	7.00	10.00	70.00	70.00	8.50
HINDU (LI)	L	2208	6.25	8.70	54.37	71.84	7.47
HINDU (LI)	R	2208	6.70	8.55	57.28	78.36	7.62
GOL BA IT	L	2007	8.10	10.70	86.67	75.70	9.40

UPPER PM3 H. SAPIENS

		N	L(M-D)	B(B-L)	L*B	L/B	L+B/2
MELOLO	L	2026	7.70	10.30	79.31	74.76	9.00
MELOLO	R	2027	7.50	9.70	72.75	77.32	8.60
MELOLO	L	2028	7.30	9.60	70.08	76.04	8.45
MELOLO	R	2029	7.80	10.10	78.78	77.23	8.95
MELOLO	L	2030	7.90	10.20	80.58	77.45	9.05
MELOLO	R	2031	6.50	8.20	53.30	79.27	7.35
MELOLO	R	2032	7.00	9.10	63.70	76.92	8.05
MELOLO	L	2033	7.70	9.50	73.15	81.05	8.60
MELOLO	R	2034	7.80	10.50	81.90	74.29	9.15
MELOLO	L	2035	7.80	10.40	81.12	75.00	9.10
SAINT CRUZ M	L	2204	7.30	10.10	73.73	72.28	8.70
SAINT CRUZ M	R	2204	7.30	10.50	76.65	69.52	8.90
SAINT CRUZ F	L	2205	7.00	10.00	70.00	70.00	8.50
SAINT CRUZ F	R	2205	6.70	9.20	61.64	72.83	7.95
CHANG YANG		2203	7.40	10.60	78.44	69.81	9.00
HAIDA	L	1406	7.30	8.70	63.51	83.91	8.00
HAIDA	R	1406	7.20	8.60	61.92	83.72	7.90
MINNESOTA MAN	L	1419	7.70	10.00	77.00	77.00	8.85
MINNESOTA MAN	R	1419	7.70	10.50	80.85	73.33	9.10
PUNIN (EQUADOR)	L	1420	9.30	11.40	106.02	81.58	10.35
PUNIN (EQUADOR)	R	1420	8.50	11.50	97.75	73.91	10.00
ILLINOIS PK2-B1	L	1426	7.30	10.20	74.46	71.57	8.75
ILLINOIS PK2-B1	R	1426	7.00	10.20	71.40	68.63	8.60
ILLINOIS T25-2	L	1427	7.10	9.00	63.90	78.89	8.05
ILLINOIS T25-2	R	1427	7.35	9.00	66.15	81.67	8.17
ILLINOIS A-2732	L	1429	6.80	8.90	60.52	76.40	7.85
ILLINOIS A-2732	R	1429	6.35	9.00	57.15	70.56	7.67
ILLINOIS A-6890	L	1430	6.55	9.00	58.95	72.78	7.77
ILLINOIS A-6890	R	1430	6.70	9.40	62.98	71.28	8.05
ILLINOIS A-4921	L	1431	7.70	9.80	75.46	78.57	8.75
ILLINOIS A-4921	R	1431	7.25	10.00	72.50	72.50	8.62
ILLINOIS PK9-B4	L	1432	7.45	9.40	70.03	79.26	8.42
ILLINOIS PK9-B4	R	1432	6.95	9.20	63.94	75.54	8.07
ILLINOIS BR19-3	L	1434	8.45	9.90	83.65	85.35	9.17
ILLINOIS BR19-3	R	1434	7.85	10.00	78.50	78.50	8.92
ILLINOIS BLUFFS	L	1435	7.40	9.90	73.26	74.75	8.65
DICKSON MOUND	L	1501	7.62	9.70	73.91	78.56	8.66
DICKSON MOUND	R	1501	7.00	9.65	67.55	72.54	8.32
DICKSON MD 242	L	1505	8.30	10.20	84.66	81.37	9.25
DICKSON MD 242	R	1505	8.00	10.30	82.40	77.67	9.15
DICKSON MD 256	L	1506	7.45	9.10	67.79	81.87	8.27
DICKSON MD 256	R	1506	7.20	9.10	65.52	79.12	8.15
DICKSON MD 261	L	1508	7.20	9.80	70.56	73.47	8.50
DICKSON MD 261	R	1508	7.35	10.10	74.23	72.77	8.72
DICKSON MD 266	L	1510	8.00	10.00	80.00	80.00	9.00
DICKSON MD 276	L	1514	8.00	11.40	91.20	70.18	9.70
DICKSON MD 276	R	1514	8.05	11.50	92.57	70.00	9.77
DICKSON MD 287	L	1516	6.75	9.65	65.14	69.95	8.20
DICKSON MD 287	R	1516	7.00	9.35	65.45	74.87	8.17
DICKSON MD 291	R	1518	7.80	9.80	76.44	79.59	8.80

UPPER PM3 H. SAPIENS

		N	L(M-D)	B(B-L)	L*B	L/B	L+B/2
DICKSON MD 297	L	1520	7.30	9.80	71.54	74.49	8.55
DICKSON MD 302	L	1521	6.90	9.50	65.55	72.63	8.20
DICKSON MD 319	L	1523	7.15	9.85	70.43	72.59	8.50
DICKSON MD 319	R	1523	7.10	9.60	68.16	73.96	8.35
DICKSON MD 327	L	1524	7.05	9.75	68.74	72.31	8.40
DICKSON MD 327	R	1524	7.25	9.80	71.05	73.98	8.52
DICKSON MD 334	L	1525	8.60	10.25	88.15	83.90	9.42
DICKSON MD 334	R	1525	7.20	10.05	72.36	71.64	8.62
DICKSON MD 348	R	1529	7.00	9.65	67.55	72.54	8.32
DICKSON MD 349	L	1530	6.95	9.55	66.37	72.77	8.25
DICKSON MD 349	R	1530	7.30	9.50	69.35	76.84	8.40
DICKSON MD 352	R	1533	7.90	10.20	80.58	77.45	9.05
DICKSON MD 355	L	1535	8.05	10.10	81.30	79.70	9.07
DICKSON MD 355	R	1535	8.10	10.05	81.40	80.60	9.07
DICKSON MD 361	L	1538	7.75	9.40	72.85	82.45	8.57
DICKSON MD 361	R	1538	7.55	9.20	69.46	82.07	8.37
DICKSON MD 362	L	1539	7.90	10.00	79.00	79.00	8.95
DICKSON MD 362	R	1539	7.80	10.10	78.78	77.23	8.95
DICKSON MD 365	L	1540	6.60	9.50	62.70	69.47	8.05
DICKSON MD 365	R	1540	6.90	9.20	63.48	75.00	8.05
DICKSON MD 467	L	1541	7.10	9.30	66.03	76.34	8.20
DICKSON MD 371	L	1542	8.40	10.10	84.84	83.17	9.25
DICKSON MD 371	R	1542	8.30	10.10	83.83	82.18	9.20
DICKSON MD 372	R	1543	7.30	9.95	72.63	73.37	8.62
DICKSON MD 379	L	1548	8.00	10.10	80.80	79.21	9.05
DICKSON MD 379	R	1548	7.95	9.30	73.93	85.48	8.62
DICKSON MD 380	L	1549	5.90	8.80	51.92	67.05	7.35
DICKSON MD 380	R	1549	6.70	9.25	61.97	72.43	7.97
DICKSON MD 381	L	1550	7.90	10.60	83.74	74.53	9.25
DICKSON MD 381	R	1550	7.60	10.60	80.56	71.70	9.10
DICKSON MD 380	L	1551	7.00	9.10	63.70	76.92	8.05
DICKSON MD 388	R	1552	8.10	10.70	86.67	75.70	9.40
DICKSON MD 396	L	1553	7.50	9.60	72.00	78.12	8.55
DICKSON MD 396	R	1553	7.70	9.90	76.23	77.78	8.80
DICKSON MD 397	L	1554	7.80	9.80	76.44	79.59	8.80
DICKSON MD 397	R	1554	7.80	9.80	76.44	79.59	8.80
DICKSON MD 398	R	1555	6.80	9.10	61.88	74.73	7.95
DICKSON MD 399	R	1556	6.75	9.30	62.77	72.58	8.02
DICKSON MD 406	L	1560	7.40	8.92	66.01	82.96	8.16
DICKSON MD 407	L	1561	7.50	10.03	75.22	74.78	8.76
DICKSON MD 407	R	1561	7.70	10.00	77.00	77.00	8.85
DICKSON MD 411	L	1563	8.05	10.30	82.91	78.16	9.17
DICKSON MD 411	R	1563	7.95	9.80	77.91	81.12	8.87
DICKSON MD 414	L	1564	7.17	9.20	65.96	77.93	8.18
DICKSON MD 415	L	1565	6.85	9.27	63.50	73.89	8.06
DICKSON MD 415	R	1565	7.05	9.30	65.56	75.81	8.17
DICKSON MD 432	L	1567	6.92	8.70	60.20	79.54	7.81
DICKSON MD 432	R	1567	6.75	8.70	58.72	77.59	7.72
DICKSON MD 443	R	1571	8.00	10.14	81.12	78.90	9.07
DICKSON MD 446	L	1572	7.60	9.90	75.24	76.77	8.75

UPPER PM3 H. SAPIENS

		N	L(M-D)	B(B-L)	L*B	L/B	L+B/2
DICKSON MD 464	L	1575	8.25	9.65	79.61	85.49	8.95
DICKSON MD 464	R	1575	7.85	9.70	76.14	80.93	8.77
DICKSON MD 476	L	1576	8.02	10.40	83.41	77.12	9.21
DICKSON MD 476	R	1576	8.22	10.44	85.82	78.74	9.33
DICKSON MD 480	L	1578	7.40	8.80	65.12	84.09	8.10
DICKSON MD 480	R	1578	7.20	9.10	65.52	79.12	8.15
DICKSON MD 497	L	1583	7.77	10.85	84.30	71.61	9.31
DICKSON MD 497	R	1583	7.75	10.75	83.31	72.09	9.25
DICKSON MD 503	L	1585	6.90	9.85	67.96	70.05	8.37
DICKSON MD 503	R	1585	7.20	10.25	73.80	70.24	8.72
DICKSON MD 509	L	1587	7.60	9.85	74.86	77.16	8.72
DICKSON MD 509	R	1587	6.72	9.40	63.17	71.49	8.06
DICKSON MD 535	L	1591	7.20	9.20	66.24	78.26	8.20
DICKSON MD 535	R	1591	7.37	9.50	70.01	77.58	8.43
DICKSON MD 536	L	1592	7.20	9.20	66.24	78.26	8.20
DICKSON MD 536	R	1592	6.85	9.30	63.70	73.66	8.07
DICKSON MD 545	L	1594	8.10	10.65	86.26	76.06	9.37
DICKSON MD 545	R	1594	8.15	10.60	86.39	76.89	9.37
DICKSON MD 557	L	1596	6.90	9.60	66.24	71.87	8.25
DICKSON MD 557	R	1596	7.33	9.64	70.66	76.04	8.48
DICKSON MD 561	L	1597	7.47	9.90	73.95	75.45	8.68
DICKSON MD 561	R	1597	7.60	9.90	75.24	76.77	8.75
DICKSON MD 567	L	1598	7.90	10.55	83.34	74.88	9.22
DICKSON MD 594	L	1601	7.20	9.45	68.04	76.19	8.32
DICKSON MD 594	R	1601	6.80	9.30	63.24	73.12	8.05
DICKSON MD 599	L	1602	7.10	9.85	69.93	72.08	8.47
DICKSON MD 599	R	1602	7.35	9.90	72.76	74.24	8.62
DICKSON MD 630	L	1603	7.80	9.70	75.66	80.41	8.75
DICKSON MD 630	R	1603	7.90	10.10	79.79	78.22	9.00
DICKSON MD 667	L	1614	7.43	9.66	71.77	76.92	8.54
DICKSON MD 667	R	1614	7.52	9.74	73.24	77.21	8.63
DICKSON MD 709	L	1623	6.40				
DICKSON MD 722	L	1624	7.25	10.50	76.12	69.05	8.87
DICKSON MD 722	R	1624	7.00	10.05	70.35	69.65	8.52
DICKSON MD 724	L	1627	7.54	9.85	74.27	76.55	8.69
DICKSON MD 724	R	1627	7.90	10.80	85.32	73.15	9.35
DICKSON MD 746	L	1628	7.20	9.85	70.92	73.10	8.52
DICKSON MD 746	R	1628	7.27	9.90	71.97	73.43	8.58
DICKSON MD 749	L	1629	7.55	9.80	73.99	77.04	8.67

UPPER PM4 H. SAPIENS

		N	L(M-D)	B(B-L)	L*B	L/B	L+B/2
ARCYSURCURE C9	L	1002	7.50	10.50	78.75	71.43	9.00
PREDMOST 3	L	1007	7.25	8.65	62.71	83.82	7.95
PREDMOST 3	R	1007	6.30	10.00	63.00	63.00	8.15
PREDMOST 4	L	1008	6.60	9.40	62.04	70.21	8.00
COMBE CHAPELLE	L	1017	6.00	8.50	51.00	70.59	7.25
COMBE CHAPELLE	R	1017	6.50	9.00	58.50	72.22	7.75
BRNO 3	L	1018	6.40	9.80	62.72	65.31	8.10
BRNO 3	R	1018	5.50	9.00	49.50	61.11	7.25
GRIMALDI ADOL.	L	1019	9.85	11.15	109.83	88.34	10.50
GRIMALDI ADOL.	R	1019	8.60	11.70	100.62	73.50	10.15
LA ROCHETTE A	L	1021	7.90	9.70	76.63	81.44	8.80
VESTONICE 3	L	1057	6.60	8.90	58.74	74.16	7.75
VESTONICE 3	R	1057	6.50	9.10	59.15	71.43	7.80
A CULOZ 2	L	1101	7.20	10.30	74.16	69.90	8.75
A CULOZ 2	R	1101		10.90			
ALAMANN 5	L	1102	6.50	9.00	58.50	72.22	7.75
ALAMANN 5	R	1102	7.00	9.00	63.00	77.78	8.00
ALAMANN 1288	L	1103	6.00	7.50	45.00	80.00	6.75
ALAMANN 1288	R	1103	5.50	7.00	38.50	78.57	6.25
BISCORDINE	L	1107	6.50	10.00	65.00	65.00	8.25
BUGGISON 1	L	1108	7.00	10.00	70.00	70.00	8.50
BUGGISON 1	R	1108	8.00	10.00	80.00	80.00	9.00
BUGGISON 2	L	1109	7.50	11.00	82.50	68.18	9.25
BUGGISON 2	R	1109	8.00	11.00	88.00	72.73	9.50
CAP BLAC	L	1110	6.00	9.20	55.20	65.22	7.60
CAP BLAC	R	1110	6.00	9.00	54.00	66.67	7.50
EGOLZWIL 1	L	1112	6.10				
EGOLZWIL 1	R	1112	5.20				
KABUA 1		1123	6.00	9.00	54.00	66.67	7.50
KOERHLISBEEK C1	L	1124	7.00	10.00	70.00	70.00	8.50
KOERHLISBEEK C1	R	1124	7.00	9.00	63.00	77.78	8.00
LAFAYE	L	1128	5.80	9.00	52.20	64.44	7.40
LAFAYE	R	1128	4.60	9.50	43.70	48.42	7.05
MASAT		1130	7.50	9.90	74.25	75.76	8.70
OKUZINI		1133	6.70	9.80	65.66	68.37	8.25
RHUNCA	R	1142	5.00	10.20	51.00	49.02	7.60
SVAERCBORG	R	1144	7.80	10.40	81.12	75.00	9.10
FRENCHMAN	L	1149	6.80	9.10	61.88	74.73	7.95
FRENCHMAN	R	1149	6.35	9.60	60.96	66.15	7.97
ALACA HOYUK 2		1183	6.30	9.30	58.59	67.74	7.80
ALACA HOYUK 3		1184	6.60	8.90	58.74	74.16	7.75
IRAN(SIALK)	L	1190	7.00	8.55	59.85	81.87	7.77
IRAN(SIALK)	L	1191	6.20	9.20	57.04	67.39	7.70
IRAN(SIALK)	L	1192	6.90	9.40	64.86	73.40	8.15
JARMO 2B	L	1193	7.50	10.80	81.00	69.44	9.15
JARMO 2B	R	1193	7.35	11.00	80.85	66.82	9.17
WADJAK 1		1701	7.60	11.00	83.60	69.09	9.30
WADJAK 2	L	1702	7.60	10.50	79.80	72.38	9.05
WADJAK 2	R	1702	8.00	10.80	86.40	74.07	9.40
KEILOR	R	1703	7.10	10.60	75.26	66.98	8.85

UPPER PM4 H. SAPIENS

		N	L(M-D)	B(B-L)	L*B	L/B	L+B/2
TALGAI	L	1704	8.1C	11.00	89.10	73.64	9.55
COHUNA	L	1705	8.15	11.50	93.72	70.87	9.82
COHUNA	R	1705	8.60	11.40	98.04	75.44	10.00
AUSTRALIAN 39		1708	7.00	10.40	72.80	67.31	8.70
AUSTRALIAN	L	1726	7.25	9.00	65.25	80.56	8.12
AUSTRALIAN	L	1728	7.20	9.80	70.56	73.47	8.50
AUSTRALIAN	R	1728	7.20	10.20	73.44	70.59	8.70
AUSTRALIAN 179	L	1732	7.30	9.80	71.54	74.49	8.55
AUSTRALIAN 179	R	1732	7.60	9.50	72.20	80.00	8.55
TASMANIAN 310		1754	8.00	11.00	88.00	72.73	9.50
TASMANIAN 3637	L	1755	7.30	8.95	65.33	81.56	8.12
TASMANIAN 3637	R	1755	7.50	9.70	72.75	77.32	8.60
TASMANIAN P1	R	1757	7.50				
TASMANIAN P2	L	1758	8.00	11.50	92.00	69.57	9.75
TASMANIAN P2	R	1758	8.00	11.50	92.00	69.57	9.75
TASMANIAN 2964	L	1763	8.20	11.40	93.48	71.93	9.80
TASMANIAN 2964	R	1763	8.10	11.30	91.53	71.68	9.70
ASSELAR	R	1903	6.50	9.00	58.50	72.22	7.75
CAPE FLATS	R	1904	7.00	10.50	73.50	66.67	8.75
NEGRO	L	1905	8.40	10.85	91.14	77.42	9.62
NEGRC		1914	6.70	9.10	60.97	73.63	7.90
NEGRO	L	1915	8.40	11.20	94.08	75.00	9.80
NEGRO	R	1915	9.30	11.20	104.16	83.04	10.25
NEGRO	R	1916	8.40	11.40	95.76	73.68	9.90
BANTU 1CO	L	1917	8.70	9.60	83.52	90.62	9.15
BANTU 1CO	R	1917	8.00	9.70	77.60	82.47	8.85
MAPUNGUBWE	L	1950	7.00	8.80	61.60	79.55	7.90
MAPUNGUBWE M2		1952	8.70	10.70	93.09	81.31	9.70
MAPUNGUBWE M3		1953	8.00	10.30	82.40	77.67	9.15
MAPUNGUBWE M5		1954	7.00	10.00	70.00	70.00	8.50
MAPUNGUBWE M9		1955	8.30	11.50	95.45	72.17	9.90
BAMBANDYANALO21		1957	7.00	9.90	69.30	70.71	8.45
BAMBANDYANALO29		1958	6.70	9.20	61.64	72.83	7.95
BAMBANDYANALO31		1959	8.10	9.90	80.19	81.82	9.00
BAMBANDYANALO 3		1962	7.00	9.10	63.70	76.92	8.05
BAMBANDYANALO13		1964	7.00	10.10	70.70	69.31	8.55
BAMBANDYANALO14		1965	6.20	9.30	57.66	66.67	7.75
BUSHMAN		1967	6.50	8.50	55.25	76.47	7.50
FISH HOEK	R	1972	6.20	7.00	43.40	88.57	6.60
N.BRITAIN 43127	R	1306	7.60	10.10	76.76	75.25	8.85
N.BRITAIN 43130	R	1307	7.30	10.60	77.38	68.87	8.95
N.BRITAIN 43133	L	1310	6.40	10.10	64.64	63.37	8.25
N.BRITAIN 43133	R	1310	6.60	9.70	64.02	68.04	8.15
N.BRITAIN 43134	L	1311	7.10	10.10	71.71	70.30	8.60
N.BRITAIN 43134	R	1311	7.30	10.10	73.73	72.28	8.70
N.BRITAIN 43135	L	1312	6.60	9.50	62.70	69.47	8.05
N.BRITAIN 43135	R	1312	6.60	9.50	62.70	69.47	8.05
N.BRITAIN 43136	R	1313	9.30				
N.BRITAIN 43137	L	1314	6.50	9.40	61.10	69.15	7.95
N.BRITAIN 43138	R	1315	7.00	9.70	67.90	72.16	8.35

UPPER PM4 H. SAPIENS

		N	L(M-D)	B(B-L)	L*B	L/B	L+B/2
N.BRITAIN 43139	L	1316	7.30	10.00	73.00	73.00	8.65
N.BRITAIN 43140	R	1317	6.70	9.20	61.64	72.83	7.95
N.BRITAIN 43141	L	1318	7.30	10.30	75.19	70.87	8.80
N.BRITAIN 43141	R	1318	7.40	10.10	74.74	73.27	8.75
N.BRITAIN 43142	L	1319	7.50	11.00	82.50	68.18	9.25
N.BRITAIN 43142	R	1319	7.30	11.20	81.76	65.18	9.25
N.BRITAIN 43143	L	1320	6.70	9.80	65.66	68.37	8.25
N.BRITAIN 43144	R	1321	6.60	9.80	64.68	67.35	8.20
N.BRITAIN 43146	L	1323	7.00	9.60	67.20	72.92	8.30
N.BRITAIN 43146	R	1323	7.30	9.60	70.08	76.04	8.45
N.BRITAIN 43147	L	1324	7.90	10.20	80.58	77.45	9.05
N.BRITAIN 43147	R	1324	8.20	10.00	82.00	82.00	9.10
N.BRITAIN 43149	L	1325	8.00	10.90	87.20	73.39	9.45
N.BRITAIN 43150	L	1326	7.00	10.30	72.10	67.96	8.65
N.BRITAIN 43150	R	1326	7.10	10.10	71.71	70.30	8.60
N.BRITAIN 43151	L	1327	7.20	10.20	73.44	70.59	8.70
N.BRITAIN 43151	R	1327	7.40	10.10	74.74	73.27	8.75
N.BRITAIN 43152	L	1328	6.80	10.40	70.72	65.38	8.60
N.BRITAIN 43153	R	1329	6.50	9.20	59.80	70.65	7.85
N.BRITAIN 43154	L	1330	7.60	10.70	81.32	71.03	9.15
N.BRITAIN 43154	R	1330	7.60	10.70	81.32	71.03	9.15
N.BRITAIN 43174	L	1331	7.70	10.70	82.39	71.96	9.20
N.BRITAIN 43174	R	1331	7.70	10.50	80.85	73.33	9.10
N.BRITAIN 43179	L	1332	6.30	9.70	61.11	64.95	8.00
N.BRITAIN 43179	R	1332	6.80	10.00	68.00	68.00	8.40
N.BRITAIN 43193	L	1333	7.60	9.80	74.48	77.55	8.70
N.BRITAIN 43193	R	1333	7.40	9.90	73.26	74.75	8.65
N.BRITAIN 43194	L	1334	7.30	10.60	77.38	68.87	8.95
N.BRITAIN 43194	R	1334	7.30	10.40	75.92	70.19	8.85
N.BRITAIN 43198	L	1335	7.80	10.40	81.12	75.00	9.10
N.BRITAIN 43198	R	1335	7.80	10.40	81.12	75.00	9.10
N.BRITAIN 43199	L	1336	6.70	9.70	64.99	69.07	8.20
N.BRITAIN 43199	R	1336	6.80	9.50	64.60	71.58	8.15
N.BRITAIN 43202	L	1337	7.80	11.20	87.36	69.64	9.50
N.BRITAIN 43202	R	1337	8.10	11.10	89.91	72.97	9.60
N.BRITAIN 43204	R	1338	7.50	11.30	84.75	66.37	9.40
N.BRITAIN 43226	L	1339	6.80	9.30	63.24	73.12	8.05
N.BRITAIN 43226	R	1339	6.80	9.40	63.92	72.34	8.10
N.BRITAIN 43329	R	1340	7.70	10.60	81.62	72.64	9.15
N.BRITAIN 43242	R	1341	7.20	10.10	72.72	71.29	8.65
N.BRITAIN 43290	L	1342	6.20	9.20	57.04	67.39	7.70
N.BRITAIN 43290	R	1342	6.60	9.60	63.36	68.75	8.10
N.BRITAIN 43291	L	1343	7.20	10.10	72.72	71.29	8.65
N.BRITAIN 43291	R	1343	7.20	9.50	68.40	75.79	8.35
N.BRITAIN 43295	L	1344	7.80	11.30	88.14	69.03	9.55
N.BRITAIN 43295	R	1344	8.10	10.30	83.43	78.64	9.20
N.BRITAIN	L	1346	6.60	10.10	66.66	65.35	8.35
N.BRITAIN	R	1346	6.90	9.80	67.62	70.41	8.35
HINDU (LI)	L	2208	6.70	8.30	55.61	80.72	7.50
HINDU (UI)	R	2208	6.50	8.15	52.97	79.75	7.32

UPPER PM4 H. SAPIENS

		N	L(M-D)	B(B-L)	L*B	L/B	L+B/2
GOL BA IT 98	L	2003		9.50			
MELOLC	R	2036	6.80	9.20	62.56	73.91	8.00
MELOLC	L	2037	6.90	8.80	60.72	78.41	7.85
MELOLO	L	2038	7.50	10.10	75.75	74.26	8.80
MELOLO	R	2039	7.30	10.20	74.46	71.57	8.75
MELOLO	L	2040	7.00	8.30	58.10	84.34	7.65
MELOLC	L	2041	7.20	9.10	65.52	79.12	8.15
MELOLO	R	2042	6.80	8.90	60.52	76.40	7.85
MELOLO	L	2043	7.00	9.70	67.90	72.16	8.35
MELOLO	L	2044	7.20	9.60	69.12	75.00	8.40
MELOLO	R	2045	6.80	9.30	63.24	73.12	8.05
MELOLC	R	2046	7.50	9.20	69.00	81.52	8.35
SAINT CRUZ M	L	2204	7.10	10.10	71.71	70.30	8.60
SAINT CRUZ M	R	2204	7.30	10.30	75.19	70.87	8.80
SAINT CRUZ F	L	2205	7.00	9.50	66.50	73.68	8.25
SAINT CRUZ F	R	2205	8.30	10.30	85.49	80.58	9.30
HAIDA	L	1406	6.60	8.40	55.44	78.57	7.50
HAIDA	R	1406	6.90	8.50	58.65	81.18	7.70
MINNESOTA MAN	L	1419	7.50	10.50	78.75	71.43	9.00
MINNESOTA MAN	R	1419	7.40	10.50	77.70	70.48	8.95
PUNIN (EQUADOR)	L	1420	9.85	10.55	103.92	93.36	10.20
PUNIN (EQUADOR)	R	1420	9.45	11.60	109.62	81.47	10.52
ILLINCIS PK2-B1	L	1426	6.10	9.35	57.03	65.24	7.72
ILLINCIS PK2-B1	R	1426	6.10	9.30	56.73	65.59	7.70
ILLINCIS T25-2	L	1427	6.00	8.30	49.80	72.29	7.15
ILLINCIS T25-2	R	1427	6.20	8.50	52.70	72.94	7.35
ILLINCIS A-2732	L	1429	6.70	9.20	61.64	72.83	7.95
ILLINCIS A-2732	R	1429	6.60	9.00	59.40	73.33	7.80
ILLINCIS A-6890	L	1430	6.30	9.85	62.05	63.96	8.07
ILLINCIS A-4921	L	1431	7.70	10.40	80.08	74.04	9.05
ILLINCIS A-4921	R	1431	7.35	10.30	75.70	71.36	8.82
ILLINCIS PK9-B4	L	1432	7.20	9.40	67.68	76.60	8.30
ILLINCIS PK9-B4	R	1432	7.30	9.25	67.52	78.92	8.27
ILLINCIS BR19-3	L	1434	7.15	9.80	70.07	72.96	8.47
ILLINCIS BR19-3	R	1434	6.80	9.85	66.98	69.04	8.32
ILLINCIS BLUFFS	L	1435	6.60	10.05	66.33	65.67	8.32
DICKSCN MOUND	L	1501	6.80	9.10	61.88	74.73	7.95
DICKSCN MOUND	R	1501	6.90	9.32	64.31	74.03	8.11
DICKSCN MD 242	L	1505	7.90	9.95	78.60	79.40	8.92
DICKSCN MD 242	R	1505	7.75	10.22	79.20	75.83	8.98
DICKSCN MD 256	L	1506	7.80	9.10	70.98	85.71	8.45
DICKSCN MD 256	R	1506	7.60	9.40	71.44	80.85	8.50
DICKSCN MD 261	L	1508	6.90	10.15	70.03	67.98	8.52
DICKSCN MD 261	R	1508	7.10	10.00	71.00	71.00	8.55
DICKSCN MD 266	L	1510	7.80	10.10	78.78	77.23	8.95
DICKSON MD 276	L	1514	7.70	11.30	87.01	68.14	9.50
DICKSCN MD 276	R	1514	7.90	11.35	89.66	69.60	9.62
DICKSCN MD 287	L	1516	6.65	9.10	60.51	73.08	7.87
DICKSCN MD 287	R	1516	6.80	9.20	62.56	73.91	8.00
DICKSCN MD 297	L	1520	7.55	9.80	73.99	77.04	8.67

UPPER PM4 H. SAPIENS

		N	L(M-D)	B(B-L)	L*B	L/B	L+B/2
DICKSCN MD 302	L	1521	7.00	8.65	60.55	80.92	7.82
DICKSCN MD 319	L	1523	6.55	8.90	58.29	73.60	7.72
DICKSCN MD 319	R	1523	6.95	8.95	62.20	77.65	7.95
DICKSCN MD 327	L	1524	7.10	9.80	69.58	72.45	8.45
DICKSCN MD 327	R	1524	7.70	9.85	75.84	78.17	8.77
CICKSCN MD 334	L	1525	7.35	10.35	76.07	71.01	8.85
DICKSCN MD 334	R	1525	7.30	10.25	74.82	71.22	8.77
DICKSCN MD 348	L	1529	6.50	9.30	60.45	69.89	7.90
DICKSCN MD 348	R	1529	6.65	9.25	61.51	71.89	7.95
DICKSCN MD 349	L	1530	7.83	9.35	73.21	83.74	8.59
DICKSCN MD 349	R	1530	7.90	9.35	73.86	84.49	8.62
DICKSCN MD 355	L	1535	7.60	9.80	74.48	77.55	8.70
DICKSON MD 355	R	1535	7.10	9.70	68.87	73.20	8.40
DICKSCN MD 361	L	1538	7.20	9.30	66.96	77.42	8.25
DICKSCN MD 361	R	1538	6.90	9.20	63.48	75.00	8.05
DICKSCN MD 362	L	1539	7.85	9.80	76.93	80.10	8.82
DICKSCN MD 362	R	1539	7.60	9.60	72.96	79.17	8.60
DICKSCN MD 365	L	1540	6.80	9.30	63.24	73.12	8.05
DICKSCN MD 365	R	1540	6.00	9.05	54.30	66.30	7.52
DICKSCN MD 467	L	1541	6.40	9.10	58.24	70.33	7.75
DICKSCN MD 371	L	1542	7.60	10.10	76.76	75.25	8.85
DICKSCN MD 371	R	1542	7.50	9.90	74.25	75.76	8.70
DICKSON MD 372	R	1543	7.00	9.80	68.60	71.43	8.40
DICKSCN MD 379	L	1548	7.05	9.50	66.97	74.21	8.27
DICKSCN MD 379	R	1548	7.75	9.70	75.17	79.90	8.72
DICKSCN MD 380	L	1549	5.70	8.60	49.02	66.28	7.15
DICKSCN MD 380	R	1549	5.50	8.80	48.40	62.50	7.15
DICKSON MD 381	L	1550	7.40	10.30	76.22	71.84	8.85
DICKSCN MD 381	R	1550	7.40	10.50	77.70	70.48	8.95
DICKSCN MD 380	L	1551	6.40	8.50	54.40	75.29	7.45
DICKSCN MD 380	R	1551	6.30	8.40	52.92	75.00	7.35
DICKSCN MD 396	L	1553	7.40	10.00	74.00	74.00	8.70
DICKSCN MD 396	R	1553	7.20	10.10	72.72	71.29	8.65
DICKSCN MD 397	L	1554	7.40	9.50	70.30	77.89	8.45
DICKSCN MD 397	R	1554	7.30	9.30	67.89	78.49	8.30
DICKSCN MD 398	R	1555	6.70	9.30	62.31	72.04	8.00
DICKSCN MD 399	R	1556	6.25	9.35	58.44	66.84	7.80
CICKSCN MD 406	L	1560	6.70	9.40	62.98	71.28	8.05
DICKSCN MD 407	L	1561	7.10	9.50	67.45	74.74	8.30
DICKSCN MD 407	R	1561	7.30	10.15	74.09	71.92	8.72
DICKSCN MD 411	L	1563	7.23	9.35	67.60	77.33	8.29
DICKSON MD 411	R	1563	7.10	9.55	67.80	74.35	8.32
DICKSCN MD 414	L	1564	7.12	8.90	63.37	80.00	8.01
CICKSCN MD 415	L	1565	6.10	8.00	48.80	76.25	7.05
DICKSCN MD 415	R	1565	6.48	8.90	57.67	72.81	7.69
DICKSCN MD 432	L	1567	6.10	8.00	48.80	76.25	7.05
DICKSCN MD 432	R	1567	5.90	7.98	47.08	73.93	6.94
DICKSCN MD 443	L	1571	7.30	9.85	71.90	74.11	8.57
DICKSCN MD 443	R	1571	7.75	9.70	75.17	79.90	8.72
DICKSCN MD 446	L	1572	7.30	9.20	67.16	79.35	8.25

UPPER PM4 H. SAPIENS

		N	L(M-D)	B(B-L)	L*B	L/B	L+B/2
DICKSCN MD 446	R	1572	6.98	9.50	66.31	73.47	8.24
DICKSCN MD 464	L	1575	7.25	9.15	66.34	79.23	8.20
DICKSCN MD 464	R	1575	7.20	9.10	65.52	79.12	8.15
DICKSCN MD 476	L	1576	7.94	10.50	83.37	75.62	9.22
DICKSCN MD 476	R	1576	8.11	10.70	86.78	75.79	9.40
DICKSON MD 480	L	1578	6.45	9.15	59.02	70.49	7.80
DICKSCN MD 480	R	1578	6.50	8.85	57.52	73.45	7.67
DICKSCN MD 497	L	1583	8.01	11.25	90.11	71.20	9.63
DICKSCN MD 497	R	1583	7.92	10.80	85.54	73.33	9.36
DICKSCN MD 5C3	R	1585	6.90	10.10	69.69	68.32	8.50
DICKSCN MD 509	L	1587	7.03	9.16	64.39	76.75	8.09
DICKSCN MD 5C9	R	1587	7.35	10.02	73.65	73.35	8.68
DICKSCN MD 535	L	1591	7.20	9.10	65.52	79.12	8.15
DICKSCN MD 535	R	1591	6.70	9.30	62.31	72.04	8.00
DICKSCN MD 536	L	1592	7.30	9.00	65.70	81.11	8.15
DICKSCN MD 536	R	1592	7.30	9.55	69.71	76.44	8.42
DICKSCN MD 545	L	1594	7.55	10.95	82.67	68.95	9.25
DICKSCN MD 545	R	1594	7.20	10.95	78.84	65.75	9.07
DICKSCN MD 557	L	1596	6.60	9.35	61.71	70.59	7.97
DICKSCN MD 557	R	1596	6.70	9.00	60.30	74.44	7.85
DICKSGN MD 561	L	1597	7.55	10.20	77.01	74.02	8.87
DICKSCN MD 561	R	1597	7.50	10.20	76.50	73.53	8.85
DICKSCN MD 567	L	1598	7.58	10.05	76.18	75.42	8.81
DICKSCN MD 567	R	1598	7.65	10.20	78.03	75.00	8.92
DICKSCN MD 594	L	1601	6.50	9.20	59.80	70.65	7.85
DICKSCN MD 594	R	1601	6.80	9.00	61.20	75.56	7.90
DICKSCN MD 599	L	1602	6.80	9.90	67.32	68.69	8.35
DICKSCN MD 599	R	1602	6.85	10.00	68.50	68.50	8.42
DICKSCN MD 630	L	1603	6.70	8.90	59.63	75.28	7.80
DICKSCN MD 630	R	1603	6.70	8.70	58.29	77.01	7.70
DICKSCN MD 658	L	1613		9.30			
DICKSCN MD 667	L	1614	7.80	10.00	78.00	78.00	8.90
DICKSCN MD 667	R	1614	7.74	9.86	76.32	78.50	8.80
DICKSCN MD 687	L	1616	6.30	9.20	57.96	68.48	7.75
DICKSCN MD 694	L	1617	7.30	8.80	64.24	82.95	8.05
DICKSCN MD 694	R	1617	7.80	9.10	70.98	85.71	8.45
DICKSCN MD 699	R	1618	6.80	9.35	63.58	72.73	8.07
DICKSCN MD 709	L	1623	6.46	9.50	61.37	68.00	7.98
DICKSCN MD 722	L	1624	6.90	10.20	70.38	67.65	8.55
DICKSCN MD 722	R	1624	7.00	10.25	71.75	68.29	8.62
DICKSCN MD 724	L	1627	7.30	10.25	74.82	71.22	8.77
DICKSCN MD 724	R	1627	7.60	10.85	82.46	70.05	9.22
DICKSGN MD 746	L	1628	7.00	9.70	67.90	72.16	8.35
DICKSCN MD 746	R	1628	6.92	9.82	67.95	70.47	8.37
DICKSCN MD 749	L	1629	7.20	9.40	67.68	76.60	8.30

UPPER M1 H. SAPIENS

		N	L(M-D)	B(B-L)	L*B	L/B	L+B/2
PREDMCST YOUTH	L	1061	10.25	10.70	109.67	95.79	10.47
PREDMCST YOUTH	R	1061	10.20	11.10	113.22	91.89	10.65
PREDMOST 3	L	1007	11.10	11.30	125.43	98.23	11.20
PREDMOST 3	R	1007	10.40	10.60	110.24	98.11	10.50
PREDMOST 4	L	1008	9.40	9.80	92.12	95.92	9.60
PREDMCST 4	R	1008	10.35	10.20	105.57	101.47	10.27
COMBE CHAPELLE	L	1017	10.50	12.00	126.00	87.50	11.25
COMBE CHAPELLE	R	1017	10.00	12.00	120.00	83.33	11.00
BRNO 3	L	1018	10.40	11.40	118.56	91.23	10.90
BRNO 3	R	1018	9.40	11.20	105.28	83.93	10.30
GRIMALCI ADOL.	L	1019	12.30	12.80	157.44	96.09	12.55
GRIMALCI ADOL.	R	1019	12.50	12.90	161.25	96.90	12.70
LA ROCHETTE A	L	1021	9.10	12.10	110.11	75.21	10.60
ROIS R54		1047	11.00	12.00	132.00	91.67	11.50
VESTONICE 3	L	1057	10.00	11.40	114.00	87.72	10.70
VESTONICE 3	R	1057	9.90	11.50	113.85	86.09	10.70
A CULOZ 2	L	1101	10.00	13.30	133.00	75.19	11.65
A CULOZ 2	R	1101	11.00	13.00	143.00	84.62	12.00
ALAMANN 5	L	1102	10.00	11.50	115.00	86.96	10.75
ALAMANN 1288	L	1103	9.50	10.00	95.00	95.00	9.75
ALAMANN 1288	R	1103	9.00	10.00	90.00	90.00	9.50
BISCORDINE	L	1107	10.10	12.70	128.27	79.53	11.40
BISCORDINE	R	11C7	10.30	12.50	128.75	82.40	11.40
BUGGISON 1	L	1108	12.00	12.50	150.00	96.00	12.25
BUGGISCN 1	R	1108	11.50	12.00	138.00	95.83	11.75
BUGGISON 2	L	1109	11.50	12.50	143.75	92.00	12.00
BUGGISON 2	R	1109	11.50	12.50	143.75	92.00	12.00
CAP BLAC	L	1110	10.00	11.50	115.00	86.96	10.75
CAP BLAC	R	1110	9.60	11.40	109.44	84.21	10.50
EGOLZWIL 1	L	1112	10.00	11.50	115.00	86.96	10.75
EGOLZWIL 1	R	1112	10.40	11.50	119.60	90.43	10.95
ELEMENTEITA	R	1113	13.00	13.00	169.00	100.00	13.00
KOERHUISBEEK C1	L	1124	11.00	12.50	137.50	88.00	11.75
KOERHLISBEEK C1	R	1124	10.50	12.00	126.00	87.50	11.25
LAFAYE	L	1128	9.70	12.40	120.28	78.23	11.05
LAFAYE	R	1128	9.90	13.10	129.69	75.57	11.50
MASAT		1130	10.40	11.10	115.44	93.69	10.75
OKUZINI		1133		11.30			
PAS ESTRET 4	L	1135	11.50	12.80	147.20	89.84	12.15
PAS ESTRET 4	R	1135	11.40	12.40	141.36	91.94	11.90
PAS ESTRET 8	R	1137	10.10	11.50	116.15	87.83	10.80
RHUNCA	R	1142	7.70	12.90	99.33	59.69	10.30
SVAERCBORG	R	1144	11.20	12.00	134.40	93.33	11.60
FRENCHMAN	L	1149	10.05	11.00	110.55	91.36	10.52
FRENCHMAN	R	1149	10.20	10.80	110.16	94.44	10.50
ALACA HOYUK 2		1183	10.30	11.40	117.42	90.35	10.85
ALACA HOYUK 3		1184	10.20	11.30	115.26	90.27	10.75
ALACA HOYUK 8		1185	10.40	12.20	126.88	85.25	11.30
BELT CAVE	R	1189	11.00	12.30	135.30	89.43	11.65
IRAN(SIALK)	L	1190	9.65	11.00	106.15	87.73	10.32

UPPER M1 H. SAPIENS

	Side	N	L(M-D)	B(B-L)	L*B	L/B	L+B/2
IRAN(SIALK)	L	1191	10.40	10.70	111.28	97.20	10.55
IRAN(SIALK)	L	1192	9.00	10.40	93.60	86.54	9.70
JARMO 28	L	1193	9.10	12.20	111.02	74.59	10.65
JARMO 28	R	1193	10.70	13.30	142.31	80.45	12.00
WADJAK 1		1701	11.20	13.80	154.56	81.16	12.50
WADJAK 2	L	1702	11.70	13.00	152.10	90.00	12.35
WADJAK 2	R	1702	12.00	13.00	156.00	92.31	12.50
KEILOR	R	1703	11.20	13.20	147.84	84.85	12.20
TALGAI	L	1704	12.60	13.10	165.06	96.18	12.85
TALGAI	R	1704	12.70	13.00	165.10	97.69	12.85
COHUNA	L	1705	12.70	14.50	184.15	87.59	13.60
COHUNA	R	1705	12.60	14.20	178.92	88.73	13.40
AUSTRALIAN 39		1708	10.50	13.00	136.50	80.77	11.75
AUSTRALIAN 2961	L	1725		13.30			
AUSTRALIAN	L	1726	11.55	10.80	124.74	106.94	11.17
AUSTRALIAN	L	1728	10.45	12.60	131.67	82.94	11.52
AUSTRALIAN	R	1728	10.80	11.30	122.04	95.58	11.05
AUSTRALIAN 179	L	1732	12.20	12.20	148.84	100.00	12.20
AUSTRALIAN 179	R	1732	11.70	12.10	141.57	96.69	11.90
TASMANIAN 310		1754	11.00	12.00	132.00	91.67	11.50
TASMANIAN 3637	L	1755	11.75	12.40	145.70	94.76	12.07
TASMANIAN 3637	R	1755	11.80	12.35	145.73	95.55	12.07
TASMANIAN 576	R	1756	11.00	13.00	143.00	84.62	12.00
TASMANIAN P1	R	1757	11.00				
TASMANIAN P2	L	1758	11.50	13.50	155.25	85.19	12.50
TASMANIAN P2	R	1758	11.50	13.00	149.50	88.46	12.25
TASMANIAN P3	R	1759		13.00			
TASMANIAN 2966	L	1762		12.70			
TASMANIAN 2966	R	1762		13.20			
TASMANIAN 2964	R	1763	12.00	13.30	159.60	90.23	12.65
BOSKOP		1902	10.50	12.50	131.25	84.00	11.50
ASSELAR	R	1903	10.50	13.00	136.50	80.77	11.75
CAPE FLATS	R	1904	10.00	12.50	125.00	80.00	11.25
NEGRO	L	1905	11.80	12.85	151.63	91.83	12.32
NEGRO		1914	10.20	11.00	112.20	92.73	10.60
NEGRO	L	1915	13.10	12.40	162.44	105.65	12.75
BANTU 100	L	1917	12.50	12.30	153.75	101.63	12.40
BANTU 100	R	1917	12.40	12.40	153.76	100.00	12.40
BANTU 118	L	1918	11.70	10.80	126.36	108.33	11.25
BANTU 118	R	1918	12.20	11.50	140.30	106.09	11.85
MAPUNGUBWE	L	1950	10.00				
MAPUNGUBWE	R	1950	10.90				
MAPUNGUBWE M2		1952	11.30	12.00	135.60	94.17	11.65
MAPUNGUBWE M3		1953	11.70	10.50	122.85	111.43	11.10
MAPUNGUBWE M5		1954	11.00	12.50	137.50	88.00	11.75
MAPUNGUBWE M9		1955	11.00	12.50	137.50	88.00	11.75
MAPUNGUBWE M10		1956	11.60	13.00	150.80	89.23	12.30
BAMBANDYANALO21		1957	10.40	11.80	122.72	88.14	11.10
BAMBANDYANALO29		1958	10.30	11.90	122.57	86.55	11.10
BAMBANDYANALO31		1959	11.30	12.30	138.99	91.87	11.80

UPPER M1 H. SAPIENS

	Side	N	L(M-D)	B(B-L)	L*B	L/B	L+B/2
BAMBANDYANALO 3		1962	11.70	13.00	152.10	90.00	12.35
BAMBANDYANALO13		1964	12.60	12.00	151.20	105.00	12.30
BAMBANDYANALO14		1965	10.50	11.20	117.60	93.75	10.85
ZITZIKAMA		1966	9.50	10.00	95.00	95.00	9.75
BUSHMAN		1967	9.90	10.60	104.94	93.40	10.25
FISH HOEK	R	1972	9.00	10.50	94.50	85.71	9.75
N.BRITAIN 43121	L	1301	11.40	12.00	136.80	95.00	11.70
N.BRITAIN 43123	L	1303	11.00	12.20	134.20	90.16	11.60
N.BRITAIN 43124	L	1304	10.40	11.40	118.56	91.23	10.90
N.BRITAIN 43124	R	1304	10.30	11.40	117.42	90.35	10.85
N.BRITAIN 43126	L	1305	10.70	12.40	132.68	86.29	11.55
N.BRITAIN 43126	R	1305	10.70	12.30	131.61	86.99	11.50
N.BRITAIN 43127	L	1306	10.90	11.90	129.71	91.60	11.40
N.BRITAIN 43127	R	1306	11.00	11.90	130.90	92.44	11.45
N.BRITAIN 43130	L	1307	11.00	12.60	138.60	87.30	11.80
N.BRITAIN 43130	R	1307	10.50	12.50	131.25	84.00	11.50
N.BRITAIN 43131	L	1308	11.40	12.80	145.92	89.06	12.10
N.BRITAIN 43131	R	1308	11.10	12.80	142.08	86.72	11.95
N.BRITAIN 43132	L	1309	9.90	11.90	117.81	83.19	10.90
N.BRITAIN 43132	R	1309	9.70	11.80	114.46	82.20	10.75
N.BRITAIN 43134	L	1311	11.10	12.10	134.31	91.74	11.60
N.BRITAIN 43134	R	1311	11.00	12.10	133.10	90.91	11.55
N.BRITAIN 43135	L	1312	10.60	11.20	118.72	94.64	10.90
N.BRITAIN 43135	R	1312	10.70	11.70	125.19	91.45	11.20
N.BRITAIN 43136	L	1313	10.40	11.10	115.44	93.69	10.75
N.BRITAIN 43136	R	1313	11.20	11.30	126.56	99.12	11.25
N.BRITAIN 43137	L	1314	10.80	11.90	128.52	90.76	11.35
N.BRITAIN 43137	R	1314	10.80	11.80	127.44	91.53	11.30
N.BRITAIN 43138	L	1315	10.90	11.70	127.53	93.16	11.30
N.BRITAIN 43138	R	1315	11.10	11.90	132.09	93.28	11.50
N.BRITAIN 43139	L	1316	11.30	11.70	132.21	96.58	11.50
N.BRITAIN 43139	R	1316	11.60	11.80	136.88	98.31	11.70
N.BRITAIN 43140	R	1317	10.80	12.10	130.68	89.26	11.45
N.BRITAIN 43141	L	1318	11.40	11.60	132.24	98.28	11.50
N.BRITAIN 43141	R	1318	11.20	11.50	128.80	97.39	11.35
N.BRITAIN 43142	L	1319	11.70	13.30	155.61	87.97	12.50
N.BRITAIN 43142	R	1319	12.20	13.40	163.48	91.04	12.80
N.BRITAIN 43143	L	1320	11.80	12.40	146.32	95.16	12.10
N.BRITAIN 43143	R	1320	11.60	12.50	145.00	92.80	12.05
N.BRITAIN 43144	L	1321	11.80	12.80	151.04	92.19	12.30
N.BRITAIN 43144	R	1321	12.70	12.80	162.56	99.22	12.75
N.BRITAIN 43146	L	1323	11.70	12.00	140.40	97.50	11.85
N.BRITAIN 43146	R	1323	12.10	11.80	142.78	102.54	11.95
N.BRITAIN 43147	L	1324	12.50	12.20	152.50	102.46	12.35
N.BRITAIN 43147	R	1324	12.90	12.10	156.09	106.61	12.50
N.BRITAIN 43149	R	1325	11.20	11.60	129.92	96.55	11.40
N.BRITAIN 43150	L	1326	11.30	12.60	142.38	89.68	11.95
N.BRITAIN 43150	R	1326	11.10	12.80	142.08	86.72	11.95
N.BRITAIN 43151	L	1327	11.20	11.80	132.16	94.92	11.50
N.BRITAIN 43151	R	1327	11.70	11.90	139.23	98.32	11.80

UPPER M1 H. SAPIENS

Specimen	Side	N	L(M-D)	B(B-L)	L*B	L/B	L+B/2
N.BRITAIN 43152	L	1328	11.20	12.60	141.12	88.89	11.90
N.BRITAIN 43153	L	1329	10.10	11.60	117.16	87.07	10.85
N.BRITAIN 43153	R	1329	9.90	11.30	111.87	87.61	10.60
N.BRITAIN 43154	L	1330	11.60	12.80	148.48	90.62	12.20
N.BRITAIN 43154	R	1330	11.30	12.70	143.51	88.98	12.00
N.BRITAIN 43174	L	1331	11.30	12.70	143.51	88.98	12.00
N.BRITAIN 43174	R	1331	11.40	12.70	144.78	89.76	12.05
N.BRITAIN 43179	L	1332	12.00	12.10	145.20	99.17	12.05
N.BRITAIN 43179	R	1332	11.00	12.00	132.00	91.67	11.50
N.BRITAIN 43193	L	1333	11.90	11.70	139.23	101.71	11.80
N.BRITAIN 43193	R	1333	11.50	11.80	135.70	97.46	11.65
N.BRITAIN 43194	L	1334	11.20	11.70	131.04	95.73	11.45
N.BRITAIN 43194	R	1334	11.40	11.40	129.96	100.00	11.40
N.BRITAIN 43198	L	1335	12.20	12.40	151.28	98.39	12.30
N.BRITAIN 43198	R	1335	12.00	12.70	152.40	94.49	12.35
N.BRITAIN 43199	L	1336	12.10	12.30	148.83	98.37	12.20
N.BRITAIN 43199	R	1336	12.40	12.40	153.76	100.00	12.40
N.BRITAIN 43202	L	1337	12.40	12.80	158.72	96.87	12.60
N.BRITAIN 43202	R	1337	12.60	12.50	157.50	100.80	12.55
N.BRITAIN 43204	L	1338	11.60	13.50	156.60	85.93	12.55
N.BRITAIN 43204	R	1338	11.40	13.40	152.76	85.07	12.40
N.BRITAIN 43226	L	1339	11.00	11.10	122.10	99.10	11.05
N.BRITAIN 43226	R	1339	10.90	11.20	122.08	97.32	11.05
N.BRITAIN 43329	L	1340	12.00	13.80	165.60	86.96	12.90
N.BRITAIN 43329	R	1340	13.00	13.80	179.40	94.20	13.40
N.BRITAIN 43242	L	1341	10.50	11.30	118.65	92.92	10.90
N.BRITAIN 43242	R	1341	11.50	11.60	133.40	99.14	11.55
N.BRITAIN 43290	L	1342	11.80	12.20	143.96	96.72	12.00
N.BRITAIN 43290	R	1342	11.80	12.20	143.96	96.72	12.00
N.BRITAIN 43291	L	1343	11.00	12.10	133.10	90.91	11.55
N.BRITAIN 43291	R	1343	12.10	12.00	145.20	100.83	12.05
N.BRITAIN 43295	L	1344	11.60	13.10	151.96	88.55	12.35
N.BRITAIN 43295	R	1344	12.70	13.10	166.37	96.95	12.90
N.BRITAIN	L	1346	11.15	11.50	128.22	96.96	11.32
N.BRITAIN	R	1346	10.40	11.70	121.68	88.89	11.05
HINDU (UI)	L	2208	10.15	11.30	114.69	89.82	10.72
HINDU (UI)	R	2208	10.50	11.50	120.75	91.30	11.00
HARAPPA 1	L	1801	10.00	11.50	115.00	86.96	10.75
HARAPPA 1	R	1801	9.50	11.50	109.25	82.61	10.50
HARAPPA 2	L	1802	11.00	12.00	132.00	91.67	11.50
HARAPPA 2	R	1802	10.00	10.50	105.00	95.24	10.25
HARAPPA 3	L	1803	11.00	12.00	132.00	91.67	11.50
HARAPPA 3	R	1803	10.50	11.50	120.75	91.30	11.00
HARAPPA 4	L	1804	10.00	11.50	115.00	86.96	10.75
HARAPPA 4	R	1804	9.50	11.50	109.25	82.61	10.50
HARAPPA 7	L	1806	10.00	10.50	105.00	95.24	10.25
HARAPPA 7	R	1806	10.00	11.00	110.00	90.91	10.50
HARAPPA 10	R	1807	11.00	12.00	132.00	91.67	11.50
HARAPPA 11	R	1808	10.00	10.50	105.00	95.24	10.25
HARAPPA 12	L	1809	9.50	9.00	85.50	105.56	9.25

UPPER M1 H. SAPIENS

Specimen	Side	N	L(M-D)	B(B-L)	L*B	L/B	L+B/2
HARAPPA 12	R	1809	11.00	11.00	121.00	100.00	11.00
HARAPPA 13	L	1810	10.50	11.50	120.75	91.30	11.00
HARAPPA 13	R	1810	11.00	11.00	121.00	100.00	11.00
HARAPPA 15	L	1812	10.00	11.50	115.00	86.96	10.75
HARAPPA 15	R	1812	11.00	11.50	126.50	95.65	11.25
HARAPPA 16	L	1813	11.00	12.00	132.00	91.67	11.50
HARAPPA 16	R	1813	10.00	10.50	105.00	95.24	10.25
HARAPPA 17	R	1814	10.00	10.00	100.00	100.00	10.00
HARAPPA 20	L	1816	10.00				
HARAPPA 21	L	1817	10.90	9.00	98.10	121.11	9.95
HARAPPA 21	R	1817	10.00	9.00	90.00	111.11	9.50
HARAPPA 23	L	1818	10.00	10.00	100.00	100.00	10.00
HARAPPA 23	R	1818	10.00	9.00	90.00	111.11	9.50
HARAPPA 25	L	1819	10.00	12.00	120.00	83.33	11.00
HARAPPA 25	R	1819	10.00	12.00	120.00	83.33	11.00
HARAPPA 15	L	1812	10.00	11.00	110.00	90.91	10.50
HARAPPA 15	R	1812	10.00	10.50	105.00	95.24	10.25
HARAPPA 32	L	1822	10.50	11.00	115.50	95.45	10.75
HARAPPA 32	R	1822	10.50	11.00	115.50	95.45	10.75
HARAPPA 35	L	1823	10.00	11.00	110.00	90.91	10.50
HARAPPA 35	R	1823	10.00	11.50	115.00	86.96	10.75
HARAPPA 36	L	1824	10.50	10.00	105.00	105.00	10.25
HARAPPA 36	R	1824	9.50	10.50	99.75	90.48	10.00
HARAPPA 37	L	1825	11.00	11.50	126.50	95.65	11.25
HARAPPA 37	R	1825	10.00	11.00	110.00	90.91	10.50
HARAPPA 38	L	1826	10.00	11.50	115.00	86.96	10.75
HARAPPA 38	R	1826	10.50	12.00	126.00	87.50	11.25
HARAPPA 39	L	1827	11.50	11.50	132.25	100.00	11.50
HARAPPA 39	R	1827	10.00	11.50	115.00	86.96	10.75
HARAPPA 40	L	1828	11.00	12.00	132.00	91.67	11.50
HARAPPA 40	R	1828	11.00	11.50	126.50	95.65	11.25
HARAPPA 41	R	1829	11.50	11.50	132.25	100.00	11.50
HARAPPA 42	L	1830	10.00	11.00	110.00	90.91	10.50
HARAPPA 43	R	1831	10.00	12.00	120.00	83.33	11.00
HARAPPA 44	L	1832	9.50	11.00	104.50	86.36	10.25
HARAPPA 44	R	1832	9.00	11.00	99.00	81.82	10.00
HARAPPA 45	L	1833	11.00	11.50	126.50	95.65	11.25
HARAPPA 45	R	1833	11.00	12.00	132.00	91.67	11.50
HARAPPA 46	L	1834	9.00	11.00	99.00	81.82	10.00
HARAPPA 46	R	1834	11.00	11.00	121.00	100.00	11.00
HARAPPA 47	L	1835	6.50	7.00	45.50	92.86	6.75
HARAPPA 47	R	1835	6.50	7.00	45.50	92.86	6.75
HARAPPA 49	L	1837	6.00	7.00	42.00	85.71	6.50
HARAPPA 49	R	1837	7.00	8.00	56.00	87.50	7.50
HARAPPA 51	L	1838	7.00	7.00	49.00	100.00	7.00
HARAPPA 51	R	1838	7.00	8.00	56.00	87.50	7.50
HARAPPA 52	L	1839	9.00	10.50	94.50	85.71	9.75
HARAPPA 52	R	1839	9.00	11.00	99.00	81.82	10.00
HARAPPA 53	R	1840	10.00	9.00	90.00	111.11	9.50
HARAPPA 54	L	1841	11.00	11.00	121.00	100.00	11.00

UPPER M1 H. SAPIENS

			N	L(M-D)	B(B-L)	L*B	L/B	L+B/2
HARAPPA 54		R	1841	11.00	11.00	121.00	100.00	11.00
HARAPPA 55		L	1842	7.00	8.00	56.00	87.50	7.50
HARAPPA 56		L	1843	9.00	10.50	94.50	85.71	9.75
HARAPPA 56		R	1843	9.50	11.00	104.50	86.36	10.25
HARAPPA 58		L	1844	10.00	11.00	110.00	90.91	10.50
HARAPPA 58		R	1844	10.00	11.00	110.00	90.91	10.50
HARAPPA 59		L	1845	9.50	12.00	114.00	79.17	10.75
HARAPPA 59		R	1845	10.50	12.00	126.00	87.50	11.25
HARAPPA 60		L	1846	10.00	11.50	115.00	86.96	10.75
HARAPPA 60		R	1846	10.00	12.00	120.00	83.33	11.00
HARAPPA 61		L	1847	11.50	11.00	126.50	104.55	11.25
HARAPPA 61		R	1847	11.00	10.50	115.50	104.76	10.75
HARAPPA 62		L	1848	10.00	11.00	110.00	90.91	10.50
HARAPPA 62		R	1848	10.50	11.00	115.50	95.45	10.75
HARAPPA 63		L	1849	10.00	10.00	100.00	100.00	10.00
HARAPPA 63		R	1849	10.00	10.50	105.00	95.24	10.25
HARAPPA 64		R	1850	9.00	11.50	103.50	78.26	10.25
HARAPPA 66		L	1852	11.00	11.50	126.50	95.65	11.25
HARAPPA 66		R	1852	10.50	11.50	120.75	91.30	11.00
HARAPPA 69		L	1853	10.50	12.00	126.00	87.50	11.25
HARAPPA 69		R	1853	11.00	12.50	137.50	88.00	11.75
HARAPPA 70		R	1854	11.00	12.50	137.50	88.00	11.75
HARAPPA 74		R	1857	11.00	12.00	132.00	91.67	11.50
HARAPPA 81		L	1859	10.50	11.00	115.50	95.45	10.75
HARAPPA 81		R	1859	11.00	11.00	121.00	100.00	11.00
HARAPPA 85		L	1860	10.50	11.00	115.50	95.45	10.75
HARAPPA 85		R	1860	10.00	11.50	115.00	86.96	10.75
GOL BA IT 95		L	2002		12.20			
GOL BA IT 95		R	2002		11.80			
GOL BA IT 98		L	2003		11.80			
GOL BA IT		L	2008	11.70	12.40	145.08	94.35	12.05
MELOLO		L	2047	8.80	12.20	107.36	72.13	10.50
MELOLO		L	2048	10.20	10.30	105.06	99.03	10.25
MELOLO		R	2049	9.50	12.40	117.80	76.61	10.95
MELOLO		R	2050	9.30	10.20	94.86	91.18	9.75
MELOLO		L	2051	9.80	10.30	100.94	95.15	10.05
MELOLO		L	2052	9.10	11.20	101.92	81.25	10.15
MELOLO		R	2053	10.90	11.30	123.17	96.46	11.10
MELOLO		L	2054	11.40	12.00	136.80	95.00	11.70
MELOLO		R	2055	10.90	11.00	119.90	99.09	10.95
MELOLO		L	2056	11.00	11.00	121.00	100.00	11.00
MELOLO		R	2057	10.60	11.10	117.66	95.50	10.85
MELOLO		R	2025	10.40	10.90	113.36	95.41	10.65
MELOLO		R	2059	10.80	11.30	122.04	95.58	11.05
MELOLO		R	2060	10.50	11.40	119.70	92.11	10.95
MELOLO		L	2061	10.20	11.40	116.28	89.47	10.80
MELOLO		R	2062	11.20	12.00	134.40	93.33	11.60
MELOLO		L	2063	10.50	10.70	112.35	98.13	10.60
MELOLO		L	2064	9.50	10.30	97.85	92.23	9.90
SAINT CRUZ	M	L	2204	11.40	12.20	139.08	93.44	11.80

UPPER M1 H. SAPIENS

			N	L(M-D)	B(B-L)	L*B	L/B	L+B/2
SAINT CRUZ	M	R	2204	10.90	11.90	129.71	91.60	11.40
SAINT CRUZ	F	L	2205	10.90	11.60	126.44	93.97	11.25
SAINT CRUZ	F	R	2205	10.70	11.10	118.77	96.40	10.90
CHANG YANG			2203	10.60	12.80	135.68	82.81	11.70
HAIDA		L	1406	11.80	12.20	143.96	96.72	12.00
HAIDA		R	1406	12.30	12.00	147.60	102.50	12.15
MINNESOTA MAN		L	1419	11.50	12.70	146.05	90.55	12.10
MINNESOTA MAN		R	1419	11.50	10.50	120.75	109.52	11.00
PUNIN (EQUADOR)		L	1420	11.50	12.50	143.75	92.00	12.00
PUNIN (EQUADOR)		R	1420	12.10	12.50	151.25	96.80	12.30
ILLINOIS PK2-B1		L	1426	11.00	12.60	138.60	87.30	11.80
ILLINOIS PK2-B1		R	1426	11.10	12.65	140.41	87.75	11.87
ILLINOIS T25-2		L	1427	10.50	12.60	132.30	83.33	11.55
ILLINOIS T25-2		R	1427	10.80	12.50	135.00	86.40	11.65
ILLINOIS A-2732		L	1429	10.90	11.50	125.35	94.78	11.20
ILLINOIS A-2732		R	1429	10.60	11.35	120.31	93.39	10.97
ILLINOIS A-6890		L	1430	10.50	11.40	119.70	92.11	10.95
ILLINOIS A-6890		R	1430	10.30	11.30	116.39	91.15	10.80
ILLINOIS A-4921		L	1431	10.40	12.30	127.92	84.55	11.35
ILLINOIS A-4921		R	1431	11.00	12.35	135.85	89.07	11.67
ILLINOIS PK9-B4		L	1432	11.10	11.00	122.10	100.91	11.05
ILLINOIS PK9-B4		R	1432	11.30	11.05	124.86	102.26	11.17
ILLINOIS PK9-B1		L	1433	11.00	13.50	148.50	81.48	12.25
ILLINOIS PK9-B1		R	1433	10.60	13.15	139.39	80.61	11.87
ILLINOIS BR19-3		L	1434	10.30	11.95	123.08	86.19	11.12
ILLINOIS BR19-3		R	1434	10.25	11.90	121.97	86.13	11.07
ILLINOIS BLUFFS		L	1435	10.35	12.35	127.82	83.81	11.35
ILLINOIS BLUFFS		R	1435	9.90	12.05	119.29	82.16	10.97
DICKSON MOUND		L	1501	10.65	11.90	126.73	89.50	11.27
DICKSON MOUND		R	1501	10.80	11.80	127.44	91.53	11.30
DICKSON MOUND		R	1502	10.85	12.10	131.28	89.67	11.47
DICKSON MD 242		L	1505	11.45	12.45	142.55	91.97	11.95
DICKSON MD 242		R	1505	11.60	12.55	145.58	92.43	12.07
DICKSON MD 256		L	1506	10.65	11.55	123.01	92.21	11.10
DICKSON MD 256		R	1506	10.52	11.40	119.93	92.28	10.96
DICKSON MD 258		R	1507	9.85	11.10	109.33	88.74	10.47
DICKSON MD 261		R	1508	9.90	11.15	110.38	88.79	10.52
DICKSON MD 262		L	1509	11.35	12.40	140.74	91.53	11.87
DICKSON MD 262		R	1509	11.50	12.50	143.75	92.00	12.00
DICKSON MD 266		L	1510	11.20	12.20	136.64	91.80	11.70
DICKSON MD 276		L	1514	12.30	13.83	170.11	88.94	13.06
DICKSON MD 276		R	1514	12.20	13.80	168.36	88.41	13.00
DICKSON MD 287		L	1516	11.35	12.20	138.47	93.03	11.77
DICKSON MD 287		R	1516	11.10	12.20	135.42	90.98	11.65
DICKSON MD 291		L	1518	11.50	12.05	138.57	95.44	11.77
DICKSON MD 291		R	1518	10.90	12.15	132.43	89.71	11.52
DICKSON MD 292		R	1519	10.55	11.75	123.96	89.79	11.15
DICKSON MD 297		L	1520	11.50	12.50	143.75	92.00	12.00
DICKSON MD 302		L	1521	10.00	10.85	108.50	92.17	10.42
DICKSON MD 302		R	1521	9.80	10.80	105.84	90.74	10.30

UPPER M1 H. SAPIENS

		N	L(M-D)	B(B-L)	L*B	L/B	L+B/2
DICKSCN MD	319 L	1523	11.50	11.90	136.85	96.64	11.70
DICKSCN MD	319 R	1523	11.40	11.90	135.66	95.80	11.65
DICKSON MD	327 L	1524	10.45	11.85	123.83	88.19	11.15
DICKSCN MD	327 R	1524	10.30	12.00	123.60	85.83	11.15
DICKSCN MD	334 L	1525	10.60	13.00	137.80	81.54	11.80
DICKSCN MD	334 R	1525	10.60	13.05	138.33	81.23	11.82
DICKSCN MD	342 R	1526	.20	11.30	2.26	1.77	5.75
DICKSCN MD	344 L	1527	9.45	12.00	113.40	78.75	10.72
DICKSCN MD	348 L	1529	9.60	11.00	105.60	87.27	10.30
DICKSCN MD	348 R	1529	9.70	10.85	105.24	89.40	10.27
DICKSCN MD	349 L	1530	10.55	11.50	121.32	91.74	11.02
DICKSCN MD	349 R	1530	10.55	11.55	121.85	91.34	11.05
DICKSCN MD	351 R	1532	11.65	11.65	135.72	100.00	11.65
DICKSCN MD	352 L	1533	11.30	12.00	135.60	94.17	11.65
DICKSCN MD	352 R	1533	10.90	12.25	133.52	88.98	11.57
DICKSCN MD	355 L	1535	12.10	12.00	145.20	100.83	12.05
DICKSCN MD	355 R	1535	11.45	12.20	139.69	93.85	11.82
DICKSON MD	361 L	1538	11.00	11.70	128.70	94.02	11.35
DICKSCN MD	361 R	1538	10.80	11.90	128.52	90.76	11.35
DICKSCN MD	362 L	1539	11.00	11.70	128.70	94.02	11.35
DICKSCN MD	362 R	1539	11.40	11.80	134.52	96.61	11.60
DICKSCN MD	365 L	1540	10.70	11.30	120.91	94.69	11.00
DICKSCN MD	365 R	1540	10.50	11.80	123.90	88.98	11.15
DICKSCN MD	467 L	1541	9.50	12.10	114.95	78.51	10.80
DICKSCN MD	371 L	1542	10.40	12.20	126.88	85.25	11.30
DICKSCN MD	371 R	1542	10.70	12.00	128.40	89.17	11.35
DICKSCN MD	372 L	1543	10.70	11.90	127.33	89.92	11.30
DICKSCN MD	372 R	1543	10.70	12.40	132.68	86.29	11.55
DICKSCN MD	378 L	1547	9.90	10.70	105.93	92.52	10.30
DICKSCN MD	379 L	1548	10.80	12.10	130.68	89.26	11.45
DICKSCN MD	379 R	1548	11.30	12.15	137.29	93.00	11.72
DICKSCN MD	380 L	1549	9.90	11.90	117.81	83.19	10.90
DICKSCN MD	380 R	1549	10.60	11.70	124.02	90.60	11.15
DICKSCN MD	381 L	1550	10.60	12.20	129.32	86.89	11.40
DICKSCN MD	381 R	1550	10.70	12.10	129.47	88.43	11.40
DICKSCN MD	380 L	1551	9.30	10.40	96.72	89.42	9.85
DICKSCN MD	380 R	1551	9.20	10.00	92.00	92.00	9.60
DICKSCN MD	388 R	1552	11.30	12.40	140.12	91.13	11.85
DICKSCN MD	396 L	1553	11.60	12.80	148.48	90.62	12.20
DICKSCN MD	396 R	1553	11.20	12.70	142.24	88.19	11.95
DICKSCN MD	397 L	1554	12.30	12.50	153.75	98.40	12.40
DICKSCN MD	397 R	1554	11.10	12.90	143.19	86.05	12.00
DICKSCN MD	398 L	1555	10.10	11.20	113.12	90.18	10.65
DICKSCN MD	398 R	1555	9.50	11.20	106.40	84.82	10.35
DICKSCN MD	399 L	1556	9.50	11.60	110.20	81.90	10.55
DICKSCN MD	399 R	1556	10.00	11.00	110.00	90.91	10.50
DICKSCN MD	402 L	1557	13.00	13.10	170.30	99.24	13.05
DICKSCN MD	402 R	1557	10.70	13.40	143.38	79.85	12.05
DICKSCN MD	406 L	1560	9.90	11.30	111.87	87.61	10.60
DICKSCN MD	407 L	1561	11.20	12.25	137.20	91.43	11.72

UPPER M1 H. SAPIENS

		N	L(M-D)	B(B-L)	L*B	L/B	L+B/2
DICKSON MD	407 L	1561	11.20	12.25	137.20	91.43	11.72
DICKSON MD	407 R	1561	11.45	12.30	140.83	93.09	11.87
DICKSON MD	411 L	1563	11.45	11.55	132.25	99.13	11.50
DICKSON MD	411 R	1563	11.64	11.85	137.93	98.23	11.74
DICKSON MD	414 L	1564	10.22	11.35	116.00	90.04	10.78
DICKSCN MD	415 L	1565	10.70	12.05	128.93	88.80	11.37
DICKSCN MD	415 R	1565	10.80	11.90	128.52	90.76	11.35
DICKSON MD	426 L	1566	10.25	11.55	118.39	88.74	10.90
DICKSCN MD	426 R	1566	10.34	11.22	116.01	92.16	10.78
DICKSON MD	432 L	1567	9.35	10.80	100.98	86.57	10.07
DICKSON MD	432 R	1567	9.20	10.95	100.74	84.02	10.07
DICKSCN MD	441 L	1569	11.55	11.40	131.67	101.32	11.47
DICKSON MD	443 L	1571	11.70	12.60	147.42	92.86	12.15
DICKSCN MD	443 R	1571	11.85	12.55	148.72	94.42	12.20
DICKSCN MD	446 L	1572	10.40	11.70	121.68	88.89	11.05
DICKSCN MD	447 L	1573	9.70	11.30	109.61	85.84	10.50
DICKSCN MD	447 R	1573	10.35	11.20	115.92	92.41	10.77
DICKSCN MD	448 L	1574	10.60	11.12	117.87	95.32	10.86
DICKSON MD	448 R	1574	10.90	10.90	118.81	100.00	10.90
DICKSON MD	464 L	1575	11.00	12.15	133.65	90.53	11.57
DICKSCN MD	464 R	1575	10.25	12.30	126.07	83.33	11.27
DICKSCN MD	476 L	1576	11.50	12.30	141.45	93.50	11.90
DICKSCN MD	476 R	1576	11.30	12.20	137.86	92.62	11.75
DICKSCN MD	478 L	1577	12.45	12.42	154.63	100.24	12.43
DICKSON MD	480 L	1578	10.40	10.70	111.28	97.20	10.55
DICKSCN MD	480 R	1578	10.80	10.85	117.18	99.54	10.82
DICKSCN MD	497 L	1583	11.85	12.68	150.26	93.45	12.26
DICKSON MD	497 R	1583	11.50	13.10	150.65	87.79	12.30
DICKSCN MD	503 L	1585	11.00	12.75	140.25	86.27	11.87
DICKSCN MD	503 R	1585	10.15	12.40	125.86	81.85	11.27
DICKSCN MD	509 L	1587	11.20	12.30	137.76	91.06	11.75
DICKSON MD	509 R	1587	11.32	12.30	139.24	92.03	11.81
DICKSCN MD	535 L	1591	11.10	12.00	133.20	92.50	11.55
DICKSCN MD	536 L	1592	11.10	12.00	133.20	92.50	11.55
DICKSON MD	536 R	1592	10.80	12.00	129.60	90.00	11.40
DICKSCN MD	545 L	1594	11.60	12.95	150.22	89.58	12.27
DICKSCN MD	545 R	1594	11.10	12.80	142.08	86.72	11.95
DICKSCN MD	557 L	1596	10.30	11.70	120.51	88.03	11.00
DICKSCN MD	557 R	1596	10.60	11.30	119.78	93.81	10.95
DICKSON MD	561 L	1597	10.65	12.50	133.12	85.20	11.57
DICKSCN MD	561 R	1597	10.90	12.60	137.34	86.51	11.75
DICKSCN MD	567 L	1598	11.50	12.35	142.02	93.12	11.92
DICKSCN MD	567 R	1598	11.00	12.35	135.85	89.07	11.67
DICKSON MD	594 L	1601	9.80	11.80	115.64	83.05	10.80
DICKSON MD	594 R	1601	10.35	11.60	120.06	89.22	10.97
DICKSON MD	599 L	1602	10.45	12.45	130.10	83.94	11.45
DICKSCN MD	630 L	1603	11.60	12.40	143.84	93.55	12.00
DICKSCN MD	630 R	1603	11.40	12.60	143.64	90.48	12.00
DICKSCN MD	633 R	1604	9.70	11.50	111.55	84.35	10.60
DICKSON MD	642 L	1607	11.00	12.00	132.00	91.67	11.50

UPPER M1   H. SAPIENS

		N	L(M-D)	B(B-L)	L*B	L/B	L+B/2
DICKSCN MD	643 L	1608	9.70	11.90	115.43	81.51	10.80
DICKSCN MD	651 L	1610	9.90	10.90	107.91	90.83	10.40
DICKSCN MD	651 R	1610	9.93	10.90	108.24	91.10	10.41
DICKSCN MD	652 R	1611	10.90	12.00	130.80	90.83	11.45
DICKSCN MD	658 L	1613	10.50	11.90	124.95	88.24	11.20
DICKSCN MD	667 L	1614	10.88	12.47	135.67	87.25	11.67
DICKSCN MD	667 R	1614	10.80	12.60	136.08	85.71	11.70
DICKSCN MD	687 L	1616	9.60	11.00	105.60	87.27	10.30
DICKSCN MD	687 R	1616	9.90	11.50	113.85	86.09	10.70
DICKSCN MD	694 L	1617	10.60	11.00	116.60	96.36	10.80
DICKSCN MD	694 R	1617	10.30	11.20	115.36	91.96	10.75
DICKSCN MD	699 R	1618	11.00	12.30	135.30	89.43	11.65
DICKSCN MD	724 L	1627	10.80	11.75	126.90	91.91	11.27
DICKSCN MD	724 R	1627	10.45	12.15	126.97	86.01	11.30
DICKSCN MD	746 L	1628	10.70	12.20	130.54	87.70	11.45
DICKSCN MD	746 R	1628	10.55	11.90	125.54	88.66	11.22
DICKSCN MD	749 L	1629	11.00	12.05	132.55	91.29	11.52
DICKSCN MD	749 R	1629	10.15	11.90	120.78	85.29	11.02

UPPER M2   H. SAPIENS

		N	L(M-D)	B(B-L)	L*B	L/B	L+B/2
PREDMCST 3	L	1007	10.90	10.15	110.63	107.39	10.52
PREDMOST 3	R	1007	10.80	11.90	128.52	90.76	11.35
PREDMCST 4	L	1008	8.65	9.50	82.17	91.05	9.07
PREDMOST 4	R	1008	9.80	10.20	99.96	96.08	10.00
COMBE CHAPELLE	L	1017	10.80	12.00	129.60	90.00	11.40
COMBE CHAPELLE	R	1017	10.50	12.00	126.00	87.50	11.25
BRNO 3	L	1018	9.60	11.40	109.44	84.21	10.50
BRNO 3	R	1018	9.00	10.90	98.10	82.57	9.95
GRIMALDI ADOL.	L	1019	11.10	13.30	147.63	83.46	12.20
GRIMALDI ADOL.	R	1019	11.20	13.30	148.96	84.21	12.25
LA ROCHETTE A	L	1021	11.50	12.00	138.00	95.83	11.75
VESTONICE 3	L	1057	9.80	11.50	112.70	85.22	10.65
VESTONICE 3	R	1057	9.80	11.40	111.72	85.96	10.60
A CULOZ 2	L	1101	10.20	12.00	122.40	85.00	11.10
A CULOZ 2	R	1101	10.00	12.00	120.00	83.33	11.00
ALAMANN 1288	L	1103	7.50	10.00	75.00	75.00	8.75
ALAMANN 1288	R	1103	7.00	9.00	63.00	77.78	8.00
BISCORDINE	L	1107	9.60	13.00	124.80	73.85	11.30
BISCORDINE	R	1107	9.80	13.10	128.38	74.81	11.45
BUGGISON 1	L	1108	10.00	12.00	120.00	83.33	11.00
BUGGISON 1	R	1108	10.50	12.00	126.00	87.50	11.25
BUGGISON 2	L	1109	10.00	11.50	115.00	86.96	10.75
BUGGISON 2	R	1109	11.00	12.00	132.00	91.67	11.50
CAP BLAC	L	1110	9.80	12.00	117.60	81.67	10.90
CAP BLAC	R	1110	9.00	11.20	100.80	80.36	10.10
EGOLZWIL 1	L	1112	8.60	10.70	92.02	80.37	9.65
EGOLZWIL 1	R	1112	8.30	10.50	87.15	79.05	9.40
ISTURITZ 2		1121	11.00	12.00	132.00	91.67	11.50
KOERHUISBEEK C1	L	1124	10.50	13.00	136.50	80.77	11.75
KOERHUISBEEK C1	R	1124	10.00	12.00	120.00	83.33	11.00
LAFAYE	L	1128	9.30	12.70	118.11	73.23	11.00
MASAT		1130	9.80	11.20	109.76	87.50	10.50
RHUNCA	R	1142	9.60	12.40	119.04	77.42	11.00
SVAERCBORG	R	1144	10.40	11.60	120.64	89.66	11.00
FRENCHMAN	L	1149	8.40	10.90	91.56	77.06	9.65
FRENCHMAN	R	1149	9.05	11.00	99.55	82.27	10.02
ALACA HOYUK 2		1183	9.70	11.00	106.70	88.18	10.35
ALACA HOYUK 3		1184	10.00	11.30	113.00	88.50	10.65
BELT CAVE	R	1189	10.40	12.00	124.80	86.67	11.20
IRAN(SIALK)	L	1190	7.80	11.60	90.48	67.24	9.70
IRAN(SIALK)	L	1191	8.20	9.00	73.80	91.11	8.60
IRAN(SIALK)	L	1192	9.10	10.40	94.64	87.50	9.75
JARMO 28	L	1193	10.65	11.90	126.73	89.50	11.27
JARMO 28	R	1193	10.80	12.40	133.92	87.10	11.60
WADJAK 1		1701	10.60	14.20	150.52	74.65	12.40
WADJAK 2	L	1702	10.30	13.40	138.02	76.87	11.85
WADJAK 2	R	1702	11.00	13.50	148.50	81.48	12.25
KEILOR	R	1703	9.90	13.00	128.70	76.15	11.45
TALGAI	L	1704	11.30	13.50	152.55	83.70	12.40
TALGAI	R	1704	11.60	14.10	163.56	82.27	12.85

UPPER M2 H. SAPIENS

		N	L(M-D)	B(B-L)	L*B	L/B	L+B/2
COHUNA	L	1705	12.00	14.50	174.00	82.76	13.25
COHUNA	R	1705	12.10	14.40	174.24	84.03	13.25
AUSTRALIAN 39		1708	10.20	13.00	132.60	78.46	11.60
AUSTRALIAN 2961	R	1725		13.10			
AUSTRALIAN	L	1726	10.25	10.30	105.57	99.51	10.27
AUSTRALIAN	L	1728	10.20	12.00	122.40	85.00	11.10
AUSTRALIAN	R	1728	10.30	10.50	108.15	98.10	10.40
AUSTRALIAN 179	L	1732	11.40	10.60	120.84	107.55	11.00
AUSTRALIAN 179	R	1732	11.40	11.00	125.40	103.64	11.20
TASMANIAN 310		1754	11.00	12.00	132.00	91.67	11.50
TASMANIAN 3637	L	1755	10.40	13.50	140.40	77.04	11.95
TASMANIAN 3637	R	1755	10.55	13.70	144.53	77.01	12.12
TASMANIAN 576	R	1756	11.50	13.50	155.25	85.19	12.50
TASMANIAN P1	R	1757	11.00	13.50	148.50	81.48	12.25
TASMANIAN P2	L	1758	11.50	14.50	166.75	79.31	13.00
TASMANIAN P2	R	1758	11.50	14.00	161.00	82.14	12.75
TASMANIAN P3	R	1759		13.00			
TASMANIAN 2965	L	1761	9.60	11.30	108.48	84.96	10.45
TASMANIAN 2966	L	1762		13.70			
TASMANIAN 2966	R	1762		13.50			
TASMANIAN 2964	L	1763	11.10	13.90	154.29	79.86	12.50
TASMANIAN 2964	R	1763	11.40	13.70	156.18	83.21	12.55
BOSKOP		1902	10.50	12.50	131.25	84.00	11.50
ASSELAR	R	1903	11.00	13.00	143.00	84.62	12.00
NEGRO	L	1905	11.80	13.30	156.94	88.72	12.55
NEGRO		1914	10.00	11.60	116.00	86.21	10.80
NEGRO	L	1915	14.10	13.70	193.17	102.92	13.90
NEGRO	R	1915	13.70	14.30	195.91	95.80	14.00
NEGRO	L	1916	13.00	13.60	176.80	95.59	13.30
NEGRO	R	1916	12.80	13.60	174.08	94.12	13.20
MAPUNGUBWE	L	1950	10.00	11.00	110.00	90.91	10.50
MAPUNGUBWE	R	1950	9.90	10.30	101.97	96.12	10.10
MAPUNGUBWE M2		1952	10.50	12.00	126.00	87.50	11.25
MAPUNGUBWE M3		1953	11.00	12.20	134.20	90.16	11.60
MAPUNGUBWE M5		1954	10.50	13.00	136.50	80.77	11.75
MAPUNGUBWE M9		1955	10.30	13.00	133.90	79.23	11.65
MAPUNGUBWE M10		1956	11.00	13.00	143.00	84.62	12.00
BAMBANDYANALO21		1957	9.90	10.70	105.93	92.52	10.30
BAMBANDYANALO29		1958	10.00	11.90	119.00	84.03	10.95
BAMBANDYANALO31		1959	12.20	12.00	146.40	101.67	12.10
BAMBANDYANALO33	R	1960	11.20	12.20	136.64	91.80	11.70
BAMBANDYANALO 3		1962	10.30	12.50	128.75	82.40	11.40
BAMBANDYANALO13		1964	11.60	12.10	140.36	95.87	11.85
BAMBANDYANALO14		1965	10.30	11.40	117.42	90.35	10.85
ZITZIKAMA		1966	9.50	10.00	95.00	95.00	9.75
BUSHMAN		1967	9.70	10.60	102.82	91.51	10.15
FISH HOEK	R	1972	10.00	11.00	110.00	90.91	10.50
GOUNGOU C	R	1976		12.60			
N.BRITAIN 43121	L	1301	9.50	11.60	110.20	81.90	10.55
N.BRITAIN 43123	R	1303	10.60	12.30	130.38	86.18	11.45

UPPER M2 H. SAPIENS

		N	L(M-D)	B(B-L)	L*B	L/B	L+B/2
N.BRITAIN 43124	L	1304	10.80	11.30	122.04	95.58	11.05
N.BRITAIN 43124	R	1304	10.60	11.90	126.14	89.08	11.25
N.BRITAIN 43126	R	1305	9.00	12.00	108.00	75.00	10.50
N.BRITAIN 43127	L	1306	10.10	12.40	125.24	81.45	11.25
N.BRITAIN 43127	R	1306	10.00	12.00	120.00	83.33	11.00
N.BRITAIN 43130	L	1307	10.70	13.50	144.45	79.26	12.10
N.BRITAIN 43131	L	1308	11.10	13.30	147.63	83.46	12.20
N.BRITAIN 43132	L	1309	9.90	12.20	120.78	81.15	11.05
N.BRITAIN 43132	R	1309	10.20	12.10	123.42	84.30	11.15
N.BRITAIN 43134	L	1311	9.90	12.70	125.73	77.95	11.30
N.BRITAIN 43134	R	1311	10.00	12.70	127.00	78.74	11.35
N.BRITAIN 43135	L	1312	9.40	11.20	105.28	83.93	10.30
N.BRITAIN 43135	R	1312	9.90	11.20	110.88	88.39	10.55
N.BRITAIN 43136	L	1313	9.50	11.50	109.25	82.61	10.50
N.BRITAIN 43136	R	1313	10.00	11.10	111.00	90.09	10.55
N.BRITAIN 43137	R	1314	10.30	11.80	121.54	87.29	11.05
N.BRITAIN 43138	L	1315		11.30			
N.BRITAIN 43138	R	1315	10.10	11.60	117.16	87.07	10.85
N.BRITAIN 43139	L	1316	10.70	11.90	127.33	89.92	11.30
N.BRITAIN 43139	R	1316	11.40	12.20	139.08	93.44	11.80
N.BRITAIN 43140	R	1317	10.00	11.50	115.00	86.96	10.75
N.BRITAIN 43141	L	1318	10.00	11.20	112.00	89.29	10.60
N.BRITAIN 43141	R	1318	9.70	11.10	107.67	87.39	10.40
N.BRITAIN 43142	L	1319	10.30	12.80	131.84	80.47	11.55
N.BRITAIN 43142	R	1319	10.60	13.00	137.80	81.54	11.80
N.BRITAIN 43143	L	1320	9.70	12.10	117.37	80.17	10.90
N.BRITAIN 43143	R	1320	9.50	11.90	113.05	79.83	10.70
N.BRITAIN 43146	L	1323	10.10	12.10	122.21	83.47	11.10
N.BRITAIN 43146	R	1323	11.00	12.20	134.20	90.16	11.60
N.BRITAIN 43147	L	1324	11.40	11.80	134.52	96.61	11.60
N.BRITAIN 43147	R	1324	11.30	11.80	133.34	95.76	11.55
N.BRITAIN 43149	R	1325	8.40	12.80	107.52	65.62	10.60
N.BRITAIN 43150	L	1326	10.30	12.60	129.78	81.75	11.45
N.BRITAIN 43150	R	1326	9.80	12.60	123.48	77.78	11.20
N.BRITAIN 43151	L	1327	10.20	11.50	117.30	88.70	10.85
N.BRITAIN 43151	R	1327	11.00	11.40	125.40	96.49	11.20
N.BRITAIN 43152	L	1328	9.30	12.60	117.18	73.81	10.95
N.BRITAIN 43152	R	1328	10.00	12.80	128.00	78.12	11.40
N.BRITAIN 43153	L	1329	10.80	11.40	123.12	94.74	11.10
N.BRITAIN 43153	R	1329	10.30	11.40	117.42	90.35	10.85
N.BRITAIN 43154	L	1330	11.10	13.30	147.63	83.46	12.20
N.BRITAIN 43154	R	1330	11.10	13.50	149.85	82.22	12.30
N.BRITAIN 43174	L	1331	11.30	13.00	146.90	86.92	12.15
N.BRITAIN 43174	R	1331	11.30	13.00	146.90	86.92	12.15
N.BRITAIN 43179	L	1332	10.70	12.20	130.54	87.70	11.45
N.BRITAIN 43179	R	1332	10.50	12.40	130.20	84.68	11.45
N.BRITAIN 43193	L	1333	9.00	11.80	106.20	76.27	10.40
N.BRITAIN 43194	L	1334	11.00	11.70	128.70	94.02	11.35
N.BRITAIN 43194	R	1334	11.00	11.70	128.70	94.02	11.35
N.BRITAIN 43198	L	1335	11.00	12.30	135.30	89.43	11.65

UPPER M2 H. SAPIENS

		N	L(M-D)	B(B-L)	L*B	L/B	L+B/2
N.BRITAIN 43198	R	1335	10.90	12.70	138.43	85.83	11.80
N.BRITAIN 43199	L	1336	10.60	12.00	127.20	88.33	11.30
N.BRITAIN 43199	R	1336	9.60	11.20	107.52	85.71	10.40
N.BRITAIN 43202	L	1337	10.90	13.10	142.79	83.21	12.00
N.BRITAIN 43204	L	1338	11.10	13.90	154.29	79.86	12.50
N.BRITAIN 43204	R	1338	11.00	14.00	154.00	78.57	12.50
N.BRITAIN 43226	R	1339	9.80	11.20	109.76	87.50	10.50
N.BRITAIN 43329	L	1340	11.80	14.00	165.20	84.29	12.90
N.BRITAIN 43329	R	1340	11.50	13.90	159.85	82.73	12.70
N.BRITAIN 43242	L	1341	9.80	11.60	113.68	84.48	10.70
N.BRITAIN 43242	R	1341	10.40	12.10	125.84	85.95	11.25
N.BRITAIN 43290	L	1342	10.00	11.00	110.00	90.91	10.50
N.BRITAIN 43290	R	1342	9.70	11.60	112.52	83.62	10.65
N.BRITAIN 43291	L	1343	10.90				
N.BRITAIN 43291	R	1343	10.70	12.20	130.54	87.70	11.45
N.BRITAIN 43295	L	1344	11.10	13.40	148.74	82.84	12.25
N.BRITAIN 43295	R	1344	10.80	14.00	151.20	77.14	12.40
N.BRITAIN	L	1346	9.30	11.00	102.30	84.55	10.15
N.BRITAIN	R	1346	9.90	10.75	106.42	92.09	10.32
HINDU (UI)	L	2208	8.75	10.90	95.37	80.28	9.82
HINDU (UI)	R	2208	9.75	11.10	108.22	87.84	10.42
HARAPPA 1	L	1801	7.50	11.00	82.50	68.18	9.25
HARAPPA 1	R	1801	9.50	12.00	114.00	79.17	10.75
HARAPPA 2	L	1802	10.00	11.50	115.00	86.96	10.75
HARAPPA 2	R	1802	10.00	12.00	120.00	83.33	11.00
HARAPPA 3	L	1803	10.00	10.50	105.00	95.24	10.25
HARAPPA 3	R	1803	10.50	10.00	105.00	105.00	10.25
HARAPPA 4	L	1804	10.50	11.50	120.75	91.30	11.00
HARAPPA 4	R	1804	10.50	11.50	120.75	91.30	11.00
HARAPPA 5	R	1805	10.50	11.50	120.75	91.30	11.00
HARAPPA 7	L	1806	10.00	10.50	105.00	95.24	10.25
HARAPPA 7	R	1806	10.50	11.00	115.50	95.45	10.75
HARAPPA 10	L	1807	10.00	10.50	105.00	95.24	10.25
HARAPPA 10	R	1807	10.00	11.50	115.00	86.96	10.75
HARAPPA 11	R	1808	10.00	10.50	105.00	95.24	10.25
HARAPPA 12	L	1809	9.00	9.00	81.00	100.00	9.00
HARAPPA 12	R	1809	10.50	11.00	115.50	95.45	10.75
HARAPPA 13	L	1810	10.00	12.50	125.00	80.00	11.25
HARAPPA 13	R	1810		10.50			
HARAPPA 15	L	1812	9.00	11.00	99.00	81.82	10.00
HARAPPA 15	R	1812	8.50	10.00	85.00	85.00	9.25
HARAPPA 16	L	1813	9.50	10.00	95.00	95.00	9.75
HARAPPA 17	R	1814	9.50	9.00	85.50	105.56	9.25
HARAPPA 18	L	1815	9.00	8.00	72.00	112.50	8.50
HARAPPA 20	L	1816	8.50	10.00	85.00	85.00	9.25
HARAPPA 20	R	1816	10.00	9.00	90.00	111.11	9.50
HARAPPA 21	L	1817	7.00	8.00	56.00	87.50	7.50
HARAPPA 21	R	1817	9.00	8.00	72.00	112.50	8.50
HARAPPA 23	L	1818	10.00	10.00	100.00	100.00	10.00
HARAPPA 23	R	1818	9.00	10.00	90.00	90.00	9.50

UPPER M2 H. SAPIENS

		N	L(M-D)	B(B-L)	L*B	L/B	L+B/2
HARAPPA 25	L	1819	11.00	11.50	126.50	95.65	11.25
HARAPPA 25	R	1819	10.00	11.00	110.00	90.91	10.50
HARAPPA 15	L	1812	10.00	10.50	105.00	95.24	10.25
HARAPPA 15	R	1812	10.00	10.00	100.00	100.00	10.00
HARAPPA 32	L	1822	11.50	11.00	126.50	104.55	11.25
HARAPPA 32	R	1822	10.00	11.50	115.00	86.96	10.75
HARAPPA 35	L	1823	9.50	11.00	104.50	86.36	10.25
HARAPPA 35	R	1823	9.50	10.50	99.75	90.48	10.00
HARAPPA 36	L	1824	9.50	10.00	95.00	95.00	9.75
HARAPPA 36	R	1824	9.50	10.00	95.00	95.00	9.75
HARAPPA 37	L	1825	11.00				
HARAPPA 37	R	1825	10.00	12.50	125.00	80.00	11.25
HARAPPA 38	L	1826	11.00	10.00	110.00	110.00	10.50
HARAPPA 38	R	1826	9.50	11.00	104.50	86.36	10.25
HARAPPA 39	L	1827	10.00	10.50	105.00	95.24	10.25
HARAPPA 39	R	1827	9.00	11.00	99.00	81.82	10.00
HARAPPA 40	L	1828	9.50	11.50	109.25	82.61	10.50
HARAPPA 40	R	1828	11.00	12.00	132.00	91.67	11.50
HARAPPA 41	R	1829	10.00	11.50	115.00	86.96	10.75
HARAPPA 42	L	1830	10.50	11.50	120.75	91.30	11.00
HARAPPA 42	R	1830	10.00	12.00	120.00	83.33	11.00
HARAPPA 43	L	1831	10.00	11.00	110.00	90.91	10.50
HARAPPA 43	R	1831	9.00	10.00	90.00	90.00	9.50
HARAPPA 44	L	1832	9.50	11.50	109.25	82.61	10.50
HARAPPA 44	R	1832	8.50	11.50	97.75	73.91	10.00
HARAPPA 45	L	1833	10.00	11.00	110.00	90.91	10.50
HARAPPA 45	R	1833	9.50	12.00	114.00	79.17	10.75
HARAPPA 46	L	1834	11.00	11.00	121.00	100.00	11.00
HARAPPA 46	R	1834	9.00	11.00	99.00	81.82	10.00
HARAPPA 47	L	1835	8.00	7.00	56.00	114.29	7.50
HARAPPA 47	R	1835	8.00	7.50	60.00	106.67	7.75
HARAPPA 48	L	1836	9.00	10.00	90.00	90.00	9.50
HARAPPA 49	L	1837	9.00	8.50	76.50	105.88	8.75
HARAPPA 51	L	1838	9.00	8.50	76.50	105.88	8.75
HARAPPA 51	R	1838	9.50	8.00	76.00	118.75	8.75
HARAPPA 53	R	1840	8.50	10.00	85.00	85.00	9.25
HARAPPA 54	L	1841	11.00	9.00	99.00	122.22	10.00
HARAPPA 54	R	1841	9.00	10.00	90.00	90.00	9.50
HARAPPA 55	L	1842	9.00	8.00	72.00	112.50	8.50
HARAPPA 56	L	1843	9.50	10.50	99.75	90.48	10.00
HARAPPA 56	R	1843	9.00	10.50	94.50	85.71	9.75
HARAPPA 58	L	1844	10.00	10.50	105.00	95.24	10.25
HARAPPA 58	R	1844	9.00	10.50	94.50	85.71	9.75
HARAPPA 59	L	1845	9.00	11.50	103.50	78.26	10.25
HARAPPA 59	R	1845	8.50	11.00	93.50	77.27	9.75
HARAPPA 60	L	1846	9.00	10.00	90.00	90.00	9.50
HARAPPA 60	R	1846	9.50	10.50	99.75	90.48	10.00
HARAPPA 61	L	1847	9.50	10.00	95.00	95.00	9.75
HARAPPA 61	R	1847	11.00	10.00	110.00	110.00	10.50
HARAPPA 62	L	1848	8.50	10.50	89.25	80.95	9.50

UPPER M2 H. SAPIENS

		N	L(M-D)	B(B-L)	L*B	L/B	L+B/2
HARAPPA 62	R	1848	8.50	11.00	93.50	77.27	9.75
HARAPPA 63	L	1849.	8.00	11.00	88.00	72.73	9.50
HARAPPA 63	R	1849	9.00	11.50	103.50	78.26	10.25
HARAPPA 64	R	1850	10.50	10.00	105.00	105.00	10.25
HARAPPA 65	L	1851	10.00	9.00	90.00	111.11	9.50
HARAPPA 66	L	1852	10.00	10.00	100.00	100.00	10.00
HARAPPA 66	R	1852	9.00	11.00	99.00	81.82	10.00
HARAPPA 69	R	1853	9.50	12.50	118.75	76.00	11.00
HARAPPA 70	L	1854	10.00	12.00	120.00	83.33	11.00
HARAPPA 70	R	1854	11.00	11.50	126.50	95.65	11.25
HARAPPA 74	R	1857	9.50	11.00	104.50	86.36	10.25
HARAPPA 81	L	1859	10.00	11.00	110.00	90.91	10.50
HARAPPA 85	L	1860	11.00	11.50	126.50	95.65	11.25
HARAPPA 85	R	1860	10.50	12.00	126.00	87.50	11.25
GOL BA IT 98	L	2003		11.30			
GOL BA IT	L	2009	10.20	11.70	119.34	87.18	10.95
MELOLO	L	2065	8.30	11.20	92.96	74.11	9.75
MELOLO	R	2066	8.70	10.20	88.74	85.29	9.45
MELOLO	L	2067	8.80	11.80	103.84	74.58	10.30
MELOLO	L	2068	9.80	11.50	112.70	85.22	10.65
MELOLO	R	2069	9.90	11.30	111.87	87.61	10.60
MELOLO	L	2070	10.00	12.20	122.00	81.97	11.10
MELOLO	R	2071	9.80	11.50	112.70	85.22	10.65
MELOLO	L	2072	11.10	11.70	129.87	94.87	11.40
MELOLO	R	2073	10.20	12.40	126.48	82.26	11.30
MELOLO	L	2074	10.60	11.00	116.60	96.36	10.80
MELOLO	R	2075	10.60	11.20	118.72	94.64	10.90
MELOLO	L	2076	9.90	10.70	105.93	92.52	10.30
MELOLO	L	2077	9.50	10.70	101.65	88.79	10.10
MELOLO	R	2078	10.00	12.20	122.00	81.97	11.10
MELOLO	L	2079	10.30	12.20	125.66	84.43	11.25
MELOLO	R	2080	9.00	10.90	98.10	82.57	9.95
SAINT CRUZ M	L	2204	10.40	12.00	124.80	86.67	11.20
SAINT CRUZ M	R	2204	10.40	11.80	122.72	88.14	11.10
SAINT CRUZ F	L	2205	10.30	11.60	119.48	88.79	10.95
SAINT CRUZ F	R	2205	9.80	11.50	112.70	85.22	10.65
CHANG YANG		2203	8.30	10.60	87.98	78.30	9.45
HAICA	L	1406	11.80	11.10	130.98	106.31	11.45
HAICA	R	1406	11.50	11.20	128.80	102.68	11.35
MINNESOTA MAN	L	1419	10.20	12.80	130.56	79.69	11.50
MINNESOTA MAN	R	1419	10.00	12.40	124.00	80.65	11.20
PUNIN (EQUADOR)	L	1420	10.70	12.50	133.75	85.60	11.60
PUNIN (EQUADOR)	R	1420	11.80	12.70	149.86	92.91	12.25
ILLINOIS PK2-B1	L	1426	10.10	12.40	125.24	81.45	11.25
ILLINOIS PK2-B1	R	1426	9.80	12.40	121.52	79.03	11.10
ILLINOIS T25-2	L	1427	10.00	11.60	116.00	86.21	10.80
ILLINOIS T25-2	R	1427	9.20	11.95	109.94	76.99	10.57
ILLINOIS A-2732	L	1429	10.20	11.50	117.30	88.70	10.85
ILLINOIS A-2732	R	1429	9.90	11.35	112.36	87.22	10.62
ILLINOIS A-6890	L	1430	9.10	11.20	101.92	81.25	10.15

UPPER M2 H. SAPIENS

		N	L(M-D)	B(B-L)	L*B	L/B	L+B/2
ILLINOIS A-6890	R	1430	8.80	10.75	94.60	81.86	9.77
ILLINOIS A-4921	L	1431	9.90	12.10	119.79	81.82	11.00
ILLINOIS A-4921	R	1431	10.40	12.10	125.84	85.95	11.25
ILLINOIS PK9-B4	L	1432	9.80	10.80	105.84	90.74	10.30
ILLINOIS PK9-B4	R	1432	9.55	11.20	106.96	85.27	10.37
ILLINOIS PK9-B1	L	1433	10.50	13.40	140.70	78.36	11.95
ILLINOIS PK9-B1	R	1433	11.00	13.30	146.30	82.71	12.15
ILLINOIS BR19-3	L	1434	9.70	11.10	107.67	87.39	10.40
ILLINOIS BR19-3	R	1434	9.55	10.90	104.09	87.61	10.22
ILLINOIS BLUFFS	L	1435	9.60	13.05	125.28	73.56	11.32
ILLINOIS BLUFFS	R	1435	9.50	12.55	119.22	75.70	11.02
DICKSON MOUND	L	1501	10.25	12.00	123.00	85.42	11.12
DICKSON MOUND	R	1501	10.40	11.62	120.85	89.50	11.01
DICKSON MOUND	R	1502	10.85	13.55	147.02	80.07	12.20
DICKSON MD 242	L	1505	11.62	12.80	148.74	90.78	12.21
DICKSON MD 242	R	1505	11.32	12.85	145.46	88.09	12.08
DICKSON MD 256	L	1506	10.00	11.20	112.00	89.29	10.60
DICKSON MD 256	R	1506	10.42	11.75	122.43	88.68	11.08
DICKSON MD 261	L	1508	10.20	11.85	120.87	86.08	11.02
DICKSON MD 261	R	1508	10.00	12.15	121.50	82.30	11.07
DICKSON MD 266	L	1510	10.95	12.20	133.59	89.75	11.57
DICKSON MD 276	L	1514	12.00	14.40	172.80	83.33	13.20
DICKSON MD 276	R	1514	12.00	14.75	177.00	81.36	13.37
DICKSON MD 287	L	1516	10.35	12.00	124.20	86.25	11.17
DICKSON MD 287	R	1516	11.30	12.03	135.94	93.93	11.66
DICKSON MD 297	L	1520	10.95	11.90	130.30	92.02	11.42
DICKSON MD 302	L	1521	10.00	11.15	111.50	89.69	10.57
DICKSON MD 302	R	1521	10.25	10.95	112.24	93.61	10.60
DICKSON MD 319	L	1523	9.90	11.80	116.82	83.90	10.85
DICKSON MD 319	R	1523	9.85	11.60	114.26	84.91	10.72
DICKSON MD 327	L	1524	10.30	12.00	123.60	85.83	11.15
DICKSON MD 327	R	1524	10.90	12.40	135.16	87.90	11.65
DICKSON MD 334	L	1525	10.90	13.50	147.15	80.74	12.20
DICKSON MD 334	R	1525	10.60	13.60	144.16	77.94	12.10
DICKSON MD 342	R	1526	9.30	11.25	104.62	82.67	10.27
DICKSON MD 344	L	1527	10.90	13.30	144.97	81.95	12.10
DICKSON MD 348	L	1529	10.30	11.15	114.84	92.38	10.72
DICKSON MD 348	R	1529	9.50	11.15	105.92	85.20	10.32
DICKSON MD 349	L	1530	10.60	11.25	119.25	94.22	10.92
DICKSON MD 349	R	1530	10.30	11.45	117.93	89.96	10.87
DICKSON MD 355	L	1535	11.80	12.10	142.78	97.52	11.95
DICKSON MD 361	L	1538	10.50	12.00	126.00	87.50	11.25
DICKSON MD 361	R	1538	10.45	12.70	132.71	82.28	11.57
DICKSON MD 362	L	1539	10.00	11.50	115.00	86.96	10.75
DICKSON MD 362	R	1539	9.55	11.45	109.35	83.41	10.50
DICKSON MD 365	L	1540	9.50	11.10	105.45	85.59	10.30
DICKSON MD 365	R	1540	9.20	11.20	103.04	82.14	10.20
DICKSON MD 371	L	1542	9.80	12.20	119.56	80.33	11.00
DICKSON MD 371	R	1542	9.90	12.65	125.23	78.26	11.27
DICKSON MD 372	L	1543	10.10	11.70	118.17	86.32	10.90

UPPER M2 H. SAPIENS

			N	L(M-D)	B(B-L)	L*B	L/B	L+B/2
DICKSCN MD	372	R	1543	9.80	11.90	116.62	82.35	10.85
DICKSCN MD	378	L	1547	8.80	10.00	88.00	88.00	9.40
DICKSCN MD	378	R	1547	8.90	10.30	91.67	86.41	9.60
DICKSON MD	379	L	1548	9.20	11.20	103.04	82.14	10.20
DICKSCN MD	379	R	1548	10.30	11.50	118.45	89.57	10.90
DICKSON MD	380	L	1549	8.90	10.70	95.23	83.18	9.80
DICKSON MD	380	R	1549	8.90	11.10	98.79	80.18	10.00
DICKSCN MD	381	L	1550	10.40	11.40	118.56	91.23	10.90
DICKSCN MD	381	R	1550	10.40	11.70	121.68	88.89	11.05
DICKSON MD	380	L	1551	9.90	11.50	113.85	86.09	10.70
DICKSCN MD	388	R	1552	11.20	12.50	140.00	89.60	11.85
DICKSON MD	396	L	1553	11.40	12.50	142.50	91.20	11.95
DICKSON MD	396	R	1553	11.00	12.60	138.60	87.30	11.80
DICKSON MD	397	L	1554	10.30	12.10	124.63	85.12	11.20
DICKSON MD	397	R	1554	10.60	12.40	131.44	85.48	11.50
DICKSCN MD	398	L	1555	9.20	10.50	96.60	87.62	9.85
DICKSON MD	398	R	1555	8.90	10.70	95.23	83.18	9.80
DICKSON MD	399	L	1556	9.40	11.60	109.04	81.03	10.50
DICKSGN MD	399	R	1556	10.00	11.35	113.50	88.11	10.67
DICKSCN MD	402	L	1557	10.70	13.40	143.38	79.85	12.05
DICKSGN MD	402	R	1557	10.50	13.40	140.70	78.36	11.95
DICKSON MD	406	L	1560	9.65	10.40	100.36	92.79	10.02
DICKSCN MD	407	L	1561	10.55	12.90	136.09	81.78	11.72
DICKSCN MD	407	R	1561	11.20	12.07	135.18	92.79	11.63
DICKSON MD	411	L	1563	10.80	11.50	124.20	93.91	11.15
DICKSCN MD	411	R	1563	10.17	11.45	116.45	88.82	10.81
DICKSCN MD	414	L	1564	9.80	11.35	111.23	86.34	10.57
DICKSON MD	415	L	1565	9.00	11.35	102.15	79.30	10.17
DICKSCN MD	415	R	1565	9.10	10.80	98.28	84.26	9.95
DICKSCN MD	426	L	1566	9.65	11.55	111.46	83.55	10.60
DICKSCN MD	426	R	1566	9.60	11.00	105.60	87.27	10.30
DICKSCN MD	432	L	1567	9.10	10.70	97.37	85.05	9.90
DICKSCN MD	432	R	1567	8.70	10.50	91.35	82.86	9.60
DICKSGN MD	443	L	1571	10.40	12.10	125.84	85.95	11.25
DICKSCN MD	443	R	1571	10.50	12.00	126.00	87.50	11.25
DICKSGN MD	446	L	1572	9.60	11.00	105.60	87.27	10.30
DICKSCN MD	464	L	1575	10.00	11.55	115.50	86.58	10.77
DICKSON MD	464	R	1575	10.20	12.30	125.46	82.93	11.25
DICKSCN MD	476	L	1576	11.10	12.25	135.97	90.61	11.67
DICKSCN MD	476	R	1576	10.39	12.20	126.76	85.16	11.29
DICKSGN MD	480	L	1578	10.20	11.50	117.30	88.70	10.85
DICKSCN MD	480	R	1578	10.35	10.10	104.53	102.48	10.22
DICKSGN MD	497	L	1583	10.85	12.90	139.96	84.11	11.87
DICKSCN MD	497	R	1583	10.60	13.05	138.33	81.23	11.82
DICKSGN MD	503	L	1585	9.40	12.00	112.80	78.33	10.70
DICKSCN MD	503	R	1585	10.20	12.05	122.91	84.65	11.12
DICKSGN MD	509	L	1587	9.70	10.60	102.82	91.51	10.15
DICKSON MD	509	R	1587	9.40	10.85	101.99	86.64	10.12
DICKSCN MD	535	L	1591	10.20	11.70	119.34	87.18	10.95
DICKSCN MD	536	L	1592	10.30	11.20	115.36	91.96	10.75

UPPER M2 H. SAPIENS

			N	L(M-D)	B(B-L)	L*B	L/B	L+B/2
DICKSCN MD	536	R	1592	10.35	11.70	121.09	88.46	11.02
DICKSCN MD	545	L	1594	10.80	13.20	142.56	81.82	12.00
DICKSCN MD	545	R	1594	10.60	12.95	137.27	81.85	11.77
DICKSCN MD	557	L	1596	10.20	11.65	118.83	87.55	10.92
DICKSCN MD	557	R	1596	10.45	11.70	122.26	89.32	11.07
DICKSCN MD	561	L	1597	10.80	12.50	135.00	86.40	11.65
DICKSCN MD	561	R	1597	10.75	12.30	132.22	87.40	11.52
DICKSCN MD	567	L	1598	10.70	12.20	130.54	87.70	11.45
DICKSGN MD	567	R	1598	10.80	12.55	135.54	86.06	11.67
DICKSCN MD	594	L	1601	9.35	11.20	104.72	83.48	10.27
DICKSCN MD	594	R	1601	9.15	11.40	104.31	80.26	10.27
DICKSGN MD	599	R	1602	10.10	12.60	127.26	80.16	11.35
DICKSCN MD	630	L	1603	10.60	12.30	130.38	86.18	11.45
DICKSGN MD	630	R	1603	10.30	12.40	127.72	83.06	11.35
DICKSCN MD	633	L	1604	9.10	11.20	101.92	81.25	10.15
DICKSCN MD	633	R	1604	9.00	11.20	100.80	80.36	10.10
DICKSCN MD	643	L	1608	10.40	12.20	126.88	85.25	11.30
DICKSCN MD	643	R	1608	10.60	12.50	132.50	84.80	11.55
DICKSON MD	667	L	1614	11.10	12.20	135.42	90.98	11.65
DICKSON MD	667	R	1614	10.82	12.50	135.25	86.56	11.66
DICKSCN MD	687	L	1616	7.90	11.20	88.48	70.54	9.55
DICKSCN MD	687	R	1616	8.60	11.30	97.18	76.11	9.95
DICKSCN MD	699	R	1618	10.25	12.00	123.00	85.42	11.12
DICKSCN MD	709	L	1623	9.70	11.75	113.97	82.55	10.72
DICKSCN MD	724	L	1627	10.90	12.40	135.16	87.90	11.65
DICKSCN MD	724	R	1627	10.50	12.25	128.62	85.71	11.37
DICKSCN MD	746	L	1628	10.40	11.95	124.28	87.03	11.17
DICKSCN MD	746	R	1628	10.00	12.13	121.30	82.44	11.06
DICKSGN MD	749	L	1629	11.85	12.35	146.35	95.95	12.10
DICKSCN MD	749	R	1629	11.56	12.40	143.34	93.23	11.98

UPPER M3 H. SAPIENS

		N	L(M-D)	B(B-L)	L*B	L/B	L+B/2
PREDMOST 3	L	1007	10.30	11.30	116.39	91.15	10.80
PREDMOST 3	R	1007	10.70	11.70	125.19	91.45	11.20
PREDMOST 4	L	1008	8.85	9.50	84.07	93.16	9.17
PREDMOST 4	R	1008	8.50	9.30	79.05	91.40	8.90
COMBE CHAPELLE	L	1017	8.20	11.00	90.20	74.55	9.60
COMBE CHAPELLE	R	1017	8.00	11.50	92.00	69.57	9.75
BRNO 3	L	1018	8.70	10.90	94.83	79.82	9.80
BRNO 3	R	1018	8.00	11.00	88.00	72.73	9.50
GRIMALDI ADOL.	L	1019	10.30	11.60	119.48	88.79	10.95
GRIMALDI ADOL.	R	1019	9.00	12.00	108.00	75.00	10.50
LA ROCHETTE A	L	1021	10.00	13.00	130.00	76.92	11.50
LA ROCHETTE A	R	1021	10.00	13.00	130.00	76.92	11.50
ROIS R50-21		1030	9.50	9.00	85.50	105.56	9.25
ROIS R51-16		1041	11.50	11.50	132.25	100.00	11.50
VESTONICE 3	L	1057	9.20	10.40	95.68	88.46	9.80
VESTONICE 3	R	1057	9.20	10.80	99.36	85.19	10.00
A CULOZ 2	L	1101	10.30	13.00	133.90	79.23	11.65
A CULOZ 2	R	1101	8.80	14.00	123.20	62.86	11.40
ALAMANN 1288	L	1103	8.00	9.00	72.00	88.89	8.50
ALAMANN 1288	R	1103	7.50	9.00	67.50	83.33	8.25
BUGGISON 1	L	1108	10.50	12.00	126.00	87.50	11.25
BUGGISON 1	R	1108	10.50	12.00	126.00	87.50	11.25
BUGGISON 2	L	1109	10.00	13.00	130.00	76.92	11.50
BUGGISON 2	R	1109	9.00	12.00	108.00	75.00	10.50
EGOLZWIL 1	L	1112	8.10	10.40	84.24	77.88	9.25
EGOLZWIL 1	R	1112	7.50	10.10	75.75	74.26	8.80
ISTURITZ 2		1121	9.00	11.50	103.50	78.26	10.25
MASAT		1130	8.30	10.40	86.32	79.81	9.35
OKUZINI		1133	7.30	10.30	75.19	70.87	8.80
RHUNCA	R	1142	9.00	11.80	106.20	76.27	10.40
FRENCHMAN	L	1149	7.50	10.80	81.00	69.44	9.15
FRENCHMAN	R	1149	8.25	10.80	89.10	76.39	9.52
IRAN(SIALK)	L	1190	7.60	11.00	83.60	69.09	9.30
IRAN(SIALK)	L	1191	9.20	10.40	95.68	88.46	9.80
IRAN(SIALK)	L	1192	7.50	10.10	75.75	74.26	8.80
JARMO 2B	L	1193	9.20	11.30	103.96	81.42	10.25
JARMO 2B	R	1193	8.00	12.40	99.20	64.52	10.20
JARMO	R	1194	8.40	10.70	89.88	78.50	9.55
WADJAK 1		1701	8.20	13.00	106.60	63.08	10.60
WADJAK 2	L	1702	10.30	13.70	141.11	75.18	12.00
WADJAK 2	R	1702	11.00	13.00	143.00	84.62	12.00
KEILOR	R	1703	9.70	12.00	116.40	80.83	10.85
COHUNA	L	1705	11.40	14.40	164.16	79.17	12.90
COHUNA	R	1705	10.60	13.70	145.22	77.37	12.15
AUSTRALIAN 39		1708	10.00	13.00	130.00	76.92	11.50
AUSTRALIAN 2961	R	1725		12.00			
AUSTRALIAN	L	1726	8.20	10.80	88.56	75.93	9.50
AUSTRALIAN	L	1728	9.50	11.20	106.40	84.82	10.35
AUSTRALIAN	R	1728	9.60	9.40	90.24	102.13	9.50
AUSTRALIAN 179	L	1732	11.40	10.30	117.42	110.68	10.85

UPPER M3 H. SAPIENS

		N	L(M-D)	B(B-L)	L*B	L/B	L+B/2
AUSTRALIAN 179	R	1732	10.50	9.80	102.90	107.14	10.15
TASMANIAN 310		1754	8.00	11.00	88.00	72.73	9.50
TASMANIAN 3637	L	1755	9.70	12.30	119.31	78.86	11.00
TASMANIAN 3637	R	1755	10.00				
TASMANIAN 576	R	1756	9.50	13.00	123.50	73.08	11.25
TASMANIAN P1	R	1757	10.50	13.00	136.50	80.77	11.75
TASMANIAN P2	L	1758	11.00	14.00	154.00	78.57	12.50
TASMANIAN P2	R	1758	11.00	13.00	143.00	84.62	12.00
TASMANIAN P3	R	1759		13.00			
TASMANIAN 2965	L	1761	8.00	11.10	88.80	72.07	9.55
TASMANIAN 2966	L	1762		11.90			
TASMANIAN 2964	L	1763	10.30	13.90	143.17	74.10	12.10
TASMANIAN 2964	R	1763	11.40	13.50	153.90	84.44	12.45
FLORISBAD	R	1901	10.20	11.90	121.38	85.71	11.05
ASSELAR	R	1903	10.50	12.50	131.25	84.00	11.50
NEGRO	L	1905	10.80	11.85	127.98	91.14	11.32
NEGRO		1914	9.00	11.00	99.00	81.82	10.00
NEGRO	L	1915	12.60				
NEGRO	R	1915	12.00				
NEGRO	L	1916	12.60	13.10	165.06	96.18	12.85
NEGRO	R	1916	13.30	13.00	172.90	102.31	13.15
MAPUNGUBWE	R	1950	9.70				
MAPUNGUBWE M5		1954	9.00	11.00	99.00	81.82	10.00
MAPUNGUBWE M9		1955	9.00	13.00	117.00	69.23	11.00
BAMBANDYANALO21		1957	8.20	10.00	82.00	82.00	9.10
BAMBANDYANALO31		1959	9.80	12.00	117.60	81.67	10.90
BAMBANDYANALO33	R	1960	11.30	12.30	138.99	91.87	11.80
BAMBANDYANALO 3		1962	8.70	11.70	101.79	74.36	10.20
BAMBANDYANALO13		1964	10.00	12.60	126.00	79.37	11.30
BAMBANDYANALO14		1965	8.60	11.00	94.60	78.18	9.80
ZITZIKAMA		1966	9.60	8.00	76.80	120.00	8.80
BUSHMAN		1967	8.20	10.30	84.46	79.61	9.25
FISH HOEK	R	1972	8.00	9.00	72.00	88.89	8.50
N.BRITAIN 43121	L	1301	10.00	11.40	114.00	87.72	10.70
N.BRITAIN 43123	R	1303	9.40	12.70	119.38	74.02	11.05
N.BRITAIN 43126	R	1305	8.70	11.40	99.18	76.32	10.05
N.BRITAIN 43127	L	1306	9.20	11.60	106.72	79.31	10.40
N.BRITAIN 43127	R	1306	9.40	11.00	103.40	85.45	10.20
N.BRITAIN 43130	L	1307	8.60	12.00	103.20	71.67	10.30
N.BRITAIN 43130	R	1307	9.60	11.70	112.32	82.05	10.65
N.BRITAIN 43134	R	1311	8.30	11.30	93.79	73.45	9.80
N.BRITAIN 43135	R	1312	9.00	10.90	98.10	82.57	9.95
N.BRITAIN 43138	L	1315		10.80			
N.BRITAIN 43138	R	1315	9.20	11.30	103.96	81.42	10.25
N.BRITAIN 43139	L	1316	11.30	11.80	133.34	95.76	11.55
N.BRITAIN 43139	R	1316	11.40	11.80	134.52	96.61	11.60
N.BRITAIN 43140	R	1317	10.00	11.40	114.00	87.72	10.70
N.BRITAIN 43141	L	1318	9.00	10.70	96.30	84.11	9.85
N.BRITAIN 43141	R	1318	9.60	10.60	101.76	90.57	10.10
N.BRITAIN 43142	L	1319		12.70			

UPPER M3 H. SAPIENS

		N	L(M-D)	B(B-L)	L*B	L/B	L+B/2
N.BRITAIN 43142	R	1319	10.00	12.60	126.00	79.37	11.30
N.BRITAIN 43143	R	1320	9.00	12.30	110.70	73.17	10.65
N.BRITAIN 43146	L	1323	9.00	11.10	99.90	81.08	10.05
N.BRITAIN 43146	R	1323	9.30	10.20	94.86	91.18	9.75
N.BRITAIN 43147	R	1324	10.00	13.40	134.00	74.63	11.70
N.BRITAIN 43149	L	1325	8.90	11.10	98.79	80.18	10.00
N.BRITAIN 43149	R	1325	9.10	12.20	111.02	74.59	10.65
N.BRITAIN 43150	L	1326	7.80	11.20	87.36	69.64	9.50
N.BRITAIN 43151	L	1327	9.60	10.90	104.64	88.07	10.25
N.BRITAIN 43152	L	1328	12.00	12.50	150.00	96.00	12.25
N.BRITAIN 43152	R	1328	10.20	12.30	125.46	82.93	11.25
N.BRITAIN 43153	L	1329		10.00			
N.BRITAIN 43153	R	1329	8.70	10.40	90.48	83.65	9.55
N.BRITAIN 43154	L	1330	8.90	13.30	118.37	66.92	11.10
N.BRITAIN 43154	R	1330	9.60	13.10	125.76	73.28	11.35
N.BRITAIN 43174	L	1331	8.60	11.10	95.46	77.48	9.85
N.BRITAIN 43174	R	1331	8.40	11.40	95.76	73.68	9.90
N.BRITAIN 43179	L	1332	10.30	12.00	123.60	85.83	11.15
N.BRITAIN 43179	R	1332	9.60	10.60	101.76	90.57	10.10
N.BRITAIN 43194	L	1334	8.80	11.30	99.44	77.88	10.05
N.BRITAIN 43194	R	1334	8.80	11.40	100.32	77.19	10.10
N.BRITAIN 43198	L	1335	9.70	11.70	113.49	82.91	10.70
N.BRITAIN 43198	R	1335	10.20	12.30	125.46	82.93	11.25
N.BRITAIN 43199	L	1336	9.80	12.20	119.56	80.33	11.00
N.BRITAIN 43204	L	1338	9.40	12.60	118.44	74.60	11.00
N.BRITAIN 43204	R	1338	9.40	12.90	121.26	72.87	11.15
N.BRITAIN 43329	L	1340	10.10	13.40	135.34	75.37	11.75
N.BRITAIN 43329	R	1340	10.20	13.60	138.72	75.00	11.90
N.BRITAIN 43242	L	1341	9.00	11.20	100.80	80.36	10.10
N.BRITAIN 43242	R	1341	9.20	11.00	101.20	83.64	10.10
N.BRITAIN 43290	L	1342	9.30	11.70	108.81	79.49	10.50
N.BRITAIN 43290	R	1342	8.70	11.20	97.44	77.68	9.95
N.BRITAIN 43291	L	1343	10.40	11.80	122.72	88.14	11.10
N.BRITAIN 43291	R	1343	9.60	11.60	111.36	82.76	10.60
N.BRITAIN 43295	L	1344	9.40	11.80	110.92	79.66	10.60
N.BRITAIN 43295	R	1344	9.00	11.60	104.40	77.59	10.30
N.BRITAIN	L	1346	8.80	10.40	91.52	84.62	9.60
N.BRITAIN	R	1346	8.80	10.10	88.88	87.13	9.45
HINDL (LI)	L	2208	9.50	11.50	109.25	82.61	10.50
HINDL (LI)	R	2208	9.30	11.80	109.74	78.81	10.55
HARAPPA 1	L	1801	8.50	11.00	93.50	77.27	9.75
HARAPPA 1	R	1801	9.50	11.00	104.50	86.36	10.25
HARAPPA 2	L	1802	10.00	12.00	120.00	83.33	11.00
HARAPPA 2	R	1802	11.00	12.00	132.00	91.67	11.50
HARAPPA 3	L	1803	10.00	11.00	110.00	90.91	10.50
HARAPPA 3	R	1803	9.50	10.50	99.75	90.48	10.00
HARAPPA 5	R	1805	10.50	11.00	115.50	95.45	10.75
HARAPPA 7	R	1806	8.50	9.50	80.75	89.47	9.00
HARAPPA 11	R	1808	7.50	10.00	75.00	75.00	8.75
HARAPPA 13	R	1810	9.00	10.50	94.50	85.71	9.75

UPPER M3 H. SAPIENS

		N	L(M-D)	B(B-L)	L*B	L/B	L+B/2
HARAPPA 17	L	1814	8.50	8.00	68.00	106.25	8.25
HARAPPA 18	L	1815	7.00	6.50	45.50	107.69	6.75
HARAPPA 20	L	1816	8.50	10.50	89.25	80.95	9.50
HARAPPA 20	R	1816	9.00	9.00	81.00	100.00	9.00
HARAPPA 21	L	1817	7.00	7.50	52.50	93.33	7.25
HARAPPA 21	R	1817	8.00	7.00	56.00	114.29	7.50
HARAPPA 23	L	1818	10.00	10.00	100.00	100.00	10.00
HARAPPA 23	R	1818	10.00	10.00	100.00	100.00	10.00
HARAPPA 25	L	1819	9.00	9.00	81.00	100.00	9.00
HARAPPA 25	R	1819	9.00	10.00	90.00	90.00	9.50
HARAPPA 15	L	1812	8.00	8.00	64.00	100.00	8.00
HARAPPA 15	R	1812	8.00	8.50	68.00	94.12	8.25
HARAPPA 37	R	1825	9.50	11.00	104.50	86.36	10.25
HARAPPA 38	L	1826	9.50	8.50	80.75	111.76	9.00
HARAPPA 38	R	1826	8.50	10.00	85.00	85.00	9.25
HARAPPA 39	L	1827	9.50	12.00	114.00	79.17	10.75
HARAPPA 39	R	1827	9.50	12.00	114.00	79.17	10.75
HARAPPA 40	L	1828	8.50	10.00	85.00	85.00	9.25
HARAPPA 40	R	1828	9.50	10.50	99.75	90.48	10.00
HARAPPA 41	L	1829	8.50	7.50	63.75	113.33	8.00
HARAPPA 41	R	1829	7.50	10.50	78.75	71.43	9.00
HARAPPA 42	L	1830	9.00	10.00	90.00	90.00	9.50
HARAPPA 42	R	1830	8.50	9.50	80.75	89.47	9.00
HARAPPA 43	L	1831	8.50	10.50	89.25	80.95	9.50
HARAPPA 44	L	1832	8.50	12.50	106.25	68.00	10.50
HARAPPA 44	R	1832	8.00	11.50	92.00	69.57	9.75
HARAPPA 45	R	1833	10.00	11.00	110.00	90.91	10.50
HARAPPA 48	L	1836	10.00	10.00	100.00	100.00	10.00
HARAPPA 48	R	1836	10.00	9.00	90.00	111.11	9.50
HARAPPA 51	L	1838	9.50	8.50	80.75	111.76	9.00
HARAPPA 51	R	1838	10.00	9.00	90.00	111.11	9.50
HARAPPA 56	R	1843	8.50	9.50	80.75	89.47	9.00
HARAPPA 58	L	1844	9.00	10.50	94.50	85.71	9.75
HARAPPA 58	R	1844	9.50	9.00	85.50	105.56	9.25
HARAPPA 59	L	1845	9.00	11.00	99.00	81.82	10.00
HARAPPA 59	R	1845	7.50	10.50	78.75	71.43	9.00
HARAPPA 60	L	1846	8.00	10.50	84.00	76.19	9.25
HARAPPA 60	R	1846	9.00	10.00	90.00	90.00	9.50
HARAPPA 61	L	1847	9.50	8.50	80.75	111.76	9.00
HARAPPA 61	R	1847	9.50	10.50	99.75	90.48	10.00
HARAPPA 62	L	1848	8.50	10.00	85.00	85.00	9.25
HARAPPA 62	R	1848	8.50	10.50	89.25	80.95	9.50
HARAPPA 63	R	1849	9.00	10.00	90.00	90.00	9.50
HARAPPA 64	R	1850	10.00	10.00	100.00	100.00	10.00
HARAPPA 65	L	1851	8.00	9.50	76.00	84.21	8.75
HARAPPA 66	L	1852	8.00	9.00	72.00	88.89	8.50
HARAPPA 66	R	1852	8.00	9.00	72.00	88.89	8.50
HARAPPA 69	L	1853	10.50	11.50	120.75	91.30	11.00
HARAPPA 69	R	1853	8.50	11.50	97.75	73.91	10.00
HARAPPA 70	L	1854	9.00	11.00	99.00	81.82	10.00

UPPER M3 H. SAPIENS

		N	L(M-D)	B(B-L)	L*B	L/B	L+B/2
HARAPPA 81	L	1859	9.00	10.00	90.00	90.00	9.50
GOL BA IT 95	R	2002		11.80			
GOL BA IT 98	L	2003		11.30			
MELOLO	L	2081	8.50	12.00	102.00	70.83	10.25
MELOLC	L	2082	8.60	11.00	94.60	78.18	9.80
MELOLC	R	2083	9.50	10.50	99.75	90.48	10.00
MELOLC	L	2084	10.20	10.40	106.08	98.08	10.30
MELOLO	L	2085	10.00	10.90	109.00	91.74	10.45
SAINT CRUZ M	L	2204	9.90	11.40	112.86	86.84	10.65
SAINT CRUZ M	R	2204	9.40	11.80	110.92	79.66	10.60
SAINT CRUZ F	R	2205	9.00	10.40	93.60	86.54	9.70
HAICA	L	1406	10.70	11.90	127.33	89.92	11.30
HAICA	R	1406	10.50	10.90	114.45	96.33	10.70
MINNESOTA MAN	L	1419	10.00	11.80	118.00	84.75	10.90
MINNESOTA MAN	R	1419	10.00	11.70	117.00	85.47	10.85
ILLINCIS T25-2	L	1427	9.60	9.55	91.68	100.52	9.57
ILLINCIS A-2732	R	1429	9.80	10.30	100.94	95.15	10.05
ILLINCIS A-6890	R	1430	9.80	11.00	107.80	89.09	10.40
ILLINCIS A-4921	L	1431	8.50	11.40	96.90	74.56	9.95
ILLINCIS A-4921	R	1431	9.35	11.85	110.80	78.90	10.60
ILLINCIS PK9-B4	L	1432	7.40	9.30	68.82	79.57	8.35
ILLINCIS PK9-B4	R	1432	7.90	9.70	76.63	81.44	8.80
ILLINCIS PK9-B1	R	1433	9.20	12.60	115.92	73.02	10.90
ILLINCIS BR19-3	L	1434	10.30	11.45	117.93	89.96	10.87
ILLINCIS BR19-3	R	1434	9.15	11.00	100.65	83.18	10.07
DICKSCN MOUND	L	1501	9.40	11.55	108.57	81.39	10.47
DICKSCN MOUND	R	1501	8.70	11.00	95.70	79.09	9.85
DICKSON MOUND	R	1502	10.00	13.43	134.30	74.46	11.71
DICKSCN MD 276	L	1514	9.45	11.85	111.98	79.75	10.65
DICKSCN MD 276	R	1514	9.00	11.10	99.90	81.08	10.05
DICKSCN MD 287	L	1516	8.60	11.90	102.34	72.27	10.25
DICKSCN MD 287	R	1516	8.90	10.75	95.67	82.79	9.82
DICKSCN MD 297	L	1520	9.25	11.00	101.75	84.09	10.12
DICKSCN MD 302	L	1521	8.80	10.95	96.36	80.37	9.87
DICKSCN MD 302	R	1521	9.45	10.70	101.11	88.32	10.07
DICKSCN MD 319	L	1523	8.75	10.65	93.19	82.16	9.70
DICKSCN MD 319	R	1523	8.10	10.80	87.48	75.00	9.45
DICKSON MD 327	L	1524	10.00	11.30	113.00	88.50	10.65
DICKSCN MD 327	R	1524	10.05	11.70	117.58	85.90	10.87
DICKSCN MD 342	R	1526	.10	11.00	1.10	.91	5.55
DICKSCN MD 344	L	1527	11.75	11.60	136.30	101.29	11.67
DICKSCN MD 344	R	1527	9.30	11.90	110.67	78.15	10.60
DICKSCN MD 349	L	1530	9.20	10.50	96.60	87.62	9.85
DICKSCN MD 349	R	1530	9.25	10.45	96.66	88.52	9.85
DICKSCN MD 361	L	1538	9.40	11.60	109.04	81.03	10.50
DICKSCN MD 361	R	1538	8.80	11.05	97.24	79.64	9.92
DICKSON MD 362	L	1539	9.35	10.60	99.11	88.21	9.97
DICKSON MD 362	R	1539	9.30	9.30	86.49	100.00	9.30
DICKSCN MD 365	L	1540	7.90	11.10	87.69	71.17	9.50
DICKSCN MD 365	R	1540	7.85	10.70	83.99	73.36	9.27

UPPER M3 H. SAPIENS

		N	L(M-D)	B(B-L)	L*B	L/B	L+B/2
DICKSCN MD 371	L	1542	8.90	11.50	102.35	77.39	10.20
DICKSCN MD 371	R	1542	9.50	11.70	111.15	81.20	10.60
DICKSCN MD 378	L	1547	8.00	9.70	77.60	82.47	8.85
DICKSCN MD 378	R	1547	8.75	9.80	85.75	89.29	9.27
DICKSCN MD 379	L	1548	10.00	12.45	124.50	80.32	11.22
DICKSCN MD 379	R	1548	10.30	11.70	120.51	88.03	11.00
DICKSCN MD 380	L	1549	7.60	10.10	76.76	75.25	8.85
DICKSCN MD 380	R	1549	7.60	10.00	76.00	76.00	8.80
DICKSON MD 381	L	1550	10.00	11.00	110.00	90.91	10.50
DICKSCN MD 381	R	1550	9.10	10.40	94.64	87.50	9.75
DICKSCN MD 380	L	1551	7.40	9.80	72.52	75.51	8.60
DICKSCN MD 380	R	1551	7.20	8.90	64.08	80.90	8.05
DICKSCN MD 396	L	1553	9.70	11.50	111.55	84.35	10.60
DICKSON MD 396	R	1553	9.20	11.50	105.80	80.00	10.35
DICKSCN MD 397	R	1554	9.50	11.60	110.20	81.90	10.55
DICKSCN MD 398	L	1555	7.90	11.65	92.03	67.81	9.77
DICKSCN MD 398	R	1555	8.20	10.70	87.74	76.64	9.45
DICKSON MD 399	L	1556	9.25	11.15	103.14	82.96	10.20
DICKSCN MD 399	R	1556	8.95	11.45	102.48	78.17	10.20
DICKSCN MD 402	L	1557	11.10	12.80	142.08	86.72	11.95
DICKSCN MD 402	R	1557	11.80	13.80	162.84	85.51	12.80
DICKSCN MD 406	L	1560	7.85	10.75	84.39	73.02	9.30
DICKSCN MD 407	L	1561	9.40	11.80	110.92	79.66	10.60
DICKSCN MD 407	R	1561	9.73	12.00	116.76	81.08	10.86
DICKSCN MD 411	L	1563	9.52	11.43	108.81	83.29	10.47
DICKSCN MD 411	R	1563	9.50	10.90	103.55	87.16	10.20
DICKSCN MD 414	L	1564	7.92	9.80	77.62	80.82	8.86
DICKSON MD 426	L	1566	8.46	9.95	84.18	85.03	9.20
DICKSCN MD 426	R	1566	8.60	9.85	84.71	87.31	9.22
DICKSCN MD 443	L	1571	11.00	11.00	121.00	100.00	11.00
DICKSCN MD 443	R	1571	9.47	11.15	105.59	84.93	10.31
DICKSCN MD 446	L	1572	8.65	10.95	94.72	79.00	9.80
DICKSCN MD 464	R	1575	8.30	9.70	80.51	85.57	9.00
DICKSON MD 476	L	1576	10.00	12.25	122.50	81.63	11.12
DICKSCN MD 476	R	1576	9.60	11.85	113.76	81.01	10.72
DICKSCN MD 480	L	1578	8.18	9.95	81.39	82.21	9.06
DICKSCN MD 480	R	1578	7.85	9.60	75.36	81.77	8.72
DICKSCN MD 497	L	1583	9.40	11.43	107.44	82.24	10.41
DICKSCN MD 497	R	1583	9.57	11.90	113.88	80.42	10.73
DICKSCN MD 503	L	1585		10.10			
DICKSCN MD 535	L	1591	9.30	10.80	100.44	86.11	10.05
DICKSCN MD 535	R	1591	8.70	10.15	88.30	85.71	9.42
DICKSCN MD 536	L	1592	9.70	10.20	98.94	95.10	9.95
DICKSCN MD 536	R	1592	8.55	9.85	84.22	86.80	9.20
DICKSCN MD 557	L	1596	9.00	11.10	99.90	81.08	10.05
DICKSCN MD 557	R	1596	8.83	10.85	95.81	81.38	9.84
DICKSCN MD 561	R	1597	9.20	10.45	96.14	88.04	9.82
DICKSON MD 567	L	1598	10.00	12.25	122.50	81.63	11.12
DICKSCN MD 567	R	1598	10.15	12.00	121.80	84.58	11.07
DICKSCN MD 594	L	1601	8.90	10.65	94.78	83.57	9.77

UPPER M3 H. SAPIENS

	N	L(M-D)	B(B-L)	L*B	L/B	L+B/2
DICKSCN MD 594 R	1601	8.60	9.95	85.57	86.43	9.27
DICKSCN MD 599 L	1602	10.05	12.20	122.61	82.38	11.12
DICKSCN MD 599 R	1602	9.52	11.95	113.76	79.67	10.73
DICKSON MD 63C L	1603	11.20	12.70	142.24	88.19	11.95
DICKSON MD 630 R	1603	10.30	12.20	125.66	84.43	11.25
DICKSCN MD 633 R	16C4	8.30	10.70	88.81	77.57	9.50
DICKSCN MD 643 L	1608	9.50	11.60	110.20	81.90	10.55
DICKSCN MD 643 R	1608	10.10	11.80	119.18	85.59	10.95
DICKSON MD 658 R	1613	8.40	10.00	84.00	84.00	9.20
DICKSCN MD 709 L	1623	9.20	11.20	103.04	82.14	10.20
DICKSON MD 724 L	1627	9.45	11.54	109.05	81.89	10.49
DICKSCN MD 724 R	1627	9.78	11.25	110.02	86.93	10.51
DICKSCN MD 746 L	1628	8.85	10.80	95.58	81.94	9.82
DICKSON MD 746 R	1628	8.88	11.25	99.90	78.93	10.06